Advances in Treatment and Management in Surgical Endocrinology

Advances in Treatment and Management in Surgical Endocrinology

EDITED BY

ALEXANDER L. SHIFRIN, MD, FACS, FACE, ECNU, FEBS (ENDOCRINE), FISS
Director of Endocrine Oncology at
Hackensack Meridian Health of Monmouth and Ocean Counties
Neptune, NJ, United States

Surgical Director
Center for Thyroid, Parathyroid and Adrenal Diseases
Jersey Shore University Medical Center
Neptune, NJ, United States

Clinical Associate Professor of Surgery
Rutgers RWJ Medical School
New Brunswick, NJ, United States

Associate Professor of Surgery
Hackensack Meridian School of Medicine at Seton Hall University
Nutley, NJ, United States

ELSEVIER

Publisher: Dolores Meloni
Acquisition Editor: Nancy Duffy
Editorial Project Manager: Sandra Harron
Production Project Manager: Sreejith Viswanathan
Cover Designer: Miles Hitchen

3251 Riverport Lane
St. Louis, Missouri 63043

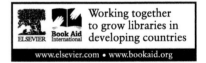

List of Contributors

Elliot A. Asare, MD, MS
Department of Surgical Oncology
The University of Texas MD Anderson Cancer Center
Houston, TX, United States

Harrison X. Bai, MD
Interventional Radiology Fellow
Interventional Radiology
Perelman School of Medicine at the University of
    Pennsylvania
Philadelphia, PA, United States

Irina Bancos, MD
Assistant Professor
Endocrinology
Mayo Clinic
Rochester, MN, United States

Andrew J. Bauer, MD
Director
The Thyroid Center
Division of Endocrinology and Diabetes
Children's Hospital of Philadelphia
Philadelphia, PA, United States

Associate Professor of Pediatrics
Department of Pediatrics
The Perelman School of Medicine
The University of Pennsylvania
Philadelphia, PA, United States

De Crea Carmela
Associate Professor of Surgery
Centro Dipartimentale di Chirurgia Endocrina
    e dell'Obesità
Fondazione Policlinico Universitario Agostino Gemelli
    IRCCS
Istituto di Semeiotica Chirurgica
Università Cattolica del Sacro Cuore
Rome, Italy

Yufei Chen, MD
Staff Physician
Endocrine Surgery
Department of Surgery
Cedars-Sinai Medical Center
Los Angeles, CA, United States

Danae Delivanis, MD, PHD
Mayo Clinic
Rochester, MN, United States

Henning Dralle, MD, PhD
University Hospital Essen
Head of the Section of Endocrine Surgery
Department of General, Visceral and
    Transplantation Surgery
Essen, Nordrhein-Westfalen, Germany

Quan-Yang Duh, MD
Professor
Chief
Section of Endocrine Surgery
Surgery
University of California
San Francisco, CA, United States

Attending Surgery
Surgery
VA Medical Center
San Francisco, CA, United States

Thomas J. Fahey, III MD
Johnson and Johnson Professor and Vice-Chair
Department of Surgery
Chief, Endocrine Surgery
Director, Endocrine Oncology Program
New York Presbyterian Hospital
Weill Cornell Medicine
New York, NY, United States

Gustavo G. Fernandez Ranvier, MD, PhD
Division of Metabolic
Endocrine and Minimally Invasive Surgery
Department of Surgery
Mount Sinai Hospital
Icahn School of Medicine at Mount Sinai
New York, NY, Unites States

Brendan M. Finnerty, MD
Assistant Professor of Surgery
Division of Endocrine Surgery
New York Presbyterian Hospital
Weill Cornell Medicine
New York, NY, United States

Sarah B. Fisher, MD, MS
Department of Surgical Oncology
The University of Texas MD Anderson Cancer Center
Houston, TX, United States

Pennestrì Francesco
Centro Dipartimentale di Chirurgia Endocrina
    e dell'Obesità
Fondazione Policlinico Universitario Agostino Gemelli
    IRCCS
Istituto di Semeiotica Chirurgica
Università Cattolica del Sacro Cuore
Rome, Italy

Mouhammed Amir Habra, MD
Department of Endocrine Neoplasia and Hormonal
    Disorders
The University of Texas MD Anderson Cancer Center
Houston, TX, United States

Joan Hallman, BSN, RN, OCN
Oncology Nurse Navigator
Hackensack Meridian Health Cancer Care
Jersey Shore University Medical Center
Neptune, NJ, United States

Jordan N. Halsey, MD
Rutgers-New Jersey Medical School Division of Plastic
    Surgery
Newark, NJ, United States

Oksana Hamidi, DO
UT Southwestern Medical Center
Dallas, TX, United States

William B. Inabnet, III MD
Eugene W Friedman Professor of Surgery
Icahn School of Medicine at Mount Sinai
System Chief
Endocrine Surgery
New York, NY, United States

Yasuhiro Ito, MD, PhD
Department of Surgery
Kuma Hospital
Chuo-ku, Kobe
Japan

Electron Kebebew, MD, FACS
Professor and Chief
Surgery
Stanford University
Stanford, CA, United States

Svetlana L. Krasnova, BSN, RN, CNOR
Monmouth University
West Long Branch, NJ, United States

Hackensack Meridian Health Jersey Shore University
    Medical Center
Neptune, NJ, United States

Schelto Kruijff, MD, PhD
Endocrine and Oncological Surgeon
Department of Surgery
University Medical Center Groningen
University of Groningen
Groningen, the Netherlands

Amanda M. Laird, MD, FACS
Chief
Section of Endocrine Surgery
Surgical Oncology
Rutgers Cancer Institute of New Jersey
Associate Professor of Surgery
Surgery
Rutgers Robert Wood Johnson Medical School
New Brunswick, NJ, United States

James A. Lee, MD
Chief of Endocrine Surgery
Columbia University Medical Center
New York, NY, United States

Steven K. Libutti, MD, FACS
Director
Rutgers Cancer Institute of New Jersey
Professor of Surgery
Rutgers Robert Wood Johnson Medical School
New Brunswick, NJ, United States

Irene Lou, MD
Endocrine Surgery Fellow
Surgery
The Mount Sinai Hospital
New York, NY, United States

Andreas Machens, MD
Associate Professor
Department of Visceral
Vascular and Endocrine Surgery
Martin Luther University Halle-Wittenberg
Halle (Saale), Germany

William W. Maggio, MD, FACS, FAANS
Neurosurgeon
Hackensack Meridian Health Medical Group
Jersey Shore University Medical Center
Neurosurgery
Neptune, NJ, United States

Vice Chairman
Assistant Professor
Department of Neurosurgery
Hackensack Meridian School of Medicine at
    Seton Hall University
Nutley, NJ, United States

Andrea R. Marcadis, MD
Department of Surgery
Head and Neck Service
Memorial Sloan Kettering Cancer Center
New York, NY, United States

Marco Raffaelli, MD
Associate Professor of Surgery
Centro Dipartimentale di Chirurgia Endocrina
    e dell'Obesità
Fondazione Policlinico Universitario Agostino
    Gemelli IRCCS

Professor
Istituto di Semeiotica Chirurgica
Università Cattolica del Sacro Cuore
Rome, Italy

Haggi Mazeh, MD, FACS, FISA
Chief-of-Surgery
Endocrine and General Surgery
Hadassah-Hebrew University Medical Center
Jerusalem, Israel

**Maureen McCartney-Anderson, DNP,
    CRNA/APN-Anesthesia**
Assistant Professor
Rutgers School of Nursing Anesthesia Program
Newark, NJ, United States

Michal Mekel, MD, MHA
Department of Surgery
Rambam - Health Care Campus
Haifa, Israel

Aryan Meknat, MD
Research Fellow
Department of Surgery
Mount Sinai Hospital
Icahn School of Medicine at Mount Sinai
New York, NY, United States

Akira Miyauchi, MD, PhD
Department of Surgery
Kuma Hospital
Chuo-ku, Kobe, Japan

Priscilla Nobecourt, MD
Department of Surgery
Resident
University of Texas Medical Branch
Galveston, TX, United States

Tushar R. Patel, MD, FACS
Assistant Professor
Plastic and Reconstructive Surgery
Seton Hall University School of Medicine
South Orange, NJ, United States

Clinical Instructor
Department of Surgery
Rutgers Robert Wood Johnson Medical School
Piscataway, NJ, United States

Plastic and Reconstructive Surgeon
The Institute for Advanced Reconstruction
The Plastic Surgery Center
Shrewsbury, NJ, United States

Sarah S. Pearlstein, MD
Resident Surgery
Northwell Health Lenox Hill Hospital
New York, NY, United States

Department of Surgery
Lenox Hill Hospital
New York, NY, United States

Nancy D. Perrier, MD, FACS
Professor of Surgery
Chief of Surgical Endocrinology
MD Anderson Cancer Center
University of Texas
Houston, Texas, United States

Lombardi Celestino Pio
Associate Professor of Surgery
Centro Dipartimentale di Chirurgia Endocrina
    e dell'Obesità
Fondazione Policlinico Universitario Agostino
    Gemelli IRCCS
Istituto di Semeiotica Chirurgica
Università Cattolica del Sacro Cuore
Rome, Italy

Bellantone Rocco
Professor of Surgery
Centro Dipartimentale di Chirurgia Endocrina
    e dell'Obesità
Fondazione Policlinico Universitario Agostino Gemelli
    IRCCS
Istituto di Semeiotica Chirurgica
Università Cattolica del Sacro Cuore
Rome, Italy

Kurt Werner Schmid, MD, PhD
Professor and Chairman
Department of Pathology
University Hospital Essen
Essen, Nordrhein-Westfalen, Germany

Meera Shah, MD
Mayo Clinic
Rochester, MN, United States

Ashok R. Shaha, MD, FACS
Professor of Surgery
Department of Surgery
Head and Neck Service
Memorial Sloan Kettering Cancer Center
New York, NY, United States

Josef Shargorodsky, MD, MPH, FAAOA
Otolaryngologist
Coastal Ear Nose and Throat
Neptune, NJ, United States

Clinical Assistant Professor
Department of Otolaryngology
Hackensack Meridian School of Medicine at Seton Hall
    University
Nutley, NJ, United States

Codirector
Skull Base Center
Jersey Shore Medical Center
Neptune, NJ, United States

Anu Sharma, MBBS
University of Utah School of Medicine
University of Texas
Salt Lake City, United States

**Alexander L. Shifrin, MD, FACS, FACE, ECNU,
    FEBS, FISS**
Director of Endocrine Oncology at
Hackensack Meridian Health of Monmouth and
    Ocean Counties
Neptune, NJ, United States

Surgical Director
Center for Thyroid, Parathyroid and Adrenal Diseases
Jersey Shore University Medical Center
Neptune, NJ, United States

Clinical Associate Professor of Surgery
Rutgers RWJ Medical School
New Brunswick, NJ, United States

Associate Professor of Surgery
Hackensack Meridian School of Medicine
    at Seton Hall University
Nutley, NJ, United States

Angelica M. Silva-Figueroa, MD
Assistant Professor
Department of Surgery
Universidad Finis Terrae
Santiago, Chile

Department of Head and Neck Surgery
Hospital Barros Luco-Trudeau
Santiago, Chile

Tiffany J. Sinclair, MD
General Surgery Resident
Stanford University
Stanford, CA, United States

Constantine A. Stratakis, MD, PHD
Scientific Director
National Institute of Child and Human Development
National Institutes of Health
Bethesda, MD, United States

Mari Suzuki, MD
Clinical Fellow
Endocrinology
National Institute of Diabetes
Digestive and Kidney Diseases

National Institutes of Health
Bethesda, MD, United States

Associate Investigator
Genetics and Endocrinology
National Institute of Child and Human Development
Bethesda, MD, United States

Scott O. Trerotola, MD
Associate Chair and Chief of Interventional Radiology
Vice Chair for Quality
Department of Radiology
Perelman School of Medicine at the University of
    Pennsylvania
Philadelphia, PA, United States

Willemijn Y. van der Plas, BSc, PhD
Department of Surgery
University Medical Center Groningen

University of Groningen
Groningen, the Netherlands

Liffert Vogt, MD, PhD
Department of Internal Medicine
Section Nephrology
Amsterdam Cardiovascular Sciences
University Medical Center Amsterdam
University of Amsterdam
Amsterdam, the Netherlands

Tal Yalon, MD
Department of General and Oncological Surgery -
    Surgery C
Chaim Sheba Medical Center
Ramat Gan, Israel

Contents

CHAPTER 1

Advances in the Diagnosis and Management of Papillary Thyroid Microcarcinoma

YASUHIRO ITO, MD, PHD • AKIRA MIYAUCHI, MD, PHD

INTRODUCTION

Papillary thyroid microcarcinoma (PTMC) refers to papillary thyroid carcinoma (PTC) measuring ≤10 mm regardless of whether lymph node metastasis, distant metastasis, or significant extrathyroid extension is present. Therefore, PTMC includes PTC ≤10 mm with a wide range of biological characteristics. Recently, PTMC without aggressive characteristics (low-risk PTMC) has been focused on as a strong candidate for active surveillance without immediate surgery. Active surveillance for low-risk PTMC was first proposed in 1993 by Akira Miyauchi (the present president and chief operating officer of Kuma Hospital [Kobe, Japan]) and is currently adopted as a management strategy for low-risk PTMC in Japanese guidelines developed by the Japan Association of Endocrine Surgeons and Japanese Society of Thyroid Surgery.[1] Similarly, active surveillance is in use by the American Thyroid Association (ATA) guidelines.[2] In this chapter, the history, outcomes, knowledge, and information gathered to date on active surveillance for low-risk PTMC are described.

BACKGROUND OF ACTIVE SURVEILLANCE FOR LOW-RISK PAPILLARY THYROID MICROCARCINOMA

Papillary thyroid microcarcinoma was detected as a latent carcinoma during autopsy of patients who died of diseases other than thyroid carcinoma. According to previous studies, the incidence of latent PTMC, measuring 3−10 mm, that are detectable by ultrasound ranged from 0.5% to 5.2%,[3] indicating that many adults unknowingly live with PTMC. Clinically, Takebe et al. reported that 3.5% of women aged 30 years or older had thyroid carcinoma detected by ultrasound and diagnosed by ultrasound-guided fine needle aspiration cytology (FNAC).[4] Among these, 85% were PTC measuring 15 mm or smaller. This incidence, which was consistent with findings from autopsy studies, was more than 1000 times the prevalence of clinical thyroid carcinoma in Japanese women (3.1 per 100,000 populations) at that time.

INCREASE IN THE INCIDENCE AND STABLE MORTALITY OF THYROID CARCINOMA PATIENTS

In 2002 and 2014, Davies et al. reported that the incidence of thyroid carcinoma increased 2.4-fold from 1973 to 2002, and 2.9-fold from 1975 to 2009 because of the increased detection and diagnosis of small PTCs, including PTMCs, by imaging studies and ultrasound-guided FNAC.[5,6] More surprisingly, in South Korea, the incidence of thyroid carcinoma showed a 15-fold increase between 1993 and 2011.[7] Similar results were reported from other countries, including Italy, France, the United Kingdom, Australia, and Nordic countries.[8] The most important issue is that in all these countries, the mortality rate of thyroid carcinoma did not change during the surveillance periods. These results strongly suggested overdiagnosis and overtreatment of PTMCs.

Advances in Treatment and Management in Surgical Endocrinology. https://doi.org/10.1016/B978-0-323-66195-9.00001-7

UNFAVORABLE EVENTS OF SURGERY FOR PAPILLARY THYROID MICROCARCINOMA

Indeed, surgery for low-risk PTMC is not difficult. However, in South Korea, it was reported that the number of patients with common unfavorable events of surgery, such as hypothyroidism and vocal cord paralysis, increased.[7] Oda et al. studied the incidence of unfavorable events in patients who underwent immediate surgery and in those who underwent active surveillance.[9] They reported that the immediate surgery group suffered a significantly higher incidence of transient vocal cord paralysis and transient and permanent hypoparathyroidism than the active surveillance group (4.1% vs. 0.6%, $P < .0001$; 16.7% vs. 2.8%, $P < .0001$; and 1.6% vs. 0.08%, $P < .0001$, respectively). Permanent vocal cord paralysis occurred in two patients (0.2%) in the immediate surgery group while it occurred in no patients in the active surveillance group. The proportion of patients, treated with L-thyroxine as supplements or for thyroid stimulating hormone (TSH) suppression, was significantly higher in the immediate surgery group than in the active surveillance group (66.1% vs. 20.7%, $P < .0001$). Kuma Hospital is a special center for thyroid, and all the attending surgeons are experts in thyroid surgery. If patients were treated by nonexperts, the incidence of these unfavorable events would be even much higher. Thus, it is important to discuss which management, whether active surveillance or immediate surgery, of low-risk PTMC is more appropriate.

INITIATION OF ACTIVE SURVEILLANCE FOR LOW-RISK PAPILLARY THYROID MICROCARCINOMA

PTMC was frequently detected if screened by ultrasound and ultrasound-guided FNAC or if searched during autopsy. The incidence was much higher than the prevalence of clinical thyroid carcinoma. These findings strongly suggest that most PTMCs stay small and are harmless throughout a person's life. Based on these, Akira Miyauchi in 1993, proposed the need for active surveillance for low-risk PTMC. This proposal was based on the hypotheses that (1) only a small fraction of PTMCs have growth activity and (2) surgery soon after the detection of progression signs, such as apparent enlargement and appearance of lymph node metastasis, is not too late. In addition, only active surveillance can discriminate PTMCs having constantly growing activity from those that do not, or those growing slowly. The proposal adopted at the medical meeting of Kuma Hospital and the active surveillance

started in 1993. In 1995, Cancer Institute Hospital (Tokyo, Japan) also commenced active surveillance using the same concept.

CONTRAINDICATIONS FOR ACTIVE SURVEILLANCE

There are some contraindications to active surveillance as shown in Table 1.1. These contraindications fall under three categories. The first one is patients' background characteristics. There is insufficient evidence on the natural course of PTMCs in children and adolescents. We therefore do not recommend active surveillance for patients in these age groups. In addition, patients who cannot undergo regular checkups with constant visits for PTMCs are not suitable for active surveillance. The second category concerns the presence of high-risk features. PTMC with clinical lymph node metastasis and/or distant metastasis (although very rarely) with evidence from imaging studies, should undergo immediate treatment. In addition, immediate surgery should be recommended for patients with symptomatic PTMC having recurrent laryngeal nerve (RLN) paralysis or tracheal invasion, which is classified as high risk. Although rarely reported, PTMC with cytology reading of high-grade malignancy, for example, tall cell variant and poorly differentiated carcinoma are not suitable for active surveillance. These cases must undergo surgery and if indicated, ablation or therapy using radioactive iodine.

Lastly, PTMCs attached to the trachea or located in the course of the RLN can be candidates for immediate surgical treatment. It is unknown at the time of diagnosis, whether or not such PTMCs grow and invade

---

TABLE 1.1

Contraindications for the Active Surveillance of Papillary Microcarcinoma.

1. Patients' background characteristics
   a. Children and adolescents
   b. Patients who cannot undergo regular checkups.
2. Presence of high-risk features
   a. Presence of clinical node metastasis and/or distant metastasis (very rare)
   b. Signs or symptoms of invasion to the recurrent laryngeal nerve or trachea
   c. High-grade malignancy on cytology (very rare)
3. Presence of features unsuitable for observation
   a. Tumors attaching to the trachea (Fig. 1.1)
   b. Tumors located in the course of the recurrent laryngeal nerve

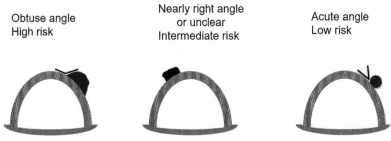

FIG. 1.1 Schema of the relationship between angles formed by the tracheal cartilage and tumor surface.

these organs; thus, they should undergo surgical treatment for safety reasons. For evaluation of tracheal invasion, the angle formed by the tracheal cartilage and tumor surface is useful (Fig. 1.1).[10] In our series, none of the PTMCs <7 mm showed invasion to the trachea. Among patients with PTMCs ≥7 mm demonstrating obtuse angles between tracheal cartilage and tumor surface, 24% showed tracheal invasion requiring laminate dissection or dissection of tracheal cartilage and mucosa, whereas none of the other patients showed significant tracheal invasion, although, some needed shaving of the tracheal adventitia. For the evaluation of RLN invasion by PTMCs located in its course, it is important to know whether or not the normal rim of the thyroid is present or not between the tumor and the thyroid surface. Nine percent of PTMCs ≥7 mm lacking a normal rim were positive for significant RLN invasion and required partial layer resection or segmental resection of RLN with reconstruction of the resected RLN, whereas none of the other patients showed significant RLN invasion.

Other important issues that were not included in the contraindication of active surveillance are the family history of thyroid carcinoma and carcinoma multiplicity. These characteristics may have prognostic significance to some extent. However, if these patients were enrolled for surgery based on these contraindications, the patients would undergo total thyroidectomy, resulting in increased severe adverse events such as vocal cord paralysis and permanent hypoparathyroidism. Thus, these were not included in the contraindications for the initiation of our trial of active surveillance.

These contraindications adopted since 1993 have not changed up till now.

TRENDS IN THE IMPLEMENTATION OF ACTIVE SURVEILLANCE IN KUMA HOSPITAL

Even though active surveillance started after the approval at Kuma Hospital, it was not accepted immediately and equally among the doctors.[11] Between 1993 and 1997, only 30% of patients underwent active surveillance. Although the incidence increased to 51% between 1997 and 2002, it decreased to 42% between 2003 and 2006. It is strange because the first publication on active surveillance came out in 2003. The incidence increased again to 64% between 2007 and 2013, and reached 88% after 2014. These increases were enhanced by important studies on active surveillance that were published after 2014. The incidence of patients who underwent active surveillance also varied according to the physicians, and even after the accumulation of published evidence that active surveillance is a safe and beneficial strategy for patients, some surgeons still adhered to the practice of immediate surgery. These trends may also occur when an institution newly commences new management strategies, including active surveillance for low-risk PTMC.

PRACTICE OF ACTIVE SURVEILLANCE FOR LOW-RISK PAPILLARY THYROID MICROCARCINOMA

In Kuma Hospital, all patients having small nodules suspected of PTMC underwent ultrasound-guided FNAC for the diagnosis, in principle. In contrast, ATA guidelines do not recommend FNAC for nodules smaller than 10 mm with suspicious ultrasound features, unless there are symptoms and aggressive signs such as clinical node and/or distant metastasis and RLN paralysis.[2] This may be, however, due to the possibility that many patients in the United States do not accept the choice of living with untreated carcinoma. In contrast, in Japan, if patients were not diagnosed as PTMC by cytology, they might see other doctors in other hospitals who might diagnose PTMC and offer unnecessary surgery.

Until recently, we presented two options, namely active surveillance and immediate surgery, equally for patients who were diagnosed with low-risk PTMC and allowed the patients to determine their choice of treatment. However, at present, we recommend active surveillance as the first line of management,[12,13] because of the accumulation of evidences of favorable outcomes among patients who underwent active surveillance.

Patients who chose active surveillance were asked to come for follow-up visit at Kuma Hospital 6 months later for checking whether the sizes of PTMCs changed and whether lymph nodes suspected of metastasis appeared. Patients without progression signs such as enlargement and novel appearance of node metastasis continue to undergo active surveillance essentially, yearly. We regard tumors as enlarged when their maximal diameter increased by 3 mm or larger. If enlargement was detected, we might recommend surgery. However, we often continue active surveillance based on patients' request until the size reaches 13 mm, because change in size of PTMC often fluctuates. For the diagnosis of lymph node metastasis, we perform FNAC for suspicious nodes and also measure the thyroglobulin level of the wash-out of the FNAC needles. For patients whose lymph nodes were diagnosed as metastasis of PTC, total thyroidectomy with therapeutic lymph node dissection is recommended. One may think that these patients were cured only by immediate hemithyroidectomy after diagnosis. However, for such patients, completion total thyroidectomy with therapeutic lymph node dissection would be necessary as the second surgery at the time of lymph node recurrence. Active surveillance until the appearance of the node metastasis ensures that the patients undergo curative surgery just once. Therefore, we conclude that active surveillance until the novel appearance of lymph node metastasis is an appropriate strategy.

RESULTS OF ACTIVE SURVEILLANCE FOR LOW-RISK PAPILLARY THYROID MICROCARCINOMA IN JAPAN

In 2003, our first report was published demonstrating that at each follow-up, more than 70% of PTMCs were stable without progression signs.[14] In the second report published in 2010, we reported the rates of PTMC progression using the Kaplan–Meier method.[15] In 2014, a study enrolling 1235 patients who underwent active surveillance (average follow-up period was 60 months) was published. Enlargement observed among participants were 4.9% at 5 years and 8.0% at 10 years. Only 1.7% and 3.8% of patients showed novel appearance of lymph node metastasis at 5-year and 10-year observations, respectively.[16] In this study, not only

univariate but also multivariate analysis for the enlargement and novel node metastasis was performed. The most important finding of this study was the inverse relationship between PTMC progression and patient age. Interestingly, young age (40 years or younger) was regarded as an independent predictor of PTMC progression in the multivariate analysis. In contrast, PTMC in elderly patients, aged 60 years or older, were most unlikely to progress. It is well known that old age significantly affects the prognosis of PTC patients. In addition, in our series, being 55 years or older was an independent and strong prognostic factor of cause-specific survival and overall survival in clinical PTC patients.[17] Therefore, the relationship between patient age and PTMC progression was completely in contrast to the relationship between age and clinical PTC progression. At the initiation of active surveillance, there was concern that PTMC in elderly patients may rapidly grow. However, these findings suggest that PTMCs in elderly patients are the most suitable for active surveillance. In the multivariate analysis, carcinoma multiplicity and family history of differentiated thyroid carcinoma were not regarded as having predictive values for PTMC progression.[16] These factors were not regarded as contraindications in our protocol of active surveillance from the beginning, which was described under "Indications and contraindications for active surveillance." These findings strongly suggest that our primary setup for contraindication of active surveillance was appropriate.

Miyauchi et al. enrolled 1211 patients aged 20–79 years and estimated the lifetime probability of PTMC progression during active surveillance for each age-decade subset from the 20–29 to the 70–79 years age groups, and calculated the progression rates at 10-yearly active surveillance periods for each age-decade subset under the following three hypotheses.[18] Hypothesis A was that PTMCs progress according to the age-decade-specific disease progression rates throughout the patient's lifetime. Hypothesis B was that patients who show disease progression during the initial 10-year period undergo surgical treatment, while the remaining patients have only tumors that are not progressive in nature. Hypothesis C was that the actual probability lies between the values estimated by hypotheses A and B. Among the three, hypothesis C was the most likely, and according to this hypothesis, the estimated lifetime probability of PMC progression was 48.6% for patients who were aged 20–29 years at presentation, 25.3% for 30–39 years, 20.9% for 40–49 years, 10.3% for 50–59 years, 8.2% for 60–69 years, and 3.5% for 70–79 years. One may consider the lifetime probability of PTMC progression of 48.6% in 20−29-year-old patients as being too high to accept active surveillance. However, these values indicate that more than half of patients could avoid surgical treatment in their lifetime. Considering that surgery in patients who underwent active surveillance after the detection of progression signs is not too late, 20−29-year-old patients should not be excluded from these candidates for active surveillance. PTMC in older patients are less likely to undergo surgery during their lifetime, and they are, of course, candidates for active surveillance.

When young female patients undergo active surveillance, pregnancy is a very important issue. In the early phase of pregnancy, human chorionic gonadotropin (hCG) is produced. hCG shares a common alpha subunit with TSH and has a weak TSH activity. Thus, the effect of pregnancy on the progression of PTMC during active surveillance is an important issue to consider. If pregnancy should bring about PTMC progression, prophylactic surgery before pregnancy would be desirable for young female patients who have the possibility of pregnancy. In our first report on selected cases, PTMC in four of nine patients during pregnancy became enlarged.[19] However, after rechecking our entire series, we found that only 4 of the 51 (8%) patients showed enlargement of their PTMCs during pregnancy and none of the patients showed the novel lymph node metastasis appearance.[20] Among the four patients whose PTMC was enlarged, two underwent surgery after delivery, and to date, no recurrence of PTC was detected. The remaining two still underwent active surveillance because their PTMCs did not enlarge any further after delivery. Therefore, it was concluded that the incidence of PTMC growth during pregnancy is very low, and even though it grew, surgery after delivery is adequate.

Our studies showed that "young" patients with low-risk PTMC are candidates for active surveillance, but we have no evidence that children and adolescents with PTMCs are candidates of active surveillance. Further studies are necessary to elucidate this point, but at this stage, we recommend surgery for children with PTMCs (Table 1.1).

From the aspect of medical economy, Oda et al. showed the total cost of immediate surgery with postoperative managements for 10 years as 928,097 yen/patient according to the Japanese Health Care Insurance System.[21] This is 4.1 times higher than the total cost of active surveillance for 10 years, which was 225,695 yen/patient. The total cost included cost for the conversion surgery in the active surveillance group, the postoperative management, and reoperation for recurrence in the immediate surgery group. Although medical costs of active surveillance and immediate surgery vary widely according to countries, active surveillance is much more economical than immediate surgery at least in Japan. From Hong Kong, similar data were published.[22]

The Cancer Institute Hospital commenced active surveillance in 1995 and published some important findings. Although they did not perform analysis using time sequence, they showed that, of 300 PTMCs in 230 patients, only 7% showed enlargement while 1% showed an appearance of nodal metastasis during active surveillance.[23] These data were not discrepant with ours. They also focused on ultrasound findings and showed that a rich blood supply in the tumor and a lack of strong calcification predict the growth of PTMC. They also showed that rich vascularity in the tumor often decreases over time, and concluded that PTMC with rich vascularity should also be a candidate of active surveillance.[24] They also claimed the lack of relationship between the level of TSH value and PTMC progression.[25]

Table 1.2 summarizes the findings regarding outcomes of active surveillance for low-risk PTMC patients in Japan.

RESULTS OF ACTIVE SURVEILLANCE FOR LOW-RISK PAPILLARY THYROID MICROCARCINOMA OUTSIDE JAPAN

After the adoption of active surveillance in the ATA guidelines 2015, Brito et al. proposed a clinical framework for risk stratification based on tumor/neck ultrasound characteristics, patient, and medical team characteristics in collaboration with us.[26] Risk stratification consisted of the ideal, the appropriate, and the inappropriate. Patients classified as inappropriate for active surveillance were those having evidence of aggressive cytology on FNAC, subcapsular location adjacent to RLN, evidence of extrathyroid extension, clinical evidence of invasion of RLN or trachea, N1 disease, M1 disease, and documented increase in size ≥3 mm in a confirmed papillary thyroid cancer tumor on tumor/neck ultrasound characteristics. Moreover, young patients aged less than 18 years were classified as inappropriate for active surveillance. These exclusion criteria for active surveillance are very similar to ours, as shown in Table 1.1. Two studies from Australia demonstrated concerns about active surveillance based on questionnaires and interviews of physicians and patients, suggesting that physicians are not ready to accept active surveillance because strong evidence has

TABLE 1.2
Knowledge About Active Surveillance for Low-Risk PTMC Obtained From Japanese Studies.

1. Most low-risk PTMC do not grow, or grow very slowly. Some PTMCs even shrink over time.
2. None of the patients had distant metastasis or died of thyroid carcinoma during active surveillance, and none of the patients who underwent conversion surgery after the detection of progression signs showed life-threatening recurrence or died of thyroid carcinoma.
3. Low-risk PTMC in old patients is not likely to progress and is a good candidate for active surveillance.
4. PTMC progression during pregnancy is not a common event, and although PTMC progresses, surgery after delivery is adequate.
5. The incidences of unfavorable events, such as recurrent laryngeal nerve paralysis and hypoparathyroidism, were much higher in patients who underwent immediate surgery than in those who underwent active surveillance, although experts (thyroid surgeons) performed the surgery.
6. Based on the Japanese medical insurance system, medical costs for immediate surgery with 10-year postoperative management were 4.1 times the total costs of the active surveillance for 10 years.
7. Estimated lifetime probability of PTMC progression significantly decreased with age at presentation.

not been available.[27,28] They also claim that overdiagnosis of PTMC and guideline recommendations should be clearly communicated to patients and that intervention to reduce unnecessary cytological diagnosis is required. However, their studies were performed before our report on the higher incidences of unfavorable events in the immediate surgery group than the active surveillance group,[8] which convinced all physicians at Kuma Hospital of the superiority of active surveillance over immediate surgery. Their hesitation and concern to accept active surveillance, a new management, is understandable because Kuma Hospital also experienced the same.

In 2017, Tuttle et al. published the first prospective study for active surveillance in the United States.[29] They reported that younger age at diagnosis and risk category at presentation was independently associated with the likelihood of tumor growth, which was consistent with findings in our previous study. All Japanese studies evaluated PTMC only on the maximum diameter; however, they proposed the evaluation of tumor volume by the calculation of the three dimensions. They demonstrated that, of the 284 patients with a median active surveillance period of 25 months, tumor volumes increased by >50% in 12.7%, were stable in 80.2%, and decreased by >50% in 6.7%. In contrast, increases in tumor diameter ≥3 mm were detected in only 3.8% of the patients. Based on these findings, they concluded that serial measurements of tumor volumes can keenly reflect tumor growth and facilitate the identification of tumors with a strong growing activity, resulting in early surgical treatment.

They cooperated with Korean teams to develop the Thyroid Cancer Treatment Choice, consisting of several cards describing the two managements of PTMC, using the conversation aid for the patients.[30] They performed prospective and comparative study between one clinic, using this conversation aid, and another clinic, with usual care. They showed that patients in the conversation aid clinic were more likely to choose active surveillance than patients in the usual care clinic, indicating the relevance of such a conversation aid in enhancing the understanding of patients concerning the merits of active surveillance.

There are a few retrospective studies from South Korea. In contrast to the study from the United States, patients enrolled in this study did not undergo immediate surgery because they refused surgery despite the recommendation of surgery by the physician, had other malignancies that could not be cured, or were at high risk of general anesthesia. Therefore, these study designs should be called "passive surveillance" instead of "active surveillance." Kwon et al. enrolled 192 patients and showed that tumor volume increased by 50% in 27 (14%) patients with a median follow-up time of 30 months.[31] As a result, 24 (13%) patients underwent delayed thyroid surgery at a median of 31.2 months while 7 (29%) were positive for pathological lymph node metastasis. As only 4 (2.1%) patients showed the maximum tumor size increase at 3 mm or more, they concluded that the change in tumor volume was more sensitive for detecting tumor progression than the change in the maximum tumor diameter. Another manuscript, published in 2018 from the same institution, enrolled 127 PTMC patients who underwent "passive surveillance". They classified patients into groups with the highest, middle, and lowest time-weighted average of TSH (TW-TSH). During a median follow-up of 26 months, PTMC in 28 (19.8%) patients progressed, and the adjusted hazard ratio for PTMC progression in the highest TW-TSH group was significantly higher, while that in the middle TW-TSH group was not.[32] They therefore concluded that sustained elevation of serum TSH levels during active surveillance is associated with PTMC progression, which is in sharp contrast to the report from Cancer Institute Hospital in Tokyo.[25]

Recently, the study protocol of a multicenter prospective cohort study of active surveillance in Korea was published.[33] They enrolled 290 patients who chose active surveillance and 149 patients who chose immediate surgery. Their exclusion criteria for active surveillance were (1) suspected organ involvement, (2) clinical suspicion or pathological diagnosis of lymph node/distant metastasis, (3) poorly differentiated histology or a variant with poor prognosis such as tall cell, diffuse sclerosing, columnar cell, or solid variant, and (4) presence of Graves' disease with an indication of radioactive iodine therapy or surgery. Their definitions of disease progression were (1) size increase of ≥3 mm at least in one dimension, or ≥2 mm in at least two dimensions, (2) suspected organ involvement during the follow-up, and (3) pathological diagnosis of lymph node/distant metastasis.

Sawka et al. published a manuscript introducing the protocol for a Canadian prospective study on active surveillance.[34] The subjects in this study were low-risk PTC less than 2 cm in adult patients, including low-risk PTMC. The aim of this study was to conduct a detailed prospective evaluation of decision-making related to the choice of active surveillance or immediate surgery and secondary outcomes such as psychological distress, disease-specific quality of life, fear of disease progression, and body image satisfaction.

DISCUSSION

It is now about 25 years since active surveillance for low-risk PTMC started in Kuma Hospital. This management was adopted in Japanese guidelines conducted by the Japan Association of Endocrine Surgeons and the Japanese Society of Thyroid Surgery[1] in 2010 and the guidelines conducted by the ATA[2] in 2015. Before 2015, manuscripts demonstrating the outcomes of patients who underwent active surveillance were published exclusively from the two institutions in Japan, Kuma Hospital and Cancer Institute Hospital. However, after the publishing of the newest ATA guidelines, movements outside Japan became active. However, to date, only one prospective study on active surveillance from the Memorial Sloan Kettering Cancer Center has

been published.[29] Furthermore, protocols of the study on active surveillance were published from South Korea and Canada.[3,34] Publishing of the prospective studies is expected from these countries in the near future.

There are some important issues on active surveillance for low-risk PTMC. The most important one is how to evaluate the change in PTMC at each measurement. Our institution measured three dimensions where possible, but adopted only the maximum diameter for evaluation. Tuttle et al. demonstrated that during active surveillance, tumor volume based on three dimensions increased by >50% in 12.7%, while increase in tumor diameter of ≥3 mm was detected only in 3.8% of patients.[29] However, there are some concerns about this issue. Similar to clinical PTC, PTMCs often have strong calcifications. For these, it is impossible to measure the height. Second, their definition might be too sensitive to convert active surveillance to rescue surgery. For example, increase of a tumor with 6 mm diameter to 7 mm diameter implies a 59% increase in its tumor volume. Third, evaluation on three dimensions should reflect observer variations more strongly than that based on the maximum diameter. If PTMCs are always evaluated by the same technician, observer variation might be held to a minimum, but it is not possible by all institutions worldwide. Besides, the size of PTMCs often fluctuates, and not all PTMCs enlarged during the period of active surveillance continue to grow with time. This issue is still debatable, but at least in our institution, none of the patients showed distant metastasis or died of PTC during active surveillance and none of the patients who underwent surgery after the detection of progression of signs showed significant recurrence or died of thyroid carcinoma. In our opinion, it is considered desirable that active surveillance can be done comprehensively not only by foundation hospitals that specialized in thyroid carcinoma but also by general clinics. For this purpose, evaluation on maximum diameter could be easier to accept for physicians, who are trying to active surveillance.

We demonstrated that patient age was significantly related to PTMC progression, and in contrast to clinical PTC, PTMC at a young age is more likely to progress.[17] However, none of the patients, including the 20–29-year-old patients, underwent surgery after the detection of the progression of signs showing significant recurrences, and none died of thyroid carcinoma. Computationally, more than half, 51.4%, of 20–29-year-old patients do not require surgery due to PTMC progression in their lifetimes.[18] Additionally, only a small portion of PTMC in young females progress during pregnancy. Therefore, there are no reasons to actively recommend immediate surgery for young patients.

As indicated earlier, there are discrepant findings between patients' TSH level and their PTMCs' progression.[22,32] Although no comparative studies are available, we often administer L-thyroxine for young patients with PTMC to set TSH level to low normal. To date, none of the patients administered with L-thyroxine showed the growth of their PTMCs.[16] Therefore, mild TSH suppression by L-thyroxine administration may be an effective strategy for PTMC, especially for young patients, to prevent progression.

At the initiation of active surveillance, Miyauchi thought it to be the only strategy to discriminate PTMCs having high growing activity from others. Unfortunately, the circumstances have not changed even now. Clinical PTC with a TERT mutation showed significantly poor prognosis,[35] but Yabuta et al. showed that none of the 15 PTMCs that showed size increase or novel appearance of nodal metastasis showed a TERT mutation.[36] Hirokawa et al. demonstrated that Ki-67 labeling index values > 5% were detected in 50% of PTMCs with tumor enlargement while only 8% of those with stable disease and 9.1% of those that showed novel nodal metastasis during active surveillance.[37] These findings suggest that cell-proliferating activities in PTMC enlarging over time were significantly higher than that in PTMC with a stable size. However, the results of this study cannot be applied at the time of decision whether a PTMC should be observed or immediately operated. To date, no biological or molecular markers predicting PTMC growth have been identified. Therefore, at least at present, all PTMCs should be candidates for active surveillance. If any markers of the growth of PTMC evaluated at the time of cytology are identified in future, we would be able to discriminate PTMCs that should be immediately treated from others at the stage of FNAC.

One concern relates to whether patients can remain calm following the diagnosis of carcinoma, even when it is low-risk PTMC. The newest ATA guidelines do not recommend FNAC for nodules ≤10 mm without symptoms or clinical evidence of thyroid carcinoma such as lymph node and/or distant metastasis.[2] These nodules must include low-risk PTMC in a certain probability, which may probably be because the diagnosis of PTMC was considered to bring about severe psychological burden to patients. As indicated in the "Practice of active surveillance of low-risk papillary thyroid microcarcinoma" section, our institution always diagnoses suspicious nodules as PTMC before active surveillance

to ensure that patients neither miss the follow-up nor undergo unnecessary surgery in other hospitals. It is true that patients experience shock after been diagnosed with malignancy and while undergoing active surveillance, even though they intellectually understand the indolent character of low-risk PTMC. Therefore, it is important to ease the concern of patients. It goes without saying that patients had no concern of carcinoma before they were declared as having PTMC, and physicians must be avoided as far as possible, making patients uneasy. We adopted the brochure for active surveillance for patients who are diagnosed as PTMC. The brochure includes our data on active surveillance, till date. The important issue is that we provided this before the patients with suspicious nodules underwent FNAC, rather than after being diagnosed as low-risk PTMC. This strategy is useful for patients to have accurate knowledge about low-risk PTMC and the appropriateness of active surveillance at the time of diagnosis by FNAC. We also prepared another brochure for patients who are midstream in active surveillance to reduce uneasiness. A dispassionate research from this aspect is necessary, but whether or not patients feel unease mainly depends on the attitude of attending physicians.

CONCLUSIONS

Low-risk PTMCs are generally an indolent disease, and only a portion of them have progressing activity. Most importantly, none of the patients with PTMCs underwent delayed surgery after the detection of progression signs had significant recurrence or died of PTC. Therefore, active surveillance is suitable for first-line management of low-risk PTMCs regardless of patients' backgrounds.

REFERENCES

1. Takami H, Ito Y, Okamoto T, et al. Therapeutic strategy for differentiated thyroid carcinoma in Japan based on a newly established guideline managed by Japanese Society of Thyroid Surgeons and Japanese Association of Endocrine Surgeons. *World J Surg.* 2011;35:111–121.
2. Haugen BR, Alexander EK, Bible KC, et al. 2015 American Thyroid Association management guidelines for adult patients with thyroid nodules and differentiated thyroid cancer: The American Thyroid Association Guidelines Task Force on thyroid nodules and differentiated thyroid cancer. *Thyroid.* 2016;26, 1-133.
3. Ito Y, Miyauchi A. A therapeutic strategy for incidentally detected papillary microcarcinoma of the thyroid. *Nat Clin Pract Endocrinol Metabol.* 2007;3:240–248.

4. Takebe K, Date M, Yamamoto N. Mass screening for thyroid cancer with ultrasonography [in Japanese]. *Karkinos.* 1994;7:309−317.

5. Davies L, Welch HG. Increasing incidence of thyroid cancer in the United States, 1973−2002. *J Am Med Assoc.* 2006; 295:2164−2167.

6. Davies L, Welch HG. Current thyroid cancer trends in the United States. *JAMA Otolaryngol Head Neck Surg.* 2014; 140:217−222.

7. 2014 Ahn HS, Kim HJ, Welch HG. Korea's thyroid-cancer "epidemic" − screening and overdiagnosis. *N Engl J Med.* 2014;371:1765−1767.

8. Vaccarella S, Franceschi S, Bray F, et al. Worldwide thyroid-cancer epidemic? The increasing impact at overdiagnosis. *N Engl J Med.* 2016;375:614−617.

9. Oda H, Miyauchi A, Ito Y, et al. Incidences of unfavorable events in the management of low-risk papillary microcarcinoma of the thyroid by active surveillance versus immediate surgery. *Thyroid.* 2016;26:150−158.

10. Ito Y, Miyauchi A, Oda H, et al. Revisiting low-risk thyroid papillary microcarcinomas resected without observation: was immediate surgery necessary? *World J Surg.* 2016;40: 523−528.

11. Ito Y, Miyauchi A, Kudo T, et al. Trends in the implementation of active surveillance for low-risk papillary thyroid microcarcinomas at Kuma Hospital: gradual increase and heterogeneity in the acceptance of this new management option. *Thyroid.* 2018;28:488−495.

12. Miyauchi A. Clinical trials of active surveillance of papillary microcarcinoma of the thyroid. *World J Surg.* 2016; 40:516−522.

13. Miyauchi A, Ito Y, Oda H. Insights into the management of papillary microcarcinoma of the thyroid. *Thyroid.* 2016;28: 23−31.

14. Ito Y, Uruno T, Nakano K, et al. An observation trial without surgical treatment in patients with papillary microcarcinoma of the thyroid. *Thyroid.* 2003;13: 381−387.

15. Ito Y, Miyauchi A, Inoue H, et al. An observation trial for papillary thyroid microcarcinoma in Japanese patients. *World J Surg.* 2010;34:28−35.

16. Ito Y, Miyauchi A, Kihara M, et al. Patient age is significantly related to the progression of papillary microcarcinoma of the thyroid under observation. *Thyroid.* 2014; 24:27−34.

17. Ito Y, Miyauchi A, Kihara M, et al. Overall survival of papillary thyroid carcinoma patients: a single institution long-time follow-up of 5897 patients. *World J Surg.* 2018;42: 615−622.

18. Miyauchi A, Kudo T, Ito Y, et al. Estimation of the lifetime probability of disease progression of papillary microcarcinoma of the thyroid during active surveillance. *Surgery.* 2018;163:48−52.

19. Shindo H, Amino N, Ito Y, et al. Papillary thyroid microcarcinoma might progress during pregnancy. *Thyroid.* 2014;2:840−844.

20. Ito Y, Miyauchi A, Kudo T, et al. Effects of pregnancy on papillary microcarcinoma of the thyroid re-evaluated in the entire patients series at Kuma Hospital. *Thyroid.* 2016;26:156−160.

21. Oda H, Miyauchi A, Ito Y, et al. Comparison of the costs of active surveillance and immediate surgery in the management of low-risk papillary microcarcinoma of the thyroid. *Endocr J.* 2017;64:59−64.

22. Lang BH, Wong CK. A cost-effectiveness comparison between early surgery and non-surgical approach for incidental papillary thyroid microcarcinoma. *Eur J Endocrinl.* 2014;173:367−375.

23. Sugitani I, Toda K, Yamada K, et al. Three distinctly different kinds of papillary thyroid microcarcinoma should be recognized our treatment strategies and outcomes. *World J Surg.* 2010;34:1222−1231.

24. Fukuoka O, Sugitani I, Ebina A, et al. Natural history of asymptomatic papillary thyroid microcarcinoma: time-dependent changes in calcification and vascularity during active surveillance. *World J Surg.* 2016;40:529−537.

25. Sugitani I, Fujimoto Y, Yamada K. Association between serum thyrotropin concentration and growth of asymptomatic papillary thyroid microcarcinioma. *World J Surg.* 2014;38:673−678.

26. Brito JP, Ito Y, Miyauchi A, et al. A clinical framework to facilitate risk stratification when considering an active surveillance alternative to immediate biopsy and surgery in papillary microcarcinoma. *Thyroid.* 2016;26:144−149.

27. Nickel B, Brito JP, Barratt A, et al. Clinicians' view on management and terminology for papillary thyroid microcarcinoma: a qualitative study. *Thyroid.* 2017;27(5):661−671.

28. Nickel B, Brito JP, Moynihan R, et al. Patients' experiences of diagnosis and management of papillary thyroid microcarcinoma: a qualitative study. *BMC Canc.* 2018;18:242. https://doi.org/10.1186/s12885-018-4152-9.

29. Tuttle RM, Fagin JA, Minkowitz G, et al. Natural history and tumor volume kinetics of papillary thyroid cancers during active surveillance. *JAMA Otolaryngol Head Neck Surg.* 2017;143:1015−1020.

30. Brito JP, Moon JH, Zauren R, et al. Thyroid Cancer Treatment Choice: a pilot study of a tool to facilitate conversations with patients with papillary microcarcinomas considering treatment choice. *Thyroid.* 2018. https://doi.org/10.1089/thy.2018.0105 [Epub ahead of print].

31. Kwon H, Oh HS, Kim M, et al. Active surveillance for patients with papillary thyroid microcarcinoma: a single center's experience in Korea. *J Clin Endocrinol Metab.* 2017;102:1917−1925.

32. Kim HI, Jang HW, Ahn HS, et al. High serum TSH level is associated with progression of papillary thyroid microcarcinoma during active surveillance. *J Clin Endocrinol Metab.* 2018;103:446−451.

33. Moon JH, Kim J-H, Lee EK, et al. Study protocol of multi-center prospective cohort study of active surveillance on papillary thyroid microcarcinoma (MAeSTro). *Endocrinol Metab.* 2018;33:278−286.

34. Sawka AM, Gai S, Tominson G, et al. A protocol for a Canadian prospective observational study of decision-making on active surveillance or surgery for low-risk papillary thyroid cancer. *BMJ Open*. 2018;8:e020298.

35. Xing A, Liu R, Liu X, et al. BRAF V600E and TERT promoter mutations cooperatively identify the most aggressive papillary thyroid cancer with highest recurrence. *J Clin Oncol*. 2014;32:2718−2726.

36. Yabuta T, Matsuse M, Hirokawa M, et al. TERT promoter mutations were not found in papillary thyroid microcarcinomas that showed disease progression on active surveillance. *Thyroid*. 2017;27:1206−1207.

37. Hirokawa M, Kudo T, Ota H, et al. Pathological characteristics of low-risk papillary thyroid microcarcinoma with progression during active surveillance. *Endocr J*. 2016;63:805−810.

CHAPTER 2

Advances in the Diagnosis and Surgical Management of Medullary Thyroid Carcinomas

ANDREAS MACHENS, MD, PHD • KURT WERNER SCHMID, MD, PHD • HENNING DRALLE, MD, PHD

INTRODUCTION

Medullary thyroid cancer (MTC) is a neuroendocrine malignancy notorious for early spread to neck lymph nodes. MTC differs in many ways from follicular-cell-derived papillary and follicular thyroid cancer, such as embryological background, morphology, and tumor biology. MTC cells do not express the sodium-iodine symporter, which makes radioiodine therapy futile because of the tumor's inability to concentrate iodine.[1]

MTC cells synthesize, deposit in dense-cored granules, and secrete procalcitonin and its posttranslational processing product calcitonin.[2,3] In addition, MTC constantly releases carcinoembryonic antigen (CEA), a membrane-bound protein, into the circulation. Procalcitonin, calcitonin, and CEA serum levels reflect overall tumor burden fairly well, in particular primary tumor diameter, lymph node, and distant metastases.[2,4−6] Some 0.83% of MTCs discharge calcitonin into the bloodstream in quantities that are completely out of proportion to tumor cell mass.[7] Furthermore, <1% of MTCs, typically in the context of bulky disease, cause hypercortisolism, with or without secretion of cortisol-releasing hormone (CRH) or adrenocorticotrophic hormone (ACTH).[8] Profuse diarrhea is another tumor-associated symptom, affecting patients with advanced MTC.[9]

MTC comes in a sporadic (70%−75%) and a hereditary variety (25%−30%), which differ primarily in time of onset by some 20 years. Mean age-standardized incidence per year is 0.19 per 100,000 for all MTC; 0.13 per 100,000 for sporadic MTC; and 0.06 per 100,000 for hereditary MTC. The corresponding prevalence is 3.8 per 100,000 for all MTC; 2.5 per 100,000 for sporadic MTC; and 1.3 per 100,000 for hereditary MTC.[10]

Sporadic MTC

In sporadic MTC, *RET*, a receptor tyrosine kinase, and *RAS* are the predominant oncogenic drivers. Mutually exclusive somatic mutations are present in *RET* (78%−88%; 62% for *RET* M918T), *HRAS* (3%−18%), and *KRAS* (3%−5%) in >90% of sporadic MTC.[11,12] Somatic *RET* mutations, affecting 90% of advanced MTC with lymph node and distant metastasis,[13,14] indicate bleaker survival regardless of tumor stage.[13] On the contrary, small MTCs mainly harbor somatic *RAS* mutations.[15] Intriguingly, *RAS*-positive MTC and *RAS*-negative MTC display similar clinical features.[16] Somatic *RET* mutations reveal a dose-effect relationship, in which the presence of more than one somatic *RET* mutation within the same tumor portends worse clinical outcome.[17] Within the same primary tumor, *RET* mutation profiles differ in 8%, and in 20% between the thyroid primary and its metastases.[14]

MTC is characterized by strong oncogene predominance, with nearly complete activation of the *RAS* pathway signaling via somatic mutations in *RET* or in *RAS*.[11] This molecular signaling mechanism may account for differences in overall response rates to an oral tyrosine kinase inhibitor: 32% for *RET mutation-positive* and 31% for RAS mutation-positive patients, as opposed to 21% for both *RET* and RAS mutation-negative patients.[18]

Hereditary MTC

Constitutive activation of the mutated *RET* tyrosine kinase receptor ("*primary hit*") is thought to be the driver behind neoplastic hyperplasia of parafollicular C cells. Subsequent somatic mutations ("*secondary hits*") are believed to give rise to hereditary MTC. Because the accrual of somatic secondary mutations is subject to the play of chance, carriers of the same *RET* mutation, even within the same *RET* family, vary considerably in terms of tumor development and manifestation.[19] The rate of tumor causation and progression differs much across and within highest risk (ATA category HST) mutations; high risk (ATA category H) mutations; and moderate risk (ATA category MOD) mutations[20]; Fig. 2.1). Moderate risk mutations have been newly broken down into moderate-high (MOD-H) and low-moderate (L-MOD) mutations.[21] The position of the respective moderate risk mutations on the *RET* tyrosine kinase receptor results in clinically less relevant codon-specific differences: earlier (vs. later) progression to MTC when the mutation is located in the extracellular (vs. intracellular) cysteine-rich domain[22] closer to (farther from) the cell membrane.[23] This close genotype–phenotype correlation forms a firm foundation for the timing of preemptive thyroidectomy in young *RET* carriers.

The slow tumor growth, 0.4–0.5 mm (node-negative tumors) and 1.2–2.6 mm (node-positive tumors) per year,[24] gives leeway to defer preemptive thyroidectomy until basal serum calcitonin levels start exceeding the upper normal limit of the calcitonin assay. As long as basal serum calcitonin levels remain ≤30 pg/mL, total thyroidectomy alone is adequate therapy.[25]

Invasive Growth and Tumor Spread

Invasive growth emerges from within the thyroid parenchyma (extrathyroidal extension) or from within the lymphatic mesenchyma (extranodal growth).[26] Two types of locoregional soft tissue infiltrates are to be distinguished: (1) by direct extension of, and/or venous microembolization from, a primary tumor penetrating the thyroid capsule, more commonly seen in the central neck; and (2) by growth of lymph node metastases through the nodal capsule, more often found in the lateral neck.[27]

Primary tumor size >20 mm is independently associated with histology-proven lymph node recurrence. This is why tumor cells are thought to spread via lymphatic channels regardless of whether the primary thyroid tumor, breaching the thyroid capsule, extends into neighboring soft tissues or not.[27] Because each thyroid primary can contribute lymph node metastases on its own, multifocal MTC is more frequently node-positive than unifocal MTC.[28]

Thyroid primaries in the upper thyroid pole may skip the central neck compartment, invading the superior lateral lymph nodes directly. Primary tumors lodging in the inferior thyroid pole involve both the central and the inferior lateral (supraclavicular) lymph nodes.[29] Oncologically, the ipsilateral and contralateral lateral neck represents a therapeutic watershed. Lymph

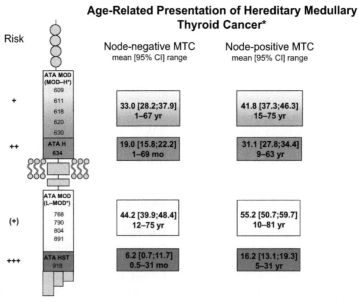

FIG. 2.1   Age-related presentation of hereditary medullary thyroid cancer*. *ATA HST, H, MOD,* American Thyroid Association Highest, High, Moderate; *MOD-H**, (moderate-high); *L-MOD**, (low-moderate); *CI,* Confidence Interval; *MTC,* Medullary Thyroid Cancer. *From Machens et al, *Hum Mutat* 2018;39:860–869.[21] (Adapted from Randolph ed., *Surgery of the Thyroid and Parathyroid Glands*, third ed., Elsevier Saunders 2019.)

node metastases limited to the ipsilateral lateral compartment denote localized disease amenable to surgical cure by systematic neck dissection. Conversely, involvement of the contralateral lateral and specifically the infrabrachiocephalic upper mediastinal compartment indicates advanced, usually systemic disease.[5] Lymphatic tumor cell dissemination conceivably progresses via posterior central lymph nodes in the paraesophageal area to ipsilateral lateral lymph nodes, or alternatively via direct lymphatic channels to the lateral jugular chain, as noted in upper thyroid pole primaries.[29]

The more lymph nodes are involved, the greater are the odds that one of the lymph node metastases happens to breach its nodal capsules to invade adjoining soft tissues.[26] Quantitative assessment of lymph node metastases, in increments of 1–10 (N1), 11–20 (N2), and >20 (N3) involved lymph nodes, is an important prognostic classifier. Of note, the number of lymph node metastases (1–10; 11–20, >20) is connected to the frequency of distant metastases (3%–4%, 13%, and 26%–30%) mainly to the lung, the axial skeleton, and the liver.[30]

DIAGNOSIS

Owing to its proclivity for lymphatic spread, it is difficult to diagnose MTC early or reliably determine the adequate extent of surgery. Many military tumor deposits defy detection by even the most advanced imaging modalities. Comparable quantities of serum calcitonin can be generated by large node-negative tumors and small node-positive tumors alike. These two conditions are not always easy to differentiate before surgery.

Presentation
Clinical disease

In patients with clinically apparent MTC, preoperative imaging for structural disease plays a central role in assessing the need for, and the extent and nature ("*curative*" or "*palliative*") of lymph node dissection. Before embarking on initial thyroidectomy, high-resolution neck ultrasonography is the imaging method of choice to spot structural neck disease but may miss lymph nodes located near or behind the thyroid gland or in the upper anterior mediastinum. In fact, more than one-third of MTC patients produce false-negative results on preoperative neck ultrasonography.[31] Such false-negative results favor the central neck (32%), in which the thyroid gland may conceal tumor deposits, more than the lateral neck (14%). Owing to scarring, the yield

of false-negative results is much worse after initial operations: 44% before reoperation for recurrent MTC, and 49% before reoperation for persistent MTC.[31] This is why surgical treatment plans should not be informed exclusively by imaging results but need to consider preoperative serum calcitonin levels as well.[5,32]

Subclinical disease

The basic tenet of a screening program is the premise that early detection of disease at an asymptomatic stage results in better clinical outcome because an intervention carried out before the disease becomes clinically apparent will be more effective than any subsequent therapy. Ideally, the disease at hand should be serious (such as MTC), and treatment of asymptomatic disease (such as early thyroidectomy) should diminish morbidity or mortality more than later treatment for symptomatic disease. The negative effects of not catching asymptomatic disease early on need to be sufficiently grave to justify the inconvenience of the screening procedure (such as a venous blood draw or imaging). The financial burden of the screening program must be acceptable to prevent or mitigate adverse clinical outcomes (such as metastatic MTC leading to persistent or recurrent disease).

Biochemical screening. The availability of sensitive calcitonin assays has changed the landscape for MTC by enabling identification of occult disease. Serum calcitonin levels, covering the entire spectrum of disease, closely correlate with tumor mass, including larger primary tumor size and more lymph node metastases, and postoperative normalization of calcitonin levels, also dubbed "biochemical cure."[5]

Earlier biochemical screening of the offspring of *RET* families and preemptive thyroidectomy of children at risk of *hereditary* MTC resulted in a fall of primary tumor size from 0.8 to 0.2 cm; a decline in the percentage of bilateral neoplasms from 100% to 13%; and a drop in the rate of lymph node metastases from 58% to 0%.[33] Freedom of these gene carriers from MTC for more than 11 years after thyroidectomy fostered the belief that regular biochemical screening and early thyroidectomy prevented metastasis and death from hereditary MTC.[34] In keeping, calcitonin screening recently proved to be more sensitive than screening for structural neck disease using high-resolution ultrasonography.[35]

Calcitonin screening likewise is an effective instrument for detecting *sporadic MTC* at a stage where it can still be cured. The cost-effectiveness of calcitonin screening for MTC is contingent on (1) the prevalence of the target disease (3.2 cases per 1000 patients with thyroid nodular disease); (2) the predictive value of the screening test (based on the respective calcitonin threshold), and (3) the existence of effective interventions (such as thyroidectomy, which removes all primary thyroid cancers together with the thyroid gland). Furthermore, the size of the structural abnormality (MTC) and the intensity of the *"background noise"* (concomitant disease causing raised serum calcitonin levels) greatly impact the accuracy of biochemical screening.

Biochemical screening for sporadic MTC has gathered momentum in patients with nodular thyroid disease, circumventing intravenous calcitonin stimulation through the use of sensitive calcitonin assays.[36–38] The revised 2015 ATA guidelines on MTC recommend neither for nor against calcitonin screening for sporadic MTC.[20] On balance, basal calcitonin thresholds of 15–25 pg/mL for women and 70–80 pg/mL for men, who have a larger C cell mass, discriminate best between reactive C cell hyperplasia and sporadic MTC.[36–38] When these calcitonin cut-off values have not been crossed, a *"wait and see"* approach, flanked by continual determination of serum calcitonin, can be a good alternative. Importantly, biochemical cure is still obtainable when preoperative basal calcitonin levels do not surpass the 100 pg/mL threshold.[5]

For screening of patients with thyroid nodules for MTC, serum procalcitonin with a cut-off of 0.155 ng/mL, having the same diagnostic accuracy, has tremendous potential as an alternative to serum calcitonin because it does not need to be kept cool on ice or frozen, making it less cumbersome to handle in primary care settings.[2,3]

DNA-based screening. DNA-based screening, involving *RET* exons 8, 10, 11, 13, 14, 15, and 16, is able to uncover genetic predisposition to hereditary MTC. Evidence of a positive *RET* gene test permits truly "prophylactic" thyroidectomies in infants and young children who still have normal thyroid glands or no more than neoplastic C cell hyperplasia.[39,40] The close genotype–phenotype correlation provides genetically encoded boundaries within which C cell hyperplasia develops into C cell cancer (MTC).[21,41,42] Molecular data alone do not pinpoint the time when malignant transformation is set to occur in a given patient. Biochemical information is very useful in defining an operative *"window of opportunity"* because the level of serum calcitonin, mirroring C cell mass, signifies progression of C cell disease fairly well. As

long as basal serum calcitonin levels remain within the reference range of the assay, MTC has not come into existence.[41,42] When serum calcitonin levels cross the upper normal limit of the calcitonin assay, typically <10 pg/mL for children aged 2 years and older,[43] malignant transformation to MTC is impending or just may have happened. This marks the last opportunity to plan for preemptive thyroidectomy without addition of central lymph node dissection. The objective is not so much to prevent malignancy from occurring in the first place but to remove the thyroid before metastasis comes into being.

Histopathology

During the descent of the thyroid anlage, C cells become dispersed among thyroid follicular cells. Most C cells are concentrated in the center of the thyroid gland, specifically within the upper lateral and posterior portion of the thyroid lobes. C cells are more scarce, or missing altogether, at the poles of the thyroid lobes, the isthmus, and the pyramidal lobe. Although it can emerge anywhere within the thyroid gland, MTC arises more frequently in areas with greater C cell concentrations.

Microscopically, C cells are hard to identify on routine hematoxylin and eosin sections but are easily spotted on calcitonin immunohistochemistry. Most C cells, sized up to 40 µm, are round or polygonal, and appear singly or group in small clusters of 3–6 cells. Some C cells are spindle-shaped and have tapered ends. Almost all C cells are situated within the follicular basement membrane. The number of C cells is higher in newborns than in adults and increases after the age of 60 years: 2.97 cells/mm^2 versus 0.99 cells/mm^2.[44] Thyroidal C cell mass typically is greater in men than women, with the former acting as a surrogate marker of larger thyroid volume. This is why sensitive calcitonin assays have gender-specific normal reference values.[36-38]

C cell hyperplasia is diagnosed on calcitonin immunohistochemistry in areas of high C cell concentration when at least 50 C cells or more than 6 C cells per thyroid follicle are found per low-power field (100-fold magnification). Morphologically, reactive C cell hyperplasia, which does not give rise to hereditary MTC, and neoplastic C cell hyperplasia are indistinguishable but only the latter progresses to hereditary MTC in an age-dependent manner. Of note, sporadic MTC, which almost always is a solitary tumor, may be accompanied by reactive C cell hyperplasia in 10% of patients.[28]

Grossly, MTC is a well-demarcated, and in rare instances a completely encapsulated firm tumor with a cut surface of greyish-white to reddish-brown color. The histopathological appearance of MTC can be diverse, mimicking a broad range of tumors of thyroid and nonthyroid origin. As a matter of policy, each unusual thyroid tumor should be stained for calcitonin to confirm, or rule out MTC.[45] Rarely, some MTC lack immunoreactivity to calcitonin, and thus are regarded as "atypical" MTC.[46] Exceptionally, large MTC, referred to as "nonsecretory MTC," do not synthesize or release calcitonin in sufficient quantities to produce increased serum calcitonin levels.[7] Immunohistochemically, these tumors harbor either a few, or only weakly staining calcitonin-positive cells, as encountered in "atypical" MTC, or numerous tumor cells with strong immunoreactivity to calcitonin.[7] Completely calcitonin-negative MTC may intensively stain for calcitonin gene-related peptide (CGRP).[47]

Histologically, MTC is characterized by a solid and compact growth pattern of nests of polygonal and spindle-shaped tumor cells that regularly invade adjacent nonneoplastic thyroid tissue. The cytoplasm of these tumor cells may appear granulated, whereas the generally uniform round-to-oval nuclei exhibit coarsely granulated, so-called *"salt-and-pepper"* chromatin. The number of mitoses can be quite variable. The tumor stroma typically is traversed by delicate bands of collagen, without or with concomitant desmoplasia (Fig. 2.2). The desmoplastic stroma reaction may be interspersed with broad fibrous bands of collagen (Fig. 2.2A), or diffuse collagen deposits surround tumor cells and tumor cell formations (Fig. 2.2B). Stromal desmoplasia, affecting 80% of MTC as a whole or only

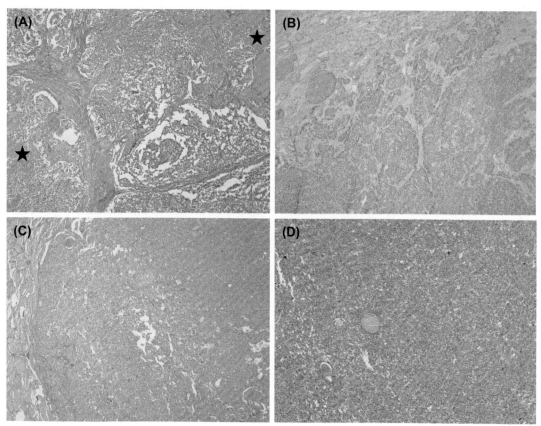

FIG. 2.2 Stromal patterns in medullary thyroid cancer (H&E) **(A)** Desmoplastic stroma reaction interspersed with broad fibrous bands of collagen. Asterisks denote amyloid deposits (×25) **(B)** Desmoplastic stroma reaction with diffuse collagen deposits surrounding tumor cells and tumor cell formations (×25) **(C)** Absence of desmoplastic stroma reaction in a 2.8 cm large node-negative MTC (serum calcitonin 4400 pg/mL; biochemical cure for >10 years; ×25). **(D)** Enlarged detail of Fig. 2.2c (×75).

focally, is significantly associated with larger tumor size, higher tumor stage, and lymph node metastases. Conversely, absence of desmoplasia (Fig. 2.2C and D) is a hallmark of node-negative MTC.[48] On receiver operating characteristic analysis, a 20% threshold of desmoplasia was found to predict lymph node metastases with a sensitivity of 96%, a specificity of 60%, a positive predictive value of 69%, and a negative predictive value of 94% (with 1 of 26 node-positive MTC exhibiting < 20% of desmoplasia).[49]

Some 60%−85% of MTC include amyloid deposits (Fig. 2.2A, asterisks). Although evidence of amyloid can be suggestive of MTC, amyloid deposits as such are nonspecific because they are present in many other conditions as well.

MTC coincides with papillary thyroid microcarcinoma in 7.0%−12.3% of patients. In all likelihood, this coincidental finding is due to greater pathological scrutiny in the search of smaller MTC.[50,51]

SURGICAL MANAGEMENT

Given the unavailability of effective nonsurgical interventions for MTC, operative clearance of the primary thyroid tumor together with its regional lymph nodes is the mainstay of therapy. Before planning a surgical procedure, the potential benefits to be gained from the operation need to be weighed against the attendant operative risks. The net benefit of surgical intervention is a continuous function of (1) the risk of morbidity if left untreated (unknown); (2) the treatment's relative risk reduction (surgical cure); and (3) the treatment's risk of harm (surgical morbidity, low in experienced hands). From a public health perspective, the one-time cost of attaining definitive cure and the cost of daily thyroxine supplementation may be smaller than the need for continual biochemical follow-up and continual imaging, some of which prompt more intervention at additional expenses. To minimize operative morbidity, the inferior parathyroid glands and recurrent laryngeal nerves are identified and preserved in situ on a vascular pedicle before dissecting the thyroid gland off the thyroid bed, keeping the line of dissection to the thyroid capsule as closely as possible.

In patients with hereditary MTC, pheochromocytoma needs to be ruled out biochemically and clinically, and, if present, removed first after having put in place an effective alpha blockade.

Initial Operation

Unless the tumor is technically irresectable or the patient is inoperable, total thyroidectomy should be pursued once the diagnosis of MTC has been established. This line of reasoning is supported by the frequent unavailability of a *RET* gene test result before the initial operation. In hereditary disease, evidenced by a positive *RET* gene test, every parafollicular C cell inside the thyroid gland has inherited the *RET* receptor mutation and may give rise to multifocal MTC, synchronously or metachronously. In sporadic disease, diagnosed with a negative *RET* gene test, there is a 10% risk of multifocal MTC, perhaps owing to intrathyroidal lymphatic spread.[28]

Minimal disease

The rapid clinical take-up of sensitive biochemical and DNA-based screening and high-resolution imaging technology has augmented tumor lead time, which is defined as the length of time between tumor detection through screening and the usual clinical manifestation of the disease.

If performed early, total thyroidectomy once and for all eliminates the potential for malignant transformation inherited by thyroid C cells while sparing young gene carriers additional morbidity from central lymph node dissection, especially postoperative hypoparathyroidism.[52,53] When operated on by experienced surgeons, younger children, including those aged ≤3 years, have no greater operative morbidity than older children,[52,53] although anatomical structures are more delicate and space constraints are greater in the former. In infants and young children, parathyroid glands are small, translucent, and hard to distinguish from adjacent soft tissues, thymus, and central lymph nodes. The thymus of infants and young children may also reach the size of a normal thyroid gland, compromising surgical exposure.[52]

Owing to the high prevalence of lymph node metastases in desmoplasia-positive MTC, total thyroidectomy typically is combined with central lymph node dissection (Fig. 2.3) when preoperative serum calcitonin levels have exceeded 30 pg/mL. Of note, as many as 6%−23.1% of 2-mm large MTC primaries, and 36.9%−43% of 10-mm large MTC primaries have already spread to lymph nodes by the time of diagnosis.[54,55]

For sporadic MTC that comes back desmoplasia-negative on frozen section, hemithyroidectomy conceptually represents adequate surgical therapy although the viability of this approach requires more research.

Advanced disease

Tumor staging takes center stage in devising treatment plans for advanced disease, which must be carefully crafted and attuned to the extent of residual disease

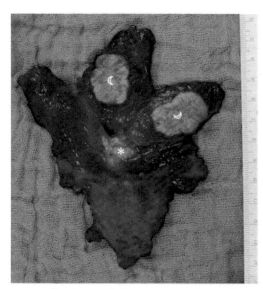

FIG. 2.3 Specimen of the central neck compartment. Primary thyroid tumor (crescent) with lymph node metastasis (asterisk).

taking into account the patient's shape. Before reoperation, it is critical to confirm the functional integrity of both recurrent laryngeal nerves. In patients with extensive locoregional disease, the aerodigestive tract should be evaluated for tumor invasion using computed tomography or magnetic resonance imaging. If technical resectability of tumor in the neck or mediastinum is doubtful, preoperative exclusion of distant metastases is of great value.

Compartment-oriented lymph node dissection.

Lymph node metastases that emerge on imaging represent the tip of the iceberg of lymphatic tumor cell dissemination. This is the rationale behind the concept of *"one positive lymph node, one involved lymph node compartment."* Miliary lymph node metastases, evading the most advanced imaging modalities, are a source of recurrence if not cleared systematically. To keep surgical morbidity low, it is advisable to use optical magnification and bipolar forceps coagulation,[56] nerve monitoring devices,[57,58] and in situ preservation of parathyroid glands, or autografting of completely devascularized parathyroid glands. Continuous intraoperative nerve monitoring heralds imminent nerve injury and enables immediate release of distressed nerves by reversing causative surgical maneuvers.

Lymph node metastases are present in the ipsilateral central and lateral neck, contralateral central neck, contralateral lateral neck, and upper mediastinum when basal calcitonin thresholds exceed 20, 50, 200, and 500 pg/mL, respectively (Fig. 2.4)[5]. The corresponding preoperative procalcitonin thresholds are 0.1, 0.25, 1.0, 1.0, and 5 ng/mL.[2] The more central lymph nodes are involved, the higher is the risk of lateral lymph node metastases in the ipsilateral and contralateral neck.[59]

Lateral lymph node dissection may be warranted for an upper thyroid pole primary, for a tumor with extensive involvement of the central compartment, and for an MTC with increased basal calcitonin level of 20−200 pg/mL (ipsilateral dissection) or >500 pg/mL (bilateral dissection) (Fig. 2.5). When basal calcitonin levels range between 200.1 and 500 pg/mL, systematic dissection of the right lateral neck is worthwhile in patients with left-sided thyroid primaries for completion, whereas it may be prudent to refrain from systematic dissection of the left lateral neck in patients with right-sided thyroid primaries absent evidence of lymph node metastases, steering clear of the thoracic duct to curb the risk of lymphatic leakage (Fig. 2.5).

Systematic bilateral compartment-oriented neck surgery can result in biochemical cure in at least half the patients with preoperative basal calcitonin levels of ≤1000 pg/mL. Lateral lymph node dissection can cause (1) left lateral lymphatic leaks, which manifest early on and are best ligated upon detection, avoiding the use of suture ligations that cut through the tender wall of the leaking lymph vessel; and (2) spinal accessory nerve injury, taking weeks to surface clinically as shoulder dysfunction.[29] Although infrequent, the cervical plexus, the sympathetic trunk, and phrenic, hypoglossal, and vagal nerves can be damaged as well, usually during resection of locoregional disease or during extensive neck dissection. Lateral (phrenic) and central neck (recurrent laryngeal) nerve palsies, working in the same direction, both aggravate breathing difficulties.[29]

Laryngotracheal and esophageal resection.

Invasion of the neck and upper anterior mediastinum greatly contributes to cancer-specific mortality. Most aerodigestive tract invasions originate from extension of the thyroid primary by continuity, reflecting the close proximity between thyroid gland and trachea.[60] With greater distance from the thyroid gland, the lymphatic system takes a more active part in aerodigestive tract invasion, specifically esophageal invasion. Tracheal invasion is believed to proceed through the pretracheal fascia, progressing around or between the cartilaginous rings, and along vessels

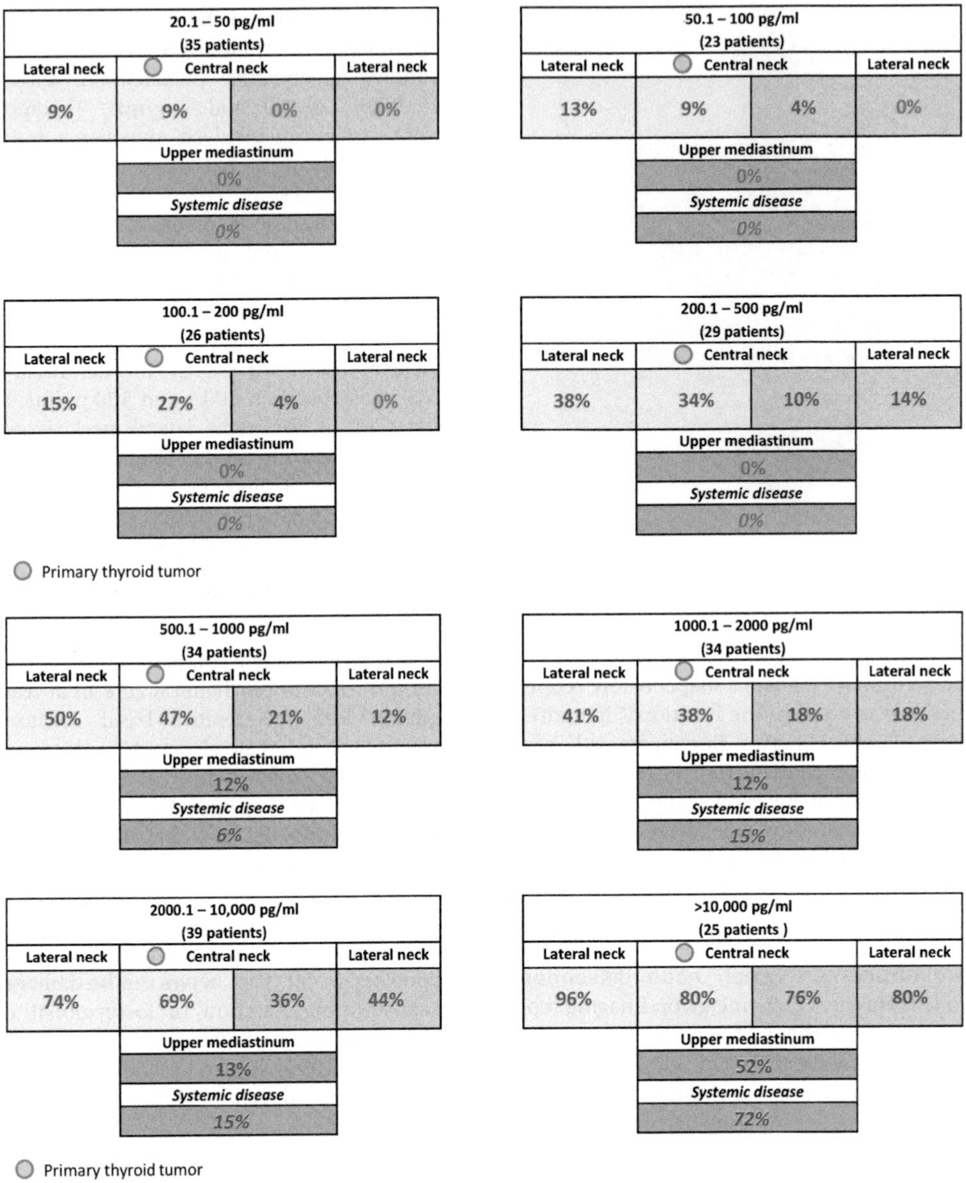

20.1 – 50 pg/ml (35 patients)			
Lateral neck	○ Central neck		Lateral neck
9%	9%	0%	0%
	Upper mediastinum		
	0%		
	Systemic disease		
	0%		

50.1 – 100 pg/ml (23 patients)			
Lateral neck	○ Central neck		Lateral neck
13%	9%	4%	0%
	Upper mediastinum		
	0%		
	Systemic disease		
	0%		

100.1 – 200 pg/ml (26 patients)			
Lateral neck	○ Central neck		Lateral neck
15%	27%	4%	0%
	Upper mediastinum		
	0%		
	Systemic disease		
	0%		

200.1 – 500 pg/ml (29 patients)			
Lateral neck	○ Central neck		Lateral neck
38%	34%	10%	14%
	Upper mediastinum		
	0%		
	Systemic disease		
	0%		

○ Primary thyroid tumor

500.1 – 1000 pg/ml (34 patients)			
Lateral neck	○ Central neck		Lateral neck
50%	47%	21%	12%
	Upper mediastinum		
	12%		
	Systemic disease		
	6%		

1000.1 – 2000 pg/ml (34 patients)			
Lateral neck	○ Central neck		Lateral neck
41%	38%	18%	18%
	Upper mediastinum		
	12%		
	Systemic disease		
	15%		

2000.1 – 10,000 pg/ml (39 patients)			
Lateral neck	○ Central neck		Lateral neck
74%	69%	36%	44%
	Upper mediastinum		
	13%		
	Systemic disease		
	15%		

>10,000 pg/ml (25 patients)			
Lateral neck	○ Central neck		Lateral neck
96%	80%	76%	80%
	Upper mediastinum		
	52%		
	Systemic disease		
	72%		

○ Primary thyroid tumor

FIG. 2.4 Spread of medullary thyroid cancer by preoperative serum calcitonin. (Based on Machens and Dralle, J Clin Endocrinol Metab 2010;95:2655–2663.[5])

penetrating the tracheal wall perpendicular to the lumen down to the tracheal mucosa.[60,61] Invasive thyroid tumors advance along the tracheal circumference, leaving the inner mucosal layer unscathed at first to penetrate it at a later time.[62]

Transsternal mediastinal lymph node dissection (Fig. 2.6) is an option for infrabrachiocephalic mediastinal lymph node metastases or primary tumors growing from the neck into the upper anterior mediastinum.

Not all patients with aerodigestive tract invasion are fit enough to undergo the extensive resection required to clear all tumors.[61,62] Although it does not yield microscopically clear surgical margins, tracheal shaving offers satisfactory disease-specific survival. For locoregional control, resection of gross tumor is of greater

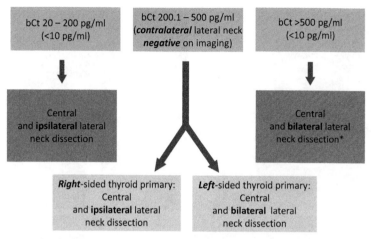

FIG. 2.5 Calcitonin-directed lateral neck dissection for medullary thyroid cancer. bCt, basal calcitonin (before initial thyroidectomy).

relevance than the type of resection. Window and sleeve resections do not differ much in operative morbidity, locoregional recurrence, and survival, so that these procedures are mostly equivalent in clinical practice. Tumors taking up more than 2 cm vertically and more than 25% of the circumference of the laryngocricoid region or the trachea are technically unsuitable for window resection. If nonetheless carried out, the frequency of tracheal leaks increases substantially. Fashioning a tracheostomy as a matter of routine is discouraged because this can promote aerodigestive tract leakage.[61,62]

Reoperation

Before planning a surgical procedure, the potential benefits to be gained from the operation (biochemical cure and locoregional control) need to be balanced with the attendant surgical risk (permanent recurrent laryngeal nerve palsy and hypoparathyroidism). This self-evident truth becomes more obvious when it comes to systematic lymph node dissection for persistent or recurrent cancer in a scarred operative field. For uncommon conditions including persistent or recurrent disease, evidence-based data facilitating this difficult trade-off are rarely, if ever, available. In experienced hands, the benefit of a reoperation for persistent or recurrent MTC usually outweighs the risk of surgical morbidity.

Exceptionally, total thyroidectomy for completion of sporadic disease after initial lobectomy is unnecessary

when serum calcitonin levels remain below the upper normal level of the calcitonin assay. Under these circumstances, barring nonsecretory MTC, compartment-oriented surgery for completion of an initial neck operation is extremely unlikely to reveal lymph node metastases or MTC deposits in the neck.

Reoperation for completion

Reoperation in the neck, involving surgery in a scarred operative field, must be well planned and approached cautiously. Because many outside pathology reports lack adequate information on the location and number of involved and dissected lymph nodes, the adequacy of past neck operations is not always straightforward to assess.[32] These details, when available, are very helpful in planning the necessary extent of reoperation.

Many patients with persistent or recurrent MTC present with significant complications from previous operations, adding to the complexity of the reoperation.[32] When the recurrent laryngeal nerve is not functioning on the side of the primary tumor, surgical completion of the other side can be challenging. In these patients, interests of safety (preservation of contralateral recurrent laryngeal nerve function) prompt modifications of an otherwise standardized surgical approach. In reoperations, there is a fine line between tumor invasion of the recurrent laryngeal nerve and soft tissue infiltrations around the recurrent laryngeal nerve. This may cause some surgeons to dissect the tumor off the nerve to preserve its function where other surgeons

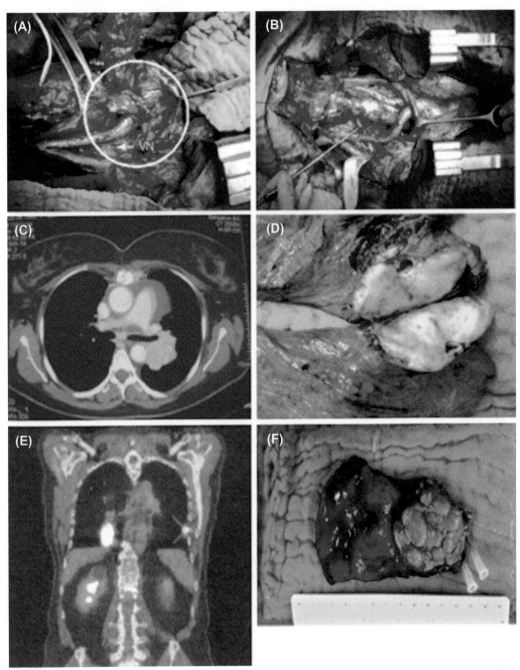

FIG. 2.6 Tackling of the "pacemaker" of recurrent MTC **(A, B)**, lung hilum with tumor obstruction of the left main bronchus **(C, D)**, and lung parenchyma **(E, F)**. (From Randolph ed., *Surgery of the Thyroid and Parathyroid Glands*, third ed., Elsevier Saunders 2019.)

would sacrifice a functional nerve to eradicate the tumor. [32]

In experienced hands, systematic lymph node dissection in patients with persistent or recurrent MTC is worthwhile and reasonably safe as long as serum calcitonin levels do not surpass 1000 pg/mL before reoperation and no more than five lymph node metastases have been cleared earlier. Systematic lymph node dissection performed for completion of an inadequate initial operation can accomplish biochemical cure in 18%–44% of patients. Once one of the aforementioned conditions (>1000 pg/mL before reoperation or >5 previous lymph node metastases) is present, biochemical cure rates are just 1%–5%. The quandary then is whether to opt for systematic lymph node dissection to optimize locoregional control, taking a higher surgical risk, or whether to go for a focused approach to target lesions, which is associated with lower surgical risk. [32] This point should be frankly discussed with the patient who will need to make a value judgment on whether to trade, or not to trade, a somewhat higher surgical risk for possible long-term improvement of locoregional control in the neck.

Targeted surgical approach

Patients with persistent or recurrent MTC who already had systematic dissections of the central and lateral neck compartments, as evidenced by operating notes and pathology reports, usually require no more than a focused surgical approach to clear a target lesion. [32] None of these patients has a realistic chance to attain biochemical cure, not even by undergoing extensive surgery. This is when the focus of treatment moves toward palliation. A targeted surgical approach is key to local control, in particular for growing target lesions that reside near the aerodigestive tract (larynx, trachea, esophagus), great vessels, or the recurrent laryngeal or vagus nerves.

Indolent distant metastases, which reflect systemic disease and seldom occur in isolation, normally do not need resection. Noteworthy exceptions include growing dominant liver and lung metastases or parahilar lymph nodes compressing or invading the bronchial tree, when nonsurgical therapies are unavailable and resection offers at least temporary relief. Bone metastases warrant surgical removal when the spinal cord, nerve roots, or the stability of the spine are in jeopardy. [63]

PROGNOSIS

Systematic lymph node dissection in the neck offers important benefits, first and foremost the chance of biochemical cure. If biochemical cure cannot be accomplished, for instance when distant metastases are present, the focus of treatment shifts to achieving tumor control. [32] Different from pathological tumor-node-metastasis (TNM) stage, which is based on tumor removed (*"what has been taken out"*), postoperative serum calcitonin levels denote the tumor burden after the operation (*"what has been left behind"*). Dynamic risk stratification, including postoperative serum calcitonin levels, is a more accurate reflection of the current situation than static initial anatomic staging. [6,64]

To identify valid surgical targets, patients are followed-up on biochemically, with high-resolution ultrasonography, computed tomography (CT), or magnetic resonance imaging (MRI) tailored to the postoperative serum calcitonin levels and/or calcitonin doubling times. [66,67] When cross-sectional imaging cannot exclude invasion of the aerodigestive tract, bronchoscopy or esophagoscopy come into play to make that determination. Axial magnetic resonance imaging and bone scintigraphy, being complementary, are sensitive procedures to track down bone metastases.

An armamentarium of sophisticated imaging technologies has become available to pinpoint tumor deposits in a scarred neck: positron-emission tomography (PET) without or with simultaneous computed tomography (CT), using 2-[Fluorine-18]fluoro-2-deoxy-D-glucose (FDG), 18F-dihydroxyphenylalanine (F-DOPA), and 68Ga-DOTA-conjugated peptides binding to somatostatin receptors. [68–72] 18F-DOPA PET/CT discloses subclinical disease better than 18FDG-PET/CT, which in turn is more useful in identifying progressive disease. [72] With a positive 18FDG PET/CT scan, survival likely is lower, whatever the result of the 18F-DOPA-PET/CT scan.

Prognosis After Initial Operation

Completeness of surgery, the only curative treatment for MTC, has great impact on clinical outcome. Compartment-oriented surgery is superior to selective dissection of enlarged lymph nodes in normalizing serum calcitonin levels and reaching locoregional tumor control when the tumor is node-positive. [73] Conventional wisdom has it that the initial operation for

MTC is deemed adequate when raised calcitonin levels normalize postoperatively.[32] Histology-proven overall recurrence after compartment-oriented surgery for MTC has been estimated at 4.4% in the dissected central neck at a mean of 61.1 (range 22–116) months; at 6.3% in the dissected ipsilateral lateral neck at a mean of 45.5 (range 8–156) months; and at 2.1% in the dissected contralateral neck at a mean of 49.7 (range 19–71) months.[27] In patients who were biochemically cured after the initial operation, extranodal growth was the sole independent predictor of overall recurrence in the dissected central and lateral neck.

In patients who end up reaching biochemical cure, time to calcitonin normalization is dependent on the level of serum calcitonin before the operation, notably in patients with node-negative MTC.[52] In node-positive patients, time to calcitonin normalization is more protracted, in proportion to the number of lymph node metastases. This delay may mirror the incremental time it takes the calcitonin-enriched lymphatic fluid to advance through the locoregional venous system before emptying into the systemic circulation. Postoperative serum calcitonin usually normalizes within 1 week; and within a fortnight in patients with node-positive MTC and preoperative serum calcitonin levels of 500–1000 pg/mL. In patients with node-positive MTC and preoperative serum calcitonin levels >1000 pg/mL, and in patients with >10 lymph node metastases, time to calcitonin normalization can be increased to 8 weeks if achievable.[74] This quick systemic elimination illustrates why a >50% fall of preoperative serum calcitonin, portending postoperative calcitonin normalization, occurred in patients with node-negative MTC more frequently than in patients with node-positive MTC 30 min after total thyroidectomy and central lymph node dissection.[75]

Prognosis After Reoperation

Systematic lymph node dissection for completion of an inadequate initial operation can bring about biochemical cure in 18%–44% of patients. Once basal calcitonin level are >1000 pg/mL or >5 lymph node metastases have been removed, biochemical cure rates after reoperation are just 1%–5%.

Reoperation for persistent or recurrent MTC can prevent, or at least delay, tumor invasion of the aerodigestive tract and recurrent laryngeal and vagus nerves, preserving breathing and swallowing and helping patients to lead high-quality lives.

SUMMARY

Early detection of, and compartment-oriented surgery for, MTC that has a propensity for lymphatic and hematogenous spread is pivotal to reach biochemical cure and locoregional tumor control. For sporadic MTC, significant increases have taken place recently in the percentage of microscopic tumors (from 11.4%–19% to 25.2%–39%), in mean patient age (from 49.1–49.8 years to 53.8–57.3 years), and in biochemical cure (from 28% to 62%), paralleled by corresponding declines in the percentage of node-positive sporadic MTC (from 73% to 49%), mediastinal lymph node metastasis (from 21% to 6%) and distant metastasis (from 23% to 6%).[76,77] For hereditary MTC, the trend of presentation with early MTC has been even more extreme.[78] This trend may pick up further speed when whole genomic sequencing in neonates for monogenic disorders becomes available, disclosing genetic predisposition to MTC before the tumor comes into existence.

The advent and expansion of advanced diagnostic modalities, including high-resolution ultrasonography, biochemical screening, and DNA-based screening, caused a paradigm shift for sporadic and hereditary medullary thyroid cancer (MTC): from a *"one-size-fits-all"* approach to precision medicine. Precision medicine predicates that patients get the right treatment at the right time, with minimum ill consequences and maximum efficacy.[79] Preoperative and postoperative biomarker serum levels of procalcitonin, calcitonin, and carcinoembryonic antigen (CEA) mirror initial and residual tumor load, helping devise adequate treatment plans by informing the necessary extent of the operation and signifying a patient's prospects of biochemical cure.

Because tumors vary a great deal in biology and progression, treatment plans must be personalized to be commensurate with the extent of the disease at hand. Adequate surgery for MTC, in particular when it comes to persistent or recurrent disease, has to amalgamate technical skills with choice of procedure appropriate to the patients most likely to benefit from it, and should be performed safely and with minimal surgical invasiveness. Refined dissection techniques, supported by the use of optical magnification, bipolar forceps coagulation, and nerve monitoring devices, have been instrumental in establishing locoregional tumor control, keeping health-related quality of life at a high level despite the presence of persistent disease.

REFERENCES

1. Machens A, Dralle H. Surgical treatment of medullary thyroid cancer. *Recent Results Cancer Res.* 2015a;204:187–205.
2. Machens A, Lorenz K, Dralle H. Utility of serum procalcitonin for screening and risk stratification of medullary thyroid cancer. *J Clin Endocrinol Metab.* 2014a;99: 2986–2994.
3. Giovanella L, Imperiali M, Piccardo A, et al. Procalcitonin measurement to screen medullary thyroid carcinoma: a prospective evaluation in a series of 2705 patients with thyroid nodules. *Eur J Clin Invest.* 2018;48:e12934.
4. Machens A, Ukkat J, Hauptmann S, Dralle H. Abnormal carcinoembryonic antigen levels and medullary thyroid cancer progression: a multivariate analysis. *Arch Surg.* 2007a;142:289–293. discussion 294.
5. Machens A, Dralle H. Biomarker-based risk stratification for previously untreated medullary thyroid cancer. *J Clin Endocrinol Metab.* 2010;95:2655–2663.
6. Yip DT, Hassan M, Pazaitou-Panayiotou K, et al. Preoperative basal calcitonin and tumor stage correlate with postoperative calcitonin normalization in patients undergoing initial surgical management of medullary thyroid carcinoma. *Surgery.* 2011;150:1168–1177.
7. Frank-Raue K, Machens A, Leidig-Bruckner G, et al. Prevalence and clinical spectrum of nonsecretory medullary thyroid carcinoma in a series of 839 patients with sporadic medullary thyroid carcinoma. *Thyroid.* 2013;23: 294–300.
8. Barbosa SL, Rodien P, Leboulleux S, et al. Groupe d'Etude des Tumeurs Endocrines. Ectopic adrenocorticotropic hormone-syndrome in medullary carcinoma of the thyroid: a retrospective analysis and review of the literature. *Thyroid.* 2005;15:618–623.
9. Dadu R, Hu MI, Cleeland C, et al. Efficacy of the natural clay, calcium aluminosilicate anti-diarrheal, in reducing medullary thyroid cancer-related diarrhea and its effects on quality of life: a pilot study. *Thyroid.* 2015;25: 1085–1090.
10. Mathiesen JS, Kroustrup JP, Vestergaard P, et al. Danish Thyroid Cancer Group (DATHYRCA). Incidence and prevalence of sporadic and hereditary MTC in Denmark 1960–2014: a nationwide study. *Endocr Connect.* 2018;7: 829–839.
11. Agrawal N, Jiao Y, Sausen M, et al. Exomic sequencing of medullary thyroid cancer reveals dominant and mutually exclusive oncogenic mutations in RET and RAS. *J Clin Endocrinol Metab.* 2013;98:E364–E369.
12. Heilmann AM, Subbiah V, Wang K, et al. Comprehensive genomic profiling of clinically advanced medullary thyroid carcinoma. *Oncology.* 2016;90:339–346.
13. Elisei R, Cosci B, Romei C, et al. Prognostic significance of somatic RET oncogene mutations in sporadic medullary thyroid cancer: a 10-year follow-up study. *J Clin Endocrinol Metab.* 2008;93:682–687.
14. Romei C, Ciampi R, Casella F, et al. RET mutation heterogeneity in primary advanced medullary thyroid cancers and their metastases. *Oncotarget.* 2018;9:9875–9884.
15. Romei C, Ugolini C, Cosci B, et al. Low prevalence of the somatic M918T RET mutation in micro-medullary thyroid cancer. *Thyroid.* 2012;22:476–481.
16. Moura MM, Cavaco BM, Pinto AE, Leite V. High prevalence of RAS mutations in RET-negative sporadic medullary thyroid carcinomas. *J Clin Endocrinol Metab.* 2011;96: E863–E868.
17. Romei C, Casella F, Tacito A, et al. New insights in the molecular signature of advanced medullary thyroid cancer: evidence of a bad outcome of cases with double RET mutations. *J Med Genet.* 2016;53:729–734.
18. Sherman SI, Clary DO, Elisei R, et al. Correlative analyses of RET and RAS mutations in a phase 3 trial of cabozantinib in patients with progressive, metastatic medullary thyroid cancer. *Cancer.* 2016;122:3856–3864.
19. Machens A, Dralle H. Advances in risk-oriented surgery for multiple endocrine neoplasia type 2. *Endocr Relat Cancer.* 2018;25:T41–T52.
20. Wells Jr SA, Asa SL, Dralle H, et al. American Thyroid Association Guidelines Task Force on Medullary Thyroid Carcinoma. Revised American Thyroid Association guidelines for the management of medullary thyroid carcinoma. *Thyroid.* 2015;25:567–610.
21. Machens A, Lorenz K, Weber F, Dralle H. Genotype-specific progression of hereditary medullary thyroid cancer. *Hum Mutat.* 2018a;39:860–869.
22. Rich TA, Feng L, Busaidy N, et al. Prevalence by age and predictors of medullary thyroid cancer in patients with lower risk germline RET proto-oncogene mutations. *Thyroid.* 2014;24:1096–1106.
23. Machens A, Hauptmann S, Dralle H. Modification of multiple endocrine neoplasia 2A phenotype by cell membrane proximity of RET mutations in exon 10. *Endocr Relat Cancer.* 2009a;16:171–177.
24. Machens A, Lorenz K, Dralle H. Progression of medullary thyroid cancer in RET carriers of ATA class A and C mutations. *J Clin Endocrinol Metab.* 2014b;99: E286–E292.
25. Rohmer V, Vidal-Trecan G, Bourdelot A, et al. Groupe Français des Tumeurs Endocrines. Prognostic factors of disease-free survival after thyroidectomy in 170 young patients with a RET germline mutation: a multicenter study of the Groupe Francais d'Etude des Tumeurs Endocrines. *J Clin Endocrinol Metab.* 2011;96:E509–E518.
26. Machens A, Dralle H. Breach of the thyroid capsule and lymph node capsule in node-positive papillary and medullary thyroid cancer: different biology. *Eur J Surg Oncol.* 2015b;41:766–772.
27. Machens A, Lorenz K, Dralle H. Histology-proven recurrence in the lateral or central neck after systematic neck

dissection for medullary thyroid cancer. *Endocrine.* 2018b; 61:428–439.

28. Machens A, Hauptmann S, Dralle H. Increased risk of lymph node metastasis in multifocal hereditary and sporadic medullary thyroid cancer. *World J Surg.* 2007b;31: 1960–1965.

29. Dralle H, Machens A. Surgical management of the lateral neck compartment for metastatic thyroid cancer. *Curr Opin Oncol.* 2013;25:20–26.

30. Machens A, Dralle H. Prognostic impact of N staging in 715 medullary thyroid cancer patients: proposal for a revised staging system. *Ann Surg.* 2013a;257:323–329.

31. Kouvaraki MA, Shapiro SE, Fornage BD, et al. Role of preoperative ultrasonography in the surgical management of patients with thyroid cancer. *Surgery.* 2003;134:946–954. discussion 954–955.

32. Machens A, Dralle H. Benefit-risk balance of reoperation for persistent medullary thyroid cancer. *Ann Surg.* 2013b; 257:751–757.

33. Graze K, Spiler IJ, Tashjian Jr AH, et al. Natural history of familial medullary thyroid carcinoma: effect of a program for early diagnosis. *N Engl J Med.* 1978;299:980–985.

34. Gagel RF, Tashjian Jr AH, Cummings T, et al. The clinical outcome of prospective screening for multiple endocrine neoplasia type 2a. An 18-year experience. *N Engl J Med.* 1988;318:478–484.

35. Morris LF, Waguespack SG, Edeiken-Monroe BS, et al. Ultrasonography should not guide the timing of thyroidectomy in pediatric patients diagnosed with multiple endocrine neoplasia syndrome 2A through genetic screening. *Ann Surg Oncol.* 2013;20:53–59.

36. Machens A, Hoffmann F, Sekulla C, Dralle H. Importance of gender-specific calcitonin thresholds in screening for occult sporadic medullary thyroid cancer. *Endocr Relat Cancer.* 2009b;16:1291–1298.

37. Ahmed SR, Ball DW. Clinical review: incidentally discovered medullary thyroid cancer: diagnostic strategies and treatment. *J Clin Endocrinol Metab.* 2011;96: 1237–1245.

38. Mian C, Perrino M, Colombo C, et al. Refining calcium test for the diagnosis of medullary thyroid cancer: cutoffs, procedures, and safety. *J Clin Endocrinol Metab.* 2014;99: 1656–1664.

39. Machens A, Niccoli-Sire P, Hoegel J, et al. European Multiple Endocrine Neoplasia (EUROMEN) Study Group. Early malignant progression of hereditary medullary thyroid cancer. *N Engl J Med.* 2003;349:1517–1525.

40. Skinner MA, Moley JA, Dilley WG, Owzar K, Debenedetti MK, Wells Jr SA. Prophylactic thyroidectomy in multiple endocrine neoplasia type 2A. *N Engl J Med.* 2005;353:1105–1113.

41. Machens A, Lorenz K, Dralle H. Individualization of lymph node dissection in RET (rearranged during transfection) carriers at risk for medullary thyroid cancer: value of pretherapeutic calcitonin levels. *Ann Surg.* 2009c;250: 305–310.

42. Elisei R, Romei C, Renzini G, et al. The timing of total thyroidectomy in RET gene mutation carriers could be

personalized and safely planned on the basis of serum calcitonin: 18 years experience at one single center. *J Clin Endocrinol Metab.* 2012;97:426–435.

43. Castagna MG, Fugazzola L, Maino F, et al. Reference range of serum calcitonin in pediatric population. *J Clin Endocrinol Metab.* 2015;100:1780–1784.

44. O'Toole K, Fenoglio-Preiser C, Pushparaj N. Endocrine changes associated with the human aging process: III. Effect of age on the number of calcitonin immunoreactive cells in the thyroid gland. *Hum Pathol.* 1985;16: 991–1000.

45. Schmid KW. Histopathology of C cells and medullary thyroid carcinoma. *Recent Results Cancer Res.* 2015;204: 41–60.

46. Schmid KW, Ensinger C. "Atypical" medullary thyroid carcinoma with little or no calcitonin expression. *Virchows Arch.* 1998;433:209–215.

47. Nakazawa T, Cameselle-Teijeiro J, Vinagre J, et al. C-cell-derived calcitonin-free neuroendocrine carcinoma of the thyroid: the diagnostic importance of CGRP immunoreactivity. *Int J Surg Pathol.* 2014;22:530–535.

48. Koperek O, Scheuba C, Cherenko M, et al. Desmoplasia in medullary thyroid carcinoma: a reliable indicator of metastatic potential. *Histopathology.* 2008;52:623–630.

49. Aubert S, Berdelou A, Gnemmi V, et al. Large sporadic thyroid medullary carcinomas: predictive factors for lymph node involvement. *Virchows Arch.* 2018;472:461–468.

50. Machens A, Dralle H. Simultaneous medullary and papillary thyroid cancer: a novel entity? *Ann Surg Oncol.* 2012a; 19:37–44.

51. Wong RL, Kazaure HS, Roman SA, Sosa JA. Simultaneous medullary and differentiated thyroid cancer: a population-level analysis of an increasingly common entity. *Ann Surg Oncol.* 2012;19:2635–2642.

52. Machens A, Elwerr M, Lorenz K, Weber F, Dralle H. Long-term outcome of prophylactic thyroidectomy in children carrying RET germline mutations. *Br J Surg.* 2018c;105: e150–e157.

53. Prete FP, Abdel-Aziz T, Morkane C, Brain C, Kurzawinski TR. MEN2 in Children UK Collaborative Group. Prophylactic thyroidectomy in children with multiple endocrine neoplasia type 2. *Br J Surg.* 2018;105: 1319–1327.

54. Kazaure HS, Roman SA, Sosa JA. Medullary thyroid microcarcinoma: a population-level analysis of 310 patients. *Cancer.* 2012;118:620–627.

55. Machens A, Dralle H. Biological relevance of medullary thyroid microcarcinoma. *J Clin Endocrinol Metab.* 2012b; 97:1547–1553.

56. Dralle H. Lymph node dissection and medullary thyroid carcinoma. *Br J Surg.* 2002;89:1073–1075.

57. Schneider R, Sekulla C, Machens A, Lorenz K, Nguyen Thanh P, Dralle H. Postoperative vocal fold palsy in patients undergoing thyroid surgery with continuous or intermittent nerve monitoring. *Br J Surg.* 2015;102: 1380–1387.

58. Schneider R, Machens A, Sekulla C, Lorenz K, Weber F, Dralle H. Twenty-year experience of paediatric thyroid

surgery using intraoperative nerve monitoring. *Br J Surg*. 2018;105:996–1005.

59. Machens A, Hauptmann S, Dralle H. Prediction of lateral lymph node metastases in medullary thyroid cancer. *Br J Surg*. 2008;95:586–591.

60. Machens A, Hinze R, Lautenschläger C, Thomusch O, Dralle H. Thyroid carcinoma invading the cervicovisceral axis: routes of invasion and clinical implications. *Surgery*. 2001;129:23–28.

61. Dralle H, Machens A, Brauckhof M, Thank PN. Chapter 49: surgical management of advanced thyroid cancer invading the aerodigestive tract. In: Clark OH, Duh QY, Kebebew E, Gosnell JE, Shen WT, eds. *Textbook of Endocrine Surgery*. 3rd revised edition. New Delhi: Jaypee Brothers Medical Publishers; 2016:603–626.

62. Brauckhoff M, Machens A, Thanh PN, et al. Impact of extent of resection for thyroid cancer invading the aerodigestive tract on surgical morbidity, local recurrence, and cancer-specific survival. *Surgery*. 2010;148:1257–1266.

63. Xu JY, Murphy Jr WA, Milton DR, et al. Bone metastases and skeletal-related events in medullary thyroid carcinoma. *J Clin Endocrinol Metab*. 2016;101:4871–4877.

64. Lindsey SC, Ganly I, Palmer F, Tuttle RM. Response to initial therapy predicts clinical outcomes in medullary thyroid cancer. *Thyroid*. 2015;25:242–249.

65. Yang JH, Lindsey SC, Camacho CP, et al. Integration of a postoperative calcitonin measurement into an anatomical staging system improves initial risk stratification in medullary thyroid cancer. *Clin Endocrinol*. 2015;83:938–942.

66. Laure Giraudet A, Al Ghulzan A, Aupérin A, et al. Progression of medullary thyroid carcinoma: assessment with calcitonin and carcinoembryonic antigen doubling times. *Eur J Endocrinol*. 2008;158:239–246.

67. Meijer JA, le Cessie S, van den Hout WB, et al. Calcitonin and carcinoembryonic antigen doubling times as prognostic factors in medullary thyroid carcinoma: a structured meta-analysis. *Clin Endocrinol*. 2010;72:534–542.

68. Machens A, Kotzerke J, Dralle H. Dens of axis metastasis from medullary thyroid cancer. *J Clin Endocrinol Metab*. 2012;97:721–722.

69. Verbeek HH, Plukker JT, Koopmans KP, et al. Clinical relevance of 18F-FDG PET and 18F-DOPA PET in recurrent medullary thyroid carcinoma. *J Nucl Med*. 2012;53:1863–1871.

70. Treglia G, Castaldi P, Villani MF, et al. Comparison of 18F-DOPA, 18F-FDG and 68Ga-somatostatin analogue PET/CT in patients with recurrent medullary thyroid carcinoma. *Eur J Nucl Med Mol Imaging*. 2012;39:569–580.

71. Archier A, Heimburger C, Guerin C, et al. (18)F-DOPA PET/CT in the diagnosis and localization of persistent medullary thyroid carcinoma. *Eur J Nucl Med Mol Imaging*. 2016;43:1027–1033.

72. Romero-Lluch AR, Cuenca-Cuenca JI, Guerrero-Vázquez R, et al. Diagnostic utility of PET/CT with 18F-DOPA and 18F-FDG in persistent or recurrent medullary thyroid carcinoma: the importance of calcitonin and carcinoembryonic antigen cutoff. *Eur J Nucl Med Mol Imaging*. 2017;44:2004–2013.

73. Rowland KJ, Jin LX, Moley JF. Biochemical cure after reoperations for medullary thyroid carcinoma: a meta-analysis. *Ann Surg Oncol*. 2015;22:96–102.

74. Machens A, Lorenz K, Dralle H. Time to calcitonin normalization after surgery for node-negative and node-positive medullary thyroid cancer. *Br J Surg*. 2019; **106**:412-418.

75. Faggiano A, Milone F, Ramundo V, et al. A decrease of calcitonin serum concentrations less than 50 percent 30 minutes after thyroid surgery suggests incomplete C-cell tumor tissue removal. *J Clin Endocrinol Metab*. 2010;95:E32–E36.

76. Machens A, Dralle H. Surgical cure rates of sporadic medullary thyroid cancer in the era of calcitonin screening. *Eur J Endocrinol*. 2016;175:219–228.

77. Randle RW, Balentine CJ, Leverson GE, et al. Trends in the presentation, treatment, and survival of patients with medullary thyroid cancer over the past 30 years. *Surgery*. 2017;161:137–146.

78. Machens A, Dralle H. Therapeutic effectiveness of screening for multiple endocrine neoplasia type 2A. *J Clin Endocrinol Metab*. 2015c;100:2539–2545.

79. Mirnezami R, Nicholson J, Darzi A. Preparing for precision medicine. *N Engl J Med*. 2012;366:489–491.

CHAPTER 3

Management of Undifferentiated (Anaplastic) Thyroid Cancer

ANDREA R. MARCADIS, MD • ASHOK R. SHAHA, MD, FACS

INTRODUCTION

Thyroid cancer is commonly classified based on cell of origin, with the more common cancers being of follicular cell origin, including papillary thyroid cancer (PTC), follicular thyroid cancer (FTC), and Hurthle cell cancer (HTC), and the less common cancers of neuroendocrine origin including medullary thyroid cancer (MTC).[1] Each of these variants of thyroid cancer can also be further subdivided by degree of differentiation, ranging from the common well differentiated thyroid cancers (WDTC) to poorly differentiated thyroid cancer (PDTC) and the rare undifferentiated anaplastic thyroid cancer (ATC). Although WDTCs of follicular cell origin generally have a favorable prognosis, thyroid cancers that are more undifferentiated generally carry a worse prognosis, with undifferentiated ATCs almost uniformly showing aggressive behavior with a high rate of metastasis and a rapidly fatal course, and most patients dying within 6 months of diagnosis.[2,3]

ATC is exceedingly rare. All thyroid cancers combined represent only about 3.6% of malignancies diagnosed in the United States, of which 1%–2% of those are ATCs.[4,5] ATC is slightly more common outside of the United States, representing 1%–10% of thyroid cancers diagnosed worldwide.[1] Although the incidence of ATC is low, it is the most aggressive form of thyroid cancer, and accounts for 14%–39% of deaths from thyroid cancer overall.[5,6] The peak incidence of ATC is in the 6th and 7th decades, with most patients being older than 50 years of age, with a slight female predominance (approximately 2:1 female:male).[7,8]

Interestingly, although the incidence of WDTC has increased significantly in the past 2 decades, often attributed to the diagnosis of more subcentimeter thyroid nodules and papillary microcarcinomas with the increased use of neck ultrasounds, the incidence of ATC has in fact *decreased* significantly during this time period.[4] This may be in part due to improved early treatment and surveillance of small thyroid cancers, thus preventing them from developing into ATCs, as well as increases in dietary iodine content from salt supplementation, leading to a decrease in endemic goiters that are a known risk factor for ATC.[3,9–12] Additionally, improvements in histologic diagnosis have allowed many previously diagnosed ATCs to be reclassified as other tumor types such as thyroid lymphomas or undifferentiated MTCs.[3,13]

Whether ATC arises de novo from normal thyroid cells or from dedifferentiation of a previously existing WDTC is an ongoing area of discussion, and there is scientific evidence that both processes may occur. Evidence for the "de novo" hypothesis of ATC tumorigenesis includes the fact that there are some patients (especially those < 50 years of age) who have tumors with pure ATC, and no intermediates or WDTC present. These tumors are completely undifferentiated, and oftentimes can only be recognized as thyroid cancers because of their anatomic location and absence of another primary malignancy.[3] Other studies that support the "dedifferentiation" hypothesis show the presence of WDTC within ATC tumors,[3,14] and many cite the fact that up to 80% of ATCs are diagnosed in patients with a long history of thyroid goiter as evidence for this hypothesis.[1,15] This postmalignant dedifferentiation is considered to occur not in a single step, but instead as a series of mutations that lead to progressive chromosomal instability and, thus, even more genetic alterations as the tumor progresses from WDTC to PDTC to ATC.[1] This theory is further supported by the fact that more aggressive carcinomas, such as tall cell variant of PTC, follicular thyroid cancers, and PDTCs commonly coexist with ATC.[3,16,17]

In recent years, improvements in molecular sequencing technology have allowed many questions about the dedifferentiation theory of ATC pathogenesis to be answered. Although the mutational burden in

Advances in Treatment and Management in Surgical Endocrinology. https://doi.org/10.1016/B978-0-323-66195-9.00003-0

WDTC is generally low, it is higher in PDTC, and even higher in ATC due to accumulation of multiple mutations.[18] The genetic alterations common to WDTC, such as mutations in *BRAF* and *RAS*, are found at higher frequency in ATCs that contain areas of WDTC compared to ATCs with no areas of WTDC.[3,19–22] Some genetic alterations, such as mutations in *TP53* occur as late steps in the pathogenesis of ATC and are considered to be hallmarks of the disease. *TP53* mutations occur in 50%–75% of ATCs compared to 8% in PDTCs,[18,21] and, when a tumor contains both well-differentiated and undifferentiated areas, the *TP53* mutations are only found in the undifferentiated areas.[3,23–25] This is evidence that *TP53* likely plays a role in the dedifferentiation process of ATC.[3] Mutations in the *TERT* promoter, which encodes the reverse transcriptase element of the telomerase complex, are also thought to be a late step in ATC pathogenesis, detected in 73% of ATCs compared to 40% of PDTCs, and in much smaller subclonal populations in WDTC.[18]

Other genetic alterations common to ATC include mutations in the PI3K/AKT/mTOR intracellular signaling pathway (39% in ATC compared to 11% in PDTC), genes that encode the SWI/SNF nucleosome remodeling complex (36% in ATC, 6% in PDTC), histone methyltransferases (24% in ATC, 7% in PDTC), and DNA mismatch repair pathways (12% in ATC, 2% in PDTC), among many others.[18,21] Genetic copy number alterations are also commonly observed in ATC and other advanced thyroid cancers, and may be associated with worse patient outcomes.[18,26] Conversely, although fusions involving genes known to be translocated in thyroid tumors are found frequently in PDTCs, one study showed that they are almost absent in ATCs.[18] Other work on microRNAs (miRNAs; small noncoding RNAs that participate in posttranscriptional gene regulation) show that although they are commonly overexpressed in many thyroid cancers, ATCs seem to have their own signature profile of altered miRNAs.[21,27,28] Although these improvements in histologic and molecular interpretation have improved diagnostic accuracy in ATC, the diagnosis is usually suspected based on a patient's history and physical exam alone and can be confirmed by cytology or surgical pathology specimens.

DIAGNOSIS

Almost all patients with ATC present with a rapidly enlarging thyroid mass.[15,29] The most frequent symptoms of ATC are from local compression and include hoarseness (40%), dysphagia (40%), and dyspnea or stridor (24%).[5] If the tumor hemorrhages into the thyroid parenchyma, patients can present with a thyroid mass that enlarges over hours, as well as pain and/or hemoptysis if the bleeding extends into the trachea.[3] Patients can also present with signs and symptoms of regional spread, including lymphadenopathy (54%) and/or neck pain (26%).[5] If the ATC is already metastatic at presentation (approximately 50%), patients may experience systemic symptoms such as anorexia and weight loss, or shortness of breath from pulmonary metastasis.[5,30]

In a patient who presents with signs or symptoms of ATC, it is important to obtain a complete history, paying special attention to any risk factors for ATC including older age, history of radiation to the chest or neck, longstanding goiter, and family history of thyroid pathology.[8,31] A full physical examination should be performed, with attention paid to the cervical lymph node examination as well as any signs of metastatic disease. The American Thyroid Association (ATA) guidelines recommend fine needle aspiration biopsy or core biopsy for preoperative diagnosis of ATC, and if the sample obtained from the biopsy is limited or nondiagnostic, then open biopsy should be performed to confirm the diagnosis.[32] Cytology from ATC nodules typically reveals multinucleated cells with large, bizarre nuclei and multiple atypical mitotic features, with no features of thyroid differentiation.[1]

In patients where ATC is suspected, basic laboratory studies to assess for anemia, adequacy of platelets, and infection should be performed, as well as assessment of electrolytes, liver function, and thyroid function.[32] Thyroid and neck ultrasounds should be obtained to evaluate the primary tumor and assess cervical lymph node basins for metastatic disease, as well as aid in assessing airway patency.[32] All patients with suspected ATC should undergo vocal cord evaluation with fiber optic laryngoscopy or mirror examination, and in patients with suspected airway invasion on laryngoscopy, a bronchoscopy to evaluate the trachea is helpful to determine disease extent and resectability.[32] Similarly, an esophagoscopy should be performed if there is suspected esophageal invasion.[32] Cross-sectional imaging (MRI and/or CT) of the neck and chest is recommended to assess extent of disease and evaluate for pulmonary metastasis. If available, PET-CT may be a valuable tool in evaluating for metastatic sites, especially looking for evidence of lung metastasis (present in 80% of patients with metastatic ATC), bone metastasis (6%–16%), and brain metastasis (5%–13%).[5,6,32–35] It is important that preoperative imaging is undertaken expeditiously and does not delay therapy in patients with ATC.[32] In addition, primary surgery should generally not be delayed to biopsy suspected distant metastasis, which could be performed after primary surgical treatment if necessary.[32]

Oftentimes, a suspected diagnosis of ATC is confirmed on surgical pathology, where ATCs are characterized by their aggressive features. Characteristics common to all subtypes of ATC include invasiveness, extensive necrosis, nuclear pleomorphism, and high mitotic activity (Nikiforov et al., 2012). ATC cells do not form thyroid follicles or colloid, and instead are arranged in solid sheets, though sometimes thyroid follicles can be observed in areas of WDTC or normal thyroid tissue that has been trapped by the ATC (Nikiforov et al., 2012). On surgical pathology, ATC may be further characterized by the presence of spindle, squamoid, or osteoclast-like giant cells, and the predominance of one of these cell types gives rise to a histological pattern by which the ATC can be subclassified[1] (Nikiforov et al., 2012) The most common variant of ATC is spindle cell (50%) followed by pleomorphic giant cell (30%–40%) and squamoid (<20%) (Nikiforov et al., 2012).[3] Other variants of ATC, such as paucicellular, rhabdoid, and small cell variant are more rare and are now often reclassified as other types of thyroid cancer (lymphoma, medullary thyroid cancer, PDTC).[3] Another common histological feature of ATCs is the finding of tumor-associated macrophages (TAMs) interspersed with the cancer cells. These have been found in varying degrees (22%–95%) and may form a web-like structure within the tumor that is specific to ATC and other advanced human cancers, but not observed in WDTC.[3,36–38]

In contrast to WDTCs of follicular cell origin, ATC cells usually do not retain any of the functions or features of thyroid follicular cells. For example, ATCs generally do not participate in iodine uptake, produce thyroglobulin, or respond to thyroid stimulating hormone (TSH).[3] Because of this dedifferentiation, immunohistochemistry (IHC) staining for thyroid markers (thyroglobulin, TTF1, keratins, PAX8) is generally weak and focal. PDTC, in comparison, usually has an intermediate level of IHC positivity for thyroid markers, falling somewhere between the strongly positive WDTC and weak ATC signals.[3,32]

The variable histological features and weak immunoreactivity of ATC mean that the differential diagnosis for ATC is broad, making the diagnosis difficult for pathologists. The differential diagnosis for ATC includes PDTC, WDTC with uncommon patterns, medullary thyroid cancer (which sometimes can become dedifferentiated), unusual primary thyroid cancers (lymphomas, squamous cell thyroid cancer, carcinomas with thymus-like elements), metastatic carcinomas from other sites, and Reidel's thyroiditis (can mimic paucicellular variant of ATC)[3,3a-b]. These other pathologies, however, generally do not show the high nuclear pleomorphism, necrosis, and mitotic activity observed in ATC, and the distinction can often be made based on clinical history, presence of other systemic malignancies, IHC for markers specific to the other entities in the differential, and molecular testing (DeLelis et al., 2004).[39]

Staging of ATC is based on the American Joint Committee on Cancer (AJCC) 8th edition (October 2016). As with the AJCC 7th edition, all ATCs are considered Stage IV, and are subclassified as Stage IVA (intrathyroidal tumor), IVB (gross extrathyroidal extension [ETE] or cervical lymph node metastasis), or IVC (distant metastasis).[40,41] The eighth edition staging of ATC differs slightly from the seventh edition in the "T" stage of the "TNM" system. In the seventh edition, ATC always carried a T stage of T4, however in the eighth edition, the T stage is based on tumor size and ETE, similar to other WDTCs (T1 ≤ 2 cm, T2 2–4 cm, T3 > 4 cm or gross ETE into strap muscles, T4 gross ETE into major neck structures). In the AJCC eighth edition, the "N" and "M" category staging remains the same as in the seventh edition (N0—no evidence of regional lymph node metastasis, N1—metastasis to regional nodes; M0—no distant metastasis, M1—distant metastasis).[40,41] In patients with ATC, correct staging is critical for ensuring that patients receive the treatment that will maximize their length of survival.

TREATMENT

Treatment of ATC remains an area of constant discussion as well as an area of exciting scientific discovery. The rarity of the disease, as well as its aggressive nature, and its relative refractoriness to many common chemotherapeutic agents make improving therapies for ATC difficult. Because ATC can develop and become symptomatic so quickly, its diagnosis requires immediate involvement of a multidisciplinary team of surgeons, radiation and medical oncologists, endocrinologists, pathologists, palliative care teams, and other necessary specialists.[3] The most recent ATA guidelines for the management of ATC recommend surgery, external beam radiation, and chemotherapy as the three primary pillars for the treatment of ATC, and these modalities may be used in different combinations depending on each patient's individual case.[32] As the most common cause of death from ATC is local invasion of vital neck structures, achieving local control gives the best chance for short-term palliation and survival.[42]

Surgical treatment for ATC is highly case dependent. In general, patients that have stage IVA and IVB disease (intrathyroidal or extrathyroidal ATC without aerodigestive tract invasion) should be considered for primary surgical management, when at least gross tumor resection (R1) can be achieved.[32,43] There are several studies that reveal a survival benefit in ATC if a complete resection can be achieved.[31,33,44–51] Because of the heterogeneous inclusion criteria in these studies, there is insufficient data to determine if there is a difference in disease-free survival between patients who have grossly negative margins (R1) compared to those who have microscopically negative margins (R0). The ATA guidelines recommended a thyroid lobectomy or near-total thyroidectomy with therapeutic lymph node dissection for patients with intrathyroidal (Stage IVA) disease, and recommend en-bloc resection if grossly negative margins (R1) can be achieved for patients with extrathyroidal invasion (Stage IVB).[32] It is important to note, however, that although most studies do show a survival benefit with R0 or R1 resection, only a small group of patients present with fully resectable disease, and, ultimately, it is left up to the operating surgeon as to whether a primary tumor resection can be attempted with acceptable risk and morbidity.[32] Many patients with initially unresectable disease benefit from external beam radiation (either full or partial course) or neoadjuvant chemotherapy to shrink the tumor, followed by surgical resection.[32]

Even after complete or near complete (R0 or R1) resection of ATC, many studies support the use of adjuvant radiotherapy, usually in combination with chemotherapy.[7,32,35,48,52–55] The ATA guidelines recommend that following an R0 or R1 operation for ATC, patients with good performance status and no evidence of metastasis who wish to have aggressive treatment should be offered postoperative radiation therapy (usually within 2–3 weeks after surgery) with or without concurrent chemotherapy (can begin sooner, even within 1 week of surgery if patient is sufficiently recovered).[32] External beam radiotherapy is generally given at a dose of at least 50–70 Gy and either hyperfractionated, intensity modulated radiotherapy (IMRT), or standard radiation may be used.[32] IMRT is recommended by the most recent ATA guidelines, however hyperfractionated radiation allows for a shorter overall treatment time and may improve survival compared to conventional IMRT (though with a higher toxicity profile), and some argue that it should be used as the preferred radiotherapy when possible.[56,57,32]

When treating a patient with radiation, toxicity can be a limiting factor, and some of the more common complications of radiotherapy for ATC include pharyngoesophagitis, tracheitis, skin changes, and radiation myelopathy.[57]

The most commonly used chemotherapeutic agents for ATC include taxanes (paclitaxel or docetaxel), anthracyclines (doxorubicin), and platins (cisplatin, carboplatin).[3] Although doxorubicin has been one of the most utilized drugs for ATC throughout the years, it is best when used in combination with other chemotherapies and has been shown to be more effective when used together with taxanes, platins, or bleomycin.[42,58] In contrast to doxorubicin, the taxanes paclitaxel and docetaxel have been shown to be effective for ATC even when used as single agents.[53,59–62] These chemotherapies are most often combined with radiotherapy in the adjuvant setting.[60]

In recent years, there has been a major interest in the use of targeted therapy for many cancers including ATC. Some of the most commonly used targeted therapies in ATC are multiple tyrosine kinase inhibitors (TKIs) that target the tyrosine kinase transmembrane and cytosolic cell signaling molecules which are often aberrantly activated in cancer.[3] Some of the TKIs that have been evaluated in clinical trials include imatinib, pazopanib, vemurafenib, gefitinib, axitinib, sunitinib, sorafenib, entrectinib, and lenvatinib.[3] Most of these are still undergoing Phase II clinical trials, but many show promise in improving survival in ATC patients.[63–66] Other drugs that are being evaluated in clinical trials include BRAF inhibitors, mTOR inhibitors, ALK inhibitors, MEK inhibitors, VEGF inhibitors, PD1/PDL1 inhibitors, and CTLA4 inhibitors, among others.[43] Even more targeted therapies are currently being studied in preclinical models.[43]

In patients who cannot undergo resection for curative intent, there are many palliative options, including surgery, radiation, and/or chemotherapy. In patients with large tumors that cannot be fully resected, surgical debulking has been shown to improve survival time, especially when combined with other therapies, and can help to prevent death from suffocation.[32,67] Other local treatments such as endotracheal laser excision or endotracheal stent placement may be performed to relieve obstruction from tumor compression or endotracheal invasion.[68] Low-dose palliative radiation may be used to control pain and obstructive symptoms in patients with local symptoms and poor performance status who cannot tolerate palliative debulking surgery.[32] A gastrostomy tube can be placed for enteral nutrition in patients with difficulty swallowing, and tracheostomy is occasionally used in patients that are at risk for airway compromise and who cannot undergo surgical resection.[3,32] It is important to note that tracheostomy may prolong the life of the patient, but may also prolong the patient's suffering. The tumor may grow through the tracheostomy area, or the tumor may fungate around the tracheostomy. There has been considerable debate about tracheostomy in patients with ATC. Certainly, prophylactic tracheostomy is not advocated in ATC, as it deteriorates the quality of life considerably. Some of these issues are more of an ethical concern rather than an area of scientific discussion.

PROGNOSIS

Despite improvements in treatment, most patients with ATC have aggressive disease with a median survival of 5−6 months and a median 1-year survival of 20%.[7,52] Survival in ATC is stage dependent, with an overall survival (regardless of treatment strategy) of 9 months for Stage IVA, 4.8 months for Stage IVB, and 3 months for Stage IVC disease.[69] The most common cause of death in ATC is suffocation from local disease progression,[3] and there is also a high incidence of recurrence despite appropriate treatment.[2]

Several studies evaluating prognostic factors in ATC have found that poor prognostic factors include older age (>60 years), low socioeconomic status, male sex, local tumor extension, large tumors (>5−7 cm), presence of distant metastasis, leukocytosis, acute presentation, and inability to achieve complete local resection.[3,7,32,43,70−74] Although preexisting thyroid disease or goiter is a known risk factor for ATC, it does not seem to be associated with prognosis. A retrospective study from 94 patients at 17 different hospitals in the Netherlands (1989−2009) showed similar overall survival in ATC patients with preexisting goiter or WDTC (55 days) compared to patients without a known history of thyroid disease (56 days).[75]

Many groups have created prognostic index scores for patients with ATC. In their prognostic scoring system, a Japanese group assigned one point each for acute presentation, tumor size >5 cm, presence of distant metastasis, and white blood cell count >10,000/μL, for a maximum of four points. Patients with a score of 1 or less were treated aggressively with multimodality treatment (surgery, radiation, and/or chemotherapy) and were compared to patients who had a score of 3 or 4 and did not receive aggressive treatment. The mean survival of those patients with a score of 1 or less was 442 days, compared to 113 days in those

with a score of 3 or 4.[73] A Chinese group used a slightly different scoring system, assigning points for age (>55 years—1 point), blood platelet count (>300,000/μL—1 point), white blood cell count (>10,000/μL—2 points), and stage (IVB—1 point, IVC—2 points), and found their scoring system to be an independent predictor of survival.[76] For all patients diagnosed with ATC, it is imperative that the treating physicians and the patient have multidisciplinary discussions and develop clear plans of care throughout the course of treatment. Physicians must ensure that these conversations with the patient are realistic, as overly optimistic or pessimistic messages to patients can dramatically affect their decision making.[77]

SUMMARY (DEEP DISCUSSION)

ATC is the rarest form of thyroid cancer; however, it is also the most aggressive and fatal form. In fact, ATC is one of the most rapidly growing and lethal solid tumors in humans. This is in stark contrast to WDTC that generally has an excellent prognosis, one of the best of all human tumors. In recent years, improvements in histologic staining and genomic sequencing of ATC has allowed a better understanding of its pathogenesis, which seems to suggest that most ATCs arise from dedifferentiation of a previously differentiated thyroid cancer, although they are considered to arise de novo in some cases.

In a patient with a rapidly growing thyroid mass suspicious for ATC, it is crucial to establish a diagnosis, generally by thyroid FNA, in an expeditious fashion. In the case of an equivocal FNA, core biopsy as well as molecular testing can help to establish the diagnosis. Early and multidisciplinary intervention in a patient with ATC is extremely important and can extend their life expectancy by several months. The multidisciplinary team for an ATC patient should include surgeons, medical oncologists, radiation oncologists, pathologists, psychologists, and physical and/or occupational therapists, among others. Ideally, patients should be seen at specialized centers with a high volume of advanced thyroid disease, as these centers likely have an infrastructure that can support the complex care of an ATC patient.

In recent years, treatment options for ATC have evolved significantly. Initially, the only treatment option available for ATC patients was palliative tracheostomy to prevent or delay death from asphyxiation. Currently, we attempt a curative resection whenever possible and generally avoid tracheostomy placement in ATC patients. The best chance of survival is achieved with local control (R0 or R1 resection); however, this should only be undertaken if all cervical and mediastinal disease can be resected without sacrificing major structures or causing significant morbidity. Another development in the treatment of ATC has been in the use of multimodality treatments. Radiotherapy and chemotherapy have both improved in their formulas over the past several years and are used routinely in the care of ATC patients. These treatments are increasingly more individualized and are being used in different combinations and at different treatment stages depending on each patient's particular case. This is particularly important, as ATC cells have been shown to develop chemoresistance to several known agents.

A major recent advancement in treatment of many cancers, including ATC, has been in the use of targeted therapies. For ATC, targeted therapies being utilized include TKIs, as well as inhibitors of BRAF, mTOR, ALK, MEK, VEGF, PD1/PDL1, and CTLA4. These therapies can be given in combinations tailored to the specific mutations present on each individual patient's tumor. Most of these therapies are still undergoing clinical trials; however, many have shown promising results. Even so, it is known that tumors are able to develop resistance to many targeted therapies, and this is an area that will likely be evolving over the next several decades. Despite our improvements in ATC treatment, there has still not been much progress made in ATC survival rates at a population level over the past several decades, and ATC still has a uniformly fatal outcome. In the current era where scientific breakthroughs are occurring on a daily basis; however, a new paradigm for ATC treatment may be on the horizon.

REFERENCES

1. O'Neill JP, Shaha AR. Anaplastic thyroid cancer. *Oral Oncol.* 2013;49:702–706.
2. Patel KN, Shaha AR. Poorly differentiated thyroid cancer. *Curr Opin Otolaryngol Head Neck Surg.* 2014;22:121–126.
3. Molinaro E, Romei C, Biagini A, et al. Anaplastic thyroid carcinoma: from clinicopathology to genetics and advanced therapies. *Nat Rev Endocrinol.* 2017;13:644–660.
3a. Nikiforov YE, Biddinger PW, Thompson LDR. *Diagnostic Pathology and Molecular Genetics of the Thyroid: A Comprehensive Guide for Practicing Thyroid Pathology.* 2nd ed. New York: LWW Publisher; 2012.
3b. DeLelis RA, Lloyd RV, Heitz PU, Eng C, eds. *Pathology and Genetics of Tumours of Endocrine Organs.* 3rd ed. New York: World Health Organization; 2004.
4. Davies L, Welch HG. Increasing incidence of thyroid cancer in the United States, 1973–2002. *J Am Med Assoc.* 2006; 295:2164–2167.
5. Hundahl SA, Fleming ID, Fremgen AM, Menck HR. A national cancer data base report on 53,856 cases of thyroid carcinoma treated in the U.S., 1985–1995 [see comments]. *Cancer.* 1998;83:2638–2648.
6. Besic N, Auersperg M, Us-Krasovec M, Golouh R, Frkovic-Grazio S, Vodnik A. Effect of primary treatment on survival in anaplastic thyroid carcinoma. *Eur J Surg Oncol.* 2001;27: 260–264.
7. Kebebew E, Greenspan FS, Clark OH, Woeber KA, McMillan A. Anaplastic thyroid carcinoma. Treatment outcome and prognostic factors. *Cancer.* 2005;103: 1330–1335.
8. Hundahl SA, Cady B, Cunningham MP, et al. Initial results from a prospective cohort study of 5583 cases of thyroid carcinoma treated in the United States during 1996. U.S. and German thyroid cancer study group. An American college of surgeons commission on cancer patient care evaluation study. *Cancer.* 2000;89:202–217.
9. Demeter JG, De Jong SA, Lawrence AM, Paloyan E. Anaplastic thyroid carcinoma: risk factors and outcome. *Surgery.* 1991;110:956–961. discussion 961-963.
10. Bakiri F, Djemli FK, Mokrane LA, Djidel FK. The relative roles of endemic goiter and socioeconomic development status in the prognosis of thyroid carcinoma. *Cancer.* 1998;82:1146–1153.
11. Ain KB. Anaplastic thyroid carcinoma: behavior, biology, and therapeutic approaches. *Thyroid.* 1998;8:715–726.
12. Besic N, Hocevar M, Zgajnar J. Lower incidence of anaplastic carcinoma after higher iodination of salt in Slovenia. *Thyroid.* 2010;20:623–626.
13. Myskow MW, Krajewski AS, Dewar AE, Millar EP, McLaren K, Fabre JW. The role of immunoperoxidase techniques on paraffin embedded tissue in determining the histogenesis of undifferentiated thyroid neoplasms. *Clin Endocrinol.* 1986;24:335–341.
14. Spires JR, Schwartz MR, Miller RH. Anaplastic thyroid carcinoma. Association with differentiated thyroid cancer. *Arch Otolaryngol Head Neck Surg.* 1988;114:40–44.
15. Aldinger KA, Samaan NA, Ibanez M, Hill CS. Anaplastic carcinoma of the thyroid: a review of 84 cases of spindle and giant cell carcinoma of the thyroid. *Cancer.* 1978;41: 2267–2275.
16. Bronner MP, LiVolsi VA. Spindle cell squamous carcinoma of the thyroid: an unusual anaplastic tumor associated with tall cell papillary cancer. *Mod Pathol.* 1991;4: 637–643.
17. Nikiforova MN, Nikiforov YE. Molecular diagnostics and predictors in thyroid cancer. *Thyroid.* 2009;19:1351–1361.
18. Landa I, Ibrahimpasic T, Boucai L, et al. Genomic and transcriptomic hallmarks of poorly differentiated and anaplastic thyroid cancers. *J Clin Investig.* 2016;126: 1052–1066.
19. Namba H, Nakashima M, Hayashi T, et al. Clinical implication of hot spot BRAF mutation, V599E, in papillary thyroid cancers. *J Clin Endocrinol Metab.* 2003;88:4393–4397.
20. Nikiforova MN, Kimura ET, Gandhi M, et al. BRAF mutations in thyroid tumors are restricted to papillary carcinomas and anaplastic or poorly differentiated carcinomas arising from papillary carcinomas. *J Clin Endocrinol Metab.* 2003;88:5399–5404.

21. Smallridge RC, Marlow LA, Copland JA. Anaplastic thyroid cancer: molecular pathogenesis and emerging therapies. *Endocr Relat Cancer*. 2009;16:17–44.

22. Xing M. BRAF mutation in thyroid cancer. *Endocr Relat Cancer*. 2005;12:245–262.

23. Asakawa H, Kobayashi T. Multistep carcinogenesis in anaplastic thyroid carcinoma: a case report. *Pathology*. 2002;34:94–97.

24. Nakamura T, Yana I, Kobayashi T, et al. p53 gene mutations associated with anaplastic transformation of human thyroid carcinomas. *Jpn J Cancer Res*. 1992;83: 1293–1298.

25. Donghi R, Longoni A, Pilotti S, Michieli P, Della Porta G, Pierotti MA. Gene p53 mutations are restricted to poorly differentiated and undifferentiated carcinomas of the thyroid gland. *J Clin Investig*. 1993;91:1753–1760.

26. Liu D, Xing M. Potent inhibition of thyroid cancer cells by the MEK inhibitor PD0325901 and its potentiation by suppression of the PI3K and NF-kappaB pathways. *Thyroid*. 2008;18:853–864.

27. Calin GA, Croce CM. MicroRNA signatures in human cancers. *Nat Rev Canc*. 2006;6:857–866.

28. Visone R, Pallante P, Vecchione A, et al. Specific microRNAs are downregulated in human thyroid anaplastic carcinomas. *Oncogene*. 2007;26:7590–7595.

29. Ain KB. Anaplastic thyroid carcinoma: a therapeutic challenge. *Semin Surg Oncol*. 1999;16:64–69.

30. Glaser SM, Mandish SF, Gill BS, Balasubramani GK, Clump DA, Beriwal S. Anaplastic thyroid cancer: prognostic factors, patterns of care, and overall survival. *Head Neck*. 2016;38(Suppl 1):E2083–E2090.

31. Kihara M, Miyauchi A, Yamauchi A, Yokomise H. Prognostic factors of anaplastic thyroid carcinoma. *Surg Today*. 2004;34:394–398.

32. Smallridge RC, Ain KB, Asa SL, et al. American Thyroid Association guidelines for management of patients with anaplastic thyroid cancer. *Thyroid*. 2012;22: 1104–1139.

33. Tan RK, Finley RK, Driscoll D, Bakamjian V, Hicks WL, Shedd DP. Anaplastic carcinoma of the thyroid: a 24-year experience. *Head Neck*. 1995;17:41–47. discussion 47-48.

34. Rossi R, Cady B, Meissner WA, Sedgwick CE, Werber J. Prognosis of undifferentiated carcinoma and lymphoma of the thyroid. *Am J Surg*. 1978;135:589–596.

35. Venkatesh YS, Ordonez NG, Schultz PN, Hickey RC, Goepfert H, Samaan NA. Anaplastic carcinoma of the thyroid. A clinicopathologic study of 121 cases. *Cancer*. 1990; 66:321–330.

36. Ryder M, Ghossein RA, Ricarte-Filho JCM, Knauf JA, Fagin JA. Increased density of tumor-associated macrophages is associated with decreased survival in advanced thyroid cancer. *Endocr Relat Cancer*. 2008;15: 1069–1074.

37. Caillou B, Talbot M, Weyemi U, et al. Tumor-associated macrophages (TAMs) form an interconnected cellular supportive network in anaplastic thyroid carcinoma. *PLoS One*. 2011;6:e22567.

38. Jung KY, Cho SW, Kim YA, et al. Cancers with higher density of tumor-associated macrophages were associated with poor survival rates. *J Pathol Transl Med*. 2015;49: 318–324.

39. Bellevicine C, Vigliar E, Malapelle U, et al. Lung adenocarcinoma and its thyroid metastasis characterized on fine-needle aspirates by cytomorphology, immunocytochemistry, and next-generation sequencing. *Diagn Cytopathol*. 2015;43:585–589.

40. Perrier ND, Brierley JD, Tuttle RM. Differentiated and anaplastic thyroid carcinoma: major changes in the American Joint Committee on Cancer eighth edition cancer staging manual. *CA Cancer J Clin*. 2018;68:55–63.

41. Tuttle RM, Haugen B, Perrier ND. Updated American Joint committee on cancer/tumor-node-metastasis staging system for differentiated and anaplastic thyroid cancer (eighth edition): what changed and why? *Thyroid*. 2017; 27:751–756.

42. Nagaiah G, Hossain A, Mooney CJ, Parmentier J, Remick SC. Anaplastic thyroid cancer: a review of epidemiology, pathogenesis, and treatment. *J Oncol*. 2011;2011: 1–13.

43. Tiedje V, Stuschke M, Weber F, Dralle H, Moss L, Führer D. Anaplastic thyroid carcinoma: review of treatment protocols. *Endocr Relat Cancer*. 2018;25:R153–R161.

44. De Crevoisier R, Baudin E, Bachelot A, et al. Combined treatment of anaplastic thyroid carcinoma with surgery, chemotherapy, and hyperfractionated accelerated external radiotherapy. *Int J Radiat Oncol*. 2004;60:1137–1143.

45. Baek S-K, Lee M-C, Hah JH, et al. Role of surgery in the management of anaplastic thyroid carcinoma: Korean nationwide multicenter study of 329 patients with anaplastic thyroid carcinoma, 2000 to 2012: surgical role in anaplastic thyroid carcinoma. *Head Neck*. 2017;39: 133–139.

46. Lee DY, Won J-K, Choi HS, et al. Recurrence and survival after gross total removal of resectable undifferentiated or poorly differentiated thyroid carcinoma. *Thyroid*. 2016; 26:1259–1268.

47. McIver B, Hay ID, Giuffrida DF, et al. Anaplastic thyroid carcinoma: a 50-year experience at a single institution. *Surgery*. 2001;130:1028–1034.

48. Passler C, Scheuba C, Prager G, et al. Anaplastic (undifferentiated) thyroid carcinoma (ATC). A retrospective analysis. *Langenbeck's Arch Surg*. 1999;384:284–293.

49. Pierie J-PEN, Muzikansky A, Gaz RD, Faquin WC, Ott MJ. The effect of surgery and radiotherapy on outcome of anaplastic thyroid carcinoma. *Ann Surg Oncol*. 2002;9: 57–64.

50. Swaak-Kragten AT, de Wilt JHW, Schmitz PIM, Bontenbal M, Levendag PC. Multimodality treatment for anaplastic thyroid carcinoma–treatment outcome in 75 patients. *Radiother Oncol*. 2009;92:100–104.

51. Haigh PI, Ituarte PH, Wu HS, et al. Completely resected anaplastic thyroid carcinoma combined with adjuvant chemotherapy and irradiation is associated with prolonged survival. *Cancer*. 2001;91:2335–2342.

52. Sugino K, Ito K, Mimura T, et al. The important role of operations in the management of anaplastic thyroid carcinoma. *Surgery.* 2002;131:245–248.

53. Higashiyama T, Ito Y, Hirokawa M, et al. Induction chemotherapy with weekly paclitaxel administration for anaplastic thyroid carcinoma. *Thyroid.* 2010;20:7–14.

54. Akaishi J, Sugino K, Kitagawa W, et al. Prognostic factors and treatment outcomes of 100 cases of anaplastic thyroid carcinoma. *Thyroid.* 2011;21:1183–1189.

55. Brignardello E, Gallo M, Baldi I, et al. Anaplastic thyroid carcinoma: clinical outcome of 30 consecutive patients referred to a single institution in the past 5 years. *Eur J Endocrinol.* 2007;156:425–430.

56. Tennvall J, Lundell G, Wahlberg P, et al. Anaplastic thyroid carcinoma: three protocols combining doxorubicin, hyperfractionated radiotherapy and surgery. *Br J Canc.* 2002;86:1848–1853.

57. Wang Y, Tsang R, Asa S, Dickson B, Arenovich T, Brierley J. Clinical outcome of anaplastic thyroid carcinoma treated with radiotherapy of once- and twice-daily fractionation regimens. *Cancer.* 2006;107:1786–1792.

58. Shimaoka K, Schoenfeld DA, DeWys WD, Creech RH, DeConti R. A randomized trial of doxorubicin versus doxorubicin plus cisplatin in patients with advanced thyroid carcinoma. *Cancer.* 1985;56:2155–2160.

59. Ain KB, Egorin MJ, DeSimone PA. Treatment of anaplastic thyroid carcinoma with paclitaxel: phase 2 trial using ninety-six-hour infusion. Collaborative Anaplastic Thyroid Cancer Health Intervention Trials (CATCHIT) Group. *Thyroid.* 2000;10:587–594.

60. Bhatia A, Rao A, Ang K-K, et al. Anaplastic thyroid cancer: clinical outcomes with conformal radiotherapy. *Head Neck.* 2010;32:829–836.

61. Troch M, Koperek O, Scheuba C, et al. High efficacy of concomitant treatment of undifferentiated (anaplastic) thyroid cancer with radiation and docetaxel. *J Clin Endocrinol Metab.* 2010;95:E54–E57.

62. Foote RL, Molina JR, Kasperbauer JL, et al. Enhanced survival in locoregionally confined anaplastic thyroid carcinoma: a single-institution experience using aggressive multimodal therapy. *Thyroid.* 2011;21:25–30.

63. Bible KC, Suman VJ, Menefee ME, et al. A multiinstitutional phase 2 trial of pazopanib monotherapy in advanced anaplastic thyroid cancer. *J Clin Endocrinol Metab.* 2012;97:3179–3184.

64. Savvides P, Nagaiah G, Lavertu P, et al. Phase II trial of sorafenib in patients with advanced anaplastic carcinoma of the thyroid. *Thyroid.* 2013;23:600–604.

65. Tahara M, Kiyota N, Yamazaki T, et al. Lenvatinib for anaplastic thyroid cancer. *Front Oncol.* 2017;7:25.

66. Ha HT, Lee JS, Urba S, et al. A phase II study of imatinib in patients with advanced anaplastic thyroid cancer. *Thyroid.* 2010;20:975–980.

67. Yau T, Lo CY, Epstein RJ, Lam AKY, Wan KY, Lang BH. Treatment outcomes in anaplastic thyroid carcinoma: survival improvement in young patients with localized disease treated by combination of surgery and radiotherapy. *Ann Surg Oncol.* 2008;15:2500–2505.

68. Ribechini A, Bottici V, Chella A, et al. Interventional bronchoscopy in the treatment of tracheal obstruction secondary to advanced thyroid cancer. *J Endocrinol Investig.* 2006; 29:131–135.

69. Haymart MR, Banerjee M, Yin H, Worden F, Griggs JJ. Marginal treatment benefit in anaplastic thyroid cancer: treatment of Anaplastic Thyroid Cancer. *Cancer.* 2013;119: 3133–3139.

70. Sugitani I, Kasai N, Fujimoto Y, Yanagisawa A. Prognostic factors and therapeutic strategy for anaplastic carcinoma of the thyroid. *World J Surg.* 2001;25:617–622.

71. Kim TY, Kim KW, Jung TS, et al. Prognostic factors for Korean patients with anaplastic thyroid carcinoma. *Head Neck.* 2007;29:765–772.

72. Gilliland FD, Hunt WC, Morris DM, Key CR. Prognostic factors for thyroid carcinoma. A population-based study of 15,698 cases from the Surveillance, Epidemiology and End Results (SEER) program 1973–1991. *Cancer.* 1997; 79:564–573.

73. Orita Y, Sugitani I, Amemiya T, Fujimoto Y. Prospective application of our novel prognostic index in the treatment of anaplastic thyroid carcinoma. *Surgery.* 2011;150: 1212–1219.

74. Wendler J, Kroiss M, Gast K, et al. Clinical presentation, treatment and outcome of anaplastic thyroid carcinoma: results of a multicenter study in Germany. *Eur J Endocrinol.* 2016;175:521–529.

75. Steggink LC, van Dijk BAC, Links TP, Plukker JTM. Survival in anaplastic thyroid cancer in relation to pre-existing goiter: a population-based study. *Am J Surg.* 2015;209: 1013–1019.

76. Sun C, Li Q, Hu Z, et al. Treatment and prognosis of anaplastic thyroid carcinoma: experience from a single institution in China. *PLoS One.* 2013;8:e80011.

77. Smallridge RC, Copland JA. Anaplastic thyroid carcinoma: pathogenesis and emerging therapies. *Clin Oncol.* 2010;22: 486–497.

FURTHER READING

1. Wong CS, Van Dyk J, Simpson WJ. Myelopathy following hyperfractionated accelerated radiotherapy for anaplastic thyroid carcinoma. *Radiother Oncol.* 1991;20:3–9.

CHAPTER 4

Familial Nonmedullary Thyroid Cancer

TIFFANY J. SINCLAIR, MD • ELECTRON KEBEBEW, MD, FACS

INTRODUCTION

Familial nonmedullary thyroid cancer (FNMTC) is defined by the presence of thyroid cancer of follicular cell origin in two or more first-degree relatives, in the absence of other predisposing causes. More than 95% of thyroid cancer cases are of follicular cell origin, and of these, FNMTC accounts for 3%–9% of cases.[1,2] FNMTC may occur as a component of inherited cancer syndromes (PTEN hamartoma tumor syndrome, Peutz–Jeghers syndrome, familial adenomatous polyposis, Carney complex, Pendred syndrome, DICER1 syndrome, ataxia-telangiectasia, and Werner syndrome).[1] The majority of patients with FNMTC (95%), however, have a nonsyndromic form of disease.[2] Although there are well-defined genotype–phenotype associations in syndromic FNMTC, the genetic etiology of nonsyndromic FNMTC remains controversial and not well understood.

SYNDROMIC FNMTC

PTEN Hamartoma Tumor Syndrome

PTEN hamartoma tumor syndrome (PHTS) is a complex group of disorders that are inherited in an autosomal-dominant manner and include Cowden syndrome (CS), Cowden-like syndrome (CS-like), Bannayan–Riley–Ruvalcaba syndrome (BRRS), PTEN-related Proteus syndrome (PS), and Proteus-like syndrome. Most subtypes are caused by germline inactivating mutations in the PTEN (phosphatase and tensin homolog) tumor-suppressor gene, located on chromosome 10q23.3. The PTEN gene product is an enzyme responsible for removing the phosphate group from other proteins and lipids, thereby regulating the cell-division process. According to the Human Gene Mutation Database, there are approximately 150 unique pathogenic PTEN variants found throughout the coding region of PTEN. Together, these mutations of the PTEN gene account 85% of cases of PHTS.[3]

Another well-recognized genetic alteration in PHTS is hypermethylation of the KLLN (killin) gene promoter.[4] Upstream of PTEN, killin is a TP53 target gene that shares a common promoter. Hypermethylation of KLLN downregulates its transcription and disrupts the TP53 activation of killin.[5] Additional genetic causes of PTEN hamartoma tumor syndrome include mutations in succinate dehydrogenase (SDH) genes SDHB or SDHD.[4] SDH gene mutations result in activation of the AKT and MAPK signaling pathways, similar to the effects of PTEN mutations. Mutations in PIK3CA and AKT1 have been identified in association with PHTS.[6] Finally, using whole-exome sequencing across four generations in a family with no known mutations (normal PTEN, SDH, KLLN promoter), three new culprit genes were identified: C160RF72, PTPN2, and SEC23B. SEC23B plays a role in intracellular protein transport. Functional studies revealed that a point mutation in SEC23B results in stress of the endoplasmic reticulum (ER) subsequently stimulating cell-colony formation, growth, and invasion. These data suggest a mechanism of action by which abnormal cell growth is induced by ER stress.[7]

Cowden syndrome

CS, first described in 1963,[8] is characterized by the presence of a combination of the following clinical features:
- Pathognomonic criteria: (a) dysplastic cerebellar gangliocytoma (also known as Lhermitte–Duclos disease), (b) facial trichilemmomas, (c) acral keratosis, and (d) papillomatous lesions.
- Major criteria: (a) macrocephaly, (b) breast cancer, (c) NMTC, and (d) endometrial cancer.
- Minor criteria: (a) hamartomas, (b) thyroid lesions (adenoma, multinodular goiter (MNG)), (c) mental retardation, (d) fibrocystic breast disease, (e) lipomas, (f) fibromas, (g) uterine fibroids, and (h) renal cell carcinoma (RCC)[9,10] (Table 4.1).

CS-like syndrome includes patients with features of CS that do not meet the diagnostic criteria for CS.[11]

Advances in Treatment and Management in Surgical Endocrinology. https://doi.org/10.1016/B978-0-323-66195-9.00004-2

TABLE 4.1
Familial Syndromes Associated With Nonmedullary Thyroid Cancer.

Syndrome	Susceptibility gene (s)	Chromosome location	Clinical features
APC-associated polyposis: FAP Attenuated polyposis Gardner Turcot syndrome II	*APC*	5q21-q22	• At least 100 colorectal adenomatous polyps occurring before age 40 or fewer than 100 adenomatous polyps and a relative with FAP associated with fibromas, desmoid tumors, epithelial cysts, hypertrophic retinal pigment epithelium, upper GI tract hamartomas, supernumerary teeth, hepatoblastoma, and benign and malignant thyroid disease. • No family member with >100 polyps before age 30 AND at least two individuals with 10–99 adenomas after age 30 OR one member with 10–99 polyps after 30yo and a first-degree relative with colorectal cancer with a few adenomas. • Colonic polyposis associated with osteomas and epidermoid cysts, desmoid tumors. • Colonic polyps associated with CNS tumors, usually medulloblastoma.
PTEN hamartoma tumor syndrome: Cowden Bannayan–Riley– Ruvalcaba PTEN-related proteus Proteus-like	PTEN—80% SDHB/ D—10% Other: *KILLIN, PIK3CA, AKT*	10q23.31	• *Pathognomonic criteria* such as Lhermitte–Duclos disease, facial trichilemmomas, acral keratosis, papillomatous lesions; *major criteria* such as macrocephaly, breast cancer, NMTC, endometrial cancer, and *minor criteria* such GI hamartomas, thyroid lesions (adenoma, MNG), mental retardation, breast fibrocystic breast disease, lipomas, fibromas uterine fibroids, RCC, and fibromas. • Macrocephaly, hamartomatous intestinal polyposis, lipomas, and pigmented macules of the glans penis. • Distorting, progressive overgrowth, cerebriform connective tissue nevi, linear verrucous epidermal nevus, adipose dysregulation. Mosaic distribution, highly variable. • Significant clinical features of PS, but do not meet the diagnostic criteria.
Peutz–Jeghers syndrome	*STK11/LKB1*	19p13.3	• Two or more PJS-type (hamartomatous gastrointestinal polyp) intestinal polyps, mucocutaneous macules, gynecomastia in males as a result of estrogen-producing Sertoli cell testicular tumor, h/o intussusception, especially in a child or young adult.
Werner	*WRN*	8p11–p12	• Premature aging, scleroderma-like skin changes, cataracts, subcutaneous calcifications, muscular atrophy, osteoporosis, atherosclerosis, DM, skin ulcers, melanoma, sarcomas, MDS.
Pendred syndrome	*SLC26A4 (PDS)*	7q21–34	• Hearing impairment and thyroid abnormalities, including benign and malignant lesions.
Carney's complex	*PRKA1A "CNC2"*	17q22–24 2p16	• Myxomas of soft tissue, lentiginosis, blue nevi, Sertoli cell testicular tumors, psammomatous melanotic schwannomatosis, pituitary adenoma, PPNAD, and endocrine overactivity secondary to pituitary adenomas, ACTH-independent Cushing syndrome due to primary pigmented nodular adrenocortical disease (PPNAD) and thyroid abnormalities, including benign and malignant tumors.

TABLE 4.1
Familial Syndromes Associated With Nonmedullary Thyroid Cancer.—cont'd

Syndrome	Susceptibility gene (s)	Chromosome location	Clinical features
Papillary renal neoplasia	PRN1	1q21	• Papillary renal neoplasia, PTC, benign thyroid nodules
DICER 1 s-me	DICER 1	14q32.13	• Phenotypes including pleuropulmonary blastoma, ovarian sex cord-stromal tumors • (Sertoli—Leydig cell tumor, juvenile granulosa cell tumor, gynandroblastoma), cystic nephroma, thyroid gland neoplasia including MNG, adenomas, or DTC; ciliary body medulloepithelioma, botryoid-type embryonal rhabdomyosarcoma of the cervix or other sites, nasal chondromesenchymal hamartoma, pituitary blastoma, pineoblastoma.
Ataxia-telangiectasia	ATM	11q22—23	• Progressive cerebellar ataxia with onset between ages one and four years, oculomotor apraxia, choreoathetosis, telangiectasias of the conjunctivae, immunodeficiency, frequent infections, and an increased risk for malignancy, particularly leukemia and lymphoma.

Thyroid diseases, both benign and malignant, are the most common extracutaneous manifestations of CS—affecting up to 68% of patients.[12,13] After breast cancer, NMTC is the second-most-common cancer in patients with CS (3%—14% of cases)[12,14] with a lifetime thyroid cancer risk as high as 35.2%.[10] In patients with CS and CS-like, follicular thyroid cancer (FTC) is more common than papillary thyroid cancer (PTC), most likely due to the prevalence of the *PTEN* mutation in these patients.[12,13,15] Thyroid cancer has a female predominance in this population and usually presents in the third decade of life.[4,13,15–18] Although cases have been reported as early as age seven, based on analysis of 664 patients with CS and CS-like, only 2.9% were diagnosed before 18 years of age.[4]

Bannayan—Riley—Ruvalcaba Syndrome
BRRS has an array of phenotypic traits[19,20] and is believed to be on a spectrum of disease with CS and CS-like. Features of BRRS include macrocephaly, hamartomatous intestinal polyps, increased linear growth, dysmorphic features, joint hyperextensibility, pectus excavatum, scoliosis, café au lait spots, lipomas, and pigmented penile macules. Additional features include developmental delay, large birth weight, and proximal muscles myopathy[20,21] (Table 4.1).

BRRS has been associated with MNG, follicular/Hürthle cell adenomas, FTC, and PTC.[20,22] Similar to CS and CS-like, patients with BRRS have a higher prevalence of FTC compared to PTC. In one case series, the average age at diagnosis of FTC was 14 years old.[22]

Given the rarity of PHTS, there are no high-quality data to use for evidence-based recommendations but clinical care can be guided by the case series described in the literature. The high incidence of thyroid pathology in patients with CS warrants routine screening with physical exam and thyroid ultrasound (US) in at-risk family members and patients.[10,17,23] For *PTEN* mutation-positive patients, baseline and annual thyroid US evaluation should be initiated after 18 years of age. For families with a history of early onset cancer, however, screening may be initiated 5—10 years before the youngest age of thyroid cancer diagnosis in the family.[24] In addition, given that *SDHx*-positive *PTEN*-negative CS/CS-like patients may have a significantly increased risk of breast, thyroid, and kidney cancers, active screening is also recommended.[11]

Peutz—Jeghers Syndrome
Peutz—Jeghers syndrome (PJS) is an autosomal-dominant disorder caused by germline mutations in the *STK11* gene (also known as *LKB1*) located on chromosome 19p13.3.[25] *STK11* is a tumor-suppressor gene that, in PJS, undergoes an inactivating mutation disrupting its ability to regulate cell division. This increased cellular proliferation signal leads to the development of noncancerous hamartomatous polyps in the gastrointestinal tract. In particular, mutations spanning the STK11 protein kinase domain are associated with a higher incidence of gastrointestinal polyp dysplasia (90%) compared to 11.8% in individuals with pathogenic variants in other regions of the gene.[26] There is

conflicting data on whether or not the pathogenic variant of *STK11* is associated with an increased incidence of cancer.[27,28] Some studies have found that in addition to having a higher polyp count, patients with pathogenic variants of *STK11* also have a greater risk of melanoma.[29,30]

PJS is characterized by the presence of small bowel hamartomatous polyposis, mucocutaneous hyperpigmentation, and, most likely, a predisposition to a wide variety of epithelial malignancies including in the pancreas, breast, uterus, ovary, and testes[31] (Table 4.1). Most patients present in the first decade of life with complications, such as mechanical obstruction, from growing intestinal polyps.[25]

Although NMTC is not a part of the known typical PJS spectrum, there are seven reported cases of differentiated thyroid cancer (DTC) in patients with PJS.[25,31−36] The age of diagnosis ranged between 6 and 30 years and the most common histopathological subtype was PTC (5 of 7 cases).[25,31−36]

There is insufficient data to recommend for or against screening for thyroid cancer in patients with PJS. Some authors suggest that early thyroid US may be recommended because thyroid cancer, when present, occurs at a young age in PJS patients.[31] Once a diagnosis is established, treatment should follow the standard treatment guidelines for the thyroid pathology.[37]

Familial Adenomatous Polyposis

Familial adenomatous polyposis (FAP) is a predominantly autosomal-dominant syndrome caused by germline mutations in the adenomatous polyposis coli (*APC*) gene on chromosome 5q21.[38,39] Most *APC* mutations are either frame-shift or nonsense mutations leading to a truncated protein.[40] The APC protein is part of the regulatory β-catenin destruction complex that regulates cell proliferation. *APC* inactivating mutations leads to loss of the β-catenin destruction complex and upregulation of cell division.[41,42] An autosomal-recessive form of this disease was identified in patients with mutations in the *MUTYH* gene that affects the ability of cells to repair errors made during DNA replication.[43]

APC-associated polyposis includes the overlapping, often indistinguishable phenotypes of FAP, attenuated FAP, Gardner syndrome, and Turcot syndrome.[44] Patients with FAP have a nearly 100% lifetime risk of colorectal cancer secondary to numerous intestinal polyps.[45] Extracolonic manifestations include hepatoblastoma, medulloblastoma, osteomas, supernumerary teeth or missing teeth, congenital hypertrophy of retinal pigment epithelium, desmoid tumors, fibromas, and thyroid abnormalities (Table 4.1). Attenuated FAP (autosomal-recessive variant) has a similar phenotype to FAP but fewer polyps.[46] Gardner's syndrome (GS)

is a clinical variant of FAP associated with the characteristic triad of desmoid tumors, osteomas, and epidermoid cysts (Table 4.1). Turcot syndrome includes patients with FAP who have central nervous system (CNS) tumors, usually medulloblastoma.[23]

Although up to 38% of patients with FAP may be found to have thyroid nodules, the rate of malignancy is much lower.[47] PTC is the most common type of NMTC among patients with FAP/GS patients. Frequency of PTC ranges from 0.7% to 12%.[46−50] However, based on two large cohorts of patients with FAP, the prevalence of PTC was closer to 1%−2%[51,52] Patients with attenuated FAP with *MUTYH* mutations have a similar risk for NMTC.[53,54]

A diagnosis of NMTC can precede a diagnosis of FAP in up to one-third of patients. Most patients with FAP and NMTC present in the second to third decades of life (18−40 years)[17,46] and are predominantly female (86%). Patients with FAP have an estimated 100−160-fold higher risk of NMTC compared to the general population.[50,55−57] Further patients of Japanese descent may be at particularly higher risk.[58]

NMTC in patients with FAP is frequently multifocal (66%−100%) and bilateral (42%−66.6%), with rare metastases and a prognosis similar to sporadic PTC.[46,48,59] There are distinct histologic features in NMTC associated with FAP, including a cribriform pattern with solid areas and a spindle-cell component with marked fibrosis.[48,60] The cribriform-morular variant represents more than 90% of PTC in patients with FAP despite being a very rare variant in sporadic PTC (0.1%−0.2%).[48] The typical histologic features of sporadic PTC, such as nuclear grooving, overlapping, intranuclear inclusions, and clear nuclei, are rare or absent in the cribriform-morular type.[59−61] Isolated FTC can be found in 9% of FAP patients, and concomitant PTC and FTC have also been described. The prognosis for FAP-related NMTC after surgical treatment is excellent with low morbidity and mortality.

There are no clear recommendations regarding NMTC screening among patients with APC-associated polyposis. Annual surveillance with a physical exam or thyroid US for all patients with FAP has been recommended.[45,47,49,50] According to the American College of Gastroenterology,[17] an annual thyroid US is recommended in individuals with FAP, *MUTYH*-associated polyposis, and attenuated polyposis (a conditional recommendation, low quality of evidence). Conversely, as the cribriform-morular form of PTC is rare and usually associated with FAP, each patient with this variant of PTC should be screened for FAP[23] (Table 4.2). Once a diagnosis of NMTC associated with FAP is made, the treatment should follow standard treatment guidelines sporadic thyroid cancer.[37]

TABLE 4.2
Characteristics of Syndromic Familial Nonmedullary Thyroid Cancer (FNMTC).

Syndrome	Frequency of thyroid cancer	Type of thyroid cancer	Clinical characteristics
APC-associated polyposis: • FAP • Attenuated FAP • Gardner • Turcot syndrome, type 2	0.7%–12%; 100–160-fold risk of TC compared to normal individuals	PTC, cribriform morular or classical PTC with sclerosis	Female predominance; second to third decade of life; TC: multifocal, bilateral, rare metastases; prognosis is similar to sporadic PTC.
PTEN-hamartoma tumor syndrome: • Cowden • Bannayan–Riley–Ruvalcaba Cowden-like syndrome	3%–14%, Lifetime risk: 35.2%	FTC associated with numerous adenomatous nodules and FAs	Female predominance; third decade of life; possible early onset in childhood at 7–13yo; prognosis is unknown.
Werner	Relative risk of TC 8.9% among Japanese WS patients	PTC, FTC, ATC, especially increased FTC and ATC	In Japanese WS patients: average age 39yo; F:M ratio 2.3:1.
Carney's complex	Up to 10%	FTC, PTC	Up to 60% have TNs; 2/3 among children and adolescents; TNs appear during the first 10 years of life.
Papillary renal neoplasia	Prevalence unknown	PTC, classic variant	Limited data.
DICER 1 s-me	Prevalence unknown	PTC, FTC	Young age; not aggressive features in TC.
Pendred syndrome	1%	FTC	Prognosis is unknown.
Ataxia-telangiectasia	Prevalence unclear	PTC, FTC	Only females were described; age 9.3–35.8 years; prognosis unknown.
Peutz–Jeghers syndrome	Prevalence is unknown	PTC	Age 21–30 years; prognosis is unknown.

DTC, differentiated thyroid cancer; FA, follicular adenomas; FNA, fine-needle aspiration; NMTC, nonmedullary thyroid cancer; TC, thyroid cancer; TN, thyroid nodules.

Carney Complex

Carney complex is an autosomal-dominant disease most commonly caused by a germline mutation in the *PRKAR1A* gene located on either chromosome 17q24.2 (type 1) or chromosome 2p16 (type 2).[62–65] The *PRKAR1A* gene codes for a regulatory alpha subunit of protein kinase A, an enzyme that promotes cell growth. Most *PRKAR1A* gene mutations (82%) produce nonsense mRNA, which is eventually degraded, ultimately resulting in constitutive activation of protein kinase A and upregulation of cell proliferation.[66,67] Based on linkage analysis, a site on the chromosome 2p16 locus may be associated with this disease—though no candidate gene has been identified.[68,69]

Carney complex is a clinical spectrum of disorders characterized by lentigines, atrial myxoma, mucocutaneous myxoma, blue nevi or nevi, myxoid neurofibroma, and endocrinopathies such as growth hormone–secreting pituitary adenomas, ACTH-independent Cushing syndrome due to primary pigmented nodular adrenocortical disease, and thyroid abnormalities.[70]

Either the presence of NMTC (at any age) or multiple hypoechogenic nodules on thyroid US in a prepubertal age are the major diagnostic criteria for Carney complex.[71] Up to 60% of all individuals with Carney complex may have thyroid nodules detected by US, and two-thirds of those present in childhood or adolescence.[62,72] Typically, thyroid nodules appear during the first 10 years of life.[73] Nonspecific cystic disease can be seen in up to 75% of cases, and follicular adenomas are seen in 25% of patients.[66,72,74] Both PTC and FTC are present in about 10% of patients with Carney complex.[71,75] In general, patients with Carney complex have a decreased life span, with the majority (57%) dying from cardiovascular complications of the disease. Fourteen percent of patients die of cancer progression, but thyroid cancer as a cause of death has not been reported.[71]

In patients with Carney complex, a screening thyroid US is recommended as a baseline in childhood and should be repeated in regular intervals as needed.[71] The value of thyroid US in older patients remains questionable.[62,76] A fine-needle aspiration biopsy of all suspicious nodules is recommended, and as with the other inherited disorders, NMTC management should follow the standard treatment algorithm for sporadic NMTC.[72]

Pendred Syndrome

Pendred syndrome is an autosomal-recessive disorder that is primarily caused by germline mutations in one of three genes: *SLC26A4*, *FOXI1*, and *KCNJ10*. More than half of patients with Pendred syndrome likely harbor pathogenic variants in the *SLC26A4* gene.[77,78] SLC26A4 is a cell membrane transport protein for negatively charged ions and mutations lead to intracellular ionic imbalance. Mutations in the other two genes, *FOXI1* and *KCNJ10*, are less common, accounting for less than 1% of cases of Pendred syndrome.[79]

Pendred syndrome is characterized by hearing impairment and a variety of thyroid pathology ranging from benign MNG to thyroid cancer.[23] Most thyroid pathology in Pendred syndrome is benign with the rate of NMTC in Pendred syndrome and is estimated to be 1%. FTC is the most common histologic subtype,[80] but a follicular variant of PTC, metastatic FTC, and anaplastic transformation from FTC have all been reported.[81–84] It is possible that NMTC in patients with Pendred syndrome may result from untreated congenital hypothyroidism and chronic stimulation by thyroid-stimulating hormone.[23] Genetic analysis of the Pendred-associated follicular variant of PTC showed a TP53 somatic mutation, supporting the proposal that the development of NMTC in these patients requires additional genetic alteration in addition to hormonal overstimulation.[82]

Thyroid US evaluation and routine thyroid examination in patients with hypothyroidism and Pendred syndrome are recommended. Given the potential association with NMTC, thyroidectomy may be considered in hypothyroid patients with thyroid nodules.[23] Once diagnosed, NMTC should be managed according to the current treatment guidelines of sporadic NMTC.[37]

DICER1 Syndrome

DICER1 syndrome is an autosomal-dominant disorder caused by germline mutations in the *DICER1* gene, located on chromosome 14q32.13. Somatic and germline mutations in *DICER1* have been found in PTC.[85] Germline *DICER1* mutations are associated with dysregulated gene expression of five miRNAs (miR-345, let-7a, miR-99b, miR-133, and miR-194).[86]

DICER1 syndrome, or the pleuropulmonary blastoma (PPB) familial tumor and dysplasia syndrome, is characterized by PPB, cystic nephroma, Sertoli–Leydig cell tumors, embryonal rhabdomyosarcomas, MNG, and Wilms tumors (WT)[87] (Table 4.1).

MNG is common in patients with *DICER1* germline mutations.[85,86] DTC has also been described in DICER1 patients, though infrequently.[85,87] The development of a somatic RNase IIIb *DICER1* mutation in addition to the *DICER1* germline mutations is suggested as a second hit for thyroid carcinogenesis in these patients.[87] It has been proposed that treatment for PPB with chemotherapy or bone marrow transplantation for pleuropulmonary may also be a predisposing risk factor for DTC in patients with *DICER1* germline mutations.[87,88] Five cases of DTC associated with a history of high-dose chemotherapy have been reported[85,87] but DTC unrelated to chemotherapy has also been documented in these patients.

Guidelines for baseline and routine surveillance thyroid US screening in patients with germline *DICER1* mutations have not been established. The International PPB registries suggest that a thyroid physical exam should be performed annually.[89] Thyroid US is recommended for any abnormality detected on physical exam, or if the patient has previously received or is anticipated to receive chemotherapy or repeated upper-body radiological imaging.[89] A thyroid US could be repeated every 3–5 years if no nodule is detected.[89] Other investigators recommend annual thyroid US during childhood and adolescence.[87] NMTC, once detected, should be treated according to the standard management guidelines.[37]

Ataxia-Telangiectasia

Ataxia-telangiectasia is a rare autosomal-recessive disorder caused by mutations in the ataxia-telangiectasia mutated (*ATM*) gene, located on chromosome 11q22–23.[90] Mutations in this gene disrupt the function of the serine-threonine kinase of ATM resulting in cell-cycle checkpoint defects and chromosomal instability. The *ATM* gene is critical for normal development of the nervous and immune systems. More than 800 unique pathogenic variants of *ATM* have been identified, and many of them are known to be associated with a higher risk of cancer.[91]

Ataxia-telangiectasia is characterized by early-onset progressive cerebellar ataxia, apraxia of eye movements, oculo-cutaneous telangiectasia, the absence or rudimentary appearance of a thymus, immunodeficiency, lymphoid tumors, insulin-resistant diabetes, and radiosensitivity.[92] The rate of cancer is approximately 100 times greater than the general population.[93] Five cases of DTC have been reported in patients with ataxia-telangiectasia—four had PTC and one patient had FTC.[93] All occurred in women and presented before age 36.

The risk of NMTC in patients with ataxia-telangiectasia is unclear, but the early age of onset of NMTC in the reported cases suggests that it may be higher than the general population. There is a lack of data regarding screening and prognosis of ataxia-telangiectasia associated NMTC. Clinicians should have a low threshold for thyroid evaluation, and if NMTC is diagnosed, it should be treated according to standard treatment guidelines.[11]

Papillary Renal Neoplasia

The genetic cause as well as the mode of inheritance of papillary renal neoplasia (PRN) is not known. There is a single case report describing the association of PTC and PRN in one kindred with five family members diagnosed with PTC, two with PRN, and one with renal oncocytoma.[94]

In addition to renal neoplasia, PRN is associated with PTC and benign thyroid nodules. On pathology, patients with PRN had a classical variant of PTC. Interestingly, PRN has similar histologic features to PTC.[94] Immunostaining for thyroglobulin can distinguish PTC from PRN metastases if this is suspected. All identified family members with PTC had tumors larger than 3 cm, and many had coexisting benign thyroid nodules.[94]

Due to the extreme rarity of this disease, there is neither management nor screening recommendations for patients with PRN, but evaluation and treatment should be similar to sporadic thyroid nodules and NMTC.

Werner Syndrome

Werner syndrome, or adult progeria, is an autosomal-recessive disorder that is associated with mutations of the *WRN* gene, located on chromosome 8p11-p12.[95] The *WRN* gene is critical in replicating and repairing DNA. Mutations in the *WRN* gene lead to truncated nonfunctional WRN proteins, ultimately resulting in decreased cell proliferation.

Werner syndrome is a characterized by premature aging that starts in the third decade, with a median life expectancy of 54 years.[70,96,97] Clinical presentation includes thin skin, wrinkles, alopecia, muscle atrophy, short stature due to an absence of pubertal growth period, age-related disorders such as diabetes, osteoporosis, cataracts, and peripheral vascular disease, and various malignant tumors (Table 4.1).[96,97]

Patients with Werner syndrome have an increased risk of both benign and malignant thyroid diseases.[48] In a study of Japanese patients with Werner syndrome, the age of DTC diagnosis was 10 years earlier and had a disproportionate number of affected males compared to the general Japanese population.[98] PTC has been associated with an N-terminal variant in *WNT*, whereas FTC is more frequently observed with a C-terminal variant.[98] These patients have an unusual distribution of histologic subtypes of DTC with higher rates of FTC (48% in Werner syndrome vs. 14% in the general Japanese population) and anaplastic thyroid cancer (13% vs. 2%, respectively), and a lower rate of classic PTC (35% vs. 78%, respectively).[98] Overall, the risk of developing NMTC is estimated to be 8.9%—16.1% for patients with Werner syndrome.[99]

Given the prevalence of NMTC in Werner syndrome and the high rate of aggressive subtypes such as FTC and ATC, screening and surveillance for thyroid pathology in this population is justified.[100] The diagnostic evaluation and treatment of thyroid disease associated with Werner syndrome should reflect standard management guidelines.

Although for most syndromic FNMTC there appears to be an increased risk of NMTC, the penetrance is low, and there is great phenotypic heterogeneity. There are limited data on the role of screening and surveillance, as well as the natural history of NMTC in syndromic FNMTC. With future studies addressing these critical issues, including the discovery of any genotype-phenotype association, it may be possible to refine the management of syndromic FNMTC and optimize patient outcome.

NONSYNDROMIC FNMTC

In 1955, Robinson and Orr reported PTC occurring in monozygotic twins. Since this report, there have been numerous case reports and case series that have led to the recognition of nonsyndromic FNMTC as a distinct clinical entity [110]. FNMTC is characterized by an autosomal-dominant pattern of inheritance with incomplete penetrance. Patients with FNMTC also have a higher rate of thyroid diseases (follicular adenoma, MNG, thyroiditis), up to 45%–55%.[101–106] Several different genetic susceptibility loci and genes have been reported, but few causative genes have been found that account for most cases of nonsyndromic FNMTC. The forkhead box E1 (*FOXE1*) gene is located at chromosome 9q22.33. It encodes for the FOXE1 transcription factor and is also known as thyroid transcription factor 2 (*TTF2*). It regulates thyroid morphogenesis. A genome-wide association study in both sporadic PTC and FTC cases identified two single nucleotide polymorphisms, rs944289 and rs965513, and was subsequently validated by target sequencing in an independent cohort.[107,108] Sequencing of the whole *FOXE1* gene showed several germline variants in the promoter region and coding sequence.[109,110] Molecular functional studies with the *FOXE1* A248G resulted in increased cellular proliferation in rat normal thyroid and human PTC cell lines as compared with to wild type, suggesting a role of *FOXE1* as a susceptibility gene for nonsyndromic FNMTC.[110] The Hyaluronan-binding protein 2 (*HABP2*) gene, located on chromosome 10q25.3, was identified as a susceptibility gene for FNMTC by a study utilizing whole-exome sequencing in a large kindred with seven affected members (six PTC and one follicular adenoma).[111] The *HABP2* G534E variant segregated with all seven affected members. Molecular functional studies suggested that the *HABP2* G534E variant functioned as a dominant negative tumor-suppressor gene. This study was validated by another group, which identified the same germline variant (G534E) of *HABP2* in four kindred with FNMTC out of 29 kindred.[112] However, other studies have either found incomplete segregation of the *HABP2* G534E variant in affected members with FNMTC or no difference in the frequency of the variant between those with cancer and "control" groups.[113–119] The tumor cell oxyphilia 1 locus on chromosome 19p13.2 was a linkage site in one French family with FNMTC.[120] Subsequent analysis in 22 families confirmed the involvement of the *TCO1* locus in only one French Canadian family.[121] Additionally, loss of heterozygosity has been shown at the *TCO1*

locus in cases of sporadic thyroid cancer as well as FNMTC, suggesting the presence of a tumor-suppressor gene in this region but the gene itself is unknown.[122,123] Cases of FNMTC have a significantly shorter germline telomere length, higher *hTERT* gene amplification, and higher hTERT mRNA expression as compared to sporadic PTC.[124] Unfortunately, these have not been validated by other investigators. Only shorter germline telomere length has been observed in affected members with FNMTC.[125,126]

Genome-wide linkage analysis using SNP arrays in a family with 13 affected members involving three generations found a strong association on chromosome 4q32.[127] Molecular functional studies showed that the 4q32 A > C mutation affected the binding of transcription factors POU2F1 and YY1.[127] The multinodular goiter 1 (*MNG1*) locus was identified as a potential locus on chromosome 14q32 in a family with 18 cases of MNG and two cases of PTC.[128] Unfortunately, other investigators have not found any linkage at the *MNG1* locus in FNMTC.[121,129–131] The familial *PTC/PRN* locus on chromosome 1q21 was identified in large, three-generation kindred with PTC and PRN.[94] The same locus was independently validated in a separate cohort of FNMTC but without PRN.[132] Unfortunately, other investigators have not found any association between this locus and nonsyndromic FNMTC.[121,133] A genome-wide scan followed by a haplotype analysis in a large Tasmanian pedigree with eight cases of NMTC (four classical PTC, four follicular-variant PTC) identified a locus on 2q21.[134] Subsequent studies in 80 pedigrees also showed significant linkage at the 2q21 locus with FNMTC, particularly for the follicular variant of PTC.[134] In another study focused on 10 FNMTC, the locus was also found to be a linkage site.[135] However, other investigators did not find linkage at this locus and FNMTC.[131,133] A study in 20 patients with PTC and history of MNG and 329 controls found the presence of a germline mutation (A339V) in *TTF-1/NKX2.1* on chromosome 14q13 in four PTC patients.[136] TTF is a thyroid transcription factor that regulates the transcription of thyroglobulin, thyroperoxidase, and thyrotropin receptor. However, this association was not found by other groups.[137]

FNMTC is present in 3.2%–9.6% of all the thyroid cancer patients.[1,101,138,139] It is estimated that sporadic disease accounts for 45%–69% of cases in which families have only two affected family members.[140] The likelihood of a truly inherited cancer is much higher when three or more first-degree relatives are affected with NMTC.[106,140] The most common histologic subtype of thyroid cancer is PTC similar. Women are affected by FNMTC approximately two to three times more frequently than men, but this may be due to cases of sporadic disease being considered as familial (family with only two first-degree relatives).[140,141] The age at diagnosis in FNMTC is younger than sporadic cases (39−43 years vs. 46−49 years).[101,102,138] Capezzone and colleagues have observed "clinical anticipation" with the second generation having more aggressive disease at younger age.[142] In contrast, there are several studies that did not find a difference in age at diagnosis between sporadic cases and FNMTC.[103,139,143−145]

Screening of all first-degree relatives of affected members has been proposed for FNMTC.[146] To our knowledge, there is only one prospective study, focused on determining the benefits of screening in FNMTC.[106,147] Based on this study, PTC was detected by screening at a lower rate in kindred with two first-degree relatives affected as compared to kindred who had three or more first-degree relatives affected (4.6% vs. 22.7%, respectively).[106] Several retrospective studies support this finding. For example, McDonald and associates found more aggressive behavior in kindred with three or more members affected as compared with families with two members affected.[148]

Most studies suggest that FNMTC is associated with earlier age of onset, higher rate of multifocality, extrathyroidal extension, lymph node metastases, higher recurrence rate, and decreased disease-free survival.[102,103,139,149−153] A meta-analysis (12 studies with a total of 12,741 patients with follow-up time of 1.5−12.1 years) evaluated if the extent of disease was different between sporadic cases and FNMTC.[154] The analysis was based on five studies conducted in Asia,[103,139,143,145,155] four in North America,[138,144,148,149] two in Europe,[142,156] and one in a combined U.S. and Japanese cohort.[102] The authors found higher rate of recurrence (OR 1.72, 95% CI: 1.34−2.20) and decreased disease-free survival (HR 1.83, 95% CI: 1.34−2.52) as compared to sporadic disease.[154] The investigators also found younger age at diagnosis, higher rate of multifocal tumor, bilateral disease, extrathyroidal invasion and lymph node metastases.[154]

As the susceptibility gene is not known for most FNMTC cases, genetic testing cannot be used to identify at-risk individuals in kindred with FNMTC. Thus, screening is based on clinical and imaging exams. In the prospective cohort study focused on screening in FNMTC families, thyroid nodules were detected by physical examination in 12.7% of patients as compared to 50.5% by neck US.[106] Therefore, the use of thyroid

US is a useful and cost-effective tool for screening of asymptomatic family members of kindred with FNMTC, as it enables an earlier detection of nonpalpable thyroid nodules.[157] US-guided fine-needle aspiration biopsy and cytologic examination is the most accurate diagnostic tool for thyroid nodules. However, the accuracy of fine-needle aspiration biopsy may be lower in patients with FNMTC, with a false-negative rate of up to 12% reported as compared to 4% in matched controls.[158] Patients with FNMTC and a thyroid nodule greater than 1 cm should have US-guided fine-needle aspiration.[37]

There are no studies addressing the cost-effectiveness of screening in kindred with FNMTC. There is insufficient evidence to strongly recommend for or against screening, as data on its potential long-term beneficial effects on survival and cost-effectiveness are still lacking. However, several studies do suggest that screening results in the detection of an earlier stage of disease, which may be associated with a lower cost of treatment and better long-term outcomes. We believe screening with thyroid US should be performed in FNMTC kindred with at least three first-degree relatives affected. We believe the most optimal age to start screening is in the teenage years, as almost 10% of patients with FNMTC are diagnosed between the age of 18 and 20 years old.[106]

REFERENCES

1. Vriens MR, Suh I, Moses W, Kebebew E. Clinical features and genetic predisposition to hereditary nonmedullary thyroid cancer. *Thyroid.* 2009;19(12):1343−1349.
2. Peiling Yang S, Ngeow J. Familial non-medullary thyroid cancer: unraveling the genetic maze. *Endocr Relat Cancer.* 2016;23(12):R577−R595.
3. Marsh DJ, Coulon V, Lunetta KL, et al. Mutation spectrum and genotype-phenotype analyses in Cowden disease and Bannayan-Zonana syndrome, two hamartoma syndromes with germline PTEN mutation. *Hum Mol Genet.* 1998;7(3):507−515.
4. Ngeow J, Mester J, Rybicki LA, Ni Y, Milas M, Eng C. Incidence and clinical characteristics of thyroid cancer in prospective series of individuals with Cowden and Cowden-like syndrome characterized by germline PTEN, SDH, or KLLN alterations. *J Clin Endocrinol Metab.* 2011;96(12):E2063−E2071.
5. Bennett KL, Mester J, Eng C. Germline epigenetic regulation of KILLIN in Cowden and Cowden-like syndrome. *J Am Med Assoc.* 2010;304(24):2724−2731.
6. Orloff MS, He X, Peterson C, et al. Germline PIK3CA and AKT1 mutations in Cowden and Cowden-like syndromes. *Am J Hum Genet.* 2013;92(1):76−80.

7. Yehia L, Niazi F, Ni Y, et al. Germline heterozygous variants in SEC23B are associated with Cowden syndrome and enriched in apparently sporadic thyroid cancer. *Am J Hum Genet.* 2015;97(5):661–676.

8. Lloyd 2nd KM, Dennis M. Cowden's disease. A possible new symptom complex with multiple system involvement. *Ann Intern Med.* 1963;58:136–142.

9. Pilarski R, Burt R, Kohlman W, Pho L, Shannon KM, Swisher E. Cowden syndrome and the PTEN hamartoma tumor syndrome: systematic review and revised diagnostic criteria. *J Natl Cancer Inst.* 2013;105(21):1607–1616.

10. Ngeow J, Eng C. PTEN hamartoma tumor syndrome: clinical risk assessment and management protocol. *Methods.* 2015;77–78:11–19.

11. Thyroid cancer. A comprehensive guide to clinical management. Third edition. *Anticancer Res.* 2017;37(1):361.

12. Pilarski R. Cowden syndrome: a critical review of the clinical literature. *J Genet Couns.* 2009;18(1):13–27.

13. Starink TM, van der Veen JP, Arwert F, et al. The Cowden syndrome: a clinical and genetic study in 21 patients. *Clin Genet.* 1986;29(3):222–233.

14. Eng C. Cowden syndrome. *J Genet Couns.* 1997;6(2):181–192.

15. Hanssen AM, Fryns JP. Cowden syndrome. *J Med Genet.* 1995;32(2):117–119.

16. Milas M, Mester J, Metzger R, et al. Should patients with Cowden syndrome undergo prophylactic thyroidectomy? *Surgery.* 2012;152(6):1201–1210.

17. Syngal S, Brand RE, Church JM, et al. ACG clinical guideline: genetic testing and management of hereditary gastrointestinal cancer syndromes. *Am J Gastroenterol.* 2015;110(2):223–262. quiz 263.

18. Smith JR, Marqusee E, Webb S, et al. Thyroid nodules and cancer in children with PTEN hamartoma tumor syndrome. *J Clin Endocrinol Metab.* 2011;96(1):34–37.

19. Marsh DJ, Kum JB, Lunetta KL, et al. PTEN mutation spectrum and genotype-phenotype correlations in Bannayan-Riley-Ruvalcaba syndrome suggest a single entity with Cowden syndrome. *Hum Mol Genet.* 1999;8(8):1461–1472.

20. Peiretti V, Mussa A, Feyles F, et al. Thyroid involvement in two patients with Bannayan-Riley-Ruvalcaba syndrome. *J Clin Res Pediatr Endocrinol.* 2013;5(4):261–265.

21. Bannayan GA. Lipomatosis, angiomatosis, and macrencephalia. A previously undescribed congenital syndrome. *Arch Pathol.* 1971;92(1):1–5.

22. Laury AR, Bongiovanni M, Tille JC, Kozakewich H, Nose V. Thyroid pathology in PTEN-hamartoma tumor syndrome: characteristic findings of a distinct entity. *Thyroid.* 2011;21(2):135–144.

23. Richards ML. Familial syndromes associated with thyroid cancer in the era of personalized medicine. *Thyroid.* 2010;20(7):707–713.

24. Eng C. PTEN hamartoma tumor syndrome. In: Pagon RA, Adam MP, Ardinger HH, et al., eds. *GeneReviews(R).* 1993. Seattle (WA).

25. Zirilli L, Benatti P, Romano S, et al. Differentiated thyroid carcinoma (DTC) in a young woman with Peutz-Jeghers syndrome: are these two conditions associated? *Exp Clin Endocrinol Diabetes.* 2009;117(5):234–239.

26. Wang Z, Wu B, Mosig RA, et al. STK11 domain XI mutations: candidate genetic drivers leading to the development of dysplastic polyps in Peutz-Jeghers syndrome. *Hum Mutat.* 2014;35(7):851–858.

27. Lim W, Olschwang S, Keller JJ, et al. Relative frequency and morphology of cancers in STK11 mutation carriers. *Gastroenterology.* 2004;126(7):1788–1794.

28. Hearle N, Schumacher V, Menko FH, et al. STK11 status and intussusception risk in Peutz-Jeghers syndrome. *J Med Genet.* 2006;43(8):e41.

29. Amos CI, Keitheri-Cheteri MB, Sabripour M, et al. Genotype-phenotype correlations in Peutz-Jeghers syndrome. *J Med Genet.* 2004;41(5):327–333.

30. Salloch H, Reinacher-Schick A, Schulmann K, et al. Truncating mutations in Peutz-Jeghers syndrome are associated with more polyps, surgical interventions and cancers. *Int J Colorectal Dis.* 2010;25(1):97–107.

31. Triggiani V, Guastamacchia E, Renzulli G, et al. Papillary thyroid carcinoma in Peutz-Jeghers syndrome. *Thyroid.* 2011;21(11):1273–1277.

32. Yamamoto M, Hoshino H, Onizuka T, Ichikawa M, Kawakubo A, Hayakawa S. Thyroid papillary adenocarcinoma in a woman with Peutz-Jeghers syndrome. *Intern Med.* 1992;31(9):1117–1119.

33. Yalcin S, Kirli E, Ciftci AO, et al. The association of adrenocortical carcinoma and thyroid cancer in a child with Peutz-Jeghers syndrome. *J Pediatr Surg.* 2011;46(3):570–573.

34. Spigelman AD, Murday V, Phillips RK. Cancer and the Peutz-Jeghers syndrome. *Gut.* 1989;30(11):1588–1590.

35. Reed MW, Harris SC, Quayle AR, Talbot CH. The association between thyroid neoplasia and intestinal polyps. *Ann R Coll Surg Engl.* 1990;72(6):357–359.

36. Boardman LA, Thibodeau SN, Schaid DJ, et al. Increased risk for cancer in patients with the Peutz-Jeghers syndrome. *Ann Intern Med.* 1998;128(11):896–899.

37. Haugen BR, Alexander EK, Bible KC, et al. 2015 American thyroid association management guidelines for adult patients with thyroid nodules and differentiated thyroid cancer: the American thyroid association guidelines task force on thyroid nodules and differentiated thyroid cancer. *Thyroid.* 2016;26(1):1–133.

38. Cottrell S, Bicknell D, Kaklamanis L, Bodmer WF. Molecular analysis of APC mutations in familial adenomatous polyposis and sporadic colon carcinomas. *Lancet.* 1992;340(8820):626–630.

39. Nagase H, Nakamura Y. Mutations of the APC (adenomatous polyposis coli) gene. *Hum Mutat.* 1993;2(6):425–434.

40. Beroud C, Soussi T. APC gene: database of germline and somatic mutations in human tumors and cell lines. *Nucleic Acids Res.* 1996;24(1):121–124.

41. Veeman MT, Axelrod JD, Moon RT. A second canon. Functions and mechanisms of beta-catenin-independent Wnt signaling. *Dev Cell.* 2003;5(3):367−377.

42. Giannelli SM, McPhaul L, Nakamoto J, Gianoukakis AG. Familial adenomatous polyposis-associated, cribriform morular variant of papillary thyroid carcinoma harboring a K-RAS mutation: case presentation and review of molecular mechanisms. *Thyroid.* 2014;24(7):1184−1189.

43. Claes K, Dahan K, Tejpar S, et al. The genetics of familial adenomatous polyposis (FAP) and MutYH-associated polyposis (MAP). *Acta Gastroenterol Belg.* 2011;74(3): 421−426.

44. Jasperson KW, Burt RW. APC-associated polyposis conditions. In: Pagon RA, Adam MP, Ardinger HH, et al., eds. *GeneReviews(R).* 1993. Seattle (WA).

45. Septer S, Slowik V, Morgan R, Dai H, Attard T. Thyroid cancer complicating familial adenomatous polyposis: mutation spectrum of at-risk individuals. *Hered Cancer Clin Pract.* 2013;11(1):13.

46. Punatar SB, Noronha V, Joshi A, Prabhash K. Thyroid cancer in Gardner's syndrome: case report and review of literature. *South Asian J Cancer.* 2012;1(1):43−47.

47. Jarrar AM, Milas M, Mitchell J, et al. Screening for thyroid cancer in patients with familial adenomatous polyposis. *Ann Surg.* 2011;253(3):515−521.

48. Nose V. Familial thyroid cancer: a review. *Mod Pathol.* 2011;24(suppl 2):S19−S33.

49. Herraiz M, Barbesino G, Faquin W, et al. Prevalence of thyroid cancer in familial adenomatous polyposis syndrome and the role of screening ultrasound examinations. *Clin Gastroenterol Hepatol.* 2007;5(3): 367−373.

50. Plail RO, Bussey HJ, Glazer G, Thomson JP. Adenomatous polyposis: an association with carcinoma of the thyroid. *Br J Surg.* 1987;74(5):377−380.

51. Bulow S, Holm NV, Mellemgaard A. Papillary thyroid carcinoma in Danish patients with familial adenomatous polyposis. *Int J Colorectal Dis.* 1988;3(1):29−31.

52. Truta B, Allen BA, Conrad PG, et al. Genotype and phenotype of patients with both familial adenomatous polyposis and thyroid carcinoma. *Fam Cancer.* 2003;2(2): 95−99.

53. Burt RW, Leppert MF, Slattery ML, et al. Genetic testing and phenotype in a large kindred with attenuated familial adenomatous polyposis. *Gastroenterology.* 2004; 127(2):444−451.

54. Jasperson KW, Tuohy TM, Neklason DW, Burt RW. Hereditary and familial colon cancer. *Gastroenterology.* 2010;138(6):2044−2058.

55. Adams MS, Bronner-Fraser M. Review: the role of neural crest cells in the endocrine system. *Endocr Pathol.* 2009; 20(2):92−100.

56. Cetta F, Curia MC, Montalto G, et al. Thyroid carcinoma usually occurs in patients with familial adenomatous polyposis in the absence of biallelic inactivation of the adenomatous polyposis coli gene. *J Clin Endocrinol Metab.* 2001;86(1):427−432.

57. Cetta F, Olschwang S, Petracci M, et al. Genetic alterations in thyroid carcinoma associated with familial adenomatous polyposis: clinical implications and suggestions for early detection. *World J Surg.* 1998;22(12): 1231−1236.

58. Iwama T, Mishima Y, Utsunomiya J. The impact of familial adenomatous polyposis on the tumorigenesis and mortality at the several organs. Its rational treatment. *Ann Surg.* 1993;217(2):101−108.

59. Soravia C, Sugg SL, Berk T, et al. Familial adenomatous polyposis-associated thyroid cancer: a clinical, pathological, and molecular genetics study. *Am J Pathol.* 1999; 154(1):127−135.

60. Harach HR, Williams GT, Williams ED. Familial adenomatous polyposis associated thyroid carcinoma: a distinct type of follicular cell neoplasm. *Histopathology.* 1994;25(6):549−561.

61. Cameselle-Teijeiro J, Chan JK. Cribriform-morular variant of papillary carcinoma: a distinctive variant representing the sporadic counterpart of familial adenomatous polyposis-associated thyroid carcinoma? *Mod Pathol.* 1999;12(4):400−411.

62. Stratakis CA, Courcoutsakis NA, Abati A, et al. Thyroid gland abnormalities in patients with the syndrome of spotty skin pigmentation, myxomas, endocrine overactivity, and schwannomas (Carney complex). *J Clin Endocrinol Metab.* 1997;82(7):2037−2043.

63. Matyakhina L, Pack S, Kirschner LS, et al. Chromosome 2 (2p16) abnormalities in Carney complex tumours. *J Med Genet.* 2003;40(4):268−277.

64. Pan L, Peng L, Jean-Gilles J, et al. Novel PRKAR1A gene mutations in carney complex. *Int J Clin Exp Pathol.* 2010;3(5):545−548.

65. Kirschner LS, Sandrini F, Monbo J, Lin JP, Carney JA, Stratakis CA. Genetic heterogeneity and spectrum of mutations of the PRKAR1A gene in patients with the carney complex. *Hum Mol Genet.* 2000;9(20):3037−3046.

66. Bertherat J, Horvath A, Groussin L, et al. Mutations in regulatory subunit type 1A of cyclic adenosine 5′-monophosphate-dependent protein kinase (PRKAR1A): phenotype analysis in 353 patients and 80 different genotypes. *J Clin Endocrinol Metab.* 2009;94(6): 2085−2091.

67. Almeida MQ, Stratakis CA. Carney complex and other conditions associated with micronodular adrenal hyperplasias. *Best Pract Res Clin Endocrinol Metabol.* 2010;24(6):907−914.

68. Stratakis CA, Carney JA, Lin JP, et al. Carney complex, a familial multiple neoplasia and lentiginosis syndrome. Analysis of 11 kindreds and linkage to the short arm of chromosome 2. *J Clin Investig.* 1996; 97(3):699−705.

69. Casey M, Mah C, Merliss AD, et al. Identification of a novel genetic locus for familial cardiac myxomas and Carney complex. *Circulation.* 1998;98(23):2560−2566.

70. Son EJ, Nose V. Familial follicular cell-derived thyroid carcinoma. *Front Endocrinol.* 2012;3:61.

71. Stratakis CA, Kirschner LS, Carney JA. Clinical and molecular features of the Carney complex: diagnostic criteria and recommendations for patient evaluation. *J Clin Endocrinol Metab.* 2001;86(9):4041–4046.

72. Correa R, Salpea P, Stratakis CA. Carney complex: an update. *Eur J Endocrinol.* 2015;173(4):M85–M97.

73. Rothenbuhler A, Stratakis CA. Clinical and molecular genetics of Carney complex. *Best Pract Res Clin Endocrinol Metabol.* 2010;24(3):389–399.

74. Sandrini F, Stratakis C. Clinical and molecular genetics of Carney complex. *Mol Genet Metabol.* 2003;78(2):83–92.

75. Bossis I, Voutetakis A, Bei T, Sandrini F, Griffin KJ, Stratakis CA. Protein kinase A and its role in human neoplasia: the Carney complex paradigm. *Endocr Relat Cancer.* 2004;11(2):265–280.

76. Stratakis CA, Kirschner LS, Carney JA. Carney complex: diagnosis and management of the complex of spotty skin pigmentation, myxomas, endocrine overactivity, and schwannomas. *Am J Med Genet.* 1998;80(2):183–185.

77. Taylor JP, Metcalfe RA, Watson PF, Weetman AP, Trembath RC. Mutations of the PDS gene, encoding pendrin, are associated with protein mislocalization and loss of iodide efflux: implications for thyroid dysfunction in Pendred syndrome. *J Clin Endocrinol Metab.* 2002;87(4):1778–1784.

78. Pera A, Villamar M, Vinuela A, et al. A mutational analysis of the SLC26A4 gene in Spanish hearing-impaired families provides new insights into the genetic causes of Pendred syndrome and DFNB4 hearing loss. *Eur J Hum Genet.* 2008;16(8):888–896.

79. Yang T, Gurrola 2nd JG, Wu H, et al. Mutations of KCNJ10 together with mutations of SLC26A4 cause digenic nonsyndromic hearing loss associated with enlarged vestibular aqueduct syndrome. *Am J Hum Genet.* 2009;84(5):651–657.

80. Nose V. Thyroid cancer of follicular cell origin in inherited tumor syndromes. *Adv Anat Pathol.* 2010;17(6):428–436.

81. Sakurai K, Hata M, Hishinuma A, et al. Papillary thyroid carcinoma in one of identical twin patients with Pendred syndrome. *Endocr J.* 2013;60(6):805–811.

82. Tong GX, Chang Q, Hamele-Bena D, et al. Targeted next-generation sequencing analysis of a Pendred syndrome-associated thyroid carcinoma. *Endocr Pathol.* 2016;27(1):70–75.

83. Snabboon T, Plengpanich W, Saengpanich S, et al. Two common and three novel PDS mutations in Thai patients with Pendred syndrome. *J Endocrinol Investig.* 2007;30(11):907–913.

84. Camargo R, Limbert E, Gillam M, et al. Aggressive metastatic follicular thyroid carcinoma with anaplastic transformation arising from a long-standing goiter in a patient with Pendred's syndrome. *Thyroid.* 2001;11(10):981–988.

85. Rutter MM, Jha P, Schultz KA, et al. DICER1 mutations and differentiated thyroid carcinoma: evidence of a direct association. *J Clin Endocrinol Metab.* 2016;101(1):1–5.

86. Rio Frio T, Bahubeshi A, Kanellopoulou C, et al. DICER1 mutations in familial multinodular goiter with and without ovarian Sertoli-Leydig cell tumors. *J Am Med Assoc.* 2011;305(1):68–77.

87. de Kock L, Sabbaghian N, Soglio DB, et al. Exploring the association between DICER1 mutations and differentiated thyroid carcinoma. *J Clin Endocrinol Metab.* 2014;99(6):E1072–E1077.

88. Rome A, Gentet JC, Coze C, Andre N. Pediatric thyroid cancer arising as a fourth cancer in a child with pleuropulmonary blastoma. *Pediatr Blood Canc.* 2008;50(5):1081.

89. Doros L, Schultz KA, Stewart DR, et al. DICER1-Related disorders. In: Pagon RA, Adam MP, Ardinger HH, et al., eds. *GeneReviews(R).* 1993. Seattle (WA).

90. McConville CM, Stankovic T, Byrd PJ, et al. Mutations associated with variant phenotypes in ataxia-telangiectasia. *Am J Hum Genet.* 1996;59(2):320–330.

91. Concannon P, Gatti RA. Diversity of ATM gene mutations detected in patients with ataxia-telangiectasia. *Hum Mutat.* 1997;10(2):100–107.

92. Lavin MF. Ataxia-telangiectasia: from a rare disorder to a paradigm for cell signalling and cancer. *Nat Rev Mol Cell Biol.* 2008;9(10):759–769.

93. Brasseur B, Beauloye V, Chantrain C, et al. Papillary thyroid carcinoma in a 9-year-old girl with ataxia-telangiectasia. *Pediatr Blood Canc.* 2008;50(5):1058–1060.

94. Malchoff CD, Sarfarazi M, Tendler B, et al. Papillary thyroid carcinoma associated with papillary renal neoplasia: genetic linkage analysis of a distinct heritable tumor syndrome. *J Clin Endocrinol Metab.* 2000;85(5):1758–1764.

95. Yu CE, Oshima J, Fu YH, et al. Positional cloning of the Werner's syndrome gene. *Science.* 1996;272(5259):258–262.

96. Nehlin JO, Skovgaard GL, Bohr VA. The Werner syndrome. A model for the study of human aging. *Ann N Y Acad Sci.* 2000;908:167–179.

97. Muftuoglu M, Oshima J, von Kobbe C, Cheng WH, Leistritz DF, Bohr VA. The clinical characteristics of Werner syndrome: molecular and biochemical diagnosis. *Hum Genet.* 2008;124(4):369–377.

98. Ishikawa Y, Sugano H, Matsumoto T, Furuichi Y, Miller RW, Goto M. Unusual features of thyroid carcinomas in Japanese patients with Werner syndrome and possible genotype-phenotype relations to cell type and race. *Cancer.* 1999;85(6):1345–1352.

99. Lauper JM, Krause A, Vaughan TL, Monnat Jr RJ. Spectrum and risk of neoplasia in Werner syndrome: a systematic review. *PLoS One.* 2013;8(4):e59709.

100. Oshima J, Martin GM, Hisama FM. Werner syndrome. In: Pagon RA, Adam MP, Ardinger HH, et al., eds. *GeneReviews(R).* 1993. Seattle (WA).

101. Sturgeon C, Clark OH. Familial nonmedullary thyroid cancer. *Thyroid.* 2005;15(6):588–593.

102. Alsanea O, Wada N, Ain K, et al. Is familial nonmedullary thyroid carcinoma more aggressive than

sporadic thyroid cancer? A multicenter series. *Surgery.* 2000;128(6):1043−1050. discussion 1050-1041.

103. Uchino S, Noguchi S, Kawamoto H, et al. Familial nonmedullary thyroid carcinoma characterized by multifocality and a high recurrence rate in a large study population. *World J Surg.* 2002;26(8):897−902.

104. Pal T, Vogl FD, Chappuis PO, et al. Increased risk for nonmedullary thyroid cancer in the first degree relatives of prevalent cases of nonmedullary thyroid cancer: a hospital-based study. *J Clin Endocrinol Metab.* 2001; 86(11):5307−5312.

105. Musholt TJ, Musholt PB, Petrich T, Oetting G, Knapp WH, Klempnauer J. Familial papillary thyroid carcinoma: genetics, criteria for diagnosis, clinical features, and surgical treatment. *World J Surg.* 2000;24(11): 1409−1417.

106. Klubo-Gwiezdzinska J, Yang L, Merkel R, et al. *Screening in Familial Non-medullary Thyroid Cancer (FNMTC) Results in Detection of Low Risk Papillary Thyroid Cancer − A Prospective Cohort Study.* 2016.

107. Gudmundsson J, Sulem P, Gudbjartsson DF, et al. Common variants on 9q22.33 and 14q13.3 predispose to thyroid cancer in European populations. *Nat Genet.* 2009; 41(4):460−464.

108. Landa I, Ruiz-Llorente S, Montero-Conde C, et al. The variant rs1867277 in FOXE1 gene confers thyroid cancer susceptibility through the recruitment of USF1/USF2 transcription factors. *PLoS Genet.* 2009;5(9):e1000637.

109. Tomaz RA, Sousa I, Silva JG, et al. FOXE1 polymorphisms are associated with familial and sporadic nonmedullary thyroid cancer susceptibility. *Clin Endocrinol.* 2012; 77(6):926−933.

110. Pereira JS, da Silva JG, Tomaz RA, et al. Identification of a novel germline FOXE1 variant in patients with familial non-medullary thyroid carcinoma (FNMTC). *Endocrine.* 2015;49(1):204−214.

111. Gara SK, Jia L, Merino MJ, et al. Germline HABP2 mutation causing familial nonmedullary thyroid cancer. *N Engl J Med.* 2015;373(5):448−455.

112. Zhang T, Xing M. HABP2 G534E mutation in familial nonmedullary thyroid cancer. *J Natl Cancer Inst.* 2016; 108(6):djv415.

113. Sahasrabudhe R, Stultz J, Williamson J, et al. The HABP2 G534E variant is an unlikely cause of familial nonmedullary thyroid cancer. *J Clin Endocrinol Metab.* 2015: jc20153928.

114. Cantara S, Marzocchi C, Castagna MG, Pacini F. HABP2 G534E variation in familial non-medullary thyroid cancer: an Italian series. *J Endocrinol Investig.* 2016;40.

115. Weeks AL, Wilson SG, Ward L, Goldblatt J, Hui J, Walsh JP. HABP2 germline variants are uncommon in familial nonmedullary thyroid cancer. *BMC Med Genet.* 2016;17(1):60.

116. Ruiz-Ferrer M, Fernandez RM, Navarro E, Antinolo G, Borrego S. G534E variant in HABP2 and nonmedullary thyroid cancer. *Thyroid.* 2016;26(7):987−988.

117. Bohorquez ME, Estrada AP, Stultz J, et al. The HABP2 G534E polymorphism does not increase nonmedullary

thyroid cancer risk in Hispanics. *Endocr Connect.* 2016; 5(3):123−127.

118. Alzahrani AS, Murugan AK, Qasem E, Al-Hindi H. HABP2 gene mutations do not cause familial or sporadic nonmedullary thyroid cancer in a highly inbred middle Eastern population. *Thyroid.* 2016;26(5):667−671.

119. Tomsic J, Fultz R, Liyanarachchi S, He H, Senter L, de la Chapelle A. HABP2 G534E variant in papillary thyroid carcinoma. *PLoS One.* 2016;11(1):e0146315.

120. Canzian F, Amati P, Harach HR, et al. A gene predisposing to familial thyroid tumors with cell oxyphilia maps to chromosome 19p13.2. *Am J Hum Genet.* 1998;63(6): 1743−1748.

121. Bevan S, Pal T, Greenberg CR, et al. A comprehensive analysis of MNG1, TCO1, fPTC, PTEN, TSHR, and TRKA in familial nonmedullary thyroid cancer: confirmation of linkage to TCO1. *J Clin Endocrinol Metab.* 2001; 86(8):3701−3704.

122. Stankov K, Pastore A, Toschi L, et al. Allelic loss on chromosomes 2q21 and 19p 13.2 in oxyphilic thyroid tumors. *Int J Cancer.* 2004;111(3):463−467.

123. Prazeres HJ, Rodrigues F, Soares P, et al. Loss of heterozygosity at 19p13.2 and 2q21 in tumours from familial clusters of non-medullary thyroid carcinoma. *Fam Cancer.* 2008;7(2):141−149.

124. Capezzone M, Cantara S, Marchisotta S, et al. Short telomeres, telomerase reverse transcriptase gene amplification, and increased telomerase activity in the blood of familial papillary thyroid cancer patients. *J Clin Endocrinol Metab.* 2008;93(10):3950−3957.

125. He M, Bian B, Gesuwan K, et al. Telomere length is shorter in affected members of families with familial nonmedullary thyroid cancer. *Thyroid.* 2013;23(3): 301−307.

126. Jendrzejewski J, Tomsic J, Lozanski G, et al. Telomere length and telomerase reverse transcriptase gene copy number in patients with papillary thyroid carcinoma. *J Clin Endocrinol Metab.* 2011;96(11):E1876−E1880.

127. He H, Li W, Wu D, et al. Ultra-rare mutation in longrange enhancer predisposes to thyroid carcinoma with high penetrance. *PLoS One.* 2013;8(5):e61920.

128. Bignell GR, Canzian F, Shayeghi M, et al. Familial nontoxic multinodular thyroid goiter locus maps to chromosome 14q but does not account for familial nonmedullary thyroid cancer. *Am J Hum Genet.* 1997;61(5): 1123−1130.

129. McKay JD, Williamson J, Lesueur F, et al. At least three genes account for familial papillary thyroid carcinoma: TCO and MNG1 excluded as susceptibility loci from a large Tasmanian family. *Eur J Endocrinol.* 1999;141(2): 122−125.

130. Lesueur F, Stark M, Tocco T, et al. Genetic heterogeneity in familial nonmedullary thyroid carcinoma: exclusion of linkage to RET, MNG1, and TCO in 56 families. NMTC Consortium. *J Clin Endocrinol Metab.* 1999; 84(6):2157−2162.

131. Tsilchorozidou T, Vafiadou E, Yovos JG, et al. A Greek family with a follicular variant of familial papillary

thyroid carcinoma: TCO, MNG1, fPTC/PRN, and NMTC1 excluded as susceptibility loci. *Thyroid.* 2005;15(12): 1349−1354.

132. Suh I, Filetti S, Vriens MR, et al. Distinct loci on chromosome 1q21 and 6q22 predispose to familial nonmedullary thyroid cancer: a SNP array-based linkage analysis of 38 families. *Surgery.* 2009;146(6):1073−1080.

133. Cavaco BM, Batista PF, Martins C, et al. Familial nonmedullary thyroid carcinoma (FNMTC): analysis of fPTC/PRN, NMTC1, MNG1 and TCO susceptibility loci and identification of somatic BRAF and RAS mutations. *Endocr Relat Cancer.* 2008;15(1):207−215.

134. McKay JD, Lesueur F, Jonard L, et al. Localization of a susceptibility gene for familial nonmedullary thyroid carcinoma to chromosome 2q21. *Am J Hum Genet.* 2001; 69(2):440−446.

135. McKay JD, Thompson D, Lesueur F, et al. Evidence for interaction between the TCO and NMTC1 loci in familial non-medullary thyroid cancer. *J Med Genet.* 2004;41(6): 407−412.

136. Ngan ES, Lang BH, Liu T, et al. A germline mutation (A339V) in thyroid transcription factor-1 (TITF-1/ NKX2.1) in patients with multinodular goiter and papillary thyroid carcinoma. *J Natl Cancer Inst.* 2009;101(3): 162−175.

137. Cantara S, Capuano S, Formichi C, Pisu M, Capezzone M, Pacini F. Lack of germline A339V mutation in thyroid transcription factor-1 (TITF-1/NKX2.1) gene in familial papillary thyroid cancer. *Thyroid Res.* 2010;3(1):4.

138. Moses W, Weng J, Kebebew E. Prevalence, clinicopathologic features, and somatic genetic mutation profile in familial versus sporadic nonmedullary thyroid cancer. *Thyroid.* 2011;21(4):367−371.

139. Park YJ, Ahn HY, Choi HS, Kim KW, Park DJ, Cho BY. The long-term outcomes of the second generation of familial nonmedullary thyroid carcinoma are more aggressive than sporadic cases. *Thyroid.* 2012;22(4):356−362.

140. Charkes ND. On the prevalence of familial nonmedullary thyroid cancer in multiply affected kindreds. *Thyroid.* 2006;16(2):181−186.

141. Malchoff CD, Malchoff DM. Familial nonmedullary thyroid carcinoma. *Cancer Control.* 2006;13(2):106−110.

142. Capezzone M, Marchisotta S, Cantara S, et al. Familial non-medullary thyroid carcinoma displays the features of clinical anticipation suggestive of a distinct biological entity. *Endocr Relat Cancer.* 2008;15(4):1075−1081.

143. Robenshtok E, Tzvetov G, Grozinsky-Glasberg S, et al. Clinical characteristics and outcome of familial nonmedullary thyroid cancer: a retrospective controlled study. *Thyroid.* 2011;21(1):43−48.

144. Maxwell EL, Hall FT, Freeman JL. Familial non-medullary thyroid cancer: a matched-case control study. *Laryngoscope.* 2004;114(12):2182−2186.

145. Ito Y, Kakudo K, Hirokawa M, et al. Biological behavior and prognosis of familial papillary thyroid carcinoma. *Surgery.* 2009;145(1):100−105.

146. Navas-Carrillo D, Rios A, Rodriguez JM, Parrilla P, Orenes-Pinero E. Familial nonmedullary thyroid cancer: screening, clinical, molecular and genetic findings. *Biochim Biophys Acta.* 2014;1846(2):468−476.

147. Sadowski SM, He M, Gesuwan K, et al. Prospective screening in familial nonmedullary thyroid cancer. *Surgery.* 2013;154(6):1194−1198.

148. McDonald TJ, Driedger AA, Garcia BM, et al. Familial papillary thyroid carcinoma: a retrospective analysis. *J Oncol.* 2011;2011:948786.

149. Mazeh H, Benavidez J, Poehls JL, Youngwirth L, Chen H, Sippel RS. In patients with thyroid cancer of follicular cell origin, a family history of nonmedullary thyroid cancer in one first-degree relative is associated with more aggressive disease. *Thyroid.* 2012;22(1):3−8.

150. Jiwang L, Zhendong L, Shuchun L, Bo H, Yanguo L. Clinicopathologic characteristics of familial versus sporadic papillary thyroid carcinoma. *Acta Otorhinolaryngol Ital.* 2015;35(4):234−242.

151. Leux C, Truong T, Petit C, Baron-Dubourdieu D, Guenel P. Family history of malignant and benign thyroid diseases and risk of thyroid cancer: a population-based case-control study in New Caledonia. *Cancer Causes Control.* 2012;23(5):745−755.

152. Pitoia F, Cross G, Salvai ME, Abelleira E, Niepomniszcze H. Patients with familial non-medullary thyroid cancer have an outcome similar to that of patients with sporadic papillary thyroid tumors. *Arq Bras Endocrinol Metabol.* 2011;55(3):219−223.

153. Tavarelli M, Russo M, Terranova R, et al. Familial nonmedullary thyroid cancer represents an independent risk factor for increased cancer aggressiveness: a retrospective analysis of 74 families. *Front Endocrinol.* 2015; 6:117.

154. Wang X, Cheng W, Li J, et al. Endocrine tumours: familial nonmedullary thyroid carcinoma is a more aggressive disease: a systematic review and meta-analysis. *Eur J Endocrinol.* 2015;172(6):R253−R262.

155. Lee YM, Yoon JH, Yi O, et al. Familial history of nonmedullary thyroid cancer is an independent prognostic factor for tumor recurrence in younger patients with conventional papillary thyroid carcinoma. *J Surg Oncol.* 2014;109(2):168−173.

156. Pinto AE, Silva GL, Henrique R, et al. Familial vs sporadic papillary thyroid carcinoma: a matched-case comparative study showing similar clinical/prognostic behaviour. *Eur J Endocrinol.* 2014;170(2):321−327.

157. Uchino S, Noguchi S, Yamashita H, et al. Detection of asymptomatic differentiated thyroid carcinoma by neck ultrasonographic screening for familial nonmedullary thyroid carcinoma. *World J Surg.* 2004;28(11): 1099−1102.

158. Vriens MR, Sabanci U, Epstein HD, et al. Reliability of fine-needle aspiration in patients with familial nonmedullary thyroid cancer. *Thyroid.* 1999;9(10): 1011−1016.

CHAPTER 5

Thyroid Cancer in Children and Adolescents

ANDREW J. BAUER, MD

INTRODUCTION

Over the last several decades, there has been an increasing trend in the diagnosis of differentiated thyroid cancer in pediatric patients, with the majority of this trend secondary to papillary thyroid cancer (PTC).[1-4] Most patients will be diagnosed after discovery of an asymptomatic thyroid nodule or persistent lymphadenopathy in the mid- to lower lateral neck (levels III or IV)[5] either on physical exam or incidentally on unrelated head and neck imaging. In general, most thyroid nodules are benign; however, when a child or adolescent is found to have a thyroid nodule there is a 2–3-fold increased risk of malignancy compared to adults, ~20%–25% compared to ~10%–15%, respectively.[6,7] This risk can be more accurately determined based on the ultrasound (US) features of the thyroid nodule and cervical neck lymph nodes followed by fine-needle aspiration (FNA) of selected lesions.[8,9] There does not appear to be a correlation between how the nodule is discovered (incidental or purposeful exam of the thyroid) and the risk of malignancy; what is discovered is of greater clinical importance rather than how it was discovered. This chapter reviews the practical evaluation of pediatric thyroid nodules as well as the management of pediatric thyroid carcinoma.

ETIOLOGY

For most children and adolescents, there are no identifiable risk factors associated with the development of a thyroid nodule or thyroid cancer. For the remaining smaller cohort of patients, identifiable risk factors include exposure to ionizing radiation (inhaled, ingested, or external beam) and genetic predisposition.

Early observations about the relationship between radiation and an increased risk for developing thyroid nodules and thyroid cancer were noted after the use of low-dose external beam radiotherapy for the treatment of benign diseases, including tonsillar hypertrophy, thymic hyperplasia, acne, and tinea capitis.[10,11] As these initial reports, additional concerns have been raised over repeated exposure to diagnostic radiological imaging, exposure from radiation therapy to treat nonthyroid malignancies, and the rare occurrence of accidental exposure to ionizing radiation. The higher proliferative cellular activity in the thyroid of a child or adolescent compared to an adult is believed to explain the disparate tumorigenic effect that all forms of radiation have on the development of radiation induced thyroid disease with the greatest risk for patients <16 years old at the time of exposure.[12]

Across the various radiological imaging modalities, computed tomography (CT) scans account for approximately 47% of the total effective dose of radiation exposure from diagnostic imaging across the world.[13] Pediatric imaging protocols reduce the amount of exposure per scan but prolonged, serial CT imaging may contribute to an increased risk of thyroid nodules and cancer.[14] In patients exposed to therapeutic radiation, doses up to 20–30 Gy and exposure before 10 years old correlate with the highest risk of developing thyroid cancer with age at the time of exposure inversely correlating with latency.[12,15,16] Overall, thyroid nodules develop at a rate of about 2% annually with up to a 70-fold increased risk for radiation induced thyroid cancer that may develop as early as 3–5 years, or as late as 3–4 decades, after exposure.[17,18]

The development and use of nuclear power has also furthered our understanding of the relationship

Advances in Treatment and Management in Surgical Endocrinology. https://doi.org/10.1016/B978-0-323-66195-9.00005-4

between radiation exposure and the development of thyroid cancer. The Chernobyl nuclear power plant accident in 1986 provides the most important data on the risks of inhaled and ingested ^{131}I in the development of pediatric thyroid cancer. In the aftermath of Chernobyl, a 60-fold increased incidence of thyroid cancer in surrounding countries did not have or implement an iodine thyroid blocking plan and allowed their populations to continue to live in regions where consumption of contaminated dietary products such as milk and green leafy vegetables continued for months and years after the accident.[19] There are conflicting data if radiation induced PTC are more[20] or similarly invasive[21] compared to sporadic PTC; however, a delay in establishing a thyroid monitoring program after a population is exposed to significant radiation may be associated with a great burden of metastatic disease at diagnosis. This is most clearly demonstrated by review of the initial cohort of pediatric patients that presented with PTC approximately 5-year after Chernobyl where regional lymph node metastases and pulmonary metastases were found in 60% and 24% of patients, respectively, and 50% of tumors exhibited extrathyroidal extension (ETE).[22] In contrast, after initiation of a thyroid monitoring program and registry, the number of children diagnosed with lymph node metastasis decreased from 60% to 30%, pulmonary metastasis from 24% to 2%, and ETE from 50% to 24%.[22]

The second most common identifiable risk factor for the development of thyroid cancer is genetic predisposition that may be divided into two broad categories: nonsyndromic and syndromic (thyroid cancer associated with other tumors). Familial nonmedullary thyroid cancer (FNMTC) is defined by the presence of two or more first-degree relatives with DTC, either PTC of follicular thyroid cancer, but not associated with additional clinical findings, including no increased risk for developing additional nonthyroid tumors.[23,24] Similar to sporadic DTC, 85% of FNMTC comprises patients with PTC. The transmission pattern is most consistent with an autosomal dominant mode of inheritance; however, to date, a single, reliable germline locus has not been identified.[25,26] Compared to sporadic DTC, FNMTC presents at a younger age and exhibits clinical anticipation between generations where subsequent generation family members present with earlier and more invasive disease.[27]

Syndromic forms of thyroid cancer in which there is a familial genetic tumor predisposition to the development of thyroid malignancy and other tumors include PTEN hamartoma tumor syndrome (PHTS) (https://www.ncbi.nlm.nih.gov/books/NBK1488/), familial

adenomatous polyposis (https://www.ncbi.nlm.nih.gov/books/NBK1345/), DICER1 syndrome (https://www.ncbi.nlm.nih.gov/books/NBK196157/), Carney complex (https://www.ncbi.nlm.nih.gov/books/NBK1286/), and multiple endocrine neoplasia type 2 (https://www.ncbi.nlm.nih.gov/books/NBK1257/). The risk of developing thyroid cancer in syndromic DTC spans a range from approximately 10% in familial adenomatous polyposis[28] to 16% in DICER1-related disorders[29] and 35% in PTEN hamartoma tumor syndrome.[30] In DICER1, the risk of developing DTC with earlier onset of disease increases in patients treated with chemotherapy for pleuropulmonary blastoma.[31]

Additional factors associated with an increased risk of thyroid cancer include iodine and autoimmune thyroid disease. The role of iodine deficiency and iodine excess in thyroid cancer tumorigenesis have both been examined with current data suggesting that iodine deficiency is a weak initiator but strong promotor of DTC, in particular for follicular thyroid cancer (FTC), likely secondary to chronic thyroid stimulating hormone (TSH) stimulation. Autoimmune thyroiditis, both hypothyroidism (Hashimoto's thyroiditis)[32] and hyperthyroidism (Graves' disease),[33,34] have also been associated with increased risk.

There is ongoing debate whether patients at increased risk for developing thyroid cancer should undergo thyroid US surveillance or surveillance by physical exam alone. For oncology survivors treated with radiation, an international group published recommendations suggesting that patients and families should be counseled about the options for surveillance by either physical exam (palpation) or by ultrasound.[35] For populations exposed to radiation from a nuclear power plant accident, the World Health Organization, International Agency for Research on Cancer, published guidelines for iodine thyroid blockade (https://www.who.int/ionizing_radiation/pub_meet/iodine-thyroid-blocking/en/) as well as for establishing a thyroid monitoring program for postexposure, high-risk populations (children and adolescents and pregnant women and their offspring) (http://tmnuc.iarc.fr/en/).[36,37] In familial thyroid predisposition disorders, thyroid surveillance by US is also recommended with the goal of identifying thyroid cancer at an earlier state of metastasis in an effort to reduce the extent of treatment and potential complications of treatment associated with more extensive therapy.

Overall, the risk of performing an ultrasound is minimal when a clinician experienced in reading thyroid ultrasound images and managing pediatric thyroid nodular disease is involved in the process.

Complication from thyroid-nodule aspiration is extraordinarily low, and the rate of permanent complications from thyroid surgery should be less than 3%–5% if performed by a high-volume thyroid surgeon.[38] Thus, in high-risk populations, the benefit of performing thyroid US monitoring appears to outweigh the risk of the procedure.

DIAGNOSTIC EVALUATION OF THYROID NODULE

Physical Exam

After a thorough review of the past medical and family history, screening for potential risk factors (discussed earlier), the next step in the evaluation is a complete thyroid exam that includes inspection and palpation of the thyroid gland as well as the lateral neck cervical lymph nodes (see—https://www.youtube.com/watch?v=Z9norsLPKfU). The size, symmetry, and texture of the thyroid gland, thyroid nodule(s), and lateral neck lymph nodes should be described. The presence of a thyroid nodule with cervical lymphadenopathy is a significant predictor for malignancy, especially if lymphadenopathy is noted in levels III and IV of the lateral neck.[39,40] In contrast, symmetric level II (under the mandible) is a common finding in pediatric patients and these lymph nodes are typically larger on physical and US exam. Physical findings related to genetic syndromes should be evaluated and recorded. PHTS is associated with macrocephaly, small benign cutaneous neoplasms on the face and neck (trichilemmomas), lipomas, and freckling of the glans penis.[41–43] Carney Complex[44] and familial adenomatous polyposis[45] are associated with lentigines, and MEN 2B is associated with alacrima (an inability or decreased ability to produce tears), marfanoid facies (typically noted around 5 years old), and oral mucosal neuromas, most commonly of the lips and tongue.[46]

Laboratory Evaluation

In general, there are no laboratory tests or values that can help to discern the risk that a thyroid nodule is more likely to be benign or malignant. However, for patients diagnosed with a thyroid nodule, the most common baseline labs to obtain are the following: (1) TSH, (2) thyroxin (T4), thyroglobulin (Tg), and antithyroglobulin (TgAb). A suppressed TSH is often associated with an autonomously functioning thyroid nodule, a nodule that carries a lower risk of malignancy in both adult and pediatric patients (1%–10%).[47] The utility of a preoperative Tg in children and adolescents with thyroid nodules has not been established and there are multiple confounding variables associated with an elevated Tg, including iodine deficiency and excess[48] and thyroiditis. In adults, there are mixed reports suggesting that an elevated Tg may be predictive of thyroid malignancy[49] as well as disease burden.[50] A calcitonin level should be obtained if there is a family history of multiple endocrine neoplasia type 2 (MEN2), clinical features suggestive of MEN 2B, or if the cytology is suspicion for MTC.[51] In contrast to adults, with a low incidence of sporadic MTC in pediatrics, the cost of obtaining a preoperative calcitonin appears to be greater than the potential benefit. If a calcitonin is ordered in a young child, one needs to be aware that there is a normal, physiologic elevation in calcitonin in patients <3 years old.[52]

Radiologic Imaging

A thyroid and neck US is the best imaging modality to assess thyroid tissue morphology and lymphadenopathy. All providers involved in the evaluation and care of pediatric patients with thyroid nodules must be comfortable with reviewing and interpreting the US images to ensure that a complete US exam was performed and that the interpretation is accurate. There are early reports showing utility of both the american thyroid association (ATA) adult thyroid nodule pictorial risk classification system and the Thyroid Imaging Reporting and Data System in children and adolescents.[9] Irrespective of what system is used, the US report should describe the size, location, composition (solid, cystic, or spongiform), echogenicity (hypoechoic, isoechoic, hyperechoic, or mixed echogenicity), shape (taller than wide or not on transverse imaging), margins (regular, infiltrative or micro- or macrolobulated, and the presence or absence of extrathyroidal extension), and the presence of echogenic foci. Cystic composition is the single most reliable feature for assessing the risk of malignancy with the degree of risk based on percent, and US features of the solid portion.[6,53] The presence of ETE is most readily identified for anteriorly located nodules by review of both the still and CINE clip images where the nodule is protruding anteriorly into the perithyroidal tissue with loss of the perithyroidal echogenic line.[54] US evaluation of the lateral neck should be performed looking for the presence of abnormal lymph nodes that show features of rounded shape, increased echogenicity with loss of the hilum, cystic composition, and/or echogenic foci, and increased peripheral blood flow on Doppler imaging.[55]

The US features of the nodule should be used to stratify the nodules that should undergo FNA. Most adult criteria apply to children and adolescents with the following exceptions: (1) US features and clinical context should be used rather than size alone to identify nodules that warrant FNA,[8] (2) solid nodules may have an increased risk of malignancy in pediatric patients compared to adults, and (3) a widely invasive form of PTC called diffuse sclerosing variant PTC (dsvPTC) presents with nonnodular, diffuse infiltration of the thyroid associated with microcalcifications throughout the gland, a "snow storm" appearance on US.[56–58] In addition, dsvPTC is commonly associated with macroscopic metastasis to lateral neck lymph nodes as well as elevated TgAb. The nonnodular appearance and the presence of elevated TgAb may mimic autoimmune hypothyroidism; however, the diffuse echogenic foci and abnormal lateral neck LN should help discern between these two conditions.

For patients undergoing FNA to confirm metastatic lymph node disease, measurement of Tg in the FNA washout of the lymph node may help to confirm equivocal cytological evidence of regional metastasis.[59,60] Axial imaging with neck CT or magnetic resonance imaging (MRI) increases the sensitivity of identifying lymph node metastasis in regions of the neck that are not readily visible by preoperative US, including the deep central neck (level VI; paratracheal and retropharyngeal), subclavicular and upper mediastinum.[61]

Radioactive iodine thyroid uptake and scan may be considered for patients with a suppressed TSH; however, there does not appear to be any benefit to obtaining this if the TSH is not suppressed. With rare exception, the use of 18F-fluoro-deoxyglucose positron emission tomography (18F-FDG PET/CT) is not indicated in the initial preoperative assessment of a thyroid nodule, however, if a thyroid nodule is detected on an unrelated 18F-FDG PET/CT there is an approximate 20% risk of nodule being malignant.[62]

Fine-Needle Aspiration

Similar to adults, The Bethesda System for Reporting Thyroid Cytopathology (TBSRTC) is used to classify the FNA results in pediatrics with equal sensitivity, specificity, and overall accuracy.[6,63] However, although the results of the FNA are similarly used to stratify an appropriate management plan, there appears to be an increased risk of malignancy for pediatric patients with benign and indeterminate cytology. In adults, benign cytology is associated with a 0%–3% risk of malignancy while in pediatrics the risk of malignancy may be as high as 10%. For nodules with TBSRTC category III (atypia of undetermined significance or follicular lesion of undetermined significance), category IV (follicular or Hürthle neoplasm), or category V (suspicious for malignancy), the risk of malignancy may be as high as 28%, 58%, and 100%, respectively.[64,65] For patients with

nondiagnostic (TBSRTC category 1) cytology, repeat FNA may be considered but there should be a 3-month delay between FNAs to avoid potential post-FNA reactive cellular atypia.[66] Cytological confirmation of sample adequacy at the bedside can decrease the rate of nondiagnostic results. Nodules with category V and category VI (suspicious for malignancy and malignant) correlate with a near 100% risk of PTC.[39,65,67] TT with prophylactic central neck lymph node dissection is recommended for patients with nodules having TBSRTC category V and category VI.[8]

In an effort to decrease reliance on diagnostic surgery, there is increasing use of supplemental molecular profile testing in pediatrics following the more widespread use of oncogene panels and gene-expression classifier testing in adults. In children, the presence of a thyroid oncogene mutation or fusion (*BRAF, RET/PTC, NTRK-fusion and others*) in an indeterminate FNA specimen is associated with an increased risk of malignancy.[65,68] Based on current data, the following approach is supported: (1) oncogene panels are the only test that have clinical utility to predict an increased risk for malignancy in patients under 19 years old, (2) oncogene panels should only be ordered on samples with indeterminate cytology (TBSRTC categories III and IV), and (3) *BRAF* V600E, *RET-PTC* and *NTRK-fusions* have near 100% specificity for DTC and appear to be associated with an increased risk for invasive disease. The presence of other mutations and fusions, including *RAS, PAX8-PPARg*, and others, is associated with both benign and malignant disease (indeterminate oncogenes), and, until further data are available, diagnostic lobectomy may still be the surgery of choice for unilateral nodules with indeterminate oncogenes.[69]

SURGICAL MANAGEMENT

Thyroid surgery should be performed by a high-volume thyroid surgeon defined as a surgeon who performs 30 or more cervical endocrine procedures annually within the age group of the patient undergoing surgery in an effort to minimize the risk of operative complications.[8,38,70] Although the exact number of surgeries performed annually may not reflect the quality of the surgeon, it increases the likelihood that the surgeon understands the disease process in children and adolescents and is familiar with age-specific treatment recommendations, age-specific physiology for perioperative care, and is comfortable with managing potential complications, including hypoparathyroidism and recurrent laryngeal nerve damage.

The use of intraoperative parathyroid hormone levels may help to identify patients at risk of hypoparathyroidism in an effort to ensure early administration of calcium and calcitriol. The perioperative calcium and phosphorus must be monitored to ensure stable values before discharge from the inpatient setting.[71,72] Early identification of hypoparathyroidism with subsequent initiation of calcitriol and calcium decreases the risk of symptomatic hypokalemia as well as shortens the duration of postoperative hospitalization.[73,74]

Papillary Thyroid Cancer

The ATA pediatric guidelines recommend that most children with PTC undergo total or near-total thyroidectomy due to the increased risk of bilateral and multifocal disease in children.[8] Compared to lobectomy, total or near total thyroidectomy is associated with a lower risk of recurrence in children over 4 decades of observation, 6% versus 30%, respectively.[75] In addition, performing a total thyroidectomy improves the clinical utility of measuring Tg levels to monitor for persistent and recurrent disease. More recent data suggest that lobectomy may be considered for pediatric patients with low-invasive PTC, including encapsulated follicular-variant PTC (enc-fvPTC),[76] and is clearly adequate for noninvasive, encapsulated lesions that are designated as noninvasive follicular thyroid neoplasm with papillary-like nuclear features.[77] On ultrasound, these noninvasive nodules are typically solid, not taller than wide, and have smooth margins without evidence of microcalcifications or lymphadenopathy.

Prophylactic central neck lymph node dissection (LND) should be considered in pediatric patients undergoing surgery for nodules with cytology suspicious for, or consistent with, PTC (Bethesda category V and VI) secondary to a high risk of central neck (level VI) metastasis. In contrast to adult patients where there is concern that pursuing a central neck LND may increase the likelihood of administering radioactive iodine (RAI) without any benefit in regard to improving disease-specific mortality, this approach is currently in favor in pediatrics secondary to the increased rate of central neck LN metastasis and in an effort to identify tumors with lower invasive behavior in an effort to reduce the use of postoperative RAI. The ATA pediatric risk levels reflect this approach with patients stratified into a "low risk" of persistent postoperative disease if only a "small number" of metastatic central lymph nodes are found on histologic exam.[8] More recently, a proposed update to the ATA pediatric risk levels recommended that "less than five" metastatic lymph nodes were associated with a low risk of persistent disease where the

immediate use of RAI may not provide any greater benefit to achieve remission.[78] Although there is concern for an increased risk of surgical complications associated with central neck dissection, the rate may be significantly reduced by referral to a high-volume thyroid surgeon.[38] A therapeutic central neck dissection should be performed in all children found to have central and/or lateral neck lymph node metastases. Lateral neck dissections should only be performed in the presence of FNA-proven metastatic lateral neck disease. When nodal dissection is performed, a complete dissection of the affected compartment should be performed, rather than "berry picking."

Follicular Thyroid Cancer

In contrast to PTC, FTC is typically unifocal and exhibits hematogenous rather than lymphatic metastasis. Pediatric FTC is an uncommon malignancy and represents 10% or less of pediatric DTC patients. FTC may develop as part of PHTS, thus, there should be a high index of suspicion in children with FTC, particularly in those with macrocephaly, lipomas, freckling of the glans penis, or a suggestive family history.[41,43,79]

FTC is typically subdivided into minimally invasive FTC (miFTC) and widely invasive FTC (wiFTC) with miFTC defined as FTC with microscopic or no capsular invasion and/or limited vascular invasion (<4 vessels in or adjacent to the tumor capsule) and wiFTC defined as FTC with widespread capsular invasion, widespread vascular invasion, or extension into surrounding thyroid tissue. Invasion of four or more vessels is associated with more aggressive disease, an increased risk of distant metastases, and a poorer prognosis.[80–82]

Similar to adult patients, children ultimately diagnosed with FTC will have indeterminate FNA cytology. Thus, the majority will initially undergo diagnostic lobectomy with or without isthmusectomy with consideration of total thyroidectomy for patients with underlying thyroid disease, bilateral nodules, or a known diagnosis of a thyroid tumor predisposition syndrome, such as PHTS. Frozen section cannot be used to rule out FTC as the diagnosis is based on complete histological evaluation of the nodule capsule to determine if the nodule is a follicular adenoma (no evidence of invasion) or follicular carcinoma (evidence of capsular and vascular invasion).[83] For minimally invasive FTC < 4 cm, lobectomy with or without isthmusectomy is considered to be sufficient. For widely invasive FTC or tumors >4 cm, completion thyroidectomy should be performed along with postoperative RAI based on 123-I diagnostic whole body scan to asses for evidence of distant metastasis to the lung or bone.[84,85] Minimally invasive FTC has excellent prognosis, whereas widely invasive FTC is associated with significant morbidity and mortality in adults.[84,86,87] Due to limited data regarding pediatric FTC, further studies are needed to risk-stratify children who would benefit from extensive surgery and ^{131}I therapy.

RADIOIODINE TREATMENT

RAI is a highly effective, targeted medical therapy to treat persistent postsurgical disease. Over the 5 decades, there has been a near twofold increase in the number of patients receiving RAI without any impact on the same excellent ($\sim$98%) 20-year disease-specific survival.[88] Although there is a paucity of long-term prospective data to define the lifetime risk of radioactive iodine administered during childhood and adolescents, with increased awareness of the potential short- and long-term risks of ^{131}I therapy there are renewed efforts to identify the patients who may (ATA pediatric intermediate and high risk) or may not (ATA pediatric low risk) benefit from ^{131}I therapy.[8,89,90]

In contrast to adults with thyroid cancer, there is no staging system for children and adolescents with PTC secondary to the extremely low disease-specific mortality.[91] However, the American Joint Committee on Cancer (AJCC) Tumor, Nodes, Metastases (TNM) classification system[92] is used to describe the extent of disease and stratify the patients who may or may not benefit from RAI as well as provide guidance on postoperative surveillance. The following is an updated version of the ATA pediatric risk levels with proposed adjustments:[8,78]

1. **ATA Pediatric Low Risk:** Disease grossly confined to the thyroid with N0 (no lymph node metastasis) or less than or equal to five metastatic lymph nodes from the central neck (N1a). These patients appear to be at lowest risk for distant metastasis but may still be at risk for residual cervical disease, especially if the initial surgery did not include a central neck LND (Nx).
2. **ATA Pediatric Intermediate Risk:** Presence of ETE (microscopic or gross), unilateral, lateral neck LN metastasis (N1b) or 6–10 metastatic LNs (extensive N1a). These patients are at an increased risk for incomplete lymph node resection and persistent cervical disease as well as distant metastasis, most commonly to the lungs. The addition of ETE to the intermediate risk level is important if a central neck LN dissection was not performed as ETE has been shown to be associated with an increased risk for LN metastasis. One should also be aware that microETE was removed as criteria for T3 tumors in the 8th

edition of the AJCC TNM classification system and that the synoptic pathology report must be reviewed to identify if microETE was present to accurately interpret the risk of postoperative persistent disease.[92]
3. **ATA Pediatric High Risk:** Regionally extensive diseases, including bilateral N1b, >10 metastatic LN, locally invasive disease (T4 tumors), and patients with distant metastasis, are considered high risk for persistent postoperative disease.

Postoperative evaluation for evidence of persistent disease is typically performed within 6–12 weeks of surgery to identify the patients who may or may not benefit from further therapy, to include additional surgery or ^{131}I therapy. For ATA low-risk patients, one may consider following the TSH-suppressed Tg level with repeat neck US instead of pursuing a stimulated Tg level with diagnostic whole-body scan (DxWBS) in the immediate postoperative time frame. The stimulated Tg and DxWBS can be performed at a later time if there is an elevated Tg and no evidence of disease based on US and/or anatomic imaging (CT or MRI).[8,89,90]

For intermediate- and high-risk patients, a TSH-stimulated Tg and a ^{123}I-DxWBS are recommended to search for residual or metastatic disease.[8] The use of ^{123}I is favored over ^{131}I due to superior imaging quality, decreased radiation exposure, and prevention of stunning.[93] Two to three weeks before, the DxWBS liothyronine (LT3) or levothyroxine (LT4) is with a goal of achieving a TSH greater than 30 U/mL. In addition, the patient is also placed on a low-iodine diet (http://www.thyca.org/pap-fol/lowiodinediet/ and http://lidlifecommunity.org/). This approach optimizes the sensitivity of the WBS as well as the efficacy of the potential RAI therapy via TSH-associated increase in the expression of the sodium-iodine symporter with concurrent and temporary iodine deficiency. Recombinant-human TSH (rhTSH) rather than thyroid-hormone withdrawal has also been studied in children using the typical adult dose (0.9 mg given 24 h apart); however, there are no pediatric data on the efficacy of rhTSH in regard to treatment outcomes.[94,95] rhTSH is a good option for patients who cannot tolerate endogenous hypothyroidism or have a pituitary TSH deficiency. Children who received iodinated contrast agents should wait 2–3 months before administration of RAI, and iodine deficiency should be confirmed by measurement of a 24-h urine iodine level.[96]

The decision to administer ^{131}I therapy should be based on the TSH-stimulated Tg level as well as the data obtained from the ^{123}I-DxWBS. A TSH-stimulated Tg < 2 ng/mL has a 94.9% predictive value for the absence of postsurgical disease.[97] If TSH-stimulated Tg is 2–10 ng/mL, ^{131}I therapy should be considered for patients with thyroid bed uptake, invasive histology (dsvPTC, sPTC, and widely invasive follicular variant PTC), evidence of gross extrathyroidal extension or extranodal extension, or in patients with extensive regional metastasis (extensive N1a or any N1b disease). If the TSH-stimulated Tg is > 10 ng/mL, ^{131}I therapy is indicated. Repeat surgery before administration of ^{131}I should be pursued if there is evidence of "bulky," macroscopic, persistent disease noted during this initial postoperative time frame. The addition of single-photon emission computed tomography with integrated conventional CT (SPECT/CT) may provide more accurate anatomic localization to differentiate metastatic regional lymph node from remnant thyroid tissue.[98]

Therapeutic ^{131}I can be dosed empirically or based on bone marrow dose limited dosimetry. There are two formulas to decide on empiric dosing: (1) given as a fraction of a child's weight compared to an average sized adult (kg divided by 70 kg) multiplied by a typical adult dose used to treat similar disease extent[99,100] or (2) based on mCi/weight with a typical range between 1.0 and 3.0 mCi/kg based on the presence of regional or distant disease.[101] Dosimetry should be considered in younger children (<10 years), those with diffuse pulmonary metastases, and those who received radiation therapy for other malignancies.[102] A posttreatment WBS (RxWBS) should be obtained 5–7 days after all ^{131}I treatments and is associated with a greater sensitivity for detecting persistent disease when compared to the DxWBS.[103] The addition of SPECT/CT may help to localize residual cervical disease.[8,104]

The most common short-term side effect of radioiodine therapy is salivary gland dysfunction (sialadenitis, xerostomia, dental caries, and stomatitis) followed by ocular dryness, and nasolacrimal duct obstruction. Postpubertal males should be counseled about sperm banking if they have significant pulmonary or other distant site metastasis, where higher cumulative activities (≥400 mCi) may be administered.[8,105] Acute, transient bone marrow suppression may develop with normalization of all hematologic levels within 3 months' of RAI therapy.[106] Pulmonary fibrosis may develop in children and adolescents with pulmonary metastasis that receive frequent, high-activity RAI treatments.[107,108] Pulmonary function testing and noncontrast chest CT should be used to monitor children with diffuse pulmonary metastasis, especially if multiple ^{131}I therapy is considered.[8]

Even with efforts to limit the delivered activity and frequency of RAI, long-term follow-up studies are needed to confirm or refute previous reports on the risk of developing RAI-induced, second primary malignancies (SPM).[75,88,109,110] Although the overall numbers are small, many of the SPMs are in iodine-avid glands (i.e., salivary glands) or in nonavid tissues passively exposed to ^{131}I during physiologic clearance (bone marrow, colon, bladder, and others).[75,111] Thus, the challenge is to determine if the SPM is RAI related or associated with risk factors that led to development of the thyroid malignancy. Clinicians should not fear the use of RAI; however, there is an obligation to identify the patients who may benefit from ^{131}I therapy and the patients whose risks of RAI outweigh the benefit. In pediatrics, the goals of achieving remission and avoiding recurrence must be balanced with the risk of complications of therapy.

Follow-Up of PTC in Children

Serial serum thyroglobulin (Tg) levels and neck US are the most useful tests for monitoring patients with PTC. Tg and TgAb levels should be simultaneously measured on all samples as up to 25% of patients with DTC have detectable TgAb that can interfere with the Tg result.[112] Due to significant variability between assays, it is critical to use the same assay and laboratory for serial surveillance laboratory monitoring to reduce interassay variance and improve assessment of the Tg and/or TgAb trend.[113]

In the absence of TgAb, a basal (non-TSH stimulated) Tg level below 0.2 ng/mL is consistent with remission from disease.[114] For patients that did not receive postsurgical ^{131}I therapy, the TSH-suppressed Tg should decrease to <0.5 ng/mL within 1 year after total thyroidectomy.[114] If the Tg remains mildly elevated, between 2 and 10 ng/mL, continued monitoring may be pursued depending on the trend in Tg over time as well as evidence of persistent or recurrent disease on radiological imaging. Increasing or frankly elevated levels of Tg (>10 ng/mL) warrant further evaluation to localize disease and to decide whether additional surgery and/or ^{131}I therapy would be beneficial.[8]

The first neck US should be performed approximately 6 months after the initial surgery and then at 6–12-month intervals for ATA pediatric intermediate- and high-risk patients and at annual intervals for ATA pediatric low-risk patients. Serial chest CT at 6–12-month intervals should be used to monitor patients with known pulmonary metastasis. The use of 18F-FDG PET/CT should be limited to patients suspected to have persistent anatomic disease that is non-RAI avid based on RAI treatment and WBS imaging.[115]

No evidence of disease (NED) is defined as the absence of structural abnormalities on radiological imaging and undetectable Tg and TgAb levels. Persistent disease is defined by TSH-suppressed > 1 ng/mL or any evidence of anatomic disease on neck US, cross-sectional (CT or MRI) or functional imaging (RAI whole body scan or 18F-FDG PET/CT). Recurrent disease is characterized by the detection of new biochemical or anatomic abnormalities in patients who were previously considered to have NED.[90]

All pediatric patients with DTC should receive thyroid hormone suppressive therapy following surgery with or without ^{131}I therapy targeted to achieve a TSH of <0.5 U/L. The degree of TSH suppression should be based on the ATA pediatric risk levels[116] adjusted to avoid signs and symptoms of hyperthyroidism. Life-long surveillance is indicated in all pediatric patients because recurrence has been reported in approximately 30% of children with DTC as long as 20–40 years after initial surgery.[117]

Persistent and Recurrent Disease

Cervical lymph nodes are the most common location for residual and recurrent PTC.[117–119] If macroscopic cervical disease is identified by imaging and confirmed via FNA, surgery is preferable to ^{131}I therapy pursuing a compartmental approach.[120,121] For preoperative procedures, percutaneous, US-guided methylene blue injection of pathologic LN may increase the efficiency and accuracy of the dissection. Children with iodine-avid small volume cervical disease can be considered for therapeutic ^{131}I therapy depending on the individual risk-to-benefit ratio as well as the absence or presence of distant metastasis.[122] If the LN are located in a surgically naïve location of the neck initial, compartment-based LN dissection should be considered.

US-guided percutaneous ethanol or radiofrequency ablation may be considered as nonsurgical treatment options in patients with a limited number of neck metastasis (one to two lymph nodes) from PTC depending on the location.[122–124] The therapeutic success rates of ethanol injection and RFA have been reported to be between 70% and 98% with assessment of success determined by assessing blood flow and post-treatment size of the treated lymph node 3–6 months after the procedure.[122,123,125]

Metastasis to the lungs is the most common site for persistent or recurrent disease distal metastasis. In contrast to adults, children and adolescents with pulmonary metastasis have low disease-specific mortality most likely secondary to the pulmonary lesions maintaining RAI avidity.[108,126] Pediatric patients with a small burden of micronodular pulmonary disease are likely to achieve remission;[108,118,126] however, up to one-third of children with more significant pulmonary disease may develop stable, persistent disease that will not resolve even with repeated doses of [131]I.[108] Retreatment of ^{131}I iodine-avid pulmonary metastases should be considered in children who have demonstrated previous improvement but continue to have persistent disease based on cross-sectional imaging obtained over 1–2 years after the last RAI treatment, sooner if there is evidence of disease progression on serial imaging obtained on a 6-month interval. The timing of additional ^{131}I should be at least 12 or more months from the previous treatment with several studies demonstrating a continuous decline in serum Tg levels for 18–24 months, or longer, following the previous RAI therapy.[126,127]

Systemic Therapy for RAI-Refractory Disease

A small proportion of children and adolescents will develop progressive DTC that is refractory to [131]-I treatment. Over the last decade, an increasing number of oral systemic therapies have been incorporated into clinical practice for adults with similar disease. These agents target tyrosine-kinase receptors or constitutively activated protein kinases in the mitogen-activated protein kinase (MAPK) and phosphatidylinositol 3-kinase signaling pathways.[128] Knowledge of the somatic oncogene driver mutation in the refractory tumor is critical in selecting the drug most likely to have the greatest clinical effect. The multitargeted tyrosine kinase inhibitors, including sorafenib, lenvatinib, and others, target the vascular endothelial growth factor receptors as well as a combination of the epithelial growth factor receptors, fibroblast growth factor receptors, platelet-derived growth factor receptor, and RET. These agents are not tumoricidal but they have been shown to slow progression and to decrease tumor burden for many patients. Unfortunately, the effect is often transient and many patients experience side effects, including hypertension, diarrhea, and anorexia with weight loss, dermatitis, and fatigue.[129]

The newer selective inhibitors have increased efficacy and less toxicity compared to the multityrosine inhibitors. Several of these agents have been in clinical use for several years, repurposed from other cancers with similar molecular alterations. The most effective of these molecular targeted inhibitors have shown remarkable clinical efficacy with regression in tumors harboring *BRAF, RET, NTRK, ALK,* or *ROS1* fusion genes.[129] Larotrectinib (LOXO-101) is a selective *NTRK* inhibitor that has been approved for use down to 12 years old. Resensitization of tumors to RAI has been achieved for patients with tumors harboring either *BRAF* or *RAS* mutations after administration of selective *BRAF* as well as *MEK* inhibitors.[130] For patients with progressive MTC, there are selective *RET*-inhibitors (BLU-667 and LOXO-292) that are currently in clinical trials with very favorable response to therapy from preliminary data.[129]

Although these agents are providing clinical benefit, the majority are cytostatic, not cytotoxic. Tumors eventually develop resistance and there is limited knowledge on the best choice for a follow-on drug for salvage therapy if or when a tumor becomes refractory to the initial agent. With the potential for significant side effects, pediatric patients should be referred to centers that have experience with these drugs in the treatment of RAI-refractory (RAIR) thyroid cancer so that the timing for initiation, selection of drug, and monitoring and adjustment of therapy can be optimized while minimizing the risk of side effects.[8,129,131]

MEDULLARY THYROID CANCER

MTC is a neuroendocrine malignancy that originates from the neural crest, parafollicular C-cells of the thyroid gland.[132] Thus, in contrast to follicular-cell-derived thyroid tumors, MTC cells are not responsive to TSH, do not express the sodium-iodine symporter, and do not produce Tg, rather they secrete calcitonin and carcinoembryonic antigen (CEA), both of which serve as tumor markers of MTC. With rare exception, MTC in children and adolescents is associated with multiple endocrine neoplasia type 2, an autosomal dominant tumor predisposition syndrome associated with germline mutations in the *RET*-protooncogene, designated as either MEN 2A or 2B depending on the specific mutation.[133,134] Sporadic MTC is uncommon in the pediatric population and, similar to adults, is associated with somatic mutations of *RET* and *RAS*.[132]

The ATA divides the most common *RET* mutations into three risk categories, highest risk, high risk, and moderate risk, and bases the recommended age for initial screening, as well as the timing of prophylactic thyroidectomy, to coincide with the goal of achieving surgical remission from disease.[132] Total thyroidectomy is recommended as follows: within the first year of life for carriers of the highest risk mutation (MEN 2B, codon 918), at or before age 5 years for those with a high-risk mutation (MEN 2A, codons 634 and 883),

and for all other moderate-risk mutations when the serum calcitonin level shows an increasing upward trend or at any time if the parents or patient do not wish to continue to embark on a long period of laboratory and radiological surveillance.[132] For patients with moderate risk mutations, the course from c-cell hyperplasia to MTC may be quite indolent with MTC not developing until the 3rd, 4th, or later decades of life. A central lymph node dissection is recommended in children whose basal calcitonin is >40 ng/L or with any evidence of lymph node metastasis.[132,135] One should be aware that in children there is a normal physiologic elevation in calcitonin with values as high as 35 ng/L before 6 months old and decreasing to the adult range by approximately three years old.[136]

In contrast to MEN 2A, mutations in codon 918 (MEN 2B) are more often de novo. Thus, recognition of the early clinical signs and symptoms is critically important to diagnose the syndrome before MTC metastasis, which may occur before 1 year old or, more commonly, before 4 years old.[137] The earliest clinical signs and symptoms include alacrima (the inability or decreased ability, to make tears), constipation (associated with ganglioneuromatosis), and hypotonia (feeding difficulties with failure to thrive, club feet, hip dislocation). The more classically defining symptoms, including oral and lip mucosal neuromas and elongated, marfanoid facies, are not clinically evident until school age, around 5 years old.[46,138]

After thyroidectomy, levothyroxine is prescribed to normalize, not suppress, the TSH. Calcitonin and CEA levels should be monitored as tumor markers every 6–12 months, with decreasing frequency once remission is confirmed. Serial neck US on a similar schedule is used for surveillance of patients that had initial lymph node metastasis or that have persistently detectable calcitonin levels. If the tumor markers remain significantly elevated, or show rapid doubling time, and the neck US is not informative, additional imaging such as chest CT, contrast-enhanced liver MRI/CT, bone scan, MRI of the axial skeleton, or 18F-FDG PET/CT should be considered in an effort to identify persistent disease.

Metastatic MTC is generally incurable, but may show an indolent clinical course with stable disease over decades. A more aggressive progression and poorer prognosis can be predicted by the inability of the MTC cells to produce calcitonin, a rapidly rising CEA out of proportion to calcitonin, and a calcitonin doubling time of less than 6 months.[132,139]

For MTC patients with symptomatic or progressive metastatic disease, the treatment of molecular targeted therapies that inhibit *RET* and other receptor tyrosine kinases involved in angiogenesis is indicated. Vandetanib and cabozantinib have been FDA approved for the treatment of adults with progressive, metastatic MTC.[128,140] Limited data suggest that vandetanib is effective and well tolerated in children with advanced MTC in the setting of MEN2B.[141] The selective *RET*-inhibitors (BLU-667 and LOXO-292) are currently in clinical trials with very favorable response to therapy from preliminary data.[129] Similar to pediatric patients with RAIR, pediatric patients with advanced MTC where systemic therapy may be beneficial should be referred to centers that have experience with these drugs so that the timing for initiation, selection of drug, and monitoring and adjustment of therapy can be optimized while minimizing the risk of side effects.

Patients with hereditary MTC should receive continued and life-long follow-up including genetic counseling, psychosocial support, and prospective screening for pheochromocytoma and primary hyperparathyroidism. Annual screening for pheochromocytoma with a urine or serum fractionated metanephrine panel is initiated at 11 years old for ATA highest risk patients (918) and at 16 years for ATA high and moderate risk patients with concurrent annual screening for hyperparathyroidism for MEN 2A patients.

REFERENCES

1. Al-Qurayshi Z, et al. A national perspective of the risk, presentation, and outcomes of pediatric thyroid cancer. *JAMA Otolaryngol Head Neck Surg.* 2016;142(5): 472–478.
2. Holmes Jr L, Hossain J, Opara F. Pediatric thyroid carcinoma incidence and temporal trends in the USA (1973–2007): race or shifting diagnostic paradigm? *ISRN Oncol.* 2012;2012:906197.
3. Siegel DA, et al. Cancer incidence rates and trends among children and adolescents in the United States, 2001–2009. *Pediatrics.* 2014;134(4):e945–e955.
4. Vergamini LB, et al. Increase in the incidence of differentiated thyroid carcinoma in children, adolescents, and young adults: a population-based study. *J Pediatr.* 2014.
5. Carty SE, et al. Consensus statement on the terminology and classification of central neck dissection for thyroid cancer. *Thyroid.* 2009;19(11):1153–1158.
6. Gupta A, et al. A standardized assessment of thyroid nodules in children confirms higher cancer prevalence than in adults. *J Clin Endocrinol Metab.* 2013;98(8): 3238–3245.
7. Niedziela M. Pathogenesis, diagnosis and management of thyroid nodules in children. *Endocr Relat Cancer.* 2006;13(2):427–453.
8. Francis GL, et al. Management guidelines for children with thyroid nodules and differentiated thyroid cancer. *Thyroid.* 2015;25(7):716–759.
9. Martinez-Rios C, et al. Utility of adult-based ultrasound malignancy risk stratifications in pediatric thyroid nodules. *Pediatr Radiol.* 2018;48(1):74–84.
10. Duffy Jr BJ, Fitzgerald PJ. Thyroid cancer in childhood and adolescence; a report on 28 cases. *Cancer.* 1950; 3(6):1018–1032.
11. Winship T. Carcinoma of the thyroid in childhood. *Pediatrics.* 1956;18(3):459–466.
12. Ron E, et al. Thyroid cancer after exposure to external radiation: a pooled analysis of seven studies. *Radiat Res.* 1995;141(3):259–277.
13. Schonfeld SJ, Lee C, Berrington de Gonzalez A. Medical exposure to radiation and thyroid cancer. *Clin Oncol.* 2011;23(4):244–250.
14. Saad AG, et al. Proliferative activity of human thyroid cells in various age groups and its correlation with the risk of thyroid cancer after radiation exposure. *J Clin Endocrinol Metab.* 2006;91(7):2672–2677.
15. Meadows AT, et al. Second neoplasms in survivors of childhood cancer: findings from the childhood cancer survivor study cohort. *J Clin Oncol.* 2009;27(14): 2356–2362.
16. Ronckers CM, et al. Thyroid cancer in childhood cancer survivors: a detailed evaluation of radiation dose response and its modifiers. *Radiat Res.* 2006;166(4): 618–628.
17. Clement SC, et al. Intermediate and long-term adverse effects of radioiodine therapy for differentiated thyroid carcinoma–a systematic review. *Cancer Treat Rev.* 2015; 41(10):925–934.
18. Sinnott B, Ron E, Schneider AB. Exposing the thyroid to radiation: a review of its current extent, risks, and implications. *Endocr Rev.* 2010;31(5):756–773.
19. Ron E. Thyroid cancer incidence among people living in areas contaminated by radiation from the Chernobyl accident. *Health Phys.* 2007;93(5):502–511.
20. Bogdanova TI, et al. Comparative histopathological analysis of sporadic pediatric papillary thyroid carcinoma from Japan and Ukraine. *Endocr J.* 2017;64(10): 977–993.
21. Tuttle RM, Vaisman F, Tronko MD. Clinical presentation and clinical outcomes in Chernobyl-related paediatric thyroid cancers: what do we know now? What can we expect in the future? *Clin Oncol.* 2011;23(4):268–275.
22. Tronko MD, et al. Thyroid carcinoma in children and adolescents in Ukraine after the Chernobyl nuclear accident: statistical data and clinicomorphologic characteristics. *Cancer.* 1999;86(1):149–156.
23. Charkes ND. On the prevalence of familial nonmedullary thyroid cancer in multiply affected kindreds. *Thyroid.* 2006;16(2):181–186.
24. Mazeh H, et al. In patients with thyroid cancer of follicular cell origin, a family history of nonmedullary thyroid cancer in one first-degree relative is associated with more aggressive disease. *Thyroid.* 2012;22(1):3–8.
25. Bauer AJ. Clinical behavior and genetics of nonsyndromic, familial nonmedullary thyroid cancer. *Front Horm Res.* 2013;41:141–148.

26. Bauer AJ. Thyroid nodules and differentiated thyroid cancer. *Endocr Dev.* 2014;26:183–201.

27. Capezzone M, et al. Familial non-medullary thyroid carcinoma displays the features of clinical anticipation suggestive of a distinct biological entity. *Endocr Relat Cancer.* 2008;15(4):1075–1081.

28. Jasperson KW, Patel SG, Ahnen DJ. APC-associated polyposis conditions. *GeneReviews® [Internet];* December 18, 1998 [Updated 2017 Feb 2]; Available from: https://www.ncbi.nlm.nih.gov/books/NBK1345/.

29. Khan NE, et al. Quantification of thyroid cancer and Multinodular goiter risk in the DICER1 syndrome: a family-based cohort study. *J Clin Endocrinol Metab.* 2017; 102(5):1614–1622.

30. Eng C. PTEN hamartoma tumor syndrome. *GeneReviews®;* 2001 [Updated 2016 Jun 2]; Available from: https://www. ncbi.nlm.nih.gov/books/NBK1488/ [Internet].

31. Schultz KAP, et al. DICER1 and associated conditions: identification of at-risk individuals and recommended surveillance strategies. *Clin Cancer Res.* 2018;24(10):2251–2261.

32. Ren PY, et al. Pediatric differentiated thyroid carcinoma: the clinicopathological features and the coexistence of Hashimoto's thyroiditis. *Asian J Surg.* 2019;42(1): 112–119.

33. Kovatch KJ, et al. Pediatric thyroid carcinoma in patients with graves' disease: the role of ultrasound in selecting patients for definitive therapy. *Horm Res Paediatr.* 2015.

34. MacFarland SP, et al. Disease burden and outcome in children and young adults with concurrent graves disease and differentiated thyroid carcinoma. *J Clin Endocrinol Metab.* 2018;103(8):2918–2925.

35. Clement SC, et al. Balancing the benefits and harms of thyroid cancer surveillance in survivors of childhood, adolescent and young adult cancer: recommendations from the International Late Effects of Childhood Cancer Guideline Harmonization Group in collaboration with the PanCareSurFup Consortium. *Cancer Treat Rev.* 2018; 63:28–39.

36. Bauer AJ, Davies L. Why the data from the Fukushima health management survey after the daiichi nuclear power station accident are important. *JAMA Otolaryngol Head Neck Surg.* 2018.

37. Togawa K, et al. Long-term strategies for thyroid health monitoring after nuclear accidents: recommendations from an expert group convened by IARC. *Lancet Oncol.* 2018;19(10):1280–1283.

38. Adam MA, et al. Is there a minimum number of thyroidectomies a surgeon should perform to optimize patient outcomes? *Ann Surg.* 2017;265(2):402–407.

39. Buryk MA, et al. Can malignant thyroid nodules be distinguished from benign thyroid nodules in children and adolescents by clinical characteristics? A review of 89 pediatric patients with thyroid nodules. *Thyroid.* 2015;25(4):392–400.

40. Papendieck P, et al. Differentiated thyroid cancer in children: prevalence and predictors in a large cohort with thyroid nodules followed prospectively. *J Pediatr.* 2015; 167(1):199–201.

41. Pilarski R, et al. Cowden syndrome and the PTEN hamartoma tumor syndrome: systematic review and revised diagnostic criteria. *J Natl Cancer Inst.* 2013;105(21): 1607–1616.

42. Lauper JM, et al. Spectrum and risk of neoplasia in Werner syndrome: a systematic review. *PLoS One.* 2013; 8(4):e59709.

43. Bubien V, et al. High cumulative risks of cancer in patients with PTEN hamartoma tumour syndrome. *J Med Genet.* 2013;50(4):255–263.

44. Bertherat J, et al. Mutations in regulatory subunit type 1A of cyclic adenosine 5′-monophosphate-dependent protein kinase (PRKAR1A): phenotype analysis in 353 patients and 80 different genotypes. *J Clin Endocrinol Metab.* 2009;94(6):2085–2091.

45. Septer S, et al. Thyroid cancer complicating familial adenomatous polyposis: mutation spectrum of at-risk individuals. *Hered Cancer Clin Pract.* 2013;11(1):13.

46. Wray CJ, et al. Failure to recognize multiple endocrine neoplasia 2B: more common than we think? *Ann Surg Oncol.* 2008;15(1):293–301.

47. Ly S, et al. Features and outcome of autonomous thyroid nodules in children: 31 consecutive patients seen at a single center. *J Clin Endocrinol Metab.* 2016;101(10): 3856–3862.

48. Zimmermann MB, et al. Thyroglobulin is a sensitive measure of both deficient and excess iodine intakes in children and indicates no adverse effects on thyroid function in the UIC range of 100–299 mug/L: a UNICEF/ICCIDD study group report. *J Clin Endocrinol Metab.* 2013;98(3):1271–1280.

49. Trimboli P, Treglia G, Giovanella L. Preoperative measurement of serum thyroglobulin to predict malignancy in thyroid nodules: a systematic review. *Horm Metab Res.* 2015;47(4):247–252.

50. Oltmann SC, et al. Markedly elevated thyroglobulin levels in the preoperative thyroidectomy patient correlates with metastatic burden. *J Surg Res.* 2014;187(1): 1–5.

51. Haugen BR, et al. 2015 American thyroid association management guidelines for adult patients with thyroid nodules and differentiated thyroid cancer: The American thyroid association guidelines task force on thyroid nodules and differentiated thyroid cancer. *Thyroid.* 2016; 26(1):1–133.

52. Verga U, et al. Normal range of calcitonin in children measured by a chemiluminescent two-site immunometric assay. *Horm Res.* 2006;66(1):17–20.

53. Gannon AW, et al. Diagnostic accuracy of ultrasound with color flow Doppler in children with thyroid nodules. *J Clin Endocrinol Metab.* 2018.

54. Lee CY, et al. Predictive factors for extrathyroidal extension of papillary thyroid carcinoma based on preoperative sonography. *J Ultrasound Med.* 2014;33(2):231–238.

55. Leboulleux S, et al. Ultrasound criteria of malignancy for cervical lymph nodes in patients followed up for differentiated thyroid cancer. *J Clin Endocrinol Metab.* 2007;92(9): 3590–3594.

56. Akaishi J, et al. Clinicopathologic features and outcomes in patients with diffuse sclerosing variant of papillary thyroid carcinoma. *World J Surg.* 2015;39(7):1728–1735.

57. Koo JS, Hong S, Park CS. Diffuse sclerosing variant is a major subtype of papillary thyroid carcinoma in the young. *Thyroid.* 2009;19(11):1225–1231.

58. Lee JY, et al. Diffuse sclerosing variant of papillary carcinoma of the thyroid: imaging and cytologic findings. *Thyroid.* 2007;17(6):567–573.

59. Moon JH, et al. Thyroglobulin in washout fluid from lymph node fine-needle aspiration biopsy in papillary thyroid cancer: large-scale validation of the cutoff value to determine malignancy and evaluation of discrepant results. *J Clin Endocrinol Metab.* 2013;98(3):1061–1068.

60. Giovanella L, Bongiovanni M, Trimboli P. Diagnostic value of thyroglobulin assay in cervical lymph node fine-needle aspirations for metastatic differentiated thyroid cancer. *Curr Opin Oncol.* 2013;25(1):6–13.

61. Choi JS, et al. Preoperative staging of papillary thyroid carcinoma: comparison of ultrasound imaging and CT. *AJR Am J Roentgenol.* 2009;193(3):871–878.

62. Barrio M, et al. The incidence of thyroid cancer in focal hypermetabolic thyroid lesions: an 18F-FDG PET/CT study in more than 6000 patients. *Nucl Med Commun.* 2016;37(12):1290–1296.

63. Mussa A, et al. Predictors of malignancy in children with thyroid nodules. *J Pediatr.* 2015;167(4):886–892 e1.

64. Buryk MA, et al. Identification of unique, heterozygous germline mutation, STK11 (p.F354L), in a child with an encapsulated follicular variant of papillary thyroid carcinoma within six months of completing treatment for Neuroblastoma. *Pediatr Dev Pathol.* 2015;18(4):318–323.

65. Monaco SE, et al. Cytomorphological and molecular genetic findings in pediatric thyroid fine-needle aspiration. *Cancer Cytopathol.* 2012;120(5):342–350.

66. Baloch ZW, LiVolsi VA. Post fine-needle aspiration histologic alterations of thyroid revisited. *Am J Clin Pathol.* 1999;112(3):311–316.

67. Lale SA, et al. Fine needle aspiration of thyroid nodules in the pediatric population: a 12-year cyto-histological correlation experience at North Shore-Long Island Jewish Health System. *Diagn Cytopathol.* 2015;43(8):598–604.

68. Buryk MA, et al. Preoperative cytology with molecular analysis to help guide surgery for pediatric thyroid nodules. *Int J Pediatr Otorhinolaryngol.* 2013;77(10):1697–1700.

69. Bauer AJ. Molecular genetics of thyroid cancer in children and adolescents. *Endocrinol Metab Clin N Am.* 2017;46(2):389–403.

70. Sosa JA, et al. Clinical and economic outcomes of thyroid and parathyroid surgery in children. *J Clin Endocrinol Metab.* 2008;93(8):3058–3065.

71. Grodski S, Serpell J. Evidence for the role of perioperative PTH measurement after total thyroidectomy as a predictor of hypocalcemia. *World J Surg.* 2008;32(7):1367–1373.

72. Sam AH, et al. Serum phosphate predicts temporary hypocalcaemia following thyroidectomy. *Clin Endocrinol.* 2011;74(3):388–393.

73. Freire AV, et al. Predicting hypocalcemia after thyroidectomy in children. *Surgery.* 2014;156(1):130–136.

74. Patel NA, et al. A clinical pathway for the postoperative management of hypocalcemia after pediatric thyroidectomy reduces blood draws. *Int J Pediatr Otorhinolaryngol.* 2018;105:132–137.

75. Hay ID, et al. Long-term outcome in 215 children and adolescents with papillary thyroid cancer treated during 1940 through 2008. *World J Surg.* 2010;34(6):1192–1202.

76. Samuels SL, et al. Characteristics of follicular variant papillary thyroid carcinoma in a pediatric cohort. *J Clin Endocrinol Metab.* 2018.

77. Scharpf J, et al. The follicular variant of papillary thyroid cancer and noninvasive follicular thyroid neoplasm with papillary-like nuclear features (NIFTP). *Curr Opin Oncol.* 2017;29(1):20–24.

78. Jeon MJ, et al. Practical initial risk stratification based on lymph node metastases in pediatric and adolescent differentiated thyroid cancer. *Thyroid.* 2018;28(2):193–200.

79. Smith JR, et al. Thyroid nodules and cancer in children with PTEN hamartoma tumor syndrome. *J Clin Endocrinol Metab.* 2011;96(1):34–37.

80. Ito Y, et al. Prognostic factors of minimally invasive follicular thyroid carcinoma: extensive vascular invasion significantly affects patient prognosis. *Endocr J.* 2013;60(5):637–642.

81. Kim HJ, et al. Vascular invasion is associated with increased mortality in patients with minimally invasive follicular thyroid carcinoma but not widely invasive follicular thyroid carcinoma. *Head Neck.* 2013.

82. O'Neill CJ, et al. Management of follicular thyroid carcinoma should be individualised based on degree of capsular and vascular invasion. *Eur J Surg Oncol.* 2011;37(2):181–185.

83. LiVolsi VA, Baloch ZW. Use and abuse of frozen section in the diagnosis of follicular thyroid lesions. *Endocr Pathol.* 2005;16(4):285–293.

84. Sugino K, et al. Prognosis and prognostic factors for distant metastases and tumor mortality in follicular thyroid carcinoma. *Thyroid.* 2011;21(7):751–757.

85. Lin JD, et al. Operative strategy for follicular thyroid cancer in risk groups stratified by pTNM staging. *Surg Oncol.* 2007;16(2):107–113.

86. DeLellis RA. Pathology and genetics of thyroid carcinoma. *J Surg Oncol.* 2006;94(8):662–669.

87. Dionigi G, et al. Minimally invasive follicular thyroid cancer (MIFTC)–a consensus report of the European Society of Endocrine Surgeons (ESES). *Langenbeck's Arch Surg.* 2014;399(2):165–184.

88. Marti JL, Jain KS, Morris LG. Increased risk of second primary malignancy in pediatric and young adult patients treated with radioactive iodine for differentiated thyroid cancer. *Thyroid.* 2015;25(6):681–687.

89. Lazar L, et al. Pediatric thyroid cancer: postoperative classifications and response to initial therapy as prognostic factors. *J Clin Endocrinol Metab.* 2016;101(5):1970–1979.

90. Pires B, et al. Prognostic factors for early and long-term remission in pediatric differentiated thyroid cancer: the role of gender, age, clinical presentation and the newly proposed American Thyroid Association risk stratification system. *Thyroid*. 2016.

91. Golpanian S, et al. Pediatric papillary thyroid carcinoma: outcomes and survival predictors in 2504 surgical patients. *Pediatr Surg Int*. 2016;32(3):201–208.

92. Tuttle RMM, Haugen BRM, Perrier N. The updated AJCC/TNM staging system for differentiated and anaplastic thyroid cancer (8th edition): what changed and why? *Thyroid*. 2017.

93. Schoelwer MJ, et al. The use of 123I in diagnostic radioactive iodine scans in children with differentiated thyroid carcinoma. *Thyroid*. 2015;25(8):935–941.

94. Luster M, et al. Recombinant thyrotropin use in children and adolescents with differentiated thyroid cancer: a multicenter retrospective study. *J Clin Endocrinol Metab*. 2009;94(10):3948–3953.

95. Handkiewicz-Junak D, et al. Recombinant human thyrotropin preparation for adjuvant radioiodine treatment in children and adolescents with differentiated thyroid cancer. *Eur J Endocrinol*. 2015;173(6):873–881.

96. Sohn SY, et al. The impact of iodinated contrast agent administered during preoperative computed tomography scan on body iodine pool in patients with differentiated thyroid cancer preparing for radioactive iodine treatment. *Thyroid*. 2014;24(5):872–877.

97. Lee JI, et al. Postoperative-stimulated serum thyroglobulin measured at the time of 131I ablation is useful for the prediction of disease status in patients with differentiated thyroid carcinoma. *Surgery*. 2013;153(6):828–835.

98. Xue YL, et al. Value of ^{131}I SPECT/CT for the evaluation of differentiated thyroid cancer: a systematic review of the literature. *Eur J Nucl Med Mol Imaging*. 2013;40(5):768–778.

99. Hung W, Sarlis NJ. Current controversies in the management of pediatric patients with well-differentiated nonmedullary thyroid cancer: a review. *Thyroid*. 2002;12(8):683–702.

100. Dinauer C, Francis GL. Thyroid cancer in children. *Endocrinol Metab Clin N Am*. 2007;36(3):779–806 (vii).

101. Jarzab B, Handkiewicz-Junak D, Wloch J. Juvenile differentiated thyroid carcinoma and the role of radioiodine in its treatment: a qualitative review. *Endocr Relat Cancer*. 2005;12(4):773–803.

102. Lassmann M, et al. The use of dosimetry in the treatment of differentiated thyroid cancer. *Q J Nucl Med Mol Imaging*. 2011;55(2):107–115.

103. Urhan M, et al. Iodine-123 as a diagnostic imaging agent in differentiated thyroid carcinoma: a comparison with iodine-131 post-treatment scanning and serum thyroglobulin measurement. *Eur J Nucl Med Mol Imaging*. 2007;34(7):1012–1017.

104. Kim HY, Gelfand MJ, Sharp SE. SPECT/CT imaging in children with papillary thyroid carcinoma. *Pediatr Radiol*. 2011;41(8):1008–1012.

105. Pacini F, et al. Testicular function in patients with differentiated thyroid carcinoma treated with radioiodine. *J Nucl Med*. 1994;35(9):1418–1422.

106. Verburg FA, et al. Dosimetry-guided high-activity (131)I therapy in patients with advanced differentiated thyroid carcinoma: initial experience. *Eur J Nucl Med Mol Imaging*. 2010;37(5):896–903.

107. Thompson GB, Hay ID. Current strategies for surgical management and adjuvant treatment of childhood papillary thyroid carcinoma. *World J Surg*. 2004;28(12):1187–1198.

108. Pawelczak M, et al. Outcomes of children and adolescents with well-differentiated thyroid carcinoma and pulmonary metastases following 131I treatment: a systematic review. *Thyroid*. 2010;20(10):1095–1101.

109. Brown AP, et al. The risk of second primary malignancies up to three decades after the treatment of differentiated thyroid cancer. *J Clin Endocrinol Metab*. 2008;93(2):504–515.

110. Lee YA, et al. Pediatric patients with multifocal papillary thyroid cancer have higher recurrence rates than adult patients: a retrospective analysis of a large pediatric thyroid cancer cohort over 33 years. *J Clin Endocrinol Metab*. 2015;100(4):1619–1629.

111. Klubo-Gwiezdzinska J, et al. Salivary gland malignancy and radioiodine therapy for thyroid cancer. *Thyroid*. 2010;20(6):647–651.

112. Verburg FA, et al. Implications of thyroglobulin antibody positivity in patients with differentiated thyroid cancer: a clinical position statement. *Thyroid*. 2013;23(10):1211–1225.

113. Spencer CA. Clinical utility of thyroglobulin antibody (TgAb) measurements for patients with differentiated thyroid cancers (DTC). *J Clin Endocrinol Metab*. 2011;96(12):3615–3627.

114. Spencer C, LoPresti J, Fatemi S. How sensitive (second-generation) thyroglobulin measurement is changing paradigms for monitoring patients with differentiated thyroid cancer, in the absence or presence of thyroglobulin autoantibodies. *Curr Opin Endocrinol Diabetes Obes*. 2014;21(5):394–404.

115. Bannas P, et al. Can (18)F-FDG-PET/CT be generally recommended in patients with differentiated thyroid carcinoma and elevated thyroglobulin levels but negative I-131 whole body scan? *Ann Nucl Med*. 2012;26(1):77–85.

116. Francis GL, et al. Management guidelines for children with thyroid nodules and differentiated thyroid cancer: The American thyroid association guidelines task force on pediatric thyroid cancer. *Thyroid*. 2015. in press.

117. Hay ID, et al. Papillary thyroid microcarcinoma: a study of 900 cases observed in a 60-year period. *Surgery*. 2008;144(6):980–987. discussion 987-8.

118. Chow SM, et al. Differentiated thyroid carcinoma in childhood and adolescence-clinical course and role of radioiodine. *Pediatr Blood Canc*. 2004;42(2):176–183.

119. Handkiewicz-Junak D, et al. Total thyroidectomy and adjuvant radioiodine treatment independently decrease locoregional recurrence risk in childhood and adolescent differentiated thyroid cancer. *J Nucl Med*. 2007;48(6):879–888.

120. Clayman GL, et al. Long-term outcome of comprehensive central compartment dissection in patients with recurrent/persistent papillary thyroid carcinoma. *Thyroid.* 2011;21(12):1309–1316.

121. Clayman GL, et al. Approach and safety of comprehensive central compartment dissection in patients with recurrent papillary thyroid carcinoma. *Head Neck.* 2009; 31(9):1152–1163.

122. Hay ID, et al. Long-term outcome of ultrasound-guided percutaneous ethanol ablation of selected "recurrent" neck nodal metastases in 25 patients with TNM stages III or IVA papillary thyroid carcinoma previously treated by surgery and 131I therapy. *Surgery.* 2013;154(6): 1448–1454. discussion 1454-5.

123. Shin JE, Baek JH, Lee JH. Radiofrequency and ethanol ablation for the treatment of recurrent thyroid cancers: current status and challenges. *Curr Opin Oncol.* 2013; 25(1):14–19.

124. Heilo A, et al. Efficacy of ultrasound-guided percutaneous ethanol injection treatment in patients with a limited number of metastatic cervical lymph nodes from papillary thyroid carcinoma. *J Clin Endocrinol Metab.* 2011; 96(9):2750–2755.

125. Kim SY, et al. Long-term outcomes of ethanol injection therapy for locally recurrent papillary thyroid cancer. *Eur Arch Oto-Rhino-Laryngol.* 2017;274(9):3497–3501.

126. Biko J, et al. Favourable course of disease after incomplete remission on (131)I therapy in children with pulmonary metastases of papillary thyroid carcinoma: 10 years follow-up. *Eur J Nucl Med Mol Imaging.* 2011;38(4): 651–655.

127. Padovani RP, et al. Even without additional therapy, serum thyroglobulin concentrations often decline for years after total thyroidectomy and radioactive remnant ablation in patients with differentiated thyroid cancer. *Thyroid.* 2012;22(8):778–783.

128. Covell LL, Ganti AK. Treatment of advanced thyroid cancer: role of molecularly targeted therapies. *Targeted Oncol.* 2015;10(3):311–324.

129. Rao SN, Cabanillas ME. Navigating systemic therapy in advanced thyroid carcinoma: from standard of care to personalized therapy and beyond. *J Endocr Soc.* 2018; 2(10):1109–1130.

130. Jaber T, et al. Targeted therapy in advanced thyroid cancer to resensitize tumors to radioactive iodine. *J Clin Endocrinol Metab.* 2018;103(10):3698–3705.

131. Tuttle RM, et al. Novel concepts for initiating multitargeted kinase inhibitors in radioactive iodine refractory differentiated thyroid cancer. *Best Pract Res Clin Endocrinol Metabol.* 2017;31(3):295–305.

132. Wells Jr SA, et al. Revised American Thyroid Association guidelines for the management of medullary thyroid carcinoma. *Thyroid.* 2015;25(6):567–610.

133. Waguespack SG, et al. Management of medullary thyroid carcinoma and MEN2 syndromes in childhood. *Nat Rev Endocrinol.* 2011;7(10):596–607.

134. Margraf RL, et al. Multiple endocrine neoplasia type 2 RET protooncogene database: repository of MEN2-associated RET sequence variation and reference for genotype/phenotype correlations. *Hum Mutat.* 2009;30(4): 548–556.

135. Machens A, et al. Prospects of remission in medullary thyroid carcinoma according to basal calcitonin level. *J Clin Endocrinol Metab.* 2005;90(4):2029–2034.

136. Castagna MG, et al. Reference range of serum calcitonin in pediatric population. *J Clin Endocrinol Metab.* 2015; 100(5):1780–1784.

137. Brauckhoff M, et al. Surgical curability of medullary thyroid cancer in multiple endocrine neoplasia 2B: a changing perspective. *Ann Surg.* 2014;259(4):800–806.

138. Brauckhoff M, et al. Premonitory symptoms preceding metastatic medullary thyroid cancer in MEN 2B: an exploratory analysis. *Surgery.* 2008;144(6):1044–1050. discussion 1050-3.

139. Laure Giraudet A, et al. Progression of medullary thyroid carcinoma: assessment with calcitonin and carcinoembryonic antigen doubling times. *Eur J Endocrinol.* 2008; 158(2):239–246.

140. Weitzman SP, Cabanillas ME. The treatment landscape in thyroid cancer: a focus on cabozantinib. *Cancer Manag Res.* 2015;7:265–278.

141. Fox E, et al. Vandetanib in children and adolescents with multiple endocrine neoplasia type 2B associated medullary thyroid carcinoma. *Clin Cancer Res.* 2013;19(15): 4239–4248.

CHAPTER 6

Brief Overview of Calcium, Vitamin D, Parathyroid Hormone Metabolism, and Calcium-Sensing Receptor Function

ALEXANDER SHIFRIN, MD, FACS, FACE, ECNU, FEBS (ENDOCRINE), FISS

CALCIUM METABOLISM

Calcium, vitamin D, magnesium, phosphate, and parathyroid hormone (PTH) are involved in bone physiology and supplement each other in function. Calcium carries two major functions: it is the structural material to strengthen bones, and it serves as an important physiological and neuromuscular regulator. Bones serve as storage reservoirs for calcium. The mechanism of neuromuscular regulation by the calcium is very complex and depends on a number of factors. The plasma concentration of calcium must be kept within narrow limits, ranging between 8.8 mg/dL and 10.4 mg/dL (2.2−2.6 mmol/L), to prevent serious metabolic disequilibrium and severe physiological consequences to the body functions. The total body calcium content depends on the body's weight. In an average size adult, the normal amount of calcium is approximately 1000−1300 g. Calcium content is particularly critical in the fetus and neonates. About 99% of the calcium is within bones, and the remaining 1% is either in the intracellular form or circulating in the plasma (extracellular). There are three main fractions of calcium in the plasma: the active ionized form of calcium (free calcium), protein bound, and complex. The ionized calcium consists of approximately 50% of the total plasma calcium, 40% of plasma calcium is bound to plasma proteins, mostly albumin, and 10% is complexed with anions such as bicarbonate, sulfate, phosphate, lactate, and citrate. The concentration of ionized calcium in normal circumstances is maintained between 1.1 and 1.3 mmol/L. This very narrow range is required to maintain normal neuromuscular activity.

Total serum concentration of calcium should be corrected to the plasma albumin level. Each 1 g/dL (10 g/L) of albumin binds about 0.8 mg/dL of calcium. The reduction in serum albumin concentration will lower the total calcium concentration without affecting the ionized calcium concentration and therefore without producing any signs or symptoms of hypocalcemia. However, hypocalcemia or hypercalcemia symptoms may develop if true (corrected or ionized) calcium level decreases or increases.[1−6] Binding of calcium by albumin is pH dependent. The lower the pH, the less calcium binds to albumin (albumin has fewer binding sites for calcium). This results in the increase of free (unbound) calcium concentration. The higher the pH, the lower is the free calcium concentration.[2,7]

Calcium homeostasis involves the following mechanisms: calcium absorption in the gastrointestinal tract, excretion of the calcium within the renal tubules, and deposition into or removal of the calcium from the bone. Plasma calcium level is regulated by five main factors: PTH, active form of vitamin D (1,25(OH)2D), PTH-related peptide (PTHrP), serum phosphate, and fibroblast growth factor 23 (FGF23).[3] Calcium is primarily controlled by PTH. It is the parathyroid hormone that maintains the concentration of unbound (free) calcium within a narrow range. Active form of vitamin D (1,25(OH)2D) also plays a significant role in calcium regulation, although in lesser extent than PTH. Calcitonin and magnesium play a role in calcium regulation as well. PTHrP factors influence the calcium transport across the membranes in the gastrointestinal tract and in the renal tubules.[1−4]

Advances in Treatment and Management in Surgical Endocrinology. https://doi.org/10.1016/B978-0-323-66195-9.00006-6

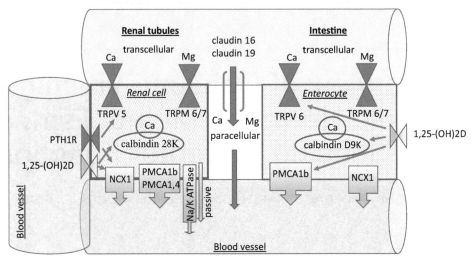

FIG. 6.1 Calcium and magnesium transport. Calcium transport and magnesium transport occur by paracellular (passive) and transcellular (active) mechanisms. In the intestine, the mechanism of calcium absorption is by paracellular and transcellular transport. Paracellular transport occurs mostly in renal tubules, and it is facilitated by the protein claudin-16 and claudin-19. Transcellular (active) transport involves three steps: entry of calcium into the cell through TRPV5 (in renal tubules) and TRPV6 (in the intestine), binding of calcium to calbindins (calbindin 28K in renal tubules, and calbindin-D9K in enterocytes) that diffuse calcium to the basolateral membrane, and then transport calcium through the basolateral membrane via ATP-dependent Ca-ATPase (PMCA1b) and a Na/Ca exchanger (NCX1) (stimulated by PTH). There is also a mechanism of passive diffusion of calcium. Transcellular magnesium absorption facilitated by TRPM6 (in renal tubules and intestinal cells) and TRPM7 (more widely distributed), and at the basolateral membrane magnesium is transported by Na/K ATPase. Active vitamin D (1,25-(OH)2D) promotes calcium-transport of ATPase and TRPV6 through its receptors on duodenal cells and stimulates the expression of calbindin-D9K and calbindin-D28K in renal tubules and enterocytes. PTH regulates NCX1 and influences the expression of TRPV5 in renal tubules. *Ca*, calcium; *Mg*, magnesium; *Na/K ATPase*, transports magnesium through basolateral membrane; *NCX1*, NA+/Ca+-exchanger; *PMCA1b*, ATP-dependent calcium transporting ATPase (transports calcium through basolateral membrane); *PTH*, parathyroid hormone; *PTH1R*, PTH receptor (also called PTH/PTHrP); *TRPM*, transient receptor potential melastatin type; *TRPV*, transient receptor potential vanilloid type.

There are two mechanisms of calcium transport: paracellular (passive) and transcellular (active) (Fig. 6.1). Paracellular (passive) transfer occurs mostly in the renal tubules. Diet, such as high sodium, protein, or acid, increases calcium excretion. Seventy percent of passive reabsorption occurs in the proximal renal tubule in conjunction with sodium, 20% is in the loop of Henle, and 5%–10% in the distal tubule.[1–3,6–8] Paracellular transfer depends on the concentration gradient, and is facilitated by proteins, called claudins, such as claudin-16 (paracellin-1) and claudin-19.[3] For example, mutations in claudin-16 result in renal magnesium wasting syndrome and impaired claudin-mediated paracellular resorption of magnesium and calcium.[7,9,10] Transcellular (active) calcium transport in renal tubules is facilitated by transient receptor potential vanilloid type 5 (TRPV5)[11,12] and calcium-binding protein calbindin 28K.[3] In conjunction with the calcium, renal tubules also facilitate passive transport of magnesium.[1–3,6–8]

In the intestine, the mechanism of calcium absorption is by passive (paracellular) and active (transcellular) transport. The main mechanism of absorption is active transport and it involves three steps: initial absorption from the intestinal lumen, transcellular transport, and transport of calcium across the basolateral membrane.[1–3,7] Transcellular transport of calcium in the enterocyte is facilitated by the calcium-binding protein, calbindin-D9K[7,13] and by transient receptor potential vanilloid type (TRPV6).[3,7,8] Furthermore, there are three steps involved in active calcium transport: entry of calcium into the cell through TRPV5 and TRPV6, binding of calcium to calbindin that diffuses it to the basolateral membrane, and transport of calcium through the basolateral membrane via an ATP-dependent Ca-ATPase (PMCA1b) and a Na/Ca exchanger (NCX1).[7,8] TRPV5 and TRPV6 channels are under the negative calcium feedback mechanism, and are downregulated by calcium influx through these channels.[7] NCX1 is expressed in different organs, including distal nephrons. It is under the direct stimulation of PTH and activated vitamin D (1,25-(OH)2D3), and it stimulates calcium reabsorption in distal nephron.[7] NCX2 and NCX3 are only present in brain and skeletal muscle.[7,14,15] PMCAs have high-affinity calcium efflux pumps that present in four different isoforms, PMCA1- 4. PMCA1 and PMCA4 (including PMCA1b) are isoforms expressed in the kidneys, while only PMCA1b is the predominant isoform expressed in the small intestine.[7] The third mechanism is by passive diffusion or extrusion of calcium-calbindin complex vesicles. Active vitamin D stimulates calcium-transporting ATPase (PMCA1b) and TRPV6 through its receptors on duodenal cells and in small intestine.[1,3,7,8]

Duodenum and upper jejunum are principal sites for the active (transcellular) calcium absorption, whereas paracellular calcium absorption occurs throughout the entire length of the intestinal track.[7,16] When food passes through the intestine, it transits the duodenum only for a short period, and the remaining time it passes through the distal part of the small intestine. When calcium intake is high, the passive (paracellular) mechanism is the predominant process of calcium absorption in the intestine. When calcium intake is low, the transcellular (active) calcium transport is the main mechanism of calcium absorption.[7,17,18]

It is important not to underestimate the influence of magnesium on calcium metabolism. Plasma magnesium is required for normal secretion of PTH. Hypomagnesemia results in inadequate PTH secretion, which cannot be corrected by calcium supplementation alone without adding magnesium. Normal plasma magnesium level is 0.7−1.2 mmol/L.[3] The process of magnesium absorption is similar to the process of calcium absorption in the small intestine. In the renal tubules, the reabsorption of magnesium is mostly passive occurring in the ascending loop of Henle, along with calcium.[3,8,19] Transcellular magnesium absorption is facilitated by two proteins, TRP melastatin type 6 (TRPM6) (in renal tubules and the intestinal cells) and TRP melastatin type 7 (TRPM7) (widely distributed, including the intestine), which are similar to the same proteins from the TRP channel family involved in calcium transport.[3,8] At basolateral surface, magnesium is transported by the Na/K ATPase.[3]

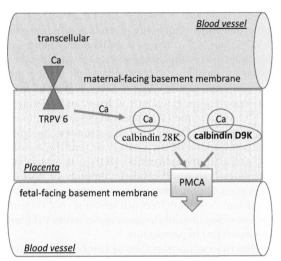

FIG. 6.2 Transcellular (active) calcium transport through the placenta. *Ca,* calcium; *PMCA,* ATP-dependent Ca−ATPase; *TRPV6,* transient receptor potential vanilloid type 6.

During pregnancy, calcium is actively transported across the placenta from the maternal circulation to the fetal circulation in late gestation by the syncytiotrophoblast cells (the epithelial layer separating the maternal and fetal circulation)[7,20] (Fig. 6.2). TRPV6 expression appears to be predominant over the TRPV5 expression.[21] Calcium diffuses across these cells by binding with both calbindin-D9K and calbindin-D28K. Then, calcium is actively transported through the fetal-facing basement membrane, specifically by a calcium-ATPase (PMCA).[22,23] The last 7 days of gestation expression of calbindin-D9K increases more than 100-fold, and PMCA over 2-fold.[24]

CALCIUM-SENSING RECEPTOR

Calcium binds to the calcium-sensing receptor (CaSR) on the parathyroid glands and alters PTH secretion. In addition to calcium, magnesium also binds to CaSR and influences the PTH secretion in a similar manner as calcium. CaSR is present and functioning not only in the parathyroid glands but in other organs as well. For example, in the gastrointestinal tract CaSR plays the role of "food sensors" by stimulating the parietal and G cells of the stomach to secrete gastric acid and gastrin. CaSR influences the exocrine pancreas secretion, regulates fluid retention in the large intestine, and affects intestinal motility through its expression in the myenteric and submucosal plexus of the enteric nervous system. The CaSR is also present in tissues such as renal tubules, bone, and cartilage. In the kidneys, it regulates the release of renin that modulates blood pressure and fluid balance.[1,3,4] In bones, it regulates the mineralization and controls the differentiation, proliferation, and activity of osteoblasts. CaSR also has a role in the central and peripheral nervous system. Lastly, it is expressed in the breast tissue, ovaries, uterus, testes, and prostate.

Mutations of the CaSR result in either activation or inactivation of the receptor. Deactivating, heterogeneous mutations of the CaSR gene result in familial hypocalciuric hypercalcemia (FHH). It causes the disabling of calcium-dependent inhibition of renal calcium reabsorption, leads to hypocalciuria, with altering of calcium-dependent feedback inhibition of PTH secretion, resulting in mild elevation in the serum PTH level and associated hypercalcemia.[1,3,4,25]

Deactivating homozygous or compound heterozygous mutations of the CaSR gene in neonates presents as neonatal severe hyperparathyroidism (NSHPT) and results in severe hypercalcemia, marked elevations in serum PTH level, and near-total loss of calcium-mediated feedback control of PTH secretion.[25,55] This results in skeletal demineralization and pathological fractures.[26,27] The bone loss will be reversed by the parathyroidectomy.[28]

There are two activating mutations of the CaSR: autosomal-dominant hypocalcemia (ADH) and Bartter Syndrome Type 5. ADH is a benign chronic condition, incidentally found on routine blood work.[29] It presents with a longstanding history of paresthesia, intermittent fasciculations, and childhood seizures. The diagnosis is made by the presence of hypocalcemia with inappropriately normal or very low serum PTH levels, and enhanced inhibition of renal calcium reabsorption resulting in hypercalciuria. Associated finding could include hypomagnesemia, hyperphosphatemia, and hypocalciuria.[30] Other findings include a reduction of the glomerular filtration rate of ionized calcium but with an intact renal calcium reabsorption mechanism.[31,32]

Bartter Syndrome Type 5 results from severe activating mutations of the CaSR with the development of the renal salt wasting syndrome, hypocalcemia, suppressed serum PTH levels, hypocalciuria, hyperphosphatemia, ectopic mineralization, and cataracts. CaSR activation on the contraluminal membrane of the thick ascending limb disables NaCl reabsorption. CaSR normally promotes phosphate retention by suppressing renal phosphate excretion and PTH-induced inhibition of phosphate reabsorption.[33–36] This syndrome is treated by giving negative modulators of the CaSR, called calcilytics.[37,38]

VITAMIN D METABOLISM

Vitamin D (Calciferol) is a fat-soluble vitamin. It functions in a role of a hormone or prohormone because of its regulatory role in calcium homeostasis and bone metabolism. It has a much lower effect on calcium homeostasis compared to PTH. Vitamin D is received in two different forms: vitamin D-2 (ergocalciferol) and vitamin D-3 (cholecalciferol). Eighty percent of the body's source of vitamin D comes from sunlight as vitamin D3, and the rest of it comes from food as vitamin D2. Both are metabolized in a similar manner, and they are equally potent. Ultraviolet light of wavelength 270–300 nm is adsorbed by the melanocytes. Its action is directed at the cholesterol precursor, 7-dehydroxycholesterol, where it breaks the B ring of the steroid molecule, creating a secosteroid. Then, by body heat action, it is converted to cholecalciferol (Vitamin D3). The peak of vitamin D3 synthesis is 6 weeks after maximal exposure to sunlight.[1–3] Darker-skinned individuals require a sixfold greater amount of sunlight exposure to synthesize the same amount of Vitamin D as a lighter-skinned individual.[39]

Vitamin D2 is received form plants and food such as fish, liver oil, fatty fish, egg yolk, liver, and milk fortified with vitamin D-2.[1–3,40] It is synthesized from ergosterol and structurally different from cholecalciferol. The process of generation of the active form of vitamin D involves three steps: synthesis, conversion to the major circulating form of vitamin D, 25-hydroxyvitamin D (25(OH)D) in the liver, and lastly conversion by the 1α-hydroxylase to the biologically active form of vitamin D, 1,25(OH)2D in the kidney (Fig. 6.3). After the synthesis, vitamin D binds to the vitamin D-binding protein (DBP), passes through the liver, where it is metabolized by cytochrome 450 enzyme to 25(OH)D, and circulates in plasma bound to DBP protein. Passing through the kidney, 25(OH) Vitamin D is metabolized by 25-hydroxyvitamin D 1 α-hydroxylase into its active hormone, 1,25(OH)2D. Activity of 1α-hydroxylase is controlled by PTH via its cAMP protein kinase action, and by hypocalcemia. Vitamin D is stored in the liver and adipose tissue. Obese people have more vitamin D into their fat store and lower circulating level of vitamin D. The primary action of 1,25(OH)2D is to stimulate the formation of calcium-binding proteins within the intestinal epithelial cells that helps absorption of calcium in the intestine[41–46] (Fig. 6.3). It also helps in phosphorus absorption. 1,25(OH)2D stimulates the expression of calbindin-D9K and NCX1in renal tubules, calbindin-D28K, PMCA1b, and enterocytes.[7]

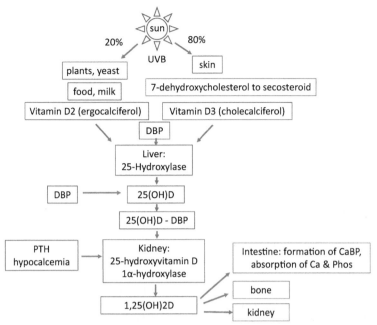

FIG. 6.3 Vitamin D metabolism. *Ca,* calcium; *CaBP,* calcium binding protein; *DBP,* vitamin D-binding protein; *Phos,* phosphorus; *PTH,* parathyroid hormone.

Optimal serum level of 25(OH) vitamin D is between 30 and 50 ng/mL.[41–46] Levels below 20 ng/mL are considered insufficient and suboptimal for skeletal health. Levels below 10 ng/mL are considered to be severely deficient. Deficiency may be the result of low dietary intake, malabsorption, target organ resistance, or impaired 1α-hydroxylation of 25(OH)D, although high level, above 50 ng/mL, may cause toxicity.[41] At high concentrations, the stimulation of osteoblasts to produce cytokines causes an increased production of osteoclasts that lead to bone resorption.[40]

PARATHYROID HORMONE METABOLISM

Parathyroid glands play a key role in maintaining the extracellular calcium concentration. The parathyroid gland is composed of two types of cells: chief and the oxyphil.[47] Parathyroid chief cells, the main type of parathyroid gland cells, produce PTH. Oxyphil cells produce PTHrP, calcitriol, and some other factors.[48] Sensitivity of the sestamibi scan depends on a radioisotope that is retained in mitochondria-rich cells, which are predominantly oxyphil cells (those that do not produce PTH). This explains the reason why the sestamibi scan is not always accurate in the identification of parathyroid adenoma. When the content of parathyroid oxyphil cells in the parathyroid adenoma is greater than 25%, the sensitivity of the sestamibi scan in the late phase of the test is much higher (sensitivity of about 78% for adenoma with more than 25% of oxyphil cells content vs. sensitivity of 33% for adenoma with 1%–25% of oxyphil cells, and sensitivity of 0% for adenoma with no oxyphil cells).[49]

PTH is 84 amino acid polypeptide synthesized from 115-amino acid polypeptide pre-pro-PTH within chief cells of the parathyroid gland. PTH synthesis is constant, and secretion is continuous through the parathyroid cell membrane, rather than sporadic, with circadian dynamics and in a pulsatile fashion.[1–3,6] Almost no hormone is stored within the glands themselves. Among 84 amino acids, only 34 amino acid terminals are required for full activity of the hormone. During episodes of hypocalcemia, PTH is secreted within seconds by exocytosis. The half-life of the PTH is approximately 3 to 4 min in the bloodstream. Maier et al. studied PTH hormone elimination kinetics during a parathyroidectomy and reported that PTH half-life was 3.43 min, while ionized calcium started to decrease only at 30 min after the adenoma was removed. PTH elimination occurs in the kidneys and in the liver. Once secreted, it is rapidly taken up mostly by the liver, cleaved into fragments, and cleared by the kidneys. The current basis for modern assays measuring of intact PTH level is the identification of these fragments in the blood stream. In the liver, PTH degrades through two mechanisms. First, by enzymatic reaction in the Kupffer cells follow a Michaelis–Mentgen kinetic (the best-known models of enzyme kinetics). Second, PTH distributes into the space of Disse (the perisinusoidal space in between a hepatocyte and a sinusoid) and intracellular space, taken up by hepatocytes where it is modulating their glucose and amino acid metabolism and does not reenter the circulation. Forty percent of PTH metabolism occurs in the kidneys, where it is filtered and then reabsorbed in the proximal tubular cells, where it is degraded without reentering the circulation. PTH works through two receptors: PTH1R and PTH2R. PTH1R (also called PTH/PTHrP receptor) binds two molecules, the PTH and PTHrP, but only, the PTH molecule binds to the PTH2R. PTH1R is predominantly expressed in bones and kidneys. PTH2R only presents in the central nervous system. The main function of PTH is to regulate calcium homeostasis. The principal target organs for PTH are bones and kidneys (through PTH1R).[1–7,50,51]

In bones, under physiological circumstances, PTH promotes bone formation via receptors on the osteoblasts. During hypocalcemia, PTH stimulates bone resorption to maintain normal calcium balance and restore normocalcemia. PTH alters the balance between the expression of the receptor activator of nuclear factor kappa-B ligand (RANKL) produced by osteoclast, and the receptor osteoprotegerin (OPG) produced by osteoblasts. PTH has either a catabolic or anabolic effect, depending on the dose and periodicity of the PTH signal. Catabolic effect on bones develops with continuous exposure to PTH, as in primary hyperparathyroidism. PTH is changing the balance between RANKL and OPG in favor of bone resorption and demineralization: the encoding for RANKL increases, and encoding for OPG mRNA decreases.[1–6] This effect of PTH on RANKL and OPG diminishes in about 1 year after a successful parathyroidectomy.[6,52] Anabolic effect develops with low doses, intermittent PTH secretion.[6]

In the proximal tubules of the kidneys nephrons, the main action of the PTH is activation of 25-hydroxyvitamin D 1α-hydroxylase that converts 25-hydroxyvitamin D (25(OH)D) to its active form, 1,25(OH)2D, which then facilitates the absorption of both calcium and phosphate from the intestines.[2,3,7,53,54] In distal tubules, it promotes reabsorption of calcium and magnesium and excretion of phosphate, by action through PTH1R receptor.[3] This mechanism of PTH binding to PTH1R involves stimulation of adenylyl cyclase and increasing cyclic AMP (cAMP) concentrations that activate phospholipase C pathway.[2] PTH also has the effect on bicarbonate and amino acid reabsorption in the proximal tubule. This results in hyperparathyroidism-related mild form of Fanconi syndrome (the generalized dysfunction of the proximal tubule presented with polyuria, hypokalemia, glycosuria, hypophosphatemia, and low molecular weight proteinuria). This is also resolved when hyperparathyroidism is reversed.[1,3,6]

REFERENCES

1. Allgrove J. Physiology of calcium, phosphate and magnesium. *Endocr Dev.* 2009;16:8−31.
2. Song L. Calcium and bone metabolism indices. *Adv Clin Chem.* 2017;82:1−46.
3. Allgrove J. Physiology of calcium, phosphate, magnesium and vitamin D. *Endocr Dev.* 2015;28:7−32.
4. Schreckenberg R, Schlüter KD. Calcium sensing receptor expression and signalling in cardiovascular physiology and disease. *Vasc Pharmacol.* 2018;107:35−42.
5. Hoenderop JG, Bindels RJ. Calciotropic and magnesiotropic TRP channels. *Physiology.* 2008;23:32−40.
6. Silva BC, Bilezikian JP. Parathyroid hormone: anabolic and catabolic actions on the skeleton. *Curr Opin Pharmacol.* June 2015;22:41−50.
7. Hoenderop JGJ, Nilius B, Bindels RJM. Calcium absorption across epithelia. *Physiol Rev.* 2005;85:373−422.
8. Lameris AL, Nevalainen PI, Reijnen D, et al. Segmental transport of Ca^{2+} and Mg^{2+} along the gastrointestinal tract. *Am J Physiol Gastrointest Liver Physiol.* 2015;308(3):G206−G216.
9. Simon DB, Lu Y, Choate KA, et al. Paracellin-1, a renal tight junction protein required for paracellular Mg^{2+} resorption. *Science.* 1999;285:103−106.
10. Wong V, Goodenough DA. Paracellular channels. *Science.* 1999;285:62.
11. Montell C, Birnbaumer L, Flockerzi V, et al. A unified nomenclature for the superfamily of TRP cation channels. *Mol Cell.* 2002;9:229−231.
12. Peng JB, Chen XZ, Berger UV, et al. Molecular cloning and characterization of a channel-like transporter mediating intestinal calcium absorption. *J Biol Chem.* 1999;274:22739−22746.
13. Yamagishi N, Yukawa YA, Ishiguro N, et al. Expression of calbindin-D9k messenger ribonucleic acid in the gastrointestinal tract of dairy cattle. *J Vet Med A Physiol Pathol Clin Med.* 2002;49:461−465.
14. Li Z, Matsuoka S, Hryshko LV, et al. Cloning of the NCX2 isoform of the plasma membrane Na -Ca2 exchanger. *J Biol Chem.* 1994;269:17434−17439.
15. Nicoll DA, Quednau BD, Qui Z, Xia YR, Lusis AJ, Philipson KD. Cloning of a third mammalian Na -Ca2 exchanger, NCX3. *J Biol Chem.* 1996;271:24914−24921.
16. Bronner F, Pansu D, Stein WD. An analysis of intestinal calcium transport across the rat intestine. *Am J Physiol Gastrointest Liver Physiol.* 1986;250:G561−G569.
17. Bronner F. Mechanisms of intestinal calcium absorption. *J Cell Biochem.* 2003;88:387−393.

18. Bronner F, Pansu D. Nutritional aspects of calcium absorption. *J Nutr.* 1999;129(9–12).
19. Schweigel M, Martens H. Magnesium transport in the gastrointestinal tract. *Front Biosci.* 2000;5:D666–D677.
20. Faulk WP, McIntyre JA. Immunological studies of human trophoblast: markers, subsets and functions. *Immunol Rev.* 1983;75:139–175.
21. Peng JB, Brown EM, Hediger MA. Structural conservation of the genes encoding CaT1, CaT2, and related cation channels. *Genomics.* 2001;76:99–109.
22. Belkacemi L, Gariepy G, Mounier C, Simoneau L, Lafond J. Calbindin-D9k (CaBP9k) localization and levels of expression in trophoblast cells from human term placenta. *Cell Tissue Res.* 2004;315:107–117.
23. Belkacemi L, Simoneau L, Lafond J. Calcium-binding proteins: distribution and implication in mammalian placenta. *Endocrine.* 2002;19:57–64.
24. Glazier JD, Atkinson DE, Thornburg KL, et al. Gestational changes in Ca^{2+} transport across rat placenta and mRNA for calbindin9K and Ca(2+)-ATPase. *Am J Physiol Regul Integr Comp Physiol.* 1992;263:R930–R935.
25. Conigrave AD. The calcium-sensing receptor and the parathyroid: past, present, future. *Front Physiol.* 2016;7:563.
26. Pollak MR, Chou YH, Marx SJ, et al. Familial hypocalciuric hypercalcemia and neonatal severe hyperparathyroidism. Effects of mutant gene dosage on phenotype. *J Clin Investig.* 1994;93:1108–1112.
27. Brown EM, Pollak M, Seidman CE, et al. Calcium-ion-sensing cell-surface receptors. *N Engl J Med.* 1995;333:234–240.
28. Marx SJ, Lasker RD, Brown EM, et al. Secretory dysfunction in parathyroid cells from a neonate with severe primary hyperparathyroidism. *J Clin Endocrinol Metab.* 1986;62:445–449.
29. Pearce SH, Williamson C, Kifor O, et al. A familial syndrome of hypocalcemia with hypercalciuria due to mutations in the calcium-sensing receptor. *N Engl J Med.* 1996;335:1115–1122.
30. Tan YM, Cardinal J, Franks AH, et al. Autosomal dominant hypocalcemia: a novel activating mutation (E604K) in the cysteine-rich domain of the calcium-sensing receptor. *J Clin Endocrinol Metab.* 2003;88:605–610.
31. Thakker RV. Diseases associated with the extracellular calcium-sensing receptor. *Cell Calcium.* 2004;35:275–282.
32. Egbuna OI, Brown EM. Hypercalcaemic and hypocalcaemic conditions due to calcium-sensing receptor mutations. *Best Pract Res Clin Rheumatol.* 2008;22:129–148.
33. Riccardi D, Brown E. Physiology and pathophysiology of the calcium-sensing receptor in the kidney. *Am J Physiol Renal Physiol.* 2010;298:F485–F499.
34. Riccardi D, Traebert M, Ward DT, et al. Dietary phosphate and parathyroid hormone alter the expression of the calcium-sensing receptor (CaR) and the Na+-dependent Pi transporter (NaPi-2) in the rat proximal tubule. *Pflügers Archiv.* 2000;441:379–387.
35. Ba J, Brown D, Friedman PA. Calcium-sensing receptor regulation of PTH-inhibitable proximal tubule phosphate transport. *Am J Physiol.* 2003;285:F1233–F1243.
36. Riccardi D, Valenti G. Localization and function of the renal calcium-sensing receptor. *Nat Rev Nephrol.* 2016;12:414–425.
37. Mayr B, Glaudo M, Schöfl C. Activating calcium-sensing receptor mutations: prospects for future treatment with calcilytics. *Trends Endocrinol Metab.* 2016;27:643–652.
38. Nemeth EF, Goodman WG. Calcimimetic and calcilytic drugs: feats, flops, and futures. *Calcif Tissue Int.* 2016;98:341–358.
39. Lo CW, Paris PW, Holick MF. Indian and Pakistani immigrants have the same capacity as Caucasians to produce vitamin D in response to ultraviolet irradiation. *Am J Clin Nutr.* 1986;44(5):683–685.
40. Winter W, Kleerekoper M. Bone and mineral metabolism. In: Risteli J, Risteli L, Burtis CA, Ashwood ER, Bruns D, eds. *Tietz Textbook of Clinical Chemistry and Molecular Diagnostics.* 5th ed. San Diego, CA: Elsevier Publishing; 2012:1765.
41. Sanders KM, Stuart AL, Williamson EJ, et al. Annual high-dose oral vitamin D and falls and fractures in older women: a randomized controlled trial. *J Am Med Assoc.* 2010;303(18):1815–1822.
42. Dawson-Hughes B. Vitamin D deficiency in adults: definition, clinical manifestations, and treatment. In: Drezner MK, Rosen CJ, eds. *UpToDate.* Waltham, MA: UpToDate; 2016 (updated: March, 2016).
43. Dawson-Hughes B, Harris SS, Krall EA, Dallal GE. Effect of calcium and vitamin D supplementation on bone density in men and women 65 years of age or older. *N Engl J Med.* 1997;337(10):670–676.
44. Chapuy MC, Pamphile R, Paris E, et al. Combined calcium and vitamin D3 supplementation in elderly women: confirmation of reversal of secondary hyperparathyroidism and hip fracture risk: the Decalyos II study. *Osteoporos Int.* 2002;13(3):257–264.
45. Trivedi DP, Doll R, Khaw KT. Effect of four monthly oral vitamin D3 (cholecalciferol) supplementation on fractures and mortality in men and women living in the community: randomised double blind controlled trial. *BMJ.* 2003;326(7387):469.
46. Bilezikian JP, Brandi ML, Eastell R, et al. Guidelines for the management of asymptomatic primary hyperparathyroidism: summary statement from the Fourth International Workshop. *Clin Endocrinol Metabol.* 2014;99(10):3561–3569.
47. Isono H, Shoumura S, Emura S. Ultrastructure of the parathyroid gland. *Histol Histopathol.* 1990;5(1):95–112.
48. Ritter CS, Haughey BH, Miller B, Brown AJ. Differential gene expression by oxyphil and chief cells of human parathyroid glands. *J Clin Endocrinol Metab.* 2012;97(8):E1499–E1505.
49. Carpentier A, Jeannotte S, Verreault J, et al. Preoperative localization of parathyroid lesions in hyperparathyroidism: relationship between technetium-99m-MIBI uptake and oxyphil cell content. *J Nucl Med.* 1998;39(8):1441–1444.
50. Zindel D, Engel S, Bottrill AR, et al. Identification of key phosphorylation sites in PTH1R that determine arrestin3 binding and fine-tune receptor signaling. *Biochem J.* 2016;473(22):4173–4192.

51. Maier GW, Kreis ME, Renn W, Pereira PL, Häring HU, Becker HD. Parathyroid hormone after adenectomy for primary hyperparathyroidism. A study of peptide hormone elimination kinetics in humans. *J Clin Endocrinol Metab.* 1998;83(11):3852–3856.

52. Stilgren LS, Rettmer E, Eriksen EF, Hegedus L, Beck-Nielsen H, Abrahamsen B. Skeletal changes in osteoprotegerin and receptor activator of nuclear factor-kappaB ligand mRNA levels in primary hyperparathyroidism: effect of parathyroidectomy and association with bone metabolism. *Bone.* 2004;35:256–265.

53. El-Hajj Fuleihan G, Brown EM. Parathyroid hormone secretion and action. In: Rosen CJ, ed. *UpToDate.* Waltham, MA: UpToDate; 2014.

54. Winter WE, Harris NS. Calcium biology and disorders. In: Clarke W, ed. *Con- Temporary Practice in Clinical Chemistry.* 2nd ed. Washington, DC: AACC Press; 2011:506.

55. Ward BK, Magno AL, Davis EA, et al. Functional deletion of the calcium-sensing receptor in a case of neonatal severe hyperparathyroidism. *J Clin Endocrinol Metab.* 2004; 89(8):3721–3730.

Advances in the Diagnosis and Surgical Management of Primary Hyperparathyroidism

ALEXANDER SHIFRIN, MD, FACS, FACE, ECNU, FEBS (ENDOCRINE), FISS

INTRODUCTION

Classic primary hyperparathyroidism (PHPT) is defined by persistent elevation of serum calcium level with corresponding elevation of serum parathyroid hormone (PTH) level. This is due to autonomous overproduction of PTH by the abnormal parathyroid gland or glands. In addition to previously mentioned classic forms of PHPT, two additional forms of PHPT have been described: normocalcemic and normohormonal. In physiological circumstances, the feedback mechanism causes suppression of either calcium or PTH when one of them is elevated. With normocalcemic PHPT, serum PTH level is elevated but serum calcium levels, both total and ionized, remain inappropriately normal (in the middle to high normal ranges) and not suppressed. To make a diagnosis of normocalcemic PHPT, secondary causes, such as vitamin D deficiency, primary hypercalciuria, chronic kidney disease, calcium malabsorption, and drugs that can potentially cause elevation of the PTH level (thiazides, lithium, anticonvulsants, bisphosphonates, and denosumab), should be excluded.[1] With an average follow-up of 4 years for patients with normocalcemic PHPT, Bilezikian et al. showed that 22% of them will become hypercalcemic. With normohormonal PHPT, serum PTH level is inappropriately normal and not suppressed compared to high serum calcium level. The presentation of PHPT became milder over the years, and severe symptoms are rarely seen.[1–4] Surgical treatment of PHPT has undergone extensive changes in the past decade shifting from a four-gland exploration to minimally invasive single gland (adenoma) directed approach (a focused resection of the single parathyroid gland) in majority of patients.[1,5,6]

DIAGNOSIS

Diagnosis of PHPT is biochemical, therefore the following measurements are essential to establish the diagnosis: serum calcium, PTH, vitamin D, phosphate, creatinine levels, glomerular filtration rate, alkaline phosphatase activity, 24-h urine calcium, and, in some instances, ionized calcium level.[1,5,6] Bone mineral density (BMD) by DEXA scan is essential to evaluate osteoporosis in the lumbar spine, femoral hip, and more importantly, at the most common site for PHPT-related osteoporosis, the wrist. Imaging studies, such as kidney ultrasonography, abdominal X-ray, or abdominal CT scan, can be used to evaluate the presence of nephrolithiasis or nephrocalcinosis.[1] In addition, specific radiological studies can be ordered to evaluate for possible bone fractures (stress fractures), if suspected. Diagnosis of normocalcemic PHPT is established by measurement of not only total serum calcium level, but also serum-ionized calcium level. In true normocalcemic PHPT, an ionized calcium level should be normal.[1–4]

Based on the recent guidelines for the management of asymptomatic PHPT from the summary statement of the Fourth International Workshop and the American Association of Endocrine Surgeons (AAES) Guidelines for Definitive Management of Primary Hyperparathyroidism, the following are indications for surgical treatment of PHPT: serum calcium 1.0 mg/dL (0.25 mmol/L) above upper limit of normal; presence of osteoporosis defined as BMD by DEXA scan, a T-score of less than −2.5 at lumbar spine, total hip, femoral neck, and especially, distal 1/3 of the radius (Z-scores should be used instead of T-scores in premenopausal women and men younger than 50 years of age);

Advances in Treatment and Management in Surgical Endocrinology. https://doi.org/10.1016/B978-0-323-66195-9.00007-8

presence of vertebral fracture by imaging studies such as X-ray, CT scan, MRI, or by the DEXA scan; 24-h urine for calcium above 400 mg/d (10 mmol/d) and increased kidney stone risk by biochemical stone risk analysis; presence of nephrolithiasis or nephrocalcinosis by X-ray, ultrasound, or CT scan; and individuals less than 50 years of age.[1,5,6]

The AAES guidelines and 4th International Workshop have recommended that patients should have genetic testing performed if there are suspicions of genetic syndrome. The patients who should be considered for genetic testing are the following: patient with hyperparathyroidism who are less than 40 years of age, patients with suspicions for familial syndromes based on positive family history, presence of multiglandular disease, and findings of parathyroid carcinoma or atypical adenoma.[1,5] It was reported that more than 10% of patients with PHPT may have one of the following familial syndromes: MEN (multiple endocrine neoplasia) type 1, MEN 2, MEN 3, MEN 4, HPT-JT (hyperparathyroidism jaw-tumor syndrome), FIHPT (familial isolated hyperparathyroidism), NSPHPT (neonatal severe PHPT), FHH (familial hypocalciuric hypercalcemia) type 1, FHH 2, FHH 3, and nsPHPT (nonsyndromic PHPT).[7,8]

What Is the Best Imaging Study to Obtain Before the Parathyroidectomy?

Approximately 85% of patients with PHPT will have a single parathyroid adenoma, and the remaining patients will have either double adenoma or hyperplasia. Radiological localization studies are obtained to help with minimally invasive surgical approach to localize the adenoma but not to establish the diagnosis of PHPT. When parathyroid adenoma is not localized by any imaging studies, but surgical criteria are met, the patient is still a candidate for the parathyroid exploration.[5] Accurate localization of parathyroid adenoma helps to achieve the following goals by using the minimally invasive approach: to minimize the risk of complications secondary to more extensive exploratory surgery, to decrease postoperative pain and discomfort, to decrease surgical operative time, and to obtain the best cosmetic result. Ultrasound is the safest imaging study for preoperative localization of parathyroid adenoma with no risk of radiation exposure (Fig. 7.1A−H). It is recommended that a designated parathyroid ultrasound, not just a neck or a thyroid gland ultrasound, always be performed before a parathyroidectomy for operative planning of all patients with PHPT. Ultrasound is the least expensive test out of all tests used

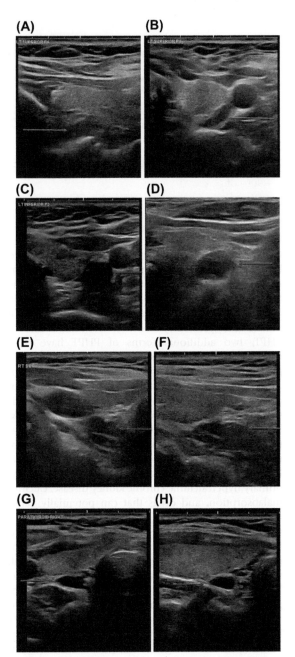

FIG. 7.1 Parathyroid ultrasound showing the parathyroid adenoma. **(A)** left superior adenoma, transverse view; **(B)** left superior adenoma, sagittal view; **(C)** left inferior adenoma, transverse view; **(D)** left inferior adenoma, sagittal view; **(E)** right superior descended adenoma, transverse view; **(F)** right superior descended adenoma, sagittal view; **(G)** right inferior adenoma, transverse view; **(H)** right inferior adenoma, sagittal view.

to localize a parathyroid adenoma. This type of test allows a practitioner to perform an evaluation of the thyroid gland to visualize the soft tissue of the neck and the parathyroid glands. Designated parathyroid ultrasound performed by an endocrine surgeon has more chances to visualize a parathyroid adenoma than those performed by a radiologist.[9-11] Sensitivity of high-resolution ultrasonography was reported between 51% and 89% if the study was interpreted by a radiologist. Surgeons performed ultrasonography correctly identified a parathyroid adenoma in 74% −90% of patients with a sensitivity 87% and specificity 88%.[10,11]

Dual-isotope subtraction single-photon emission computed tomography−computed tomography scan (SPECT-CT) is a newer diagnostic technique that showed superior result to the sestamibi scan (Fig. 7.2). Recent study showed that the sensitivity of the SPECT-CT scan was 95%, and specificity was 89% for the detection and localization of a parathyroid adenoma. The positive predictive value was estimated to be 97%, and the negative predictive value was estimated to be 83%. The accuracy of the technique was reported from 80% to 94% in detecting parathyroid adenoma

and 92% in accurate localization to the appropriate gland and not only the laterality.[1,10,12]

The surgeon should always evaluate the sestamibi scan images and not rely solely on the radiologist report (Fig. 7.3). Sensitivity of technetium-99m sestamibi scan is shown to be between 39% and 90% if the study is interpreted by the radiologist.[11] M. Zeiger et al. showed that preoperative assessment of the sestamibi scan by the surgeon, looking for subtleties or "shadows" may lead to a finding of parathyroid adenoma in imaging studies that were initially described as "negative" by the radiologist. M. Zeiger et al. reported 41% subtleties or "shadows" in patients with "negative" and in 76% of patients with "indeterminate" sestamibi scans. In this group of patients, 91% underwent successful minimally invasive parathyroidectomy with a curative rate of 99%.[13]

When the patient is presented with a truly negative sestamibi scan, the likelihood of intraoperative findings of multiglandular disease is much higher than the findings of a single adenoma. A retrospective study from Lund University in Sweden evaluated this subgroup of patients and found that those patients are also more likely to suffer from diabetes, have findings of lower

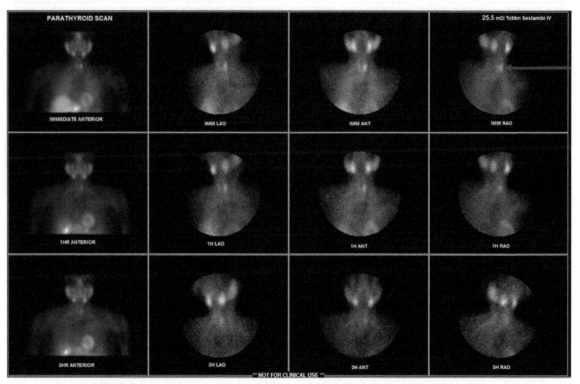

FIG. 7.2 SPECT-CT sestamibi scan showing a left inferior parathyroid adenoma (you can see a persistent uptake at 3 hour after the tracer injection - lower row of images).

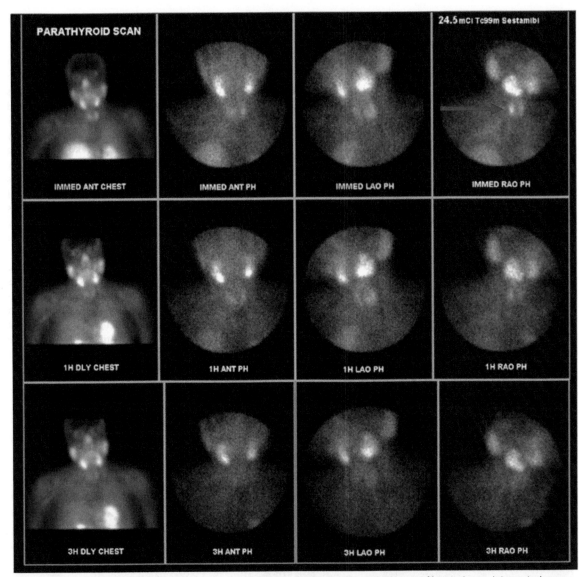

FIG. 7.3 SPECT-CT sestamibi scan showing a right superior parathyroid adenoma (the study was interpreted by the radiologist as "negative for the findings of a parathyroid adenoma").

preoperative levels of urinary calcium, and elevated level of osteocalcin.[14] Study by A. Harari et al. showed that if a preoperative sestamibi scan shows persistent uptake on one side, but preoperative US failed to localize the adenoma, then the patient is more likely to have posteriorly located upper parathyroid gland adenoma.[15] In patients with PHPT, it is important to ascertain if the patient has a history of lithium therapy or radiation exposure. Patient treated with lithium will most likely have multiglandular disease with an asymmetrical hyperplasia rather than a single adenoma.

Therefore, the preoperative imaging studies could be misleading by showing only a single adenoma. Bilateral neck exploration is therefore recommended.[16] In contrast, patient with radiation exposure will most likely be presented with a single adenoma, but metachronous disease may develop several years after a successful parathyroidectomy. Therefore, lifelong follow-up is essential.[17]

Study by N. Perrier et al., evaluated the outcome of patients who routinely underwent preoperative four-dimensional CT (4D CT) scan before surgical intervention for PHPT. The length of stay was shown to be lower in patients who underwent preoperative 4D CT scan compared to those patients who did not (0.61 vs. 0.23 days). Reason being patients with precise localization of the parathyroid adenoma by 4D CT scan underwent less extensive surgical exploration directed to the parathyroid adenoma rather than the four-gland exploration.[18] Utilizing appropriate localization studies and combination of different modalities, such as 4D CT scan and ultrasonography, helps to maximize the success of the minimally invasive approach in patients with PHPT.[9]

Thin-cut CT scan (2.5 mm cuts) is one of the well-established techniques in localization of difficult to find parathyroid adenomas (Fig. 7.4). The study by A. Harari et al. showed that patients with negative preoperative sestamibi scans, who subsequently had thin-cut CT scans, showed a sensitivity of 85% and specificity of 94% for correctly lateralizing the side of the adenoma. They also had a sensitivity of 66% and specificity of 89% for predicting the exact location of the diseased gland.[19] Our program has been using the thin-cut CT scan for over 12 years (at the same radiology location as in the article referenced earlier) with the great success. We have found that the thin-cut CT scan is very helpful in the preoperative workup of patients who have recurrent or persistent PHPT, or those patients who had negative preoperative US and sestamibi scan. Some of the patients with persistent PHPT were found to have ectopic parathyroid glands located either in the mediastinum (Fig. 7.5) or high in the lateral neck (Fig. 7.4). Therefore, the precise localization with a thin-cut CT scan has helped us to perform a focused neck exploration even in redo cases.

Summary. Ultrasound is the safest imaging study for preoperative parathyroid adenoma localization with no risk of radiation exposure. Ultrasound should always be performed for preoperative planning before a parathyroidectomy. The second confirmatory test should be either SPECT-CT sestamibi or 4D-CT scan. Performing dedicated parathyroid ultrasound by the surgeon will have more sensitivity than those performed by the radiologist. A surgeon should always evaluate the sestamibi scan before performing a parathyroidectomy, looking for subtleties or "shadows" that may lead to the findings of parathyroid adenoma in imaging studies that were initially described as "negative" by the radiologist. Thin-cut CT can be used for the patients with persistent and recurrent PHPT or in difficult to localize parathyroid adenomas.

Cost Analysis of the Imaging Studies for Parathyroid Localization

Several studies have looked at the cost utility analysis of preoperative diagnostic tests in parathyroid localization. Although the least expensive test was an ultrasound, the most cost-effective strategy to localize a parathyroid adenoma was an ultrasound followed by the SPECT-CT sestamibi scan plus/minus four-dimensional computed tomography (4D-CT) scan or ultrasound followed by 4D-CT scan. Ultrasound followed by 4D-CT scan was the least expensive strategy with an estimated cost reported as $5901.[9,20] The least cost-effective study was SPECT-CT sestamibi alone.[21]

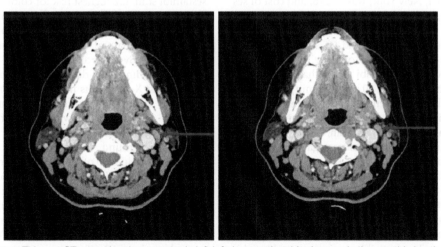

FIG. 7.4 Thin-cut CT scan showing an ectopic left inferior parathyroid adenoma in the carotid sheath at the level of 2 cm above the carotid bifurcation.

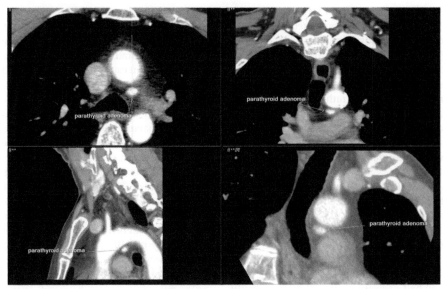

FIG. 7.5 Thin-cut CT scan showing an ectopic left inferior mediastinal parathyroid adenoma.

Preoperative 4D-CT scan does not shorten operating time and does not decrease the failure rate significantly, but was associated with shorter hospital stays.[18] The sensitivity and specificity of combination of both studies, ultrasound and SPECT-CT sestamibi scan, were reported between 91% and 96% in localization of parathyroid adenoma.[10] Positive predictive value of SPECT-CT was greater than 90% with accuracy at about 83%. It was also more accurate (36%) in predicting multiglandular disease.[22]

When comparing the cost of CT scan and sestamibi scan, the charges for dynamic CT scan (at Mount Sinai Medical Center, New York) was $1296, and cost of sestamibi scintigraphy was about $1112, ranging between $669 and $1156 depending on the type and amount of radiotracer injected. Parathyroid CT scan was also the quickest test with mean time of study less than 5 min, compared to the sestamibi scan that took about 306 min (ranges between 50 and 538 min).[23] Consider above data the recommendation can be made that the most extensive studies, such as highly sensitive thin-cut CT scan or the 4D CT scan, could be used if ultrasound and sestamibi scans are negative, and in reoperative redo cases.

The Risk of Radiation Exposure with Imaging Studies for Parathyroid Localization

It is important to understand the risk of radiation exposure associated with different radiological diagnostic tests. For example, sestamibi scan is contraindicated in pregnancy and should be used very cautiously in children.[24,25] In comparing the dose of radiation, the dynamic parathyroid CT scan delivers an effective radiation doses (ERD) of 5.56 mSv (millisievert). The mean patient's total ERD for three-phase CT scan is about 15.9 mSv, and for four-phase CT scan is between 20 and 28 mSv, which is significantly more than the dose received from the parathyroid sestamibi scan in which the ERD measure is between 3.3 and 5.6 mSv. However, the lifetime risk of cancer from these exposures was extremely low and was comparable to the incidence at baseline. The highest attributable lifetime risk for lung cancer after multiphase CT scan was about 0.03%; after sestamibi scan, the highest risk for colon cancer was reported as 0.06%.[26,27] For comparison, the average person in the United States receives an ERD of about 3 mSv per year from natural and cosmic radiation. ERD of about 0.03 mSv is received during a coast-to-coast round trip airline flight due to exposure of cosmic radiation. Chest X-ray results in ERD of 0.1 mSv, which is equal to 10 days of natural background radiation. Head CT scan with and without contrast results in ERD of 4 mSv, which is comparable to 16 months of natural background radiation. Bone densitometry (DEXA) results in ERD of 0.001 mSv, which is comparable to 3 h of natural background radiation.[28]

Summary. The least expensive and the safest test for parathyroid localization is an ultrasound. The most cost-effective strategy to localize parathyroid adenoma is an ultrasound followed by the SPECT-CT sestamibi scan plus/minus 4D-CT scan, or ultrasound followed by 4D-CT scan. The risk of radiation exposure should be considered before ordering imaging studies, especially for pregnant patients and children.

Intraoperative PTH Monitoring

PTH hormone elimination kinetics after parathyroidectomy was studied by Maier et al. PTH half-life after the adenoma removal was 3.43 min, while ionized calcium started to decrease only at 30 min after the adenoma removal. PTH elimination occurs in the kidney and liver, and it is proportional to its plasma concentration. The lowest drop of PTH level occurs at 5 h after the adenoma removal. PTH levels starts to increase again at postoperative day two.[29]

Intraoperative PTH (IOPTH) monitoring, first reported by Nussbaum in 1988 and then introduced by G. Irving et al., had revolutionized the surgical approach to PHPT. It allowed for the shift toward the minimally invasive, targeted parathyroidectomy directed toward the removal of a single parathyroid adenoma rather than the need for a bilateral neck exploration.[30−32] Since that time, parathyroidectomy became a highly successful procedure performed with a limited surgical dissection and excision of only the affected gland (or glands). It is guided by the IOPTH assessment in addition to visual morphologic characteristics that have been performed by surgeons in the past.[33] Ability to perform a rapid IOPTH assessment has become possible due to the development of a new generation of PTH assay with two monoclonal antibodies specific for the N- and C-terminal regions of the hormone (1−84)PTH, while earlier assays were directed to either N-terminal, midregion, or C-terminal.[34] Although there are some debates on the timing and the best criteria for the IOPTH assay, the 50% drop in PTH level at 5 and 10 min after the excision of the parathyroid adenoma, described by Irving's group, became the gold standard of IOPTH criteria. Despite different literature questioning the criteria, this approach has been utilized by most of endocrine, and head and neck surgeons who perform high volume parathyroidectomies.[35−37] It has been shown that IOPTH monitoring accurately predicts operative success or failure in 96.3% of patients. Some authors also recommended to use additional measurements of IOPTH level at 20 min after the parathyroidectomy, which showed 97.3% operative success rate.[38] Earlier data on IOPTH measurements established that the goal of 50% IOPTH levels drop was enough to achieve the biochemical cure, even if final IOPTH levels were still above the upper limit of normal.[39] More recent data have shown that in addition to 50% IOPTH level drop, it also must go down to normal ranges. It was therefore recommended to achieve the goal of

IOPTH level less than 40 pg/mL. Study of patients in 2 years after the parathyroidectomy has shown that patients with final IOPTH level less than 40 pg/mL had a lower rate of persistence and recurrence compared to patients with IOPTH level between 40 and 59 pg/mL. The patients with a final IOPTH level between 41 and 65 pg/mL have a higher likelihood of persistent disease due to not identifying an additional parathyroid adenoma or due to hyperplasia. Patients with final IOPTH $\geq$60 pg/mL were reported to have a recurrence rate of 5.9%, and a persistence rate of 5.4% as compared to patients with IOPTH level <40 pg/mL, which had a recurrence rate of 1.3% and the lowest persistence rate of 0.2%.[40,41] Retrospective study by H Chen et al. showed that the IOPTH level drop greater than 70% was protective against the recurrence.[42]

Treating patients with normocalcemic or normohormonal PHPT could be challenging, and relying only on the IOPTH levels may not be sufficient. It has been shown that patients presented with normocalcemic PHPT may have about 12% chances of multigland disease. Patients presented with normohormonal PHPT may have up to 58% chances of multigland disease (44% of them were reported to have hyperplasia). Therefore, bilateral parathyroid exploration could be considered in perioperative planning.[43,44] Patients with normohormonal PHPT most often had a negative sestamibi scan compared to classic PHPT (18.3% vs. 4.8%). Cure rate for normohormonal PHPT was 88% compared to 96% in the classic group. Patients with normohormonal PHPT with preoperative PTH $\leq$55 pg/mL had a cure rate of 83%, and those with preoperative PTH levels between 56 pg/mL and 65 pg/mL had a cure rate of 96%.[45] The major cause of operative failure of minimally invasive surgical approach utilizing IOPTH monitoring was not the failure of IOPTH technique itself, but rather the surgeons' misinterpretation of the IOPTH result and the failure to identify all abnormal parathyroid glands.[46]

Summary. Since introduction of IOPTH monitoring, it has become an essential part of performing a parathyroidectomy. The goal of the IOPTH assessment is to achieve an instant intraoperative conformation of biochemical cure of hyperparathyroidism. IOPTH assay facilitates a minimally invasive surgical approach by minimizing the extent of the surgery leading to minimal surgical trauma. The ideal time points for IOPTH measurements are at following: Tb—at baseline (before the parathyroidectomy); at the T0—during the parathyroid adenoma manipulation; T5—at 5 min after the adenoma removal; T10—at 10 min after the adenoma removal; T20 can be added if IOPTH levels are decreasing slowly as seen in the case of very high initial preoperative PTH level. The goal of IOPTH assessment is not only to have a 50% drop in PTH levels between pre-excision levels (T0 and Tb) and post-excision levels (T5 and T10), but also to achieve a final IOPTH value down to normal ranges and, in ideal circumstances, to less than 40 pg/mL after the parathyroidectomy.

SURGICAL APPROACH

Currently, the concept of a "minimally invasive surgery" is presented to the patient as a surgery performed through a small neck incision, or no neck incision at all, which is very appealing, especially for female patients. This concept has also become the major trend in patients' referrals. The goal of minimally invasive surgery is to minimize the surgical trauma and the ability to perform successful parathyroidectomy through a small incision.[47] The best *definition of minimally invasive parathyroid surgery* was given by the pioneer of this approach, JF Henry. He defined a minimally invasive parathyroidectomy as an operation through the incision that is less than 3 cm in length that allows for direct access to and focused dissection of the parathyroid gland. The most important point of his definition was the concept of *"surgical invasiveness"*. He stated that minimally invasive surgery is not only defined by the length and site of the skin incision, but by the extend of the dissection related to all underlying structures affected by the dissection during the procedure, by the type of anesthesia, by the duration of the operation, by postoperative pain, and by complication and success rates as a long-term outcome.[48]

The outcome of minimally invasive approach versus standard open neck exploration was studied by D. Schneider et al. in series of 1368 parathyroid surgeries for PHPT over a 10-year period. This study showed no differences in recurrence between the minimally invasive and open groups (2.5% vs. 2.1%).[49] Similar findings were reported by H. Chen et al. in their retrospective cohort of 196 patients over 10 years of follow-up.[42]

The concept of minimal dissection is especially important when we encounter the recurrent or persistent disease that was reported to occur in 2.5%–5% of patients with PHPT.[23,47] Patients who were presented for reoperative surgery with persistent or recurrent disease after initial standard four-gland neck exploration had complication rates of 44% that are significantly higher compared to 15% of patients with an initial minimally invasive parathyroidectomy.[50]

Several recent guidelines on the management of asymptomatic PHPT have established indications for surgery.[1,5] In addition, 15-year follow-up data showed that after nonsurgical observation 40% of patients develop at least one indication for the surgery.[51] Literature showed improved outcomes among patients with asymptomatic PHPT who underwent a curative parathyroidectomy, and therefore it was recommended that most patients with PHPT, even those who do not met criteria for surgery, still should be considered for a parathyroidectomy.[51,52] Therefore, The American Association of Endocrine Surgeons Guidelines for Definitive Management of Primary Hyperparathyroidism stated that parathyroidectomy is indicated for all symptomatic patients and should be considered for most asymptomatic patients. Parathyroidectomy is more cost-effective than observation or pharmacologic therapy. Parathyroidectomy is recommended regardless of the results of preoperative localizing studies for all patients who have met surgical criteria. Minimally invasive parathyroidectomy can achieve cure rate in up to 97%–99% of patients when IOPTH monitoring is used.[5] Minimally invasive approach showed no differences in recurrence compared to open technique.[49]

Over the last 2 decades, several new minimally invasive techniques of a parathyroidectomy including mini-open, video-assisted, and totally endoscopic approaches have developed. The benefits include a target surgical approach to the parathyroid adenoma, and the ability to perform a neck exploration with possible thyroid lobectomy without the need to convert to a standard open procedure. This allows for cosmetically pleasing and curative results.[53,54] Recently developed transoral endoscopic parathyroidectomy vestibular approach (TOEPVA) uses three incisions in the vestibule of the oral cavity and could be used as an option for selected patients who want to avoid a neck incision.[55] Robotic-assisted transaxillary parathyroidectomy has been described in small published series, but remained debatable in their role and benefit if any. The advantage of leaving no scar in the neck by concealing the scar in the axilla or infraclavicular area overweighed by the long procedure time and the extensive internal dissection that has to be performed to reach the parathyroid gland through such a remote approach. In contrast, robotic-assisted thoracoscopic approach would be the best surgical option to treat patients with an ectopic mediastinal parathyroid adenoma[56] (Fig. 7.5). Challenges in finding parathyroid adenoma lead to the search for different technical modalities. For example, one study has used a green fluorescence angiography to facilitate intraoperative parathyroid localization. Intravenously injected indocyanine green fluorescence angiography has helped to guide operative navigation and accurately localized the adenoma in 100% of patients in this study.[57] Near-infrared (NIR) auto-fluorescence were used first ex vivo, and then in vivo, to identify parathyroid glands during the surgery. Real-time NIR imaging based on parathyroid auto-fluorescence identified parathyroid glands in 98.8% of the cases.[58] In November 2018, U.S. Food and Drug Administration approved two devices that provide real-time location of parathyroid tissue during surgical procedure and avoid the need for a contrast agent. The Fluobeam 800 Clinic Imaging Device detects parathyroid tissue that emits a fluorescent glow when exposed to the device's light source. The Parathyroid Detection PTeye System detects parathyroid tissues in 93% of the cases by using a probe that emits fluorescence light and measures how the tissue reacts to the fluorescent light.[59]

Looking at the long-term recurrence risk after a parathyroidectomy, retrospective study by H. Chen et al. reported a 10-year recurrence rate of 14.8% with median recurrence time of 6.3 years. Forty-one percent recurrence occurred in the first 5 years after the initial parathyroidectomy; 65.5% in 10 years, and 34.5% at more than 10 years after the parathyroidectomy.[42] Oltmann et al. reported the outcome of 1371 patients after a parathyroidectomy over the period of more than 10 years. Recurrence rate was dependent on final IOPTH values. With an IOPTH drop of less than 40 pg/mL, 1 year recurrence rate was 0.5%, 2 years recurrence rate was 1.5%, and 5 years recurrence rate was 4.3%. In contrast, with IOPTH level above 60 pg/mL, the recurrence rate at 1 year was 3.7%, at 2 years was 9.5%, and at 5 years was 25.2%.[41]

Should an intraoperative frozen section be performed on the resected parathyroid adenoma? AAES Guidelines Recommendation 7-2 states that frozen section analysis may be used to confirm the resection of parathyroid tissue (weak recommendation; low-quality evidence).[5] Despite low-quality evidence stated in the guidelines, performing an intraoperative frozen section may be helpful when surgeon is not 100% convinced that what was excised was the parathyroid gland adenoma. A satellite thyroid nodule or lymph node may be visually resembling the parathyroid adenoma. Experienced pathologist can call a parathyroid adenoma on frozen section by detecting the rim of a normal parathyroid tissue surrounding the hyperplastic *intraparathyroidal* parathyroid adenoma. This facilitates in making the diagnosis of an adenoma rather than a diffuse parathyroid gland hyperplasia (although, multifocal microadenomas in all four parathyroid glands can also occur) (Fig. 7.6).

Summary. There is no difference in the long-term outcome of a minimally invasive parathyroidectomy compared to the standard open neck exploration. The cure rate of minimally invasive parathyroidectomy was achieved in 97%–99% of patients when an IOPTH monitoring was used. The concept of "minimally invasive surgery" underlines not only performing surgery through the small incision, but also achieving a *minimal surgical invasiveness*. The goals include limiting the extent of the underlying surgical dissection, decreasing the duration of surgery, minimizing postoperative pain and complication rate, and achieving long-term cure.

Surgeon' Experience and Definition of a High-Volume Surgeon

The experience of the surgeon has the most important role in the success of a parathyroidectomy. The success rate is higher and complications rate, length of stay, and cost are lower when parathyroidectomy is performed by a high volume, experienced surgeon. Recommendation 3-11 of the American Association of Endocrine Surgeons Guidelines for Definitive Management of Primary Hyperparathyroidism stated that "parathyroidectomy should be conducted by surgeons with adequate training and experience in management of PHPT." The guidelines defined that the success rate for surgeons

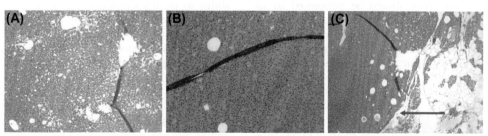

FIG. 7.6 H&E staining of the parathyroid adenoma showing the rim of tissue in between the area of the adenoma and a normal parathyroid gland (red arrow on the image "C"). **(A)** parathyroid adenoma, 100×; **(B)** parathyroid adenoma, 400×; **(C)** 40×, parathyroid adenoma to the left and normal portion of the parathyroid gland to the right.

who perform fewer than 10 parathyroidectomies per year is lower than for experienced surgeons performing more than 10 parathyroidectomies per year.[5]

Ten parathyroidectomies per year seem to be an extremely low number for the high-volume center or experienced surgeon. The earlier study by J. Sosa et al. had been more realistic in the definition of a "high-volume" surgeon. This study demonstrated that a high-volume surgeon is the one who performs more than 50 parathyroidectomies per year. The overall surgical cure rate was reported to be 95.2% after the primary operation and 82.7% after the reoperation. As predicted, the rate of intraoperative complications for a high-volume surgeon was 1.0%, which is significantly lower than 1.9% for a low-volume surgeon. The rate of reoperation was 1.5% for a high-volume surgeon and 3.8% for a low-volume surgeon. In-hospital mortality rates were lower than 0.04% for a high-volume surgeon when compared to 1.0% for a low-volume surgeon.[60] Considering hospitals volume, low-volume centers were defined as those performing less than 20 thyroidectomies/parathyroidectomies per year and high-volume centers as those performing ≥20 cases per year.[61] Similarly, H. Chen et al. defined a high-volume hospital as those performing more than 50 parathyroidectomies per year. Authors showed that high-volume centers are less likely to miss the parathyroid gland in a normal anatomic location compared to low-volume centers (13% vs. 89%).[62,63] In a study by M. Yeh et al., high-volume hospitals were defined as those performing >100 parathyroidectomies per year.[64] In more recent study published by M. Yeh et al., authors categorized hospitals by parathyroidectomy volume into a very low: 1–4 operations annually, low: 5–9, medium: 10–19, high: 20–49, and very high volume: 50 or more operations per year. Hospitals with high-volume parathyroidectomies had lower rates of complication and reoperations compared to low-volume hospitals.[65,66]

Summary. To minimize the complication rate, and decrease the rate of persistent and recurrent disease, the parathyroidectomy should be performed by an experienced high-volume parathyroid surgeon. A high-volume parathyroid surgeon is the one who is preforming more than 50 parathyroidectomies a year. This number is more realistic than 10 procedures per year stated in the recent AAES Guidelines.

Prediction and Treatment of Postoperative Hypocalcemia

Successful parathyroidectomy can result in acute serum calcium level drop after the surgery, which was reported as "temporary hypoparathyroidism" and "hungry bone syndrome." In P. Logerfo series of 1112 patients over a 17-year period published by Allendorf et al., the rate of transient hypocalcemia was reported to be 1.8%. All patients underwent bilateral neck explorations.[67] Mittendorf et al. reported the development of postparathyroidectomy hypocalcemia in 42% of patients in series of 132 patients with PHPT.[68] More recent date from Collaborative Endocrine Surgery Quality Improvement Program (CESQIP) from 2014 to 2017, summarized by J. Sosa et al., showed a 10.5% rate of hypocalcemia after remedial parathyroidectomy and 2.4% after an index parathyroidectomy.[69] Rate of permanent hypoparathyroidism is reported in up to 3.6% of patients after initial surgery, and the rate increases in patients after bilateral neck exploration.[5]

Studies showed that immediate postoperative PTH level is a predictor of the development of postoperative hypocalcemia symptoms.[70] Therefore, several studies tried to answer the question, what would be the best time point to measure the PTH level after the surgery and adequately predict postoperative hypocalcemia? A study of patients after a thyroidectomy showed that there was no statistically significant difference in predicting postoperative hypocalcemia when PTH levels when measured in 1 h after the surgery versus in 24 h after the surgery.[71] Barczyński M et al. tried to develop criteria of intraoperative IOPTH assay that would most accurately predict postoperative hypocalcemia after thyroid surgery. Their study of patients after a thyroidectomy showed that PTH levels less than 10 pg/mL at 4 h after the surgery with high accuracy predict the postoperative drop of serum calcium level below 8.02 mg/dL (2.0 mmol/L).[72] Intraoperative or early postoperative intact PTH levels less than 15 pg/mL increase the risk for symptomatic postoperative hypocalcemia. N. Crea et al. reported that 85% reduction in the IOPTH level is predictive in the development of postparathyroidectomy hypocalcemia in patients with PHPT.[73] An intact PTH level measured on postoperative day 1 after the parathyroidectomy showed the highest ability to predict temporary hypoparathyroidism, but not hungry bones syndrome. The best time for the evaluation of hungry bones syndrome was reported to be between postoperative day 5 and 7. Most centers perform the parathyroidectomy on an outpatient basis as the same day surgery; therefore, delayed assessment of PTH level is not always possible before the patient is discharged from the hospital. Due to the inability to predict the development of hungry bones syndrome and to prevent postoperative hypocalcemia, routine, empiric, prophylactic postoperative administration of oral calcium with vitamin D is recommended to avoid the development of symptoms in the early postoperative period.[5,70,74] Recent statement of the American Association of Clinical Endocrinologists and American College of Endocrinology recommended routine, prophylactic treatment with oral calcium with or without calcitriol for all patients after a parathyroidectomy to prevent transient hypocalcemia.[75] Oral calcium supplementation appeared to be the most cost-effective approach. If IOPTH value is measured at 20 min or longer after the parathyroidectomy is > 15 ng/mL, the patient can be discharged home on prophylactic oral calcium dose, which is between 500 mg and 1000 mg thrice a day. If IOPTH level <15 ng/mL, calcitriol at dose 0.5–1.0 mcg twice a day should be started in addition to calcium and, possibly, magnesium supplementation. Patient can be observed in the hospital overnight. In order for calcitriol to be effective, it may take up to 72 h. For patient who develops severe symptoms of postoperative hypocalcemia, intravenous calcium is administered as 1–2 g boluses in 50 mL of 5% dextrose infused over 20 min. If symptoms of severe hypocalcemia persist despite supplementation, then intravenous calcium infusion of a solution composed of 11 g of calcium gluconate added to normal saline or 5% dextrose water, to provide a final volume of 1000 mL, is administered at 50 mL/h intravenous infusion rate and adjusted to maintain the calcium level in the low normal range.[75]

REFERENCES

1. Bilezikian JP, Brandi ML, Eastell R, et al. Guidelines for the management of asymptomatic primary hyperparathyroidism: summary statement from the Fourth International Workshop. *J Clin Endocrinol Metab.* 2014;99(10):3561–3569.
2. Jolobe OM. Normal ionized serum calcium is a prerequisite for characterization of normocalcemic primary hyperparathyroidism. *Am J Med Sci.* 2012;343(6):512.
3. Babwah F, Buch HN. Normocalcaemic primary hyperparathyroidism: a pragmatic approach. *J Clin Pathol.* 2018;71(4):291–297.
4. Bilezikian JP, Silverberg SJ. Normocalcemic primary hyperparathyroidism. *Arq Bras Endocrinol Metabol.* 2010;54(2):106–109.
5. Wilhelm SM, Wang TS, Ruan DT, et al. The American association of endocrine surgeons guidelines for definitive management of primary hyperparathyroidism. *JAMA Surg.* 2016;151(10):959–968.
6. Udelsman R, Åkerström G, Biagini C, et al. The surgical management of asymptomatic primary hyperparathyroidism: proceedings of the Fourth International Workshop. *J Clin Endocrinol Metab.* 2014;99(10):3595–3606.
7. Eastell R, Brandi ML, Costa AG, D'Amour P, Shoback DM, Thakker RV. Diagnosis of asymptomatic primary hyperparathyroidism: proceedings of the Fourth International Workshop. *J Clin Endocrinol Metab.* 2014;99(10):3570–3579.
8. Bilezikian JP, Cusano NE, Khan AA, Liu JM, Marcocci C, Bandeira F. Primary hyperparathyroidism. *Nat Rev Dis Primers.* 2016;2:16033.
9. Solorzano CC, Carneiro-Pla D. Minimizing cost and maximizing success in the preoperative localization strategy for primary hyperparathyroidism. *Surg Clin.* 2014;94(3):587–605.
10. Arora S, Balash PR, Yoo J, Smith GS, Prinz RA. Benefits of surgeon-performed ultrasound for primary hyperparathyroidism. *Langenbeck's Arch Surg.* 2009;394(5):861–867.
11. Deutmeyer C, Weingarten M, Doyle M, Carneiro-Pla D. Case series of targeted parathyroidectomy with surgeon-performed ultrasonography as the only preoperative imaging study. *Surgery.* 2011;150(6):1153–1160.
12. Keidar Z, Solomonov E, Karry R, Frenkel A, Israel O, Mekel M. Preoperative [99mTc]MIBI SPECT/CT interpretation criteria for localization of parathyroid adenomas-correlation with surgical findings. *Mol Imag Biol.* 2017;19(2):265–270.
13. Neychev VK, Kouniavsky G, Shiue Z, et al. Chasing "shadows": discovering the subtleties of sestamibi scans to facilitate minimally invasive parathyroidectomy. *World J Surg.* 2011;35(1):140–146.
14. Thier M, Daudi S, Bergenfelz A, Almquist M. Predictors of multiglandular disease in primary hyperparathyroidism. *Langenbeck's Arch Surg.* 2018;403(1):103–109.
15. Harari A, Mitmaker E, Grogan RH, et al. Primary hyperparathyroidism patients with positive preoperative sestamibi scan and negative ultrasound are more likely to have posteriorly located upper gland adenomas (PLUGs). *Ann Surg Oncol.* 2011;18(6):1717–1722.
16. Skandarajah AR, Palazzo FF, Henry JF. Lithium-associated hyperparathyroidism: surgical strategies in the era of minimally invasive parathyroidectomy. *World J Surg.* 2011;35(11):2432–2439.
17. Ippolito G, Palazzo FF, Sebag F, Henry JF. Long-term follow-up after parathyroidectomy for radiation-induced hyperparathyroidism. *Surgery.* 2007;142(6):819–822; discussion 822.e1.
18. Abbott DE, Cantor SB, Grubbs EG, et al. Outcomes and economic analysis of routine preoperative 4-dimensional CT for surgical intervention in de novo primary hyperparathyroidism: does clinical benefit justify the cost? *J Am Coll Surg.* 2012;214(4):629–637; discussion 637-9.
19. Harari A, Zarnegar R, Lee J, Kazam E, Inabnet 3rd WB, Fahey 3rd TJ. Computed tomography can guide focused exploration in select patients with primary hyperparathyroidism and negative sestamibi scanning. *Surgery.* 2008;144(6):970–976; discussion 976-9.

20. Lubitz CC, Stephen AE, Hodin RA, Pandharipande P. Preoperative localization strategies for primary hyperparathyroidism: an economic analysis. *Ann Surg Oncol.* 2012; 19(13):4202–4209.

21. Wang TS, Cheung K, Farrokhyar F, Roman SA, Sosa JA. Would scan, but which scan? A cost-utility analysis to optimize preoperative imaging for primary hyperparathyroidism. *Surgery.* 2011;150(6):1286–1294.

22. McCoy KL, Ghodadra AG, Hiremath TG, et al. Sestamibi SPECT/CT versus SPECT only for preoperative localization in primary hyperparathyroidism: a single institution 8-year analysis. *Surgery.* 2018;163(3):643–647.

23. Madorin CA, Owen R, Coakley B, , et alLowe H, Nam K-H, Weber K, Kushnir L, Rios J, Genden E, Pawha PS, Inabnet WB. Comparison of radiation exposure and cost between dynamic computed tomography and sestamibi scintigraphy for preoperative localization of parathyroid lesions. *JAMA Surg.* 2013;148(6):500–503.

24. McMullen TP, Learoyd DL, Williams DC, Sywak MS, Sidhu SB, Delbridge LW. Hyperparathyroidism in pregnancy: options for localization and surgical therapy. *World J Surg.* 2010;34(8):1811–1816.

25. Azarbar S, Salardini A, Dahdah N, et al. A phase I-II, open-label, multicenter trial to determine the dosimetry and safety of 99mTc-sestamibi in pediatric subjects. *J Nucl Med.* 2015;56(5):728, 3.

26. Moosvi SR, Smith S, Hathorn J, Groot-Wassink. Evaluation of the radiation dose exposure and associated cancer risks in patients having preoperative parathyroid localization. *Ann R Coll Surg Engl.* 2017;99(5):363–368.

27. Hoang JK, Reiman RE, Nguyen GB, et al. Lifetime attributable risk of cancer from radiation exposure during parathyroid imaging: comparison of 4D CT and parathyroid scintigraphy. *AJR Am J Roentgenol.* 2015;204(5): W579–W585.

28. https://www.radiologyinfo.org/en/info.cfm?pg=safety-xray.

29. Maier GW, Kreis ME, Renn W, Pereira PL, Häring HU, Becker HD. Parathyroid hormone after adenectomy for primary hyperparathyroidism. A study of peptide hormone elimination kinetics in humans. *J Clin Endocrinol Metab.* 1998;83(11):3852–3856.

30. Irvin 3rd GL, Dembrow VD, Prudhomme DL. Operative monitoring of parathyroid gland hyperfunction. *Am J Surg.* 1991;162(4):299–302.

31. Irvin 3rd GL, Dembrow VD, Prudhomme DL. Clinical usefulness of an intraoperative "quick parathyroid hormone" assay. *Surgery.* 1993;114(6):1019–1022; discussion 1022-3.

32. Irvin 3rd GL, Deriso 3rd GT. A new, practical intraoperative parathyroid hormone assay. *Am J Surg.* 1994;168(5): 466–468.

33. Carneiro-Pla D. Contemporary and practical uses of intraoperative parathyroid hormone monitoring. *Endocr Pract.* 2011;17(Suppl 1):44–53.

34. Bieglmayer C, Prager G, Niederle B. Kinetic analyses of parathyroid hormone clearance as measured by three rapid immunoassays during parathyroidectomy. *Clin Chem.* 2002;48(10):1731–1738.

35. Carneiro DM, Irvin 3rd GL. New point-of-care intraoperative parathyroid hormone assay for intraoperative guidance in parathyroidectomy. *World J Surg.* 2002;26(8): 1074–1077.

36. Carneiro-Pla D. Recent findings in the use of intraoperative parathyroid hormone monitoring in parathyroid disease. *Curr Opin Oncol.* 2009;21(1):18–22.

37. Trinh G, Noureldine SI, Russell JO, et al. Characterizing the operative findings and utility of intraoperative parathyroid hormone (IOPTH) monitoring in patients with normal baseline IOPTH and normohormonal primary hyperparathyroidism. *Surgery.* 2017;161(1):78–86.

38. Calò PG, Pisano G, Loi G, et al. Intraoperative parathyroid hormone assay during focused parathyroidectomy: the importance of 20 minutes measurement. *BMC Surg.* 2013;13:36.

39. Carneiro-Pla DM, Solorzano CC, Lew JI, Irvin 3rd GL. Long-term outcome of patients with intraoperative parathyroid level remaining above the normal range during parathyroidectomy. *Surgery.* 2008;144(6):989–993; discussion 993-4.

40. Wharry LI, Yip L, Armstrong MJ, et al. The final intraoperative parathyroid hormone level: how low should it go? *World J Surg.* 2014;38(3):558–563.

41. Rajaei MH, Bentz AM, Schneider DF, Sippel RS, Chen H, Oltmann SC. Justified follow-up: a final ioPTH over 40 pg/mL is associated with an increased risk of persistence and recurrence in primary hyperparathyroidism. *Ann Surg Oncol.* 2015;22(2):454–459.

42. Lou I, Balentine C, Clarkson S, Schneider DF, Sippel RS, Chen H. How long should we follow patients after apparently curative parathyroidectomy? *Surgery.* 2017;161(1): 54–61.

43. Trinh G, Rettig E, Noureldine SI, et al. Surgical management of normocalcemic primary hyperparathyroidism and the impact of intraoperative parathyroid hormone testing on outcome. *Otolaryngol Head Neck Surg.* 2018; 159(4):630–637.

44. Javid M, Callender G, Quinn C, Carling T, Donovan P, Udelsman R. Primary hyperparathyroidism with normal baseline intraoperative parathyroid hormone: a challenging population. *Surgery.* 2017;161(2):493–498.

45. Orr LE, McKenzie TJ, Thompson GB, Farley DR, Wermers RA, Lyden ML. Surgery for primary hyperparathyroidism with normal non-suppressed parathyroid hormone can be both challenging and successful. *World J Surg.* 2018;42(2):409–414.

46. Lee S, Ryu H, Morris LF, et al. Operative failure in minimally invasive parathyroidectomy utilizing an intraoperative parathyroid hormone assay. *Ann Surg Oncol.* 2014; 21(6):1878–1883.

47. Starker LF, Fonseca AL, Tobias C, Udelsman R. Minimally invasive parathyroidectomy. *Int J Endocrinol.* 2011:1–8. Article ID 206502.

48. Henry JF. Minimally invasive thyroid and parathyroid surgery is not a question of length of the incision. *Langenbeck's Arch Surg.* September 2008;393(5):621−626.

49. Schneider D, Mazeh H, Chen H, Sippel R. Predictors of recurrence in primary hyperparathyroidism: an analysis of 1,386 cases. *Ann Surg.* 2014;259(3):563−568.

50. Morris LF, Lee S, Warneke CL, et al. Fewer adverse events after reoperative parathyroidectomy associated with initial minimally invasive parathyroidectomy. *Am J Surg.* 2014;208(5):850−855.

51. Walker MD, Silverberg SJ. Primary hyperparathyroidism. *Nat Rev Endocrinol.* 2018;14(2):115−125.

52. Stephen AE, Mannstadt M, Hodin RA. Indications for surgical management of hyperparathyroidism: a review. *JAMA Surg.* 2017;152(9):878−882.

53. Fouquet T, Germain A, Zarnegar R, et al. Totally endoscopic lateral parathyroidectomy: prospective evaluation of 200 patients. ESES 2010 Vienna presentation. *Langenbeck's Arch Surg.* 2010;395(7):935−940.

54. Bakkar S, Matteucci V, Corsini C, Pagliaro S, Miccoli P. Less is more: time to expand the indications for minimally invasive video-assisted parathyroidectomy. *J Endocrinol Investig.* 2017;40(9):979−983.

55. Sasanakietkul T, Carling T. Primary hyperparathyroidism treated by transoral endoscopic parathyroidectomy vestibular approach (TOEPVA). *Surg Endosc.* 2017;31(11):4832−4833.

56. Brunaud L, Li Z, Van Den Heede K, Cuny T, Van Slycke S. Endoscopic and robotic parathyroidectomy in patients with primary hyperparathyroidism. *Gland Surg.* 2016;5(3):352−360.

57. DeLong JC, Ward EP, Lwin TM, et al. Indocyanine green fluorescence-guided parathyroidectomy for primary hyperparathyroidism. *Surgery.* 2018;163(2):388−392.

58. De Leeuw F, Breuskin I, Abbaci M, et al. Intraoperative near-infrared imaging for parathyroid gland identification by auto-fluorescence: a feasibility study. *World J Surg.* 2016;40(9):2131−2138.

59. https://www.fda.gov/NewsEvents/Newsroom/Press Announcements/ucm624982.htm.

60. Sosa J, Powe N, Levine M, Udelsman R, Zeiger M. Profile of a clinical practice: Thresholds for surgery and surgical outcomes for patients with primary hyperparathyroidism: a national survey of endocrine surgeons. *J Clin Endocrinol Metab.* 1998;83(8):2658−2665.

61. Mitchell J, Milas M, Barbosa G, Sutton J, Berber E, Siperstein A. Avoidable reoperations for thyroid and parathyroid surgery: effect of hospital volume. *Surgery.* 2008;144(6):899−907.

62. Chen H, Wang T, Yen T, et al. Operative failures after parathyroidectomy for hyperparathyroidism: the influence of surgical volume. *Ann Surg.* 2010;252(4):691−695.

63. Zarebczan B, Chen H. Influence of surgical volume on operative failures for hyperparathyroidism. *Adv Surg.* 2011;45:237−248.

64. Yeh MW, Wiseman JE, Chu SD, et al. Population-level predictors of persistent hyperparathyroidism. *Surgery.* 2011;150:1113−1119.

65. Abdulla AG, Ituarte PH, Harari A, Wu JX, Yeh MW. Trends in the frequency and quality of parathyroid surgery: analysis of 17,082 cases over 10 years. *Ann Surg.* 2015;261(4):746−750.

66. Melfa G, Porello C, Cocorullo G, et al. Surgeon volume and hospital volume in endocrine neck surgery: how many procedures are needed for reaching a safety level and acceptable costs? A systematic narrative review. *Geka Chiryo.* 2018;39(1):5−11.

67. Allendorf J, DiGorgi M, Spanknebel K, Inabnet W, Chabot J, Logerfo P. 1112 consecutive bilateral neck explorations for primary hyperparathyroidism. *World J Surg.* 2007;31(11):2075−2080.

68. Mittendorf EA, Merlino JI, McHenry CR. Postparathyroidectomy hypocalcemia: incidence, risk factors, and management. *Am Surg.* 2004;70(2):114−119; discussion 119-20.

69. Kazaure HS, Thomas S, Scheri RP, Stang MT, Roman SA, Sosa JA. The devil is in the details: assessing treatment and outcomes of 6,795 patients undergoing remedial parathyroidectomy in the Collaborative Endocrine Surgery Quality Improvement Program. *Surgery.* 2019;165(1):242−249.

70. Kaderli RM, Riss P, Geroldinger A, Selberherr A, Scheuba C, Niederle B. Primary hyperparathyroidism: dynamic postoperative metabolic changes. *Clin Endocrinol.* 2018;88(1):129−138.

71. Yetkin G, Citgez B, Yazici P, Mihmanli M, Sit E, Uludag M. Early prediction of post-thyroidectomy hypocalcemia by early parathyroid hormone measurement. *Ann Ital Chir.* 2016;87:417−421.

72. Barczyński M, Cichoń S, Konturek A. Which criterion of intraoperative iPTH assay is the most accurate in prediction of true serum calcium levels after thyroid surgery? *Langenbeck's Arch Surg.* 2007;392(6):693−698.

73. Crea N, Pata G, Casella C, Cappelli C, Salerni B. Predictive factors for postoperative severe hypocalcaemia after parathyroidectomy for primary hyperparathyroidism. *Am Surg.* 2012;78(3):352−358.

74. Orloff LA, Wiseman SM, Bernet VJ, et al. American thyroid association statement on postoperative hypoparathyroidism: diagnosis, prevention, and management in adults. *Thyroid.* 2018;28(7):830−841.

75. Stack Jr BC, Bimston DN, Bodenner DL, et al. American Association of clinical Endocrinologists and American College of Endocrinology disease state clinical review: postoperative hypoparathyroidism - definitions and management. *Endocr Pract.* 2015;21(6):674−685.

CHAPTER 8

Advances in Diagnosis and Management of Secondary and Tertiary Hyperparathyroidism

WILLEMIJN Y. VAN DER PLAS, BSC, PHD • LIFFERT VOGT, MD, PHD • SCHELTO KRUIJFF, MD, PHD

INTRODUCTION

Hyperparathyroidism (HPT) is a condition in which the parathyroid glands produce too much of their parathyroid hormone (PTH). In primary HPT, this overproduction is in most cases caused by a single hyperplastic adenoma.[1] In contrast, secondary HPT and tertiary HPT are defined by parathyroid hormonal disturbances caused by an external stimulus. The most common cause of secondary HPT is end-stage renal disease (ESRD). Other causes include calcium malabsorption (e.g., by vitamin D deficiency, bariatric surgery, or celiac disease), the use of loop diuretics, bisphosphonates, or denosumab.[2] This chapter focuses on secondary and tertiary HPT caused by ESRD.

HPT secondary to renal failure has been described in case reports dating from the late 1930 and 1940s. At that time, however, the prognosis of ESRD was poor and patients did not live long enough to develop severe HPT. It was only after the Dutch physician Willem Johan Kolff built the first artificial dialyzer in 1943, that the life-expectancy of patients with renal failure started to increase.[3] Long-term hemodialysis was established with the development of the arteriovenous shunt in the early 1960s by Dr. Belding Scribner.[4,5] In the following years, patients lived longer, and subsequently, also started to develop novel complications secondary to chronic renal failure, which were previously not seen, including secondary HPT.

The parathyroid glands were first identified by Sir Richard Owen (1804–1892), who had been allowed to dissect and preserve all animals that died in the London Zoo.[6] In 1849, after 15 years of life in captivity, an Indian rhinoceros named Clara died during an altercation with an elephant. Sir Richard Owen spent over 12 months dissecting the 2000 kg weighing animal

investigating the cause of her tragedious death.[7] Clara appeared to have broken multiple ribs causing a pneumothorax. In his extensive anatomy report, Sir Richard Owen described "a small compact yellow glandular body attached to the thyroid."[6] Subsequently, it was the Swedish medical student Ivor Sandström (1852–1889) who named the glands after identifying the *glandulae parathyroideae* first in a canine specimen, and later in numerous other animal species, including 50 human bodies.[8]

FEEDBACK SYSTEM PARATHYROID, BONES, AND KIDNEY

Calcium and Phosphate

Calcium and phosphate homeostasis is regulated by a complex feedback system of the parathyroid glands, bone, and kidneys. Extracellular calcium comprises only 1% of the total calcium in the body as 99% is stored in bone. Calcium is of crucial importance in the coagulation cascade, signal transmission, and muscle contraction.[9] As with calcium, most phosphate is stored in the bones. Phosphate plays an important role in bone formation, neural impulse transmission, energy metabolism (as ATP), and serves as a compound of phospholipids. In healthy individuals, both serum calcium and phosphate concentrations are maintained in relatively narrow ranges. Nutrition is the only source of calcium and phosphate for humans. Calcium is mainly absorbed within the duodenum, jejunum, and ileum. The rate of absorption by the intestine is regulated by the presence of 1,25-dihydroxyvitamin D ($1,25(OH)_2D$) by influencing the permeability of calcium through the intracellular tight junctions of the intestinal lumen. In individuals with a healthy renal function, 99% of

Advances in Treatment and Management in Surgical Endocrinology. https://doi.org/10.1016/B978-0-323-66195-9.00008-X

calcium in the glomerular filtrate is reabsorbed within the renal tubules. The phosphate homeostasis is also regulated by the kidneys, by reabsorbing 80% of the filtered load, mainly within the proximal tubule. Phosphate is predominantly absorbed in the proximal small intestine, also under the influence of vitamin D.

PTH and the Parathyroid Glands

Serum calcium and phosphate levels are controlled by the influence of PTH on bones, kidneys, and the intestinal tract. In the bones, PTH binds to its receptors on osteoblasts that, via a complex ligand-dependent pathway, stimulate osteoclasts. In turn, osteoclasts enhance bone resorption through which calcium is released into the bloodstream.[10,11] PTH stimulates renal active reabsorption of calcium in the distal tubule, but has the opposite effect to phosphate. It inhibits the absorption of phosphate in the proximal tubule. Lastly, PTH enhances the activation of 25-hydroxycholecalciferol to $1,25(OH)_2D$, the active metabolite of vitamin D. As previously described, calcium absorption is regulated by $1,25(OH)_2D$ in the intestinal tract. Thus, the net effect of PTH is lowering serum phosphate levels, while increasing the serum calcium level (Fig. 8.1). Secretion of PTH by the chief parathyroid cells is strictly regulated and can alternate rapidly. The parathyroid gland is able to sense extracellular levels of calcium via the calcium-sensing receptor (CaSR) on the parathyroid cells. CaSR senses and maintains extracellular calcium concentration within a certain range by regulating parathyroid chief cell secretion of PTH.[12,13] The actions of increased extracellular levels of calcium on the CaSR lead to a reduction

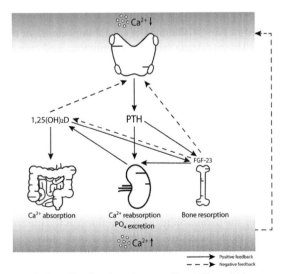

FIG. 8.1 Feedback system parathyroid/bone/kidney.

of serum calcium levels, mainly by inhibiting the release of secretary granules with PTH by the parathyroid glands, increasing urinary calcium excretion, and promoting calcitonin secretion.[14] Apart from the reduction of PTH secretion, CaSR stimulation reduces PTH synthesis in general, as well as parathyroid cell proliferation.[15] Thus, there is a direct relationship between serum PTH levels and levels of calcium illustrated by the sensitivity of the control mechanism.[16,17] The CaSR is also of importance in the kidneys, because it inhibits renal $1,25(OH)_2D$ production and calcium reabsorption by the thick ascending limb of the cortical tubule.[15] Lastly, the CaSR is present on the membrane of several cell types involved in bone metabolism and morphogenesis. In response to increased levels of $1,25(OH)_2D$, osteocytes and osteoclasts secrete the protein fibroblast growth factor (FGF) 23. In turn, FGF-23 acts on the sodium-phosphate cotransporter in the proximal tubules of the kidneys in the presence of membrane-bound protein Klotho, causing a decrease in the reabsorption and increase in excretion of phosphate. Thus, the net effect of FGF-23 is phosphatiuria.[18–20]

Definitions

The exact definitions of and distinction between secondary and tertiary HPT have been a matter of debate for many years. In general, secondary HPT is characterized by increased PTH levels in combination of hypocalcemia and hyperphosphatemia in the presence of ESRD. In tertiary HPT, patients have increased PTH levels, as well as hypercalcemia and hyperphosphatemia, due to a disturbed feedback system after prolonged period of secondary HPT. The severity of chronic kidney disease (CKD) can be divided in a 5-stage classification by the Kidney Disease Outcome Quality Initiative (K/DOQI) guidelines.[21] Stage 1 is defined by kidney damage with normal or elevated glomerular filtration rate (GFR) (>90 mL/min/1.73 m^2). Stages 2–4 represent mild-to-severe reduction in GFR. Patients with stage 5 kidney failure, also known as ESRD, have a GFR <15 mL/min/1.73 m^2, or require dialysis.

Pathogenesis of secondary and tertiary HPT

Early in the development of ESRD, hyperphosphatemia occurs due to excretion failure in the proximal tubule because of a decreased renal mass, and a failure of the kidneys to synthesize $(1,25(OH)_2D)$.[22,23] Together with a decreased serum concentration of calcium and increased levels of FGF-23, the parathyroid glands are stimulated to excrete PTH to return to homeostasis.[23]

In ESRD, the parathyroid glands are chronically exposed to this external stimulation, first leading to polyclonal, followed by monoclonal hyperplastic parathyroid tissue.[24] These morphologic changes are accompanied by a decreased expression of both the CaSR and the vitamin D receptor, although the number of secretory chief cells as well as the total number of parathyroid cells increases.[25,26]

Ultimately, this process leads to autonomous PTH synthetization and secretion, regardless of serum calcium concentrations. The parathyroid—bone—kidney feedback loop becomes irreversibly distorted. This leads to severe hypercalcemia, hyperphosphatemia, and HPT, also known as tertiary HPT. As mentioned previously, tertiary HPT is always preceded by a prolonged period of secondary HPT in ESRD patients and can be distinguished of secondary HPT by the presence of hypercalcemia. Monoclonal hyperplasia is often accompanied by nodules, further increasing the parathyroid mass. Tertiary HPT becomes most clear after successful kidney transplantation (KTx). By eliminating metabolic and biochemical disturbances with a successful KTx, the external stimulus triggering the parathyroid glands to produce and secrete PTH is removed. However, HPT only resolves spontaneously in 6 out of 10 patients after KTx, thus 40% of patients have continuous elevated PTH, calcium, and phosphate levels after KTx.[27] The exact role and timing of KTx in the treatment of secondary and tertiary HPT will be discussed further in this chapter.

Prevalence and incidence of ESRD and HPT
The worldwide prevalence of ESRD is 0.1%.[28] Since the last decade, the incidence of patients with ESRD requiring renal replacement therapy (RRT) has remained fairly stable over time.[29,30] More than 80% of the patients with a GFR rate below 20 mL/min/1.73 m², present with PTH levels above the upper limit of normal.[31] The prevalence of HPT (defined as PTH levels >300 pg/mL) in ESRD patients varies from 12% in Japan, to 54% in the United States of America.[32,33]

Clinical manifestations
Patients with severe hypercalcemia present with various serious conditions such as pruritus, bone pain, calciphylaxis, pathologic fractures, and muscle weakness. However, many patients with increased PTH and calcium levels also present with a wide range of nonspecific complaints that are less known such as concentration difficulties, feeling depressed, and forgetfulness (Fig. 8.2). In 1998, Pasieka et al. included all these symptoms in the parathyroidectomy assessment score, initially intended as a disease-specific outcome tool for patients with primary HPT undergoing parathyroidectomy.[34] Two years later, this questionnaire was also validated for patients with secondary and tertiary HPT.[35] The questionnaire consists of the following symptoms: pain in the bones, feeling tired easily, mood swings, feeling "blue" or depressed, pain in the abdomen, feeling weak, feeling irritable, pain in the joints, forgetfulness, difficulty getting out of a chair or car, headaches, itchy skin, and being thirsty.[34] In most patients, the previously described symptoms in HPT patients result in a significant decrease in quality of life.[36] On top of this, the PTH-mediated elevation of free calcium is responsible for much of the generalized organ

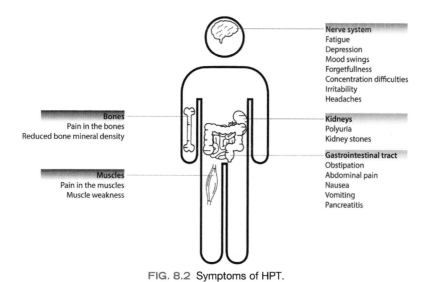

FIG. 8.2 Symptoms of HPT.

dysfunction accompanying ESRD.[37] These serious clinical manifestations may vary from progressive bone loss due to increased bone turnover to an increased risk of cardiovascular disease and mortality due to accelerated cardiovascular calcification.[38–41] The impact of long-term increased PTH, calcium, and phosphate levels on the kidney and especially on a future kidney transplant is a matter of debate. HPT in ESRD patients is an independent risk factor for renal graft loss and GFR decline after transplantation, as will be discussed further.[42,43] Lastly, both secondary and tertiary HPT have been associated with increased all-cause mortality.[41,42]

DIAGNOSIS

Diagnostic evaluation of secondary and tertiary HPT should be incorporated in the diagnostic workup for mineral and bone disorder (MBD) in every patient with CKD. According to the Kidney Disease—Improving Global Outcomes (KDIGO) guideline for CKD-MBD, physicians should start routinely measuring serum concentrations of PTH, calcium, phosphate, and alkaline phosphatase in CKD stage 3 every 6–12 months.[44] For patients with CKD stage 5, requiring RRT, serum calcium, phosphate, and PTH should be monitored every 3 months. Evidently, more frequent laboratory testing is recommended in case of rapidly progressive disease, changes in symptomatology, and during therapeutic interventions to closely monitor biochemical changes. No exact values or thresholds are currently defined by the KDIGO CKD-MBD Working Group for the diagnosis of HPT; however, it is recommended to focus particularly on the trend of the laboratory findings rather than on singular measurements to assess progression of HPT.

Serum Vitamin D

As vitamin D deficiency is common in ESRD, measurement of $25(OH)_2D$ levels is recommended and repeated testing determined by baseline values and therapeutic interventions. In practice, supplementation of $25(OH)_2D$ is usually started independent of its serum levels. The added value of repeated testing might therefore be low. Vitamin D deficiency is most commonly defined as serum $25(OH)_2D$ values below 10 ng/mL (or 25 nmol/L).[45] It should be noted that vitamin D represents both vitamin D_2 (ergocalciferol) as well as vitamin D_3 (cholecalciferol). The former is the main dietary source of vitamin D for humans. Cholecalciferol is synthesized when the skin is exposed to ultraviolet solar radiation, which contributes for 90% of human vitamin D requirements. Both vitamin D_2 and D_3 are functionally inactive,

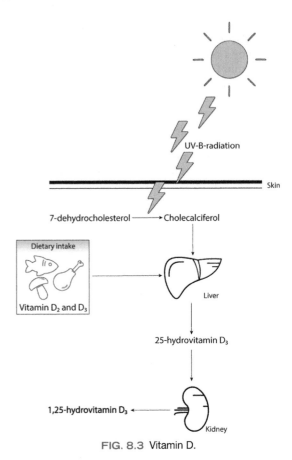

FIG. 8.3 Vitamin D.

and are only biologically available after hepatic hydroxylation into the active form of vitamin D 1,25-dihydroxycholecalcerferol ($1,25(OH)_2D$ (Fig. 8.3).[46]

Serum Calcium and Phosphate

Half of the serum calcium is bound to albumin, which makes it physiologically inactive. Serum ionized calcium is not bound to albumin and thus physiologically active. It is therefore essential to correct the measured serum calcium according to the concentration of circulating albumin. The following formula can be used to calculate corrected serum calcium:

$$corrected\ serum\ calcium(mmol/L)$$
$$= measured\ serum\ calcium(mmol/L)$$
$$+ (0.025 * (40 - [albumin\ g/L])$$

Reference range for corrected serum calcium is 8.5–10.5 mg/dL or 2.1–2.6 mmol/L. Healthy individuals maintain serum concentrations of phosphate between 2.5 and 4.5 mg/dL or 0.81 and 1.45 mmol/L. Serum calcium levels will be decreased in the early onset of secondary HPT, and increased in more severe secondary and tertiary HPT.

PTH

Modern assays for PTH measurement are increasingly accurate, detecting both the N-terminal of the 1-84-amino acid protein as well as the C-terminal. As PTH has a half-life of only a few minutes, it makes the circulating PTH level a reliable surrogate for parathyroid function in vivo. Reference range of PTH is extremely assay-dependent; however, serum PTH in healthy individuals is normally below 65 pg/mL or 7 pmol/L. In patients with ESRD, PTH levels >65 pg/mL or 7 pmol/L indicates secondary HPT. Again multiple testing is recommended to assess the progression of HPT. A tendency toward rising PTH levels suggests a higher risk of developing tertiary HPT and an increased risk of cardiovascular and bone mineral disease. The KDIGO CKD-MBD recommends treatment target levels of PTH <2−9 the upper limit of normal, which is practically impossible and maybe even undesirable. A large study using data from the international Dialysis Outcomes and Practice Patterns Study (DOPPS) investigating over 35,000 individuals on dialysis found an increased risk of all-cause mortality in patients with PTH levels above 300 pg/mL. Serum PTH levels >600 pg/mL were also found to be associated with an increased risk of cardiovascular mortality and all-cause and cardiovascular hospitalizations.[47] Nevertheless, the KDIGO CKD-MBD Working Group advices to maintain serum PTH levels between 2 and 9 times the upper limit normal of the used assay (130−585 pg/mL). The level of evidence for this recommendation is, however, weak, and the long-term effect of chronically elevated PTH levels remains unclear.

Parathyroid Imaging Studies

The confirmation of enlarged parathyroid glands with imaging studies, such as Technetium (99 mTc) sestamibi scan, computed tomography (CT), or magnetic resonance imaging (MRI), is not required and will not provide extra value confirming the diagnosis of secondary or tertiary HPT. Secondary and tertiary HPT are therefore solely biochemical diagnoses. The role of imaging during the preoperative workup when a PTx is indicated will be discussed later.

Differential Diagnosis Hyperparathyroidism and Hypercalcemia

In every ESRD patient with elevated PTH levels, primary HPT should be considered as concomitant diagnosis,

unrelated to renal failure. It is sometimes difficult to distinguish from secondary HPT, as concentrations of PTH and calcium can be elevated in both cases. However, patients with secondary HPT must have a history of initial decreased serum calcium levels in combination with increased PTH concentrations, before the development of hypercalcemia. In addition, PTH levels are often more profoundly elevated in secondary HPT patients. Other causes of secondary HPT are long-term use of the antidepressant lithium, isolated vitamin D deficiency, malabsorption (e.g., bariatric surgery or celiac disease), use of loop diuretics, bisphosphonates, or denosumab.

The differential diagnosis of hypercalcemia is much broader. Outside the hospital, primary HPT is responsible for 90% of hypercalcemia in combination with elevated PTH levels.[48] Another, much rarer, cause of PTH-dependent hypercalcemia is ectopic PTH production by small lung cancer or rare neuroendocrine tumors. Malignancy, often metastatic disease, is the predominant cause of hypercalcemia due to enhanced bone resorption in hospitalized patients.[48] In this case, the elevated serum calcium levels suppress the parathyroid glands to secrete PTH, thus measured PTH levels will be normal to low. There are several other endocrine diseases that may cause hypercalcemia such as thyrotoxicosis, pheochromocytoma, and adrenal insufficiency. Chronic granulomatous diseases such as sarcoidosis sometimes lead to elevated calcium levels, as familial hypocalciuric hypercalcemia does. Lastly, hypercalcemia can be part of hereditary endocrine syndromes such as multiple endocrine neoplasia type 1 and 2, familial isolated hyperparathyroidism and hyperparathyroidism-jaw tumor syndrome.[48]

THERAPY

The treatment of secondary HPT consists of a stepped approach according to stage of kidney failure, the severity of biochemical levels, and clinical features of the disease. The treatment options include vitamin D supplements, phosphate binders, calcimimetics, and parathyroid surgery. The management of secondary HPT remains complex as all variables in the calcium−phosphate−parathyroid hormone−vitamin D axis should be controlled. As mentioned earlier, evidence-based target levels for serum PTH concentrations are not available, and reaching target levels for calcium and phosphate is often challenging in these complex patients. Although the biochemical impact of the available treatment options is well investigated, most options lack evidence with regard to important patient outcomes such as quality of life, overall survival, progression of renal failure, and survival of kidney transplant. There are also only a handful of studies comparing the available treatment options, or combinations of them. Therefore, most of the recommendations made by the CKD-MBD KDIGO Working Group are based on level 2 (weak) and grade B or C (moderate of low quality) evidence.[44]

Vitamin D

Supplementation of vitamin D is one of the first steps in the prevention and treatment of secondary hyperparathyroidism. Vitamin D deficiency is already seen in almost 90% of predialysis patients, despite (excessive) sun exposure.[49] Different types of natural vitamin D sterols are to our availability: ergocalciferol, cholecalciferol, $25(OH)_2D$, and calcitriol. The first synthetic vitamin D was already produced for patients with rickets in 1927 by Merck and Bayer, but only became part of the treatment algorithm of secondary HPT in the 1960s. The following synthetic vitamin D_3 analogues are available: alfacalcidol, maxacalcitol, and falecalcitriol. In patients with low vitamin D levels, supplementation will prevent and treat a-dynamic bone disease, and prevents fractures, especially in postmenopausal women.[50,51] Inconsistent results have been found on the role of vitamin D supplementation in the prevention and treatment of cardiovascular diseases, endocrine disorders such as diabetes mellitus, neurologic diseases, and several forms of cancer.[46] Moreover, the effect of vitamin D supplementation in ESRD population on mortality, cardiovascular events, quality of life, but also fracture rate has never been evaluated in a prospective randomized controlled trial. Reported impact of vitamin D administration in the ESRD population is a decrease in serum concentration of PTH, a reduction of bone turnover, and reduced proteinuria.[52–55]

The KDIGO CKD-MBD guidelines recommend with a moderate level of evidence that calcitriol, or vitamin D analogs, should be used to lower the increasing PTH levels.[44] No consensus has been reached on the optimal target concentration and subsequently the optimal dosage of vitamin D supplementation in the general population, nor the ESRD population.[56] Weekly or monthly regimens are efficient to restore $25(OH)_2D$ concentrations due to the long half-life of cholecalciferol. A sum dosage of 50,000–100,000 IU per month seems adequate to normalize serum $25(OH)D$ levels in most of the patients.[56]

Overdose of vitamin D inducing toxicity (serum concentrations of $25(OH)_2D$ greater than 150 ng/mL) is very rare, but possible. This results mainly in hypercalcemia and hyperphosphatemia, and its related clinical manifestations such as nausea and vomiting, anorexia, and cardiac arrhythmias.[46,57] Therefore, the maximum dosage of vitamin D supplementation should be 4000 IU per day.[58]

Phosphate Binders

To control hyperphosphatemia, dietary restrictions (max. 800–1000 mg/day) are recommended, but appear difficult to adhere and a low phosphorus-diet alone seems insufficient. Therefore, almost every ESRD patient is administered phosphate binders. They can be divided into calcium-based phosphate binders and calcium-free phosphate binders. The first has the disadvantage of possibly inducing iatrogenic hypercalcemia; however, there is little evidence that they are superior to calcium-free phosphate binders. Calcium-based phosphate binders are, however, less costly compared to the noncalcium-containing binders. The KDIGO CKD-MBD guidelines suggest lower elevated serum phosphate concentrations toward the normal range.[44] Although hyperphosphatemia has been associated with increased mortality and morbidity, no randomized controlled trials have been conducted to investigate the effect of lowering serum phosphate levels on patient-related outcomes such as all-cause mortality, cardiovascular events, or quality of life.[59,60]

As phosphate retention is one of the earliest manifestations of renal excretion failure and secondary HPT, phosphate binders can be initiated as soon as PTH and FGF-23 levels start to rise.

Calcimimetics

Relatively new to the treatment algorithm of secondary HPT are calcimimetic agents. Calcimimetics are allosteric modulators of the CaSR, not only activating the CaSR itself, but also increasing the sensitivity of the CaSR to extracellular calcium. As a result, PTH production and excretion by the parathyroid glands is inhibited.[61] Calcimimetics are available both for oral use (cinacalcet) and for intravenous administration (etelcalcetide). To date, most secondary HPT patients are managed medically.

Cinacalcet

Cinacalcet, a second-generation calcimimetic, is available in tablets of 30, 60, and 90 mg. The initial dose is 30 mg per day, increased by using a dose titration protocol based on serum calcium and PTH levels, and side effects. Cinacalcet has half-life of 30–40 h and a steady-state is achieved in approximately 7 days. Maximum dose of cinacalcet is 180 mg a day.

Cinacalcet was approved for the treatment of secondary HPT in 2004. Initial studies showed that the treatment with cinacalcet is associated with a decrease of serum PTH, calcium, and phosphate levels, although moderately.[62] A meta-analysis comparing 24 RCTs with over 10,000 dialysis patients concluded that cinacalcet leads to a significant reduction of PTH (weighted mean difference of −206.5 pg/mL), calcium (weighted mean difference of −0.73 mg/dL), and phosphate (weighted mean difference of −0.38 mg/dL).[63] Circulating FGF-23 also decreases significantly with cinacalcet treatment. However, cinacalcet use is accompanied by various side effects such as nausea, vomiting, and diarrhea, and patients have an 8.2-fold increased risk of developing hypocalcemia when using cinacalcet (compared to placebo).[63] Drug adherence is therefore a major issue in ESRD patients who are already dealing with polypharmacy. In the real world-setting, the impact of calcimimetics on these biochemical values might therefore be less profound compared to its effect in patients enrolled in a study.[64] There are some studies suggesting that cinacalcet has a positive effect on bone resorption and formation markers, bone mineral disease, and fracture risk; however, others could not confirm these significant effects of cinacalcet.[63] Although improving biochemical levels, cinacalcet is not significantly associated with a decreased risk of all-cause and cardiovascular mortality.[63,65] Despite this, the international KDIGO CKD-MBD guidelines advise the administration of calcimimetics and/or calcitriol or vitamin D analogues for ESRD patients requiring PTH-lowering therapy.[44] Cinacalcet use has not been associated with an improvement in the quality of life of these patients. Thus, importantly, cinacalcet seems to improve biochemical values rather than clinical outcomes.[66] Finally, cinacalcet is only registered for hemodialysis patients and not for kidney transplant patients with persistent HPT, although frequently off-label prescribed.

Etelcalcetide

Twelve years after the introduction of cinacalcet, etelcalcetide was registered for the treatment of secondary HPT. In contrast to cinacalcet, the peptide etelcalcetide is a direct agonist of the CaSR, and therefore reduces circulating levels of PTH and calcium.[67] Its effect is enhanced by the presence of calcium. Etelcalcetide is available in doses of 2.5, 5, and 20 mg solutions for intravenous injection. The half-life of etelcalcetide is substantially longer than cinacalcet, exceeding 7 days. A sufficient plasma level of the drug is therefore achieved with a triweekly bolus injection that enables the administration during dialysis. This makes drug adherence easier for the ESRD patient. Etelcalcetide should be titrated with an initial dose of 2.5 or 5 mg bolus injection thrice a week, with a maximum dose of a total of 45 mg (in three gifts) a week. Etelcalcetide was both compared to placebo as to its precursor cinacalcet.[68,69] A reduction of PTH to ≤300 pg/mL was achieved in almost half of the patients who received etelcalcetide. With the introduction of a new calcimimetic drug administered intravenously, it was expected that the common side effects such as nausea, vomiting, and diarrhea would diminish by bypassing the gastrointestinal tract. However, when comparing etelcalcetide with cinacalcet, no significant difference was found in the occurrence of these adverse events.[68] Eighty percent of the patients using etelcalcetide reach an FGF-23 reduction of over 30% after 27 weeks.[69] Studies investigating the long-term effects of etelcalcetide on MBD, overall survival, and cardiovascular events are not available yet. Overall, it seems that etelcalcetide is more effective in lowering PTH levels compared to cinacalcet, which might implicate that the risk of subsequent complications of chronically elevated PTH levels is therefore also decreased. The incremental cost-effectiveness ratio of etelcalcetide compared to cinacalcet is between €24,521 (US$28,833) and €47,687 (US$56,073) per quality adjusted life years.[70] Therefore, etelcalcetide should only be prescribed for patients who do not respond sufficiently to initial cinacalcet treatment. As cinacalcet, etelcalcetide is only registered for the treatment of secondary HPT, not for tertiary HPT.

Surgical Management
Parathyroid surgery
Parathyroid surgery is the most classic available treatment for HPT. The first parathyroidectomy (PTx) was performed by Dr. Mandl in 1925 in Vienna, in a male tram car conductor with advanced osteitis fibrosa (extreme weakening of the bones due to HPT).[71] He excised an enlarged parathyroid gland, after which the patients' health improved remarkably. Perhaps, the most notable case of an HPT patient who underwent a PTx was Captain Charles Martell. Between 1926 and 1932, surgeons unsuccessfully attempted to resect his parathyroid glands six times, after which the captain himself suggested that the parathyroid gland might be located in the mediastinum.[72] Unfortunately, 6 months after a successful mediastinal exploration, Martell died of iatrogenic hypocalcemia. Surgeons started to operate on the parathyroid glands in patients with ESRD-related HPT in the early 1960s. Before the calcimimetic era, PTx was the only next step when the HPT was insufficiently

controlled by vitamin D analogues and/or phosphate binders.

Indications for PTx

PTx in only indicated in case of tertiary HPT, defined as hypercalcemia and elevated HPT levels. The aforementioned KDIGO CKD-MBD guidelines state that PTx is indicated in patients with ESRD and severe HPT who fail to respond to pharmacological treatment.[44] However, there is no consensus between nephrologists and surgeons regarding the exact indication criteria for PTx in patients on dialysis. Japanese surgical guidelines conclude that indications for PTX include the following: high levels of PTH (>500 pg/mL); detection of enlarged parathyroid glands (volume >500 m^3) by imaging; hypercalcemia (>10.2 mg/dL); hyperphosphatemia (>6.0 mg/dL).[73] Absolute criteria for PTx in ESRD patients according to the authors of the guideline are high bone turnover, osteitits fibrosa on X-ray, severe symptoms, progressive ectopic calcification, calciphylaxis, progression of bone loss, and anemia resistant to erythropoeitin.[73] An absolute contraindication is preoperative hypocalcemia.

In 2015, the European Society of Endocrine Surgeons established a consensus report regarding the surgical management of HPT in patients with ESRD.[74] According to this consensus statement, PTx is indicated when medical treatment fails to correct metabolic parameters (PTH >800 pg/mL, hypercalcemia, hyperphosphatemia). Next, PTx is valuable in those with severe symptoms such as pruritus, bone pain, and calciphylaxis.

The role of PTx in asymptomatic patients is debatable. As the PTH level >600 pg/mL has been identified as an independent risk factor for all-cause mortality, cardiovascular mortality, and all-cause and cardiovascular hospitalizations, PTx is also indicated in asymptomatic patients with PTH levels persistently exceeding 600 pg/mL.[47]

Overall, the selection of dialysis patients with tertiary HPT suitable for PTx must be individualized. Factors such as course of biochemical values over time, comorbidity, age, chance of prompt kidney transplantation, severity of biochemical status and symptoms, and patients' preference should be considered. In general, the aim of PTx should be to achieve long-term biochemical values within the recommended range, amelioration of symptoms related to HPT, and improvement of clinical outcome measures such as overall and disease-specific survival, cardiovascular risk, and fracture risk.[74]

For patients with persistent HPT after KTx, PTx has a more prominent role in the treatment algorithm, as calcimimetics are not registered for these patients (although frequently prescribed).

Preoperative imaging

The beneficial role of preoperative imaging in patients with four-gland hyperplasia that will undergo a four-gland exploration is debatable. Sensitivity of ultrasound (US) for detection of enlarged parathyroid glands is only 63%–81% in patients with secondary HPT compared to 99% in patients with one enlarged adenoma in primary HPT.[75–77] The combination of SPECT-CT and US seems to have an increased sensitivity to US alone.[76] The question is whether the preoperative identification of the parathyroid glands in the neck area by imaging has any intraoperative surgical consequences. Imaging might be of value to detect potential (intra-mediastinal) ectopic glands. Technetium sestamibi is of no value before primary surgery in patients with secondary or tertiary HPT.

Surgical anatomy

Four parathyroid glands are normally found in the superior and inferior regions posteriorly of both sides of the thyroid, although their localizations vary widely.[78] Other than being close neighbors, the thyroid and parathyroid glands are not functionally related (Fig. 8.4). The beanlike shaped soft glands weigh usually between 30 and 40 mg per gland. In 4%–18%, less than four glands are found in autopsy studies and approximately in 5% of individuals, supernumerary parathyroid glands are found.[78,79] Parathyroid glands generally receive their blood supply by the inferior thyroid arteries (Fig. 8.4). To perform a PTx, the patient requires general anesthesia. After a transverse "collar" incision, also known as Kocher's thyroid 3–5 cm incision (named after Dr. Theodor Kocher, one of the leading thyroid surgeons of the 19th century), platysma and strap muscles are divided to expose the thyroid gland and parathyroid glands. First, the parathyroid glands are searched superior and inferior of the posterior thyroid gland by mobilizing and anteriomedially retracting the thyroid gland. When not all four parathyroid glands are found in normal anatomic locations, further exploration is necessary and a thymectomy might be required.

PTx approaches

In contrast to primary HPT, in which mostly only one parathyroid gland is enlarged, all four glands are frequently hyperplastic in ESRD-related HPT.

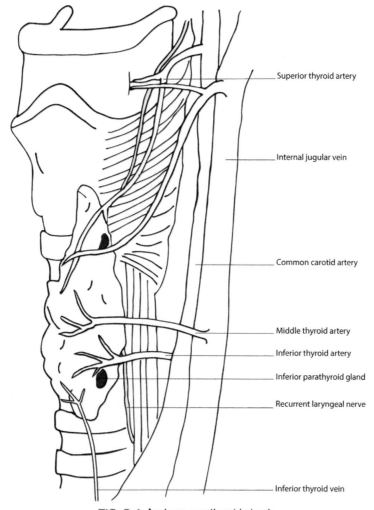

FIG. 8.4 Anatomy parathyroid glands.

Consequently, patients with ESRD patients, when referred for surgery, should undergo a four-gland exploration. Over the years, different surgical approached were described. Two surgical techniques are mostly used worldwide and are considered standard procedures for patients with ESRD-related HPT.[74,80] These strategies include subtotal PTx, resecting 3.5 of the four parathyroid glands, leaving half of the most normal-appearing gland (30–50 mg) in situ, and total PTx, resecting all four glands. For the latter, half of one the resected glands can be autotransplanted (AT) in either the sternocleidomastoid muscle or the brachioradial muscle of the nondominant forearm.

During parathyroid surgery, surgical adjuncts such as recurrent laryngeal nerve monitoring and intraoperative PTH measurements may be used. The clinical benefit of recurrent laryngeal nerve monitoring during PTx for secondary or tertiary HPT is unknown, but might especially be of assistance during difficult cases such as reoperative setting. Intraoperative PTH monitoring is possible due to the short half-life of PTH and can be of value when the surgeon is not sure whether enough parathyroid tissue is resected.[81]

Outcomes of PTx

Subtotal PTx has been shown to be a very effective and safe procedure for patients with ESRD-related HPT. PTH levels decrease immediately after surgery, with a PTH drop between 85% and 95%.[82–84] Recurrence disease occurs in between 4% and 13% of the cases and scar tissue complicates a potential reoperation in case of recurrent or persistent disease, which increases the risk of recurrent laryngeal nerve damage (7% vs. 1% after primary surgery).[80,85−87] In subtotal PTx, it is important that the remnant parathyroid tissue is still well vascularized after surgery. This appears sometimes to be a difficulty, resulting in hypoparathyroidism postoperatively. The reported rate of permanent hypoparathyroidism after subtotal PTx is approximately 2%.[74]

Total PTx with AT also effectively decreases PTH, calcium, and phosphate levels.[83,86] In 2017, a systematic review and meta-analysis was published comparing the outcomes of subtotal PTx with total PTx with AT for patients with ESRD-related HPT.[88] The authors evaluated a total of approximately 1600 patients of in total 13 studies comparing both approaches. There was no significant difference in the rate of persistent or recurrent disease (OR 1.31; 95% confidence interval 0.02−1.56, $P = .90$) between the two procedures. Next, the reoperation rate was similar for both groups.

After (sub)total PTx, serum calcium and phosphate concentrations decrease significantly to within the normal range.[83,89,90] Observational studies have shown that PTx reduces mortality, the risk of cardiovascular events and fracture risk significantly.[91−95]

Total PTx without AT has also been one of the treatment options. However, this approach leaves the patient with complete hypoparathyroidism which is, not desirable, considering the negative consequences of chronic hypoparathyroidism and hypocalcemia.

Role of KTx and timing of PTx
As chronic kidney failure is the underlying cause of secondary and tertiary HPT, the ultimate treatment for these patients is kidney transplantation. Indeed, a reduction of parathyroid functional mass has been seen after kidney transplantation.[96] However, a study investigating 1690 patients with HPT undergoing KTx showed that KTx cured HPT in 30% of the cases after 1 year, and 57% of the cases 2 years after KTx. Therefore, in patients with persistent HPT after KTx, pragmatically, it could be a fruitful strategy to wait at least 2 years after transplantation to proceed with PTx. On top of this, a decrease in graft function has been reported in patients undergoing PTx within 1 year after KTx.[97,98] On the other hand, HPT before KTx has been identified as an independent risk factor for graft loss, and all-cause mortality in transplant recipients.[42] Thus, the optimal timing of PTx with regard to KTx remains a matter of debate and should be carefully evaluated for every individual patient.

PROGNOSIS
The clinical consequences of long-term HPT in patients with ESRD are serious: an increased PTH level of >600 pg/mL has proved to be an independent risk factor of all-cause and cardiovascular mortality and hospitalization.[47] Furthermore, hypocalcemia in secondary HPT is independently associated with more rapid CKD progression.[99] Next, patients with hypercalcemia have a high risk for death compared to patients that are normocalcaemic.[100] Vascular calcification is seen more frequently in patients with increased serum phosphate concentrations.[101] In summary, HPT causes both short-term as well as long-term complications that should be adequately treated. Mild-to-moderate HPT patients will benefit from pharmacological treatment with vitamin D analogues, phosphate binders, and calcimimetics. Severe and prolonged HPT in symptomatic patients should be treated by means of PTx, which is very safe and effective in these fragile patients.

SUMMARY
HPT is a common complication secondary to ESRD. Secondary HPT is characterized by the development of increased PTH levels in response to phosphate retention, decreased vitamin D and calcium levels, and increased FGF-23 concentration due to renal excretion failure. Tertiary HPT develops after prolonged secondary HPT and is defined by an autonomous production and secretion of PTH levels in combination with increased calcium and phosphate levels. Signs and symptoms of hyperparathyroidism include abdominal pain, constipation, nausea and vomiting, pancreatitis, fatigue, depression, concentration difficulties, irritability, muscle weakness and pain, osteoporosis, and pain in the joints and bones. These clinical manifestations result in a decreased quality of life in patients with often multiple comorbidities. Long-term complications of ESRD-related HPT are increased risk of all-cause and cardiovascular mortality, vascular and extravascular calcifications, osteoporosis, increased fracture risk, and an increased risk of adverse outcomes of KTx in the future.

Diagnosis is established by the measurement of serum PTH, calcium, phosphate, and vitamin D concentrations multiple times over a longer period of time. The course of these biochemical values is essential in determining the optimal treatment for the individual patient. Imaging of the parathyroid glands is not required for establishing the diagnosis HPT, however, could be of use within the preoperative workup.

Up to 2018, the only international guidelines for the treatment of secondary and tertiary HPT available are the monodisciplinary CKD-MBD guideline of the KDIGO Working Group.[44] There is no consensus between treating nephrologists and surgeons about the use of the different available treatment options. In general, patients with kidney failure progressing toward ESRD receive vitamin D supplements to correct for their low $1,25(OH)_2D$ status. Phosphate binders should be administered in an early phase of ESRD to decrease serum phosphate concentrations in attempt to prevent progression to secondary HPT. Unfortunately, in most patients, vitamin D analogues and phosphate binders are not sufficient to prevent HPT progression. Hypocalcemia can be treated by calcium supplements. For patients with tertiary HPT (e.g., HPT in combination with hypercalcemia), calcimimetics should be prescribed as initial treatment. The oral calcimimetic cinacalcet can be administered in doses up to 180 mg daily and significantly lowers PTH and calcium concentrations.[62,63] The EVOLVE trial showed that cinacalcet does not lower the risk on all-cause and cardiovascular death.[65] Cinacalcet seems to lower mineral and bone disorder (MBD) biomarkers; however, it is unknown if this results in a decrease of the risk of fractures, and its positive impact on symptom amelioration and quality of life has not been shown.[44] The introduction of cinacalcet in 2004 has changed the treatment algorithm of ESRD-related HPT.[21,44,102] For instance, PTx rates decreased significantly since the advent of calcimimetics.[103−106] A study evaluating the impact of the introduction of cinacalcet on the treatment of ESRD-related HPT concluded that the introduction of cinacalcet led to a 2-year delay of definite surgical treatment.[107] Nevertheless, PTx is still indicated in patients with severe (>600−800 pg/mL) HPT, uncontrollable hypercalcemia, severe symptoms, and signs of MBD.[44,74] The outcomes of the preferred surgical strategies, subtotal PTx or total PTx with autotransplantation, have similar outcomes with regard to amelioration of biochemical values and risk of persistent or recurrent disease.[88] The risk of mortality and cardiovascular events, and fracture risk reduce significantly after PTx.[91−95]

There is only one randomized controlled trial comparing cinacalcet with PTx directly in patients with persistent HPT after KTx.[108] At 12 months, PTx was found to be superior compared to treatment with cinacalcet in controlling hypercalcemia and reducing PTH levels. A multicenter randomized controlled trial investigating dialysis patients is highly warranted, but not yet performed.[104,109] A systematic review comparing the effects of cinacalcet and PTx on quality of life concluded that PTx significantly improves quality of life, whereas cinacalcet does not.[66]

In the future, the treatment algorithm of ESRD-related HPT will most definitely keep evolving. The role of the new intravenous calcimimetic, etelcalcetide, is yet to be found out in the next few years. Next, improving dialysis solutions and increasing availability of donor kidneys might result in a reduction of the incidence of (severe) HPT.

REFERENCES

1. Wilhelm SM, Wang TS, Ruan DT, et al. The American association of endocrine surgeons guidelines for definitive management of primary hyperparathyroidism. *JAMA Surg.* 2016;151(10):959. https://doi.org/10.1001/jamasurg.2016.2310.
2. Rosen CJ, Bouillon R, Compston J, Rosen V. *Primer on the Metabolic Bone Diseases and Disorders of Mineral Metabolism.* Wiley-Blackwell; 2013. https://www.wiley.com/en-us/Primer+on+the+Metabolic+Bone+Diseases+and+Disorders+of+Mineral+Metabolism%2C+8th+Edition-p-9781118453889.
3. Kolff WJ. First clinical experience with the artificial kidney. *Ann Intern Med.* 1965;62(3):608. https://doi.org/10.7326/0003-4819-62-3-608.
4. Scribner BH, Buri R, Caner JE, Hegstrom R, Burnell JM. The treatment of chronic uremia by means of intermittent hemodialysis: a preliminary report. *Trans Am Soc Artif Intern Organs.* 1960;6:114−122. http://www.ncbi.nlm.nih.gov/pubmed/13749429.
5. Quinton W, Dillard D, Scribner BH. Cannulation of blood vessels for prolonged hemodialysis. *Trans Am Soc Artif Intern Organs.* 1960;6:104−113. http://www.ncbi.nlm.nih.gov/pubmed/13738750.
6. Owen S. On the anatomy of the Indian rhinoceros. *Trans Zool Soc Lond.* 1862;4(2):31−58. https://doi.org/10.1111/j.1469-7998.1862.tb08046.x.
7. Modarai B, Sawyer A, Ellis H. The glands of owen. *J R Soc Med.* 2004;97(10):494−495. https://doi.org/10.1258/jrsm.97.10.494.
8. Sandström I. Om en ny körtel hos menniskan och åtskilliga däggdjur. *Ups Läk Förh.* 1880;XV:441−471.
9. Jacobson HR, Harry R, Striker GE, Klahr S. *The Principles and Practice of Nephrology.* Mosby-Year Book; 1995.
10. Hall JE, John E, Guyton AC. *Guyton and Hall Textbook of Medical Physiology.* Saunders Elsevier; 2011.
11. Poole K, Reeve J. Parathyroid hormone — a bone anabolic and catabolic agent. *Curr Opin Pharmacol.* 2005;5(6):612−617. https://doi.org/10.1016/j.coph.2005.07.004.
12. Bräuner-Osborne H, Wellendorph P, Jensen AA. Structure, pharmacology and therapeutic prospects of family C G-protein coupled receptors. *Curr Drug Targets.* 2007;8(1):169−184. http://www.ncbi.nlm.nih.gov/pubmed/17266540.

13. Filopanti M, Corbetta S, Barbieri AM, Spada A. Pharmacology of the calcium sensing receptor. *Clin Cases Miner Bone Metab*. 2013;10(3):162–165. http://www.ncbi.nlm.nih.gov/pubmed/24554924.

14. Tfelt-Hansen J, Brown EM. The calcium-sensing receptor in normal physiology and pathophysiology: a review. *Crit Rev Clin Lab Sci*. 2005;42(1):35–70. http://www.ncbi.nlm.nih.gov/pubmed/15697170.

15. Brown EM. Clinical lessons from the calcium-sensing receptor. *Nat Clin Pract Endocrinol Metabol*. 2007;3(2): 122–133. https://doi.org/10.1038/ncpendmet0388.

16. Ward DT, Riccardi D. New concepts in calcium-sensing receptor pharmacology and signalling. *Br J Pharmacol*. 2012;165(1):35–48. https://doi.org/10.1111/j.1476-5381.2011.01511.x.

17. Mayer GP, Hurst JG. Sigmoidal relationship between parathyroid hormone secretion rate and plasma calcium concentration in calves. *Endocrinology*. 1978;102(4): 1036–1042. https://doi.org/10.1210/endo-102-4-1036.

18. Quarles LD. Role of FGF23 in vitamin D and phosphate metabolism: implications in chronic kidney disease. *Exp Cell Res*. 2012;318(9):1040–1048. https://doi.org/10.1016/j.yexcr.2012.02.027.

19. Jüppner H. Phosphate and FGF-23. *Kidney Int Suppl*. 2011; 79(121):S24–S27. https://doi.org/10.1038/ki.2011.27.

20. Razzaque MS. The FGF23–Klotho axis: endocrine regulation of phosphate homeostasis. *Nat Rev Endocrinol*. 2009; 5(11):611–619. https://doi.org/10.1038/nrendo.2009.196.

21. National Kidney Foundation. K/DOQI clinical practice guidelines for bone metabolism and disease in chronic kidney disease. *Am J Kidney Dis*. 2003; 42(4 suppl 3):S1–S201. http://www.ncbi.nlm.nih.gov/pubmed/14520607.

22. Hruska KA, Mathew S, Lund R, Qiu P, Pratt R. Hyperphosphatemia of chronic kidney disease. *Kidney Int*. 2008; 74(2):148–157. https://doi.org/10.1038/ki.2008.130.

23. Cunningham J, Locatelli F, Rodriguez M. Secondary hyperparathyroidism: pathogenesis, disease progression, and therapeutic options. *Clin J Am Soc Nephrol*. 2011; 6(4):913–921. https://doi.org/10.2215/CJN.06040710.

24. Drüeke TB. Cell biology of parathyroid gland hyperplasia in chronic renal failure. *J Am Soc Nephrol*. 2000;11: 1141–1152. http://jasn.asnjournals.org/content/11/6/1141.full.pdf.

25. Lewin E, Garfia B, Recio FL, Rodriguez M, Olgaard K. Persistent downregulation of calcium-sensing receptor mRNA in rat parathyroids when severe secondary hyperparathyroidism is reversed by an isogenic kidney transplantation. *J Am Soc Nephrol*. 2002;13(8):2110–2116. http://www.ncbi.nlm.nih.gov/pubmed/12138143.

26. Canadillas S, Canalejo A, Santamaría R, et al. Calcium-sensing receptor expression and parathyroid hormone secretion in hyperplastic parathyroid glands from humans. *J Am Soc Nephrol*. 2005;16(7):2190–2197. https://doi.org/10.1681/ASN.2004080657.

27. Lou I, Foley D, Odorico SK, et al. How well does renal transplantation cure hyperparathyroidism? *Ann Surg*. 2015;262(4):653–659. https://doi.org/10.1097/SLA.0000000000001431.

28. Hill NR, Fatoba ST, Oke JL, et al. Global prevalence of chronic kidney disease - a systematic review and meta-analysis. *PLoS One*. 2016;11(7):e0158765. https://doi.org/10.1371/journal.pone.0158765.

29. Ward MM. Changes in the incidence of endstage renal disease due to lupus nephritis in the United States, 1996–2004. *J Rheumatol*. 2009;36(1):63–67. https://doi.org/10.3899/jrheum.080625.

30. Zoccali C, Kramer A, Jager KJ. Chronic kidney disease and end-stage renal disease–a review produced to contribute to the report "the status of health in the European Union: towards a healthier Europe.". *Clin Kidney J*. 2010;3(3): 213–224. https://doi.org/10.1093/ndtplus/sfp127.

31. Levin A, Bakris GL, Molitch M, et al. Prevalence of abnormal serum vitamin D, PTH, calcium, and phosphorus in patients with chronic kidney disease: results of the study to evaluate early kidney disease. *Kidney Int*. 2007;71(1):31–38. https://doi.org/10.1038/sj.ki.5002009.

32. The Japanese Society of Dialysis and Transplant. http://www.jsdt.or.jp/index_e.html. Published 2015.

33. Arbor Research Collaborative for Health. Dialysis Outcomes Practice Patterns Study (DOPPS) Practice Montior. https://www.dopps.org/DPM/. Published 2015.

34. Pasieka JL, Parsons LL. Prospective surgical outcome study of relief of symptoms following surgery in patients with primary hyperparathyroidism. *World J Surg*. 1998; 22:513–519. https://link-springer-com.proxy-ub.rug.nl/content/pdf/10.1007%2Fs002689900428.pdf.

35. Pasieka JL, Parsons LL. A prospective surgical outcome study assessing the impact of parathyroidectomy on symptoms in patients with secondary and tertiary hyperparathyroidism. *Surgery*. 2000;128(4):531–539. https://doi.org/10.1067/MSY.2000.108117.

36. Cheng SP, Lee JJ, Liu TP, et al. Parathyroidectomy improves symptomatology and quality of life in patients with secondary hyperparathyroidism. *Surgery*. 2014;155(2):320–328. https://doi.org/10.1016/j.surg.2013.08.013.

37. Massry SG, Fadda GZ. Chronic renal failure is a state of cellular calcium toxicity. *Am J Kidney Dis*. 1993;21(1): 81–86. http://www.ncbi.nlm.nih.gov/pubmed/8418632.

38. Block GA, Klassen PS, Lazarus JM, Ofsthun N, Lowrie EG, Chertow GM. Mineral metabolism, mortality, and morbidity in maintenance hemodialysis. *J Am Soc Nephrol*. 2004;15(8):2208–2218. https://doi.org/10.1097/01.ASN.0000133041.27682.A2.

39. Danese MD, Kim J, Doan QV, Dylan M, Griffiths R, Chertow GM. PTH and the risks for hip, vertebral, and pelvic fractures among patients on dialysis. *Am J Kidney Dis*. 2006;47(1):149–156. https://doi.org/10.1053/j.ajkd.2005.09.024.

40. Davies MR, Hruska KA. Pathophysiological mechanisms of vascular calcification in end-stage renal disease. *Kidney Int.* 2001;60(2):472–479. https://doi.org/10.1046/j.1523-1755.2001.060002472.x.

41. Floege J, Kim J, Ireland E, et al. Serum iPTH, calcium and phosphate, and the risk of mortality in a European haemodialysis population. *Nephrol Dial Transplant.* 2011;26(6):1948–1955. https://doi.org/10.1093/ndt/gfq219.

42. Pihlstrøm H, Dahle DO, Mjøen G, et al. Increased risk of all-cause mortality and renal graft loss in stable renal transplant recipients with hyperparathyroidism. *Transplantation.* 2015;99(2):351–359. https://doi.org/10.1097/TP.0000000000000583.

43. Parikh S, Nagaraja H, Agarwal A, et al. Impact of post-kidney transplant parathyroidectomy on allograft function. *Clin Transplant.* 2013;27(3):397–402. https://doi.org/10.1111/ctr.12099.

44. Kidney Disease: Improving Global Outcomes (KDIGO) CKD-MBD Update Work Group. KDIGO clinical practice guideline for the diagnosis, evaluation, prevention and treatment of chronic kidney disease mineral and bone disorder (CKD-MBD). *Kidney Int Suppl.* 2017;7:1–59. https://doi.org/10.1038/ki.2009.188.

45. Hollis BW. Assessment of vitamin D status and definition of a normal circulating range of 25-hydroxyvitamin D. *Curr Opin Endocrinol Diabetes Obes.* 2008;15(6):489–494. https://doi.org/10.1097/MED.0b013e328317ca6c.

46. Haines ST, Park SK. Vitamin D supplementation: what's known, what to do, and what's needed. *Pharmacotherapy.* 2012;32(4):354–382. https://doi.org/10.1002/phar.1037.

47. Tentori F, Wang M, Bieber BA, et al. Recent changes in therapeutic approaches and association with outcomes among patients with secondary hyperparathyroidism on chronic hemodialysis: the DOPPS study. *Clin J Am Soc Nephrol.* 2015;10(1):98–109. https://doi.org/10.2215/CJN.12941213.

48. Meng QH, Wagar EA. Laboratory approaches for the diagnosis and assessment of hypercalcemia. *Crit Rev Clin Lab Sci.* 2015;52(3):107–119. https://doi.org/10.3109/10408363.2014.970266.

49. Ngai M, Lin V, Wong HC, Vathsala A, How P. Vitamin D status and its association with mineral and bone disorder in a multi-ethnic chronic kidney disease population. *Clin Nephrol.* 2014;82(4):231–239. https://doi.org/10.5414/CN108182.

50. Rachner TD, Khosla S, Hofbauer LC. Osteoporosis: now and the future. *Lancet.* 2011;377(9773):1276–1287. https://doi.org/10.1016/S0140-6736(10)62349-5.

51. Bischoff-Ferrari HA, Willett WC, Wong JB, Giovannucci E, Dietrich T, Dawson-Hughes B. Fracture prevention with vitamin D supplementation. *J Am Med Assoc.* 2005;293(18):2257. https://doi.org/10.1001/jama.293.18.2257.

52. Alvarez JA, Law J, Coakley KE, et al. High-dose cholecalciferol reduces parathyroid hormone in patients with early chronic kidney disease: a pilot, randomized, double-blind, placebo-controlled trial. *Am J Clin Nutr.* 2012;96(3):672–679. https://doi.org/10.3945/ajcn.112.040642.

53. Kandula P, Dobre M, Schold JD, Schreiber MJ, Mehrotra R, Navaneethan SD. Vitamin D supplementation in chronic kidney disease: a systematic review and meta-analysis of observational studies and randomized controlled trials. *Clin J Am Soc Nephrol.* 2011;6(1):50–62. https://doi.org/10.2215/CJN.03940510.

54. Salusky IB, Kuizon BD, Belin TR, et al. Intermittent calcitriol therapy in secondary hyperparathyroidism: a comparison between oral and intraperitoneal administration. *Kidney Int.* 1998;54(3):907–914. https://doi.org/10.1046/j.1523-1755.1998.00045.x.

55. Kim MJ, Frankel AH, Donaldson M, et al. Oral cholecalciferol decreases albuminuria and urinary TGF-β1 in patients with type 2 diabetic nephropathy on established renin–angiotensin–aldosterone system inhibition. *Kidney Int.* 2011;80(8):851–860. https://doi.org/10.1038/ki.2011.224.

56. Jean G, Souberbielle JC, Chazot C. Vitamin D in chronic kidney disease and dialysis patients. *Nutrients.* 2017;9(4). https://doi.org/10.3390/nu9040328.

57. Holick MF. Vitamin D deficiency. *N Engl J Med.* 2007;357(3):266–281. https://doi.org/10.1056/NEJMra070553.

58. Institute of Medicine (US). Committee to review dietary reference intakes for vitamin D and calcium. In: Ross AC, Taylor CL, Yaktine AL, Valle Del HB, eds. *Dietary Reference Intakes for Calcium and Vitamin D.* National Academies Press (US); 2011. https://doi.org/10.17226/13050.

59. Covic A, Kothawala P, Bernal M, Robbins S, Chalian A, Goldsmith D. Systematic review of the evidence underlying the association between mineral metabolism disturbances and risk of all-cause mortality, cardiovascular mortality and cardiovascular events in chronic kidney disease. *Nephrol Dial Transplant.* 2009;24(5):1506–1523. https://doi.org/10.1093/ndt/gfn613.

60. Tentori F, Blayney MJ, Albert JM, et al. Mortality risk for dialysis patients with different levels of serum calcium, phosphorus, and PTH: the dialysis outcomes and practice patterns study (DOPPS). *Am J Kidney Dis.* 2008;52(3):519–530. https://doi.org/10.1053/j.ajkd.2008.03.020.

61. Nemeth EF, Steffey ME, Hammerland LG, et al. Calcimimetics with potent and selective activity on the parathyroid calcium receptor. *Proc Natl Acad Sci U S A.* 1998;95(7):4040–4045. https://doi.org/10.1073/PNAS.95.7.4040.

62. Block GA, Martin KJ, de Francisco ALM, et al. Cinacalcet for secondary hyperparathyroidism in patients receiving hemodialysis. *N Engl J Med.* 2004;350(15):1516–1525. https://doi.org/10.1056/NEJMoa031633.

63. Greeviroj P, Kitrungphaiboon T, Katavetin P, et al. Cinacalcet for treatment of chronic kidney disease-mineral and bone disorder: a meta-analysis of randomized controlled trials. *Nephron.* 2018;139(3):197–210. https://doi.org/10.1159/000487546.

64. Brunaud L, Ngueyon Sime W, Filipozzi P, et al. Minimal impact of calcimimetics on the management of hyperparathyroidism in chronic dialysis. *Surgery.* 2016; 159(1):183—192. https://doi.org/10.1016/j.surg.2015. 06.058.

65. The Evolve Trial Investigators. Effect of cinacalcet on cardiovascular disease in patients undergoing dialysis. *N Engl J Med.* 2012;367(26):2482—2494. https:// doi.org/10.1056/NEJMoa1205624.

66. van der Plas WY, Dulfer RR, Engelsman AF, et al. Effect of parathyroidectomy and cinacalcet on quality of life in patients with end-stage renal disease-related hyperparathyroidism: a systematic review. *Nephrol Dial Transplant.* 2017;32(11):1902—1908. https://doi.org/10.1093/ndt/gfx044.

67. Alexander ST, Hunter T, Walter S, et al. Critical cysteine residues in both the calcium-sensing receptor and the allosteric activator AMG 416 underlie the mechanism of action. *Mol Pharmacol.* 2015;88(5):853—865. https:// doi.org/10.1124/mol.115.098392.

68. Block GA, Bushinsky DA, Cheng S, et al. Effect of etelcalcetide vs cinacalcet on serum parathyroid hormone in patients receiving hemodialysis with secondary hyperparathyroidism. *J Am Med Assoc.* 2017;317(2):156. https://doi.org/10.1001/jama.2016.19468.

69. Block GA, Bushinsky DA, Cunningham J, et al. Effect of etelcalcetide vs placebo on serum parathyroid hormone in patients receiving hemodialysis with secondary hyperparathyroidism. *J Am Med Assoc.* 2017;317(2):146. https://doi.org/10.1001/jama.2016.19456.

70. Stollenwerk B, Iannazzo S, Akehurst R, et al. A decision-analytic model to assess the cost-effectiveness of etelcalcetide vs. Cinacalcet. *Pharmacoeconomics.* 2018;36(5): 603—612. https://doi.org/10.1007/s40273-017-0605-2.

71. Mandl F. Therapeutischer Versuch bei einem Falle von Ostitis fibrosa generalisata mittels Exstirpation eines Epithelkorperchentumors. *Zentralbl f Chir.* 1926;53:260.

72. Dorairajan N, Pradeep PV. Vignette hyperparathyroidism: glimpse into its history. *Int Surg.* 2014;99(5): 528—533. https://doi.org/10.9738/INTSURG-D-13-00225.1.

73. Tominaga Y, Matsuoka S, Sato T. Surgical indications and procedures of parathyroidectomy in patients with chronic kidney disease. *Ther Apher Dial.* 2005;9(1): 44—47. https://doi.org/10.1111/j.1774-9987.2005.00213.x.

74. Lorenz K, Bartsch DK, Sancho JJ, Guigard S, Triponez F. Surgical management of secondary hyperparathyroidism in chronic kidney disease—a consensus report of the European Society of Endocrine Surgeons. *Langenbeck's Arch Surg.* 2015;400(8):907—927. https://doi.org/10.1007/s00423-015-1344-5.

75. Anari H, Bashardoust B, Pourissa M, Refahi S. The diagnostic accuracy of high resolution ultrasound imaging for detection of secondary hyperparathyroidism in patients with chronic renal failure. *Acta Med Iran.* 2011; 49(8):527—530. http://www.ncbi.nlm.nih.gov/pubmed/22009809.

76. Yuan LL, Kan Y, Ma DQ, Yang JG. Combined application of ultrasound and SPECT/CT has incremental value in detecting parathyroid tissue in SHPT patients. *Diagn Interv Imaging.* 2016;97(2):219—225. https://doi.org/10.1016/J.DIII.2015.08.007.

77. Piciucchi S, Barone D, Gavelli G, Dubini A, Oboldi D, Matteuci F. Primary hyperparathyroidism: imaging to pathology. *J Clin Imaging Sci.* 2012;2:59. https:// doi.org/10.4103/2156-7514.102053.

78. Akerström G, Malmaeus J, Bergström R. Surgical anatomy of human parathyroid glands. *Surgery.* 1984; 95(1):14—21. http://www.ncbi.nlm.nih.gov/pubmed/6691181.

79. Hibi Y, Tominaga Y, Uchida K, Tominaga Y, Uchida K, et al. Cases with fewer than four parathyroid glands in patients withRenal hyperparathyroidism at initial parathyroidectomy. *World J Surg.* 2002;26(3):314—317. https://doi.org/10.1007/s00268-001-0224-z.

80. Pitt SC, Sippel RS, Chen H. Secondary and tertiary hyperparathyroidism, state of the art surgical management. *Surg Clin.* 2009;89(5):1227—1239. https://doi.org/10.1016/j.suc.2009.06.011.

81. Kim WY, Lee JB, Kim HY. Efficacy of intraoperative parathyroid hormone monitoring to predict success of parathyroidectomy for secondary hyperparathyroidism. *J Korean Surg Soc.* 2012;83(1):1—6. https://doi.org/10.4174/jkss.2012.83.1.1.

82. Seehofer D, Rayes N, Klupp J, et al. Predictive value of intact parathyroid hormone measurement during surgery for renal hyperparathyroidism. *Langenbeck's Arch Surg.* 2005;390(3):222—229. https://doi.org/10.1007/s00423-005-0541-z.

83. Schneider R, Slater EP, Karakas E, Bartsch DK, Schlosser K. Initial parathyroid surgery in 606 patients with renal hyperparathyroidism. *World J Surg.* 2012; 36(2):318—326. https://doi.org/10.1007/s00268-011-1392-0.

84. Milas M, Weber CJ. Near-total parathyroidectomy is beneficial for patients with secondary and tertiary hyperparathyroidism. *Surgery.* 2004;136(6):1252—1260. https://doi.org/10.1016/J.SURG.2004.06.055.

85. Low T-H, Clark J, Gao K, Eris J, Shannon K, O'Brien C. Outcome of parathyroidectomy for patients with renal disease and hyperparathyroidism: predictors for recurrent hyperparathyroidism. *ANZ J Surg.* 2009;79(5):378—382. https://doi.org/10.1111/j.1445-2197.2009.04893.x.

86. Dotzenrath C, Cupisti K, Goretzki E, et al. Operative treatment of renal autonomous hyperparathyroidism: cause of persistent or recurrent disease in 304 patients. *Langenbeck's Arch Surg.* 2003;387(9—10):348—354. https://doi.org/10.1007/s00423-002-0322-x.

87. Patow CA, Norton JA, Brennan MF. Vocal cord paralysis and reoperative parathyroidectomy. A prospective study. *Ann Surg.* 1986;203(3):282—285. http://www.ncbi.nlm.nih.gov/pubmed/3954480.

88. Chen J, Jia X, Kong X, Wang Z, Cui M, Xu D. Total parathyroidectomy with autotransplantation versus subtotal parathyroidectomy for renal hyperparathyroidism: a

systematic review and meta-analysis. *Nephrology*. 2017; 22(5):388–396. https://doi.org/10.1111/nep.12801.

89. Hargrove GM, Pasieka JL, Hanley DA, Murphy MB. *Short- and Long-Term Outcome of Total Parathyroidectomy with Immediate Autografting versus Subtotal Parathyroidectomy in Patients with End-Stage Renal Disease*; 1999. https://www.karger.com/Article/Pdf/13520.

90. Gagné ER, Ureña P, Leite-Silva S, et al. Short- and long-term efficacy of total parathyroidectomy with immediate autografting compared with subtotal parathyroidectomy in hemodialysis patients. *J Am Soc Nephrol*. 1992;3(4): 1008–1017.   http://www.ncbi.nlm.nih.gov/pubmed/1450363.

91. Apetrii M, Goldsmith D, Nistor I, et al. Impact of surgical parathyroidectomy on chronic kidney disease-mineral and bone disorder (CKD-MBD) - a systematic review and meta-analysis. *PLoS One*. 2017;12(11):e0187025. https://doi.org/10.1371/journal.pone.0187025.

92. Ma T-L, Hung P-H, Jong I-C, et al. Parathyroidectomy is associated with reduced mortality in hemodialysis patients with secondary hyperparathyroidism. *BioMed Res Int*. 2015;2015:639587. https://doi.org/10.1155/2015/639587.

93. Hsu Y-H, Chen H-J, Shen S-C, Tsai W-C, Hsu C-C, Kao C-H. Reduced stroke risk after parathyroidectomy in end-stage renal disease: a 13-year population-based cohort study. *Medicine (Baltimore)*. 2015;94(23):e936. https://doi.org/10.1097/MD.0000000000000936.

94. Rudser KD, de Boer IH, Dooley A, Young B, Kestenbaum B. Fracture risk after parathyroidectomy among chronic hemodialysis patients. *J Am Soc Nephrol*. 2007;18(8): 2401–2407. https://doi.org/10.1681/ASN.2007010022.

95. Isaksson E, Ivarsson K, Akaberi S, et al. The effect of parathyroidectomy on risk of hip fracture in secondary hyperparathyroidism. *World J Surg*. 2017; 41(9):2304–2311. https://doi.org/10.1007/s00268-017-4000-0.

96. Bonarek H, Merville P, Bonarek M, et al. Reduced parathyroid functional mass after successful kidney transplantation. *Kidney Int*. 1999;56(2):642–649. https://doi.org/10.1046/J.1523-1755.1999.00589.X.

97. Littbarski SA, Kaltenborn A, Gwiasda J, et al. Timing of parathyroidectomy in kidney transplant candidates with secondary hyperparathryroidism: effect of pretransplant versus early or late post-transplant parathyroidectomy. *Surgery*.   2018;163(2):373–380.   https://doi.org/10.1016/j.surg.2017.10.016.

98. Jeon HJ, Kim YJ, Kwon HY, et al. Impact of parathyroidectomy on allograft outcomes in kidney transplantation. *Transpl Int*. 2012;25(12):1248–1256. https://doi.org/10.1111/j.1432-2277.2012.01564.x.

99. Janmaat CJ, van Diepen M, Gasparini A, et al. Lower serum calcium is independently associated with CKD progression. *Sci Rep*. 2018;8(1):5148. https://doi.org/10.1038/s41598-018-23500-5.

100. Obi Y, Mehrotra R, Rivara MB, et al. Hidden hypercalcemia and mortality risk in incident hemodialysis patients. *J Clin Endocrinol Metab*. 2016;101(6):2440–2449. https://doi.org/10.1210/jc.2016-1369.

101. Nishizawa Y, Jono S, Ishimura E, Shioi A. Hyperphosphatemia and vascular calcification in end-stage renal disease. *J Ren Nutr*. 2005;15(1):178–182. https://doi.org/10.1053/J.JRN.2004.09.027.

102. Kidney Disease: Improving Global Outcomes (KDIGO) CKD-MBD Work Group. KDIGO clinical practice guideline for the diagnosis, evaluation, prevention, and treatment of Chronic Kidney Disease-Mineral and Bone Disorder (CKD-MBD). *Kidney Int*. 2009;76(113): S1–S130. https://doi.org/10.1038/ki.2009.188.

103. Cunningham J, Danese M, Olson K, Klassen P, Chertow GM. Effects of the calcimimetic cinacalcet HCl on cardiovascular disease, fracture, and health-related quality of life in secondary hyperparathyroidism. *Kidney Int*. 2005;68(4):1793–1800. https://doi.org/10.1111/j.1523-1755.2005.00596.x.

104. Wetmore JB. Parathyroidectomy: complex decisions about a complex procedure. *Clin J Am Soc Nephrol*. 2016;11(7): 1133–1135. https://doi.org/10.2215/CJN.04950516.

105. Kim SM, Long J, Montez-Rath ME, Leonard MB, Norton JA, Chertow GM. Rates and outcomes of parathyroidectomy for secondary hyperparathyroidism in the United States. *Clin J Am Soc Nephrol*. 2016;11(7): 1260–1267. https://doi.org/10.2215/CJN.10370915.

106. van der Plas WY, Engelsman AF, Umakanthan M, et al. Treatment strategy of end-stage renal disease related hyperparathyroidism before, during and after the era of calcimimetics. *Surgery*. 2019 Jan;165(1):135–141. https://doi.org/10.1016/j.surg.2018.04.092.

107. van der Plas WY, Engelsman AF, Özyilmaz A, et al. Impact of the introduction of calcimimetics on timing of parathyroidectomy in secondary and tertiary hyperparathyroidism. *Ann Surg Oncol*. 2017;24(1): 15–22. https://doi.org/10.1245/s10434-016-5450-6.

108. Cruzado JM, Moreno P, Torregrosa JV, et al. A randomized study comparing parathyroidectomy with cinacalcet for treating hypercalcemia in kidney allograft recipients with hyperparathyroidism. *J Am Soc Nephrol*. 2016;27(8):2487–2494. https://doi.org/10.1681/ASN.2015060622.

109. Kruijff S, van der Plas WY, Dulfer RR, et al. Changing landscape of the treatment of hyperparathyroidism related to end-stage renal disease - can we turn the clock backward? *Surgery*. 2019 Feb;165(2):289–290. https://doi.org/10.1016/j.surg.2018.07.043.

CHAPTER 9

Advances in the Diagnosis and Surgical Management of Parathyroid Carcinoma

TAL YALON, MD • MICHAL MEKEL, MD, MHA • HAGGI MAZEH, MD, FACS, FISA

INTRODUCTION

Parathyroid carcinoma is a rare endocrine malignancy. It accounts for approximately 0.005% of all cancers. The vast majority of these tumors are functional, secreting parathyroid hormone (PTH); nevertheless, it is diagnosed in less than 1% of all patients with hyperparathyroidism.[1-5] The scarce number of cases and lack of large scale databases contribute to the limited understanding of the natural course of disease, diagnosis, treatment effectivity, and prognosis. Most studies are single institution, small retrospective reviews with conflicting data. Lack of proper evidence-based management guidelines and consensus statements makes this disease difficult to treat effectively.[6]

Incidence, Epidemiology, and Genetics

The first description of parathyroid carcinoma was made in 1904 by the Swiss surgeon Fritz De Quervain, who described a nonfunctioning metastatic parathyroid carcinoma.[7] Later in 1933, Millot and Sainton published the first case of a metastatic functioning parathyroid carcinoma.[8] Since these publications, more than 1000 cases were published in the English medical literature, most in rather small retrospective studies (Table 9.1).[9]

Factors contributing to the development of parathyroid carcinoma still remain unclear, with most cases considered to be sporadic. Some cases of parathyroid carcinoma were reported to be linked to genetic syndromes such as multiple endocrine neoplasm (MEN) syndrome 1 or MEN2a, isolated familial hyperparathyroidism, and hyperparathyroidism jaw tumor syndrome (HPT-JT). Somatic mutations in HRPT2 tumor suppressor genes, while uncommon in patients with sporadic parathyroid adenoma, are frequent in patients with parathyroid carcinoma, and might represent undiagnosed HPT-JT. Association with MEN1 gene mutations and germline HRPT2 mutations are rare in parathyroid carcinoma. To date, no significant predisposing factors have been reported aside from suggested association to prior neck irradiation.[1,10,11]

Parathyroid carcinoma accounts for only a minute number of all cancers (0.005%) and is diagnosed in less than 1% of all patients with hyperparathyroidism.[1,3-5,12] The highest documented incidence is in Japan, where parathyroid carcinoma diagnosis is confirmed in up to 5% of the patients with hyperparathyroidism.[2] According to studies utilizing the National Cancer Data Base (NCDB) and the National Surveillance Epidemiology and End Result cancer registry (SEER), there is an equal gender distribution, in contrast with benign parathyroid adenoma that has a female predominance of 3-4: 1.[3,4,13,14] Peak incidence is in the 5th and 6th decade of life, about a decade younger than patients with benign etiology.[1] The only additional demographic parameter found in the SEER study was ethnical distribution, with whites being affected eight times more than other races.[4]

PRESENTATION

Most parathyroid tumors are hormonally active, with the vast majority of parathyroid carcinoma cases manifesting as primary hyperparathyroidism (PHPT).[12,15] Less than 5% of cases are considered nonfunctional tumors and to date, less than 40 cases of nonfunctional parathyroid carcinoma were reported in the English medical literature. Due to lack of hormonal activity of nonfunctional tumors, their typical presentation is of a palpable neck mass, without other biochemical alterations or systemic findings. As a consequence of lack of systemic manifestations, these subsets of patients are often diagnosed at an advanced stage and the lack of biochemical profile makes both the diagnosis and follow-up challenging.[16-18]

Advances in Treatment and Management in Surgical Endocrinology. https://doi.org/10.1016/B978-0-323-66195-9.00009-1

TABLE 9.1
Large Retrospective Studies of Parathyroid Carcinoma.

Study, Year, Country	Number of Patients	Data Source	Main Conclusions
Wynne et al. 1992, USA[22]	$n = 43$	Single institution	45% palpable neck mass Mean PTH X10 the normal 60% reoperation 14% radiation therapy
Sandelin et al. 1992, Sweden[37]	$n = 95$	Swedish cancer registry	Thyroidectomy/lobectomy associated with longer OS and DSF Repeated surgical interventions are beneficial.
Hundahl et al. 1999, USA[3]	$n = 286$	NCDB	Tumor size and nodal status are significant prognostic factors.
Busaidy et al. 2004, USA[20]	$n = 27$	Single institution	22% radiotherapy—improved locoregional recurrence All deaths were hypercalcemia related.
Lee et al. 2007, USA[4]	$n = 224$	SEER	12.5% en-bloc resections—improved survival Young age, female gender, and absence of distant metastases improved survival rate.
Talat and Schulte 2010, UK[25]	$n = 330$	Multicenter	1.5–2-fold locoregional recurrence after local or no central lymphadenectomy.
Harari et al. 2011, USA[45]	$n = 37$	Single institution	Multiple surgeries resulted in high complications rate (mainly RLN injury) Distal metastasis is a strong mortality predictor Metastasectomy can control serum calcium levels Better outcomes in high-volume centers
Schaapveld et al. 2011, Netherland[28]	$n = 41$	The Netherlands cancer registry	High serum PTH, profound hypercalcemia, palpable neck mass, should alert for parathyroid carcinoma.
Villar-del-Moral et al. 2014, Spain[35]	$n = 62$	Multicenter	91% 10 years DSF and 69% 10 years RFS All recurrences in the first 5 years 71% en-bloc resection Surgeons performance and preoperative diagnosis are key factors of RFS
Sadler et al. 2014, USA[14]	$n = 1022$	NCDB	81% 5 years OS 12.6% radiotherapy—lower survival Tumor size/R_1 margins are not predictors of OS >1 surgeries did not impact OS
Asare et al. 2015, USA[13]	$n = 733$	NCDB	Nodal status is not associated with mortality Tumor size >4 cm associated with higher mortality 5- and 10-year OS 82% and 66%, respectively

NCDB, National Cancer Database Registry; *SEER,* Surveillance, Epidemiology, and End Results cancer registry; *OS,* Overall survival; *DFS,* Disease free survival; *RFS,* Recurrence free survival; *RLN,* recurrent laryngeal nerve; *PTH,* Parathyroid hormone.

Functional parathyroid tumors, whether benign or malignant, produce and secrete PTH in an unregulated manner. PTH is the key player in calcium homeostasis and exerts its affect through several mechanisms: activates osteoclasts, increases renal tubular reabsorption of calcium, increases conversion of vitamin D to its active form 1,25-dihydroxycholecalciferol in the kidney, increases phosphate renal excretion, and augments calcium absorption in the gastrointestinal tract. All result in an elevated serum calcium levels.

As opposed to many other solid organ tumors, signs and symptoms related to parathyroid tumors are mainly due to the biochemical profile of the tumor (i.e., hyperparathyroidism and hypercalcemia) rather than a mass effect of the tumor itself. Different from benign parathyroid adenoma that is hardly ever distinguishable on physical examination, parathyroid carcinoma may present as a palpable neck mass with accompanied local mass effect due to tissue compression or tumor infiltration to surrounding tissues. Symptoms such as hoarseness due to infiltration to the recurrent laryngeal nerve, dysphagia, and dyspnea have been reported in as many as 70% of cases of parathyroid carcinoma.[5,15]

In patients with PHPT, hypercalcemia manifest in a vast array of nonspecific signs and symptoms of several organ systems: renal (nephrolithiasis, chronic renal disease), musculoskeletal (osteoporosis, pathological fractures, bone pain, myalgia), neurological (depression, nervousness, memory problems, and diminished concentration), and gastrointestinal (constipation, abdominal pain, peptic ulcer disease, and pancreatitis).[1,2,19-22] These nonspecific signs and symptoms often present simultaneously in PHPT and patients with parathyroid carcinoma more often present with bone and renal involvement compared to patients with benign etiology.[15]

As opposed to benign parathyroid adenoma, in which patients often present with mild or even no symptoms, patients with parathyroid carcinoma tend to generally exhibit a more pronounced presentation as a result of higher levels of serum PTH and calcium levels.[1,5] Some patients may even present with hypercalcemic crisis (known as parathyroxicosis), which is defined as significantly elevated serum calcium level with end organ dysfunction.[23]

Data regarding lymph node involvement at presentation are insufficient. The SEER and NCDB-based papers contain unknown initial nodal status in 62.3% –75.4% of the patients.[3,4,13,14] In other studies, the presence of regional lymph node involvement upon diagnosis has been reported in up to 32% of patients.[24-26] As much as a third of patients present with distant metastasis to the lung, liver, and bones.[5,12]

DIAGNOSIS

The preoperative diagnosis of parathyroid carcinoma may be challenging in most cases as there are no specific diagnostic signs and symptoms, biochemical markers, or imaging techniques. Most patients will present with signs, symptoms, and laboratory workup that are similar to PHPT. This overlap in presentation makes the preoperative diagnosis of parathyroid carcinoma very difficult. In most cases, the suspicion for malignancy arises only during surgery and confirmed or even initially discovered only on the pathology report.[4,27] That being said, there are several factors that may raise the surgeon's suspicion before or during surgery. Extremely high preoperative levels of serum PTH and/or calcium levels, presence of a palpable neck mass, or worrisome imaging features should raise the suspicion of the possible parathyroid carcinoma diagnosis, as will be discussed in this section.

Biochemical Profile

The diagnosis of PHPT is based on its biochemical profile, and parathyroid carcinoma should be considered in the differential diagnosis depending on biochemical indices. In PHPT serum PTH levels are either high or not adequately suppressed by the elevated serum calcium levels due to unregulated hormone production and secretion. Parathyroid carcinoma typically presents with very high serum PTH and calcium levels.[15] PTH levels in parathyroid carcinoma have been typically reported to be around 3–10-fold the upper normal limit of the lab's assay.[1] Talat et al. reported a PTH level from 1 to 76-fold the upper normal lab value with an average of 4.5-fold.[25] In addition, it has been suggested that serum PTH level above 10-fold the upper normal limit should be considered highly predictive for parathyroid carcinoma (positive predictive value of 84%).[28] Serum calcium levels in patients presenting with parathyroid carcinoma far exceed those of benign etiology of PHPT, ranging from 2.2 to 6.0 mmol/L (8.8–24 mg/dL) with a mean of 3.6 mmol/L (14.4 mg/dL) upon presentation.[15,25]

Imaging

In general, imaging modalities have no role in strictly diagnosing patients with PHPT and are used for localization purposes as a part of preoperative assessment and planning. Neck ultrasound (US) done by an experienced parathyroid sonographer combined with

Technetium-99m sestamibi scanning with single photon emission computed tomography and/or four-dimensional cervical computer tomography (CT) are considered the most cost effective strategy for localization of parathyroid tumor.[15] Although no imaging modality can differentiate between a benign and malignant lesion, several characteristics may suggest the presence of an underlying malignancy. The average parathyroid carcinoma size has been reported as 3 cm, which far exceeds the size of a benign parathyroid adenoma.[13,14,25] Large tumor size upon diagnosis is an independent factor that should raise the preoperative suspicion of parathyroid carcinoma.[15] In addition to size, several other radiological features can be utilized.

- Sonographic features that might differentiate parathyroid carcinoma from a benign lesion include irregular shape, round appearance, firm noncompressible lesion, intralesion radial vessels with no clearly demonstrated supplying vessels, calcifications, structural heterogeneity, and infiltration. Tissue infiltration is considered the histopathological hallmark for diagnosis of parathyroid cancer. Sonographic surrounding tissue infiltration features include thickened, coarse capsule, or effacement of borders of the lesion with respect to neighboring solid organ and vessels.[29]
- Technetium Tc99m is the dominant radioisotope used in parathyroid scintigraphy, with its high affinity to mitochondria in the parathyroid tissue. Sestamibi scan is considered a highly specific localization study, although there are no established uptake parameters that differentiate between benign and malignant disease.[15,30] Nevertheless, sestamibi scans have been found useful in diagnosing and localizing metastatic parathyroid carcinoma.[31]
- Cross-sectional imaging such as CT and magnetic resonance imaging (MRI) can provide some useful additional information regarding the anatomical description, extent of involved surrounding organs, and identification of metastasis. These hold an important role in surgery planning when parathyroid carcinoma is suspected preoperatively, although this is not usually the case.[5] In a small series, 18F-FDG PET/CT has been reported useful both preoperatively as a useful tool for evaluation of the disease extent and presence of distant metastasis, as well as postoperatively for residual disease and recurrence evaluation.[32]

Cytology

Fine-needle aspiration (FNA) cytology is not part of the routine evaluation of PHPT nor is it recommended when parathyroid carcinoma is suspected for several reasons. First, FNA cannot reliably distinguish between parathyroid carcinoma and benign adenomas. Second, there is a theoretical risk of malignant cells seeding along the tract of biopsy. Lastly, an additional risk is noted of obscuring anatomical planes due to bleeding or infection as a consequence of the FNA.[15,33,34]

Intraoperative Findings

In addition to the previously mentioned preoperative clues, some intraoperative findings may raise the suspicion of malignancy and affect the extent of the index procedure, leading to reduced locoregional disease progression and recurrence. In addition to size and firm consistency, thick capsule, fibrotic mass, and presence of substrap adhesions (i.e., adhesions to the thyroid, strap muscles, esophagus, trachea, and fascia) were all found to be a significant predictor for the presence of malignancy.[15,27]

TREATMENT

Before discussing treatment options, it is imperative to have better understanding of the natural disease course and behavior, as it can guide and facilitate treatment goals. In most cases, parathyroid carcinoma demonstrates a slow growing indolent progressive course of disease, and only a small number of cases present with an aggressive metastatic behavior.[1,15,35] The principal cause of morbidity and mortality is the consequence of metabolic complications secondary to chronic intractable hypercalcemia rather than mass effect and organ dysfunction due to malignant cells infiltration.[12,36] Therefore, hyperparathyroidism resolution should be the main treatment objective.

By virtue of this disease being a rare endocrine cancer, reliable data are in short supply.[6] Being an orphan disease, all data gathered rely on retrospective studies, with relatively small number of subjects (Table 9.1). Although some reliable information regarding the epidemiology exists, there is no sufficient data nor is it possible to perform clinical trials that will guide toward the best course of treatment with high level of evidence.

Surgery

To date, the only consensus is that surgery is considered the mainstay of treatment, with complete tumor resection with negative histologic margins at the index procedure, and serves the best opportunity for curative results.[1,4,5,9,12,15,25,36]

When parathyroid carcinoma is suspected preoperatively or intraoperatively, most experts agree that complete en-bloc resection of the tumor (i.e., ipsilateral thyroid lobectomy, strap muscles, and any adjacent structure that are involved) with clear gross margins is considered the gold standard.[13,15] This should be done while avoiding violation of the tumor capsule with subsequent spillage and seeding of malignant cells in the area of resection.[5,15] Unfortunately, as mentioned earlier, in most instances, the presence of malignancy is detected only postoperatively; hence, most Patents undergo a suboptimal index procedure. For those circumstances, it is worth mentioning that although incomplete local excision was reported to increase the risk of recurrence 1.5−2-fold, undergoing surgical resection, regardless of its extent, was shown to be associated with improved survival compared with no surgical treatment at all.[13,25]

Although most papers have insufficient data regarding regional lymph node metastasis, such presence upon presentation is considered low, and when present, it is usually limited to the central compartment.[13,14,25,26] Currently, prophylactic lymphadenectomy is not recommended due to increased morbidity, without contributing to patient survival. However, therapeutic lymphadenectomy is indicated when involvement of cervical lymph nodes is suspected pre or intraoperatively.[15]

Reexploration

As stated, most patients are diagnosed postoperatively after undergoing a suboptimal index procedure. This raises the question whether a second neck exploration is needed and for whom. In addition, parathyroid carcinoma is a disease with recurrence rates as high as 42%−60%, with most recurrences occurring 2−5 years after the first surgery.[4,25,37,38]

Reoperation for recurrent disease is feasible, although holds a higher risk of surgical complication due to scaring and distortion of anatomical plains.[15] Repeated surgical interventions have been shown to be of limited benefit, and undergoing more than one surgery did not show to have significant impact in terms of overall survival.[4,14,37] Keeping in mind the treatment objective (i.e., controlling complications secondary to hyperparathyroidism), repeated surgery, though never curative, can have a significant role in biochemical and clinical palliation and may prolong survival. In these circumstances, localization studies must be utilized to identify size and location of resectable disease.[15,38,39]

Radiotherapy

Parathyroid carcinoma is not considered a radiosensitive tumor, and there is no evidence to support the use of external beam radiation for the primary treatment of this tumor.[1] However, the use of adjuvant radiotherapy has been suggested in several small series to reduce the rates of locoregional recurrence. Although some variable level of success in decreasing locoregional recurrence was reported, these studies lack statistical significance.[20−22,27,40] Radiotherapy was not associated with improved survival in other larger population series.[4,14] As stated, patients with parathyroid carcinoma have a high chance of reoperation and the use of postoperative radiation may increase the difficulty and morbidity of reoperation. The current recommendation made by the American Association of Endocrine Surgeons (AAES) is that external beam radiation should not be routinely given as an adjunct measure and should be reserved as a palliative option.[15]

Chemotherapy

Due to the scarcity of this disease, no effective cytotoxic agent or regimen has been proven effective for the treatment of parathyroid carcinoma, with all data obtained from anecdotal case reports. Currently, there is no established role for chemotherapy as adjuvant treatment or in the setting of non-resectable disease.[1,5,12,15,36]

Follow-up

There is no consensus in terms of patient follow-up. The current AAES recommendation is that following attempted curative surgery, patients with functional parathyroid carcinoma should be followed-up for recurrence by means of biochemical profile. Surveillance should include testing of serum calcium and PTH levels in 3−6-month intervals. Suspected recurrence should be followed by supplementary localization studies.[15] As anticipated, there are no guidelines for nonfunctional tumors and there is no role for biochemical profiling as follow-up. In these rare circumstances, repeated imaging studies such as ultrasound, CT, or MRI should be performed.

PROGNOSIS

Based on the larger population-based cancer databases, overall survival of patients with parathyroid carcinoma has been reported as 78%−85% at 5 years and 50%−66% at 10 years.[3,13,14,37] Cancer-related mortality is reported as 4.4% after 1 year and 9% at 5 years.[4]

Prognostic Factors

Over the years, several prognostic factors have been linked with worse overall survival. The presence of distant metastases (i.e., disease found beyond the central and lateral neck) was found to be a consistent strong predictor of grim outcome.[41] Older age at time of initial diagnosis and male gender have also been uniformly proposed to be negative outcome predictors. The prognostic value of tumor size, lymph node involvement, and positive resection margins remains a matter of controversy.[4,13,14,25,35,37] Intraoperative tumor rapture and spillage are also associated with increased locoregional recurrence.[35,42] In contrast, aggressive surgical resection and repeated surgical resections did not seem to improve the overall survival, probably as a consequence of related increased morbidity.[13,14] These notions should be interpreted with caution, as all studies in relation to parathyroid carcinoma are limited by small sample size and are all considered by the American Joint Comity on Cancer (AJCC) as low level of evidence III (i.e., the available level of evidence is problematic).[41]

Staging

In past years, several attempts have been made to establish a staging system that will provide standardized nomenclature and help guide clinical practice in terms of staging and prognosis. Shaha and Shah proposed in 1999 a TNM staging system that relies on the size of the tumor (for T1 and T2) and extent of surrounding tissue invasion (for T3 and T4).[43] Later, another staging system was suggested by Talat and Schulte in 2010 and subsequently validated by Schulte et al. in 2012. In their TNM staging system, primary tumor definition (T category) was based on the extent of invasion rather than its size. In addition, they further classified tumors into low- and high-risk cancers, based on local invasion. This risk stratification was based on cancer exhibiting vascular invasion, vital organ invasion, lymph node involvement or distant metastasis. Those tumors were considered high-risk tumors.[25,44] In both systems, there were no differences in terms of regional nodal status (N category) and distant metastasis (M category).

In 2017, the AJCC proposed their TNM definition of parathyroid carcinoma, which is based on the tumor level of invasion and subclassification of lymph node involvement according to their anatomical locations (Table 9.2). Due to lack of sufficient data, no anatomical stage and prognostic groups have been described for parathyroid carcinoma to date.[41]

TABLE 9.2
AJCC 2017 Proposed TNM Classification[41].

TNM CLASSIFICATION

T Category	T Criteria
Tx	Primary tumor cannot be assessed
T0	No evidence of primary tumor
Tis	Atypical parathyroid neoplasm (neoplasm of uncertain malignant potential)
T1	Localized to the parathyroid gland with extension limited to soft tissue
T2	Direct invasion into the thyroid gland
T3	Direct invasion into recurrent laryngeal nerve, esophagus, trachea, skeletal muscle, adjacent lymph nodes, or thymus
T4	Direct invasion into major blood vessel or spine

N Category	N Criteria
Nx	Regional nodes cannot be assessed
N0	No regional lymph node metastasis
N1	Regional lymph node metastasis
N1a	Metastasis to level VI (pretracheal, paratracheal, and prelaryngeal/Delphian lymph nodes) or superior mediastinal lymph nodes (level VII)
N1b	Metastasis to unilateral, bilateral, or contralateral cervical (level I, II, III, IV, or V) or retropharyngeal nodes

M Category	M Criteria
M0	No distant metastasis
M1	Distant metastasis

HISTOLOGICAL GRADE (G)

G	G Definition
LG	Low grade: Round monomorphic nuclei with only mild-to-moderate nuclear size variation, indistinct nucleoli, and chromatin characteristics resembling those of normal parathyroid or of adenoma.
HG	High grade: More pleomorphism, with a nuclear size variation greater than 4:1: prominent nuclear membrane irregularities; chromatin alterations, including hyperchromasia or margination of chromatin; and prominent nucleoli. High-grade tumors show several discrete confluent areas with nuclear changes.

SUMMARY

Parathyroid carcinoma is a rare endocrine malignancy with limited evidence-based data that are all retrospective. The signs and symptoms often resemble those of PHPT and extremely high preoperative PTH and calcium levels may be the only clues for preoperative diagnosis. Once diagnosed or suspected, en-bloc resection is recommended and constitutes to be the mainstay of treatment. Unfortunately, there are no effective known adjuvant treatments although external beam radiotherapy may be an option for palliation. The main cause of morbidity and mortality is a consequence of metabolic complications secondary to chronic intractable hypercalcemia. The overall survival is 78%–85% at 5 years and 50%–66% at 10 years.

REFERENCES

1. Shane E. *Clinical Review*. 2000;321:1000–1002.
2. Obara T, Fujimoto Y. Diagnosis and treatment of patients with parathyroid carcinoma: an update and review. *World J Surg*. 1991;15(6):738–744.
3. Hundahl SA. Two hundred eighty-six cases of parathyroid carcinoma treated in the U.S. Between 1985–1995: a National cancer data Base report. The American college of surgeons commission on cancer and the American cancer society. *Cancer*. 1999;86:538–544.
4. Lee PK. Trends in the incidence and treatment of parathyroid cancer in the United States. *Cancer*. 2007;109(9):1736–1741.
5. Al-Kurd A, Mekel M, Mazeh H. Parathyroid carcinoma. *Surg Oncol*. 2014;23(2):107–114.
6. James BC, Aschebrook-kilfoy B, Cipriani N, Kaplan EL, Angelos P, Grogan RH. The incidence and survival of rare cancers of the thyroid, parathyroid, adrenal, and pancreas. *Ann Surg Oncol*. 2016:424–433.
7. DeQuervain F. Parastruma maligna aberrata (Malignant aberrant parathyroid). *Deusche Zeitschr Chir*. 1904;100(1):334–352, 1904.
8. Sainton P, MillotMalegne J. Dun adenoma parathyroidiene eosinophile (Malignant eosinophilic parathyroid). Au cours dune de Recklinghausen. *Ann Anat Pathol*. 1933;10(1):813–814, 1933.
9. Goswamy J, Lei M, Simo R. Parathyroid carcinoma. *Curr Opin Otolaryngol Head Neck Surg*. 2016;24(2):155–162. https://doi.org/10.1097/MOO.0000000000000234.
10. Sharretts JM, Kebebew E, S WF. Parathyroid cancer. *Semin Oncol*. 2010;37(6):580–590, 2011.
11. Sharretts JM, Simonds WF. Clinical and molecular genetics of parathyroid neoplasms. *Best Pract Res Clin Endocrinol Metabol*. 2010;24(3):491–502.
12. Wei CH, Harari A. Parathyroid carcinoma: update and guidelines for management. *Curr Treat Options Oncol*. 2012;13(1):11–23.
13. Asare EA. Parathyroid carcinoma: an update on treatment outcomes and prognostic factors from the National cancer data base (NCDB). *Ann Surg Oncol*. 2015;22(12):3990–3995.
14. Sadler C, Gow KW, Beierle EA, et al. Parathyroid carcinoma in more than 1,000 patients: a population-level analysis. *Surgeon*. 2014;156(6):1622–1629.
15. Campbell MJ. The definitive management of primary hyperparathyroidism who needs an operation? *JAMA*. 2017;317(11):959–968.
16. Mazeh H, Prus D, Freund HR. Incidental non-functional parathyroid carcinoma identified during thyroidectomy. *Isr Med Assoc J*. 2008;10(9):659.
17. Wilkins BJ, Lewis JS. Non-functional parathyroid carcinoma: a review of the literature and report of a case requiring extensive surgery. *Head Neck Pathol*. 2009;3(2):140–149.
18. Wang L, Han D, Chen W, et al. Non-functional parathyroid carcinoma: a case report and review of the literature. *Cancer Biol Ther*. 2015;16(11):1569–1576.
19. Quinn CE, Healy J, Lebastchi AH, et al. Modern experience with aggressive parathyroid tumors in a high-volume New England referral center. *J Am Coll Surg*. 2015;220(6):1054–1062.
20. Busaidy NL, Jimenez C, Habra MA, et al. Parathyroid carcinoma: a 22-year experience. *Head Neck*. 2004;26(8):716–726.
21. Munson ND, Foote RL, Northcutt RC, et al. Parathyroid carcinoma: is there a role for adjuvant radiation therapy? *Cancer*. 2003;98(11):2378–2384.
22. Wynne AG, van Heerden J, Carney JA, F L. Parathyroid carcinoma: clinical and pathologic features in 43 patients. *Medicine (Baltimore)*. 1992;71(4):197–205, 1992.
23. Kebebew E, Clark O. Parathyroid adenoma, hyperplasia, and carcinoma: localization, technical details of primary neck exploration, and treatment of hypercalcemic crisis. *Surg Oncol Clin*. 1998;7(4):721–748.
24. Schulte KM, Talat N, Galata G, et al. Oncologic resection achieving r0 margins improves disease-free survival in parathyroid cancer. *Ann Surg Oncol*. 2014;21(6):1891–1897.
25. Talat N, Schulte KM. Clinical presentation, staging and long-term evolution of parathyroid cancer. *Ann Surg Oncol*. 2010;17(8):2156–2174.
26. Hsu KT, Sippel RS, Chen H, Schneider DF. Is central lymph node dissection necessary for parathyroid carcinoma? *Surgeon*. 2014;156(6):1336–1341.
27. Selvan B, Paul MJ, Seshadri MS, et al. High index of clinical suspicion with optimal surgical techniques and adjuvant radiotherapy is critical to reduce locoregional disease progression in parathyroid carcinoma. *Am J Clin Oncol Cancer Clin Trials*. 2013;36(1):64–69.
28. Schaapveld M, Jorna FH, Aben KKH, Haak HR, Plukker JTM, Links TP. Incidence and prognosis of parathyroid gland carcinoma: a population-based study in the Netherlands estimating the preoperative diagnosis. *Am J Surg*. 2011;202(5):590–597.

29. Sidhu PS, Talat N, Patel P, Mulholland NJ, Schulte KM. Ultrasound features of malignancy in the preoperative diagnosis of parathyroid cancer: a retrospective analysis of parathyroid tumours larger than 15 mm. *Eur Radiol.* 2011;21(9):1865–1873.

30. Rodgers SE, Perrier ND. Parathyroid carcinoma. *Curr Opin Oncol.* 2006;18(1):16–22.

31. Al-Sobhi S. Detection of metastatic parathyroid carcinoma with Tc-99m sestamibi imaging. *Clin Nucl Med.* 1999;24(1):21–23, 1999.

32. Evangelista L, Sorgato N, Torresan F, et al. *World J Clin Oncol.* 2011;2(10):348–354.

33. Spinelli C, Bonadio AG, Berti P, Materazzi G, Miccoli P. Cutaneous spreading of parathyroid carcinoma after fine needle aspiration cytology. *J Endocrinol Investig.* 2000;23(4):255–257.

34. Agarwal G, Dhingra S, Mishra SK, Krishnani N. Implantation of parathyroid carcinoma along fine needle aspiration track. *Langenbeck's Arch Surg.* 2006;391(6):623–626.

35. Villar Del Moral J, Jiménez-García A, Salvador-Egea P, et al. Prognostic factors and staging systems in parathyroid cancer: a multicenter cohort study. *Surgery.* 2014;156(5):1132–1144.

36. Mohebati A, Shaha A, Shah J. Parathyroid carcinoma: challenges in diagnosis and treatment. *Hematol Oncol Clin North Am.* 2012;26(6):1222–1238.

37. Sandelin K, Auer G, Bondeson L, Grimelius L, F L. Prognostic factors in parathyroid cancer: a review of 95 cases. *World J Surg.* 1992;16(4):724–731.

38. Iacobone M, Ruffolo C, Lumachi F, Favia G. Results of iterative surgery for persistent and recurrent parathyroid carcinoma. *Langenbeck's Arch Surg.* 2005;390(5):385–390.

39. Kebebew E, Arici C, Duh QY, et al. Localization and reoperation results for persistent and recurrent parathyroid carcinoma. *Arch Surg.* 2001;136(8):878–885.

40. Erovic BM. Parathyroid cancer: outcome analysis of 16 patients treated at the princess margaret hospital. *Head Neck.* 2013;35(1):35–39.

41. *American Joint Committee on Cencer (AJCC) Cancer Staging Manual.* 8th ed. 2017.

42. Rawat N, Khetan N, Williams DW, Baxter JN. Parathyroid carcinoma. *Br J Surg.* 2005;92(11):1345–1353.

43. Shaha AR, Shah JP. Parathyroid carcinoma: a diagnostic and therapeutic challenge. *Cancer.* 1999;86(3):378–380.

44. Schulte KM, Gill AJ, Barczynski M, et al. Classification of parathyroid cancer. *Ann Surg Oncol.* 2012;19(8):2620–2628.

45. Harari A, Waring A, Fernandez-Ranvier G, et al. Parathyroid carcinoma: a 43-year outcome and survival analysis. *J Clin Endocrinol Metab.* 2011;96(12):3679–3686.

CHAPTER 10

Advances in the Diagnosis and Management of Primary Hyperparathyroidism due to MEN Type 1 Syndrome

PRISCILLA NOBECOURT, MD* • ANGELICA M. SILVA-FIGUEROA, MD* • NANCY D. PERRIER, MD, FACS

INTRODUCTION

Definition

Multiple endocrine neoplasia type 1 (MEN1) syndrome also known as *Wermer syndrome*[1] was first described in 1954 by Dr. Paul Wermer as a "familial occurrence of adenomatosis of endocrine glands [...] caused by a dominant autosomal gene with a high degree of penetrance."[1] Over half a century later, we still reference Dr. Wermer—MEN1 syndrome is a hereditary syndrome with an autosomal-dominant pattern of inheritance. It is characterized by a mutation in the *MEN1* gene located on chromosome 11q13.[2] This gene is a tumor suppressor gene, which encodes the *menin* protein. This protein plays a role in transcriptional regulation, cell cycle regulation, genome stability, cell signaling, cytoskeletal structure, and epigenetic regulation.[2,3] Over 1100 germline mutations have been identified in the *MEN1* gene most of which are inactivating mutations, but new mutations keep being identified.[2,3]

Knowing this wide variety of possible mutations in the *MEN1* gene exists, it comes of no surprise that there are combinations of presentation of over 20 different endocrine and nonendocrine tumors in the MEN1 syndrome.[4] Following the recent clinical practice guidelines for MEN1, there are three approaches to diagnosing MEN1. The clinical diagnosis is made by diagnosing two of the three major MEN1-associated endocrine tumors in one patient, which are parathyroid, enteropancreatic endocrine, and pituitary tumors.

The familial diagnosis is made when in addition to the initial patient clinically diagnosed with MEN1, a first-degree relative is diagnosed with at least one of the main MEN1 tumors mentioned previously. A genetic diagnosis of MEN1 is made if a patient has a germline mutation in the *MEN1* gene and may be asymptomatic and has no evidence of tumor presence at the time of diagnosis.[5]

Epidemiology and Prognosis

MEN1 syndrome has an incidence of 1 in 30,000 births worldwide.[6] In 85% of these patients, the first manifestation of the syndrome is parathyroid tumors[3] with primary hyperparathyroidism (PHPT) being the most common endocrinopathy with nearly 100% penetrance by age 50.[5] In the other 15% of these patients, the first manifestation is most likely an insulinoma or prolactinoma.[3] PHPT, sporadic, and inherited presentations combined has an annual incidence of 100,000 cases annually in the United States.[7]

Men and women are equally affected by PHPT among MEN1 patients, and 1%—18% of patients with PHPT have MEN1 syndrome.[3,7]

Untreated patients with MEN1 have a low life expectancy with 50% risk of death by 50 years of age associated to malignancies.[3] Thymic carcinoids account for 25% of deaths in MEN1 patients, and pancreatic neuroendocrine tumors account for 60% of deaths. Therefore, prevention, early diagnosis, and treatment are essential to this disease.

---

*This author contributed equally to this work—coauthors.

Advances in Treatment and Management in Surgical Endocrinology. https://doi.org/10.1016/B978-0-323-66195-9.00010-8

PRESENTATION

As mentioned, the first manifestation of MEN1 syndrome in most of these patients is PHPT. The first clinical manifestations usually present around 20–25 years of age, which is 3 decades earlier than in patients with sporadic parathyroid adenoma.[4,7] Most commonly, the first presentation of PHPT in a patient with MEN1 syndrome is hypercalcemia, diagnosed on a routine laboratory work[7] and associated with inappropriately normal or elevated intact parathyroid hormone (PTH) levels in a patient between 20 and 30 years of age.

Patients may present with asymptomatic hypercalcemia. However, signs and symptoms of hypercalcemia can include weakness, fatigue, constipation, bone and joint pain, concentration issues, sleep disturbances, depression, decreased social interaction nephrolithiasis, decreased bone density, nausea, vomiting, polyuria, dehydration, hypertension, shortened QT interval, anorexia, or hypercalciuria among other manifestations.[8–10]

In MEN1-related PHPT, all parathyroid tissue is affected, and it is a multigland disease. It is associated with asymmetric and asynchronous four gland parathyroid growth,[11] revealing hypercellularity of the parathyroid tissue and frequently the presence of supernumerary glands.[7]

WORKUP AND DIAGNOSIS

PHPT is diagnosed biochemically with high normal or high serum calcium levels with concomitant inappropriately normal or elevated intact PTH levels. The difficulty when diagnosing PHPT is the ability to diagnose MEN1 syndrome in these patients as well. Physicians should be highly suspicious of MEN1 syndrome when PHPT is diagnosed in a young patient (less than 40 years old), there is multigland or recurrent disease, a family history or the presence of another endocrine pathology or tumor.[12] Preoperative identification of MEN1 syndrome in these patients is critical to determine the most appropriate surgical treatment and screen them for other MEN1-related pathologies.[7] Once the diagnosis of PHPT has been made and if there is a high suspicion for MEN1 syndrome, the patient should undergo genetic testing. When a presymptomatic diagnosis of MEN1 has been made, the patient should undergo surveillance with periodic serum calcium and PTH levels, in addition to bone mineral density scans until the diagnosis of PHPT can be confirmed, led to early treatment.

Certain institutions perform routine MEN1 genetic testing for pediatric patients with PHPT given the low incidence of sporadic disease in these patients. This has allowed the diagnosis of various patients whose diagnosis would have been missed based on clinical criteria alone.[7]

According to the last MEN1 Guidelines, genetic testing should be offered to every patient diagnosed with MEN1 syndrome and their first-degree relatives regardless of their symptoms.[5] This testing should be preempted by genetic counseling and performed before any other screening if a germline *MEN1* mutation has indeed been identified. Actual genetic testing methods can identify approximately 70%–95% of the patients with MEN1 syndrome[7] allowing the identification of at-risk family members and thus providing them with early treatment. Of note, there exists a sporadic-nonfamilial form of MEN1 where de novo mutations of the *MEN1* gene have been identified in about 10% of patients with MEN1.[3] If a mutation of the *MEN1* gene has been identified but is not part of the known pathogenic *MEN1* mutations, then population genetics can be of help. Additionally, when possible, any de novo mutation should be evaluated in first-degree family members to confirm the association or not with the disease. The availability of open-access genome sequencing databases is essential to validate genetic variations in patients with rare diseases.[2]

As we discuss early genetic detection of MEN1 as being essential in early treatment and improving prognosis in these patients, there is also the possibility of preimplantation genetic diagnosis for patients with known MEN1. In vitro fertilization is performed followed by blastocyst biopsy on day 5 or 6 after fertilization. Testing is performed in the embryos, and those free of abnormalities are implanted in the mother.[2] Polar body testing can also be performed in women with MEN1 syndrome before embryo formation, which some patients may prefer. Oocytes are isolated and fertilized using in vitro technique and testing is done before the division of the fertilized ovum. If the tests are negative for *MEN1* mutation, then the zygote is developed into an embryo and implanted. This technique does not allow detection of paternal abnormalities.[2]

Once a biochemical diagnosis of PHPT and a genetical diagnosis of MEN1 have been made, there is little value for imaging in these patients regarding their parathyroid disease. Preoperative studies such as neck ultrasound or 99m-technetium parathyroid scintigraphy have a limited benefit in identifying multiglandular disease or ectopic parathyroid disease due to a high false negative rate[13,14] and lack of cost-effectiveness.[15] The combination of these two imaging modalities has shown only a 30% success rate of identification of multiglandular disease.[16] The only study demonstrated to add value (defined as outcome over cost) to patient treatment is a neck ultrasound as it helps to determine concomitant thyroidal disease or the presence of extrathymic ectopic glands in most instances.[15] The treatment in these patients is dictated by bilateral cervical exploration regardless of preoperative localization studies.

Before undergoing parathyroidectomy, patients should have a baseline bone mineral density scan performed to evaluate their bone remineralization postoperatively and in the following years. Most patients already have one as it is usually ordered as part of the initial workup of PHPT.

Thymic carcinoid tumors have a prevalence of 2%–3% in MEN1 patients.[17,18] They are usually diagnosed once the disease is advanced and have poor prognosis. Therefore, it is important to screen these patients for thymic tumors once the diagnosis of MEN1 has been made. Current guidelines recommend screening for thymic carcinoids every 3–5 years starting at the age of 25[4]; however, some studies have shown rapid progression and recommend a yearly screening with a chest CT scan.[19] It is important to ensure patients do not have concomitant malignant thymic tumors before undergoing parathyroidectomy. If there is concern of concomitant thymic tumor in these patients, we recommend ordering imaging in accordance (CT or MRI of the chest) to appropriately plan the surgical procedure.

TREATMENT

The mainstay of treatment in MEN1 patients with hyperparathyroidism is parathyroidectomy. The optimal surgical timing is still debatable. The recommendations are generally based on the guidelines for asymptomatic sporadic primary hyperparathyroidism (sHPT) but are not precisely defined for MEN1-associated PHPT.[20] In general, the recommendation for surgical treatment is reserved for patients with hypercalcemia (calcium level 1 mg/dL above upper normal range accompanied by simultaneous nonsuppressed PTH levels) and symptomatic patients.[5,21] Objective symptoms of PHPT usually result from hypercalcemia and manifest as loss of bone density, decreased kidney function, nephrolithiasis, neurocognitive symptoms, and pathological fractures.[20] Some surgeons advocate close monitoring of patients until symptoms of hypercalcemia appear before operating.[5] This would help to limit repeated cervical surgeries in these patients, which expose them to higher risk of nerve injury or hypoparathyroidism.

On the other hand, early surgical intervention in this type of patient may reduce the prolonged exposure to elevated PTH levels and prevent its early complications.[22–24] Burgess JR et al. found that restoration of age appropriate bone mass is unobtainable in MEN1-associated PHPT patients with advanced osteopenia[22] and in a comparative review, Silva, A. et al. observed early bone loss in the 4th decade of life in these patients.[24] Additionally, it has been shown that kidney damage and bone density loss start early on in the disease's natural history,[10,25] and in patients considered asymptomatic but with neurocognitive symptoms, surgery has shown to improve their quality of life.[20] The authors favor early parathyroidectomy in patients with PHPT and known MEN1, as this data suggests that the negative effects of hyperparathyroidism take place well before it can be correlated with clinical manifestations and can even be irreversible.

Surgical Options

The aims of treatment for patients with MEN1-associated PHPT are the following: (1) to correct hypercalcemia for as long as possible, (2) to avoid permanent hypoparathyroidism, and (3) to facilitate the surgical exploration of recurrences, described for the first time by Carling and Udelsman.[26] So far, these remain the mainstays of surgical treatment in MEN1/HPT patients. To fulfill these therapeutic objectives, it is necessary to remove all the overactive parathyroid glands in patients with MEN1 through a bilateral cervical exploration, because the four glands are affected with hyperplasia or adenoma. To date, the association with parathyroid carcinoma has been reported in only four patients with MEN1 germline mutations,[27–29] which would involve en bloc resection.

Several therapeutic surgical options have been proposed, with controversial results that we will analyze later.

1. *Subtotal parathyroidectomy (SPx)* corresponds to the removal of at least 3–3½ parathyroid glands, preserving no more than 50 mg of parathyroid tissue from the most normal appearing parathyroid gland macroscopically. The authors favor a remnant 1.5–2 times the size of a normal parathyroid gland. The parathyroid remnant is marked with a metal clip or nonabsorbable suture, and ideally this is done away from the recurrent laryngeal nerve to prevent its injury in case of reoperation. This surgical technique aims to prevent the development of permanent hypoparathyroidism. It is also a feasible option when the fourth parathyroid gland cannot be found intraoperatively, and is even practiced in specialized

TABLE 10.1

Clinical Outcomes After Subtotal Parathyroidectomy (SPx) in Multiple Endocrine Neoplasia Type 1-Hyperparathyroidism (MEN1-HPT).

Year	Period	Patients	Mean Follow-up (years)	Persistent HPT %	Recurrent HPT %	Hypoparathy-roidism %	References
1979	1959–79	55	3.9	13	0	35	Edis et al.[33]
1983	1960–80	45	N.A	6.7	6.7	45	Van Heerden et al.[34]
1991	1986–90	18	N.A	11	0	0	Goretzki et al.[35]
1992	1982–91	34	8.9	0	27.3	12	Hellmann et al.[36]
1993	1970–91	54	10	0	16	8	O'Riordain et al.[37]
2001	1986–97	174	N.A	16.8	N.A	N.A	Goudet et al.[31]
2001	1986–98	25	4.5	N.A	12	12	Dotzenrath et al.[38]
2002	1972–2001	66	4	0	11	13	Arnalsteen et al.[39]
2003	1960–2002	63	6.1	0	33	26	Elaraj et al.[40]
2005	1973–2004	16	4	0	7	0	Lambert et al.[32]
2006	1974–2002	29	7.4	0	4.8	57	Hubbard et al.[41]
2008	1970–2005	40	7.2	12	44	10	Norton et al.[42]
2010	1980–2008	69	6.3	0	13	4.3	Salmeron et al.[43]
2011	1967–2008	17	12	7	65	18	Schreinemakers et al.[9]
2012	1990–2009	23	4.3	17		39	Pieterman et al.[44]

N.A., not applicable.

centers in this similar instance.[30–32] This surgical procedure has several technical difficulties. Carving of the remnant is a delicate task where the remaining tissue's vascularity must not be compromised—fine parathyroid vessels can be irreversibly damaged with the subsequent development of permanent post-surgical hypoparathyroidism—but where the right amount of parathyroid gland must be left behind so as to delay recurrence for as long as possible. Additionally, the manipulation of the remnant theoretically exposes the patient to a greater risk of seeding parathyroid cells, which would favor the recurrence of HPT in MEN1.

The aforementioned factors could explain the wide range of recurrence rates found in multiple studies published to date, from 7% to 65%, and the post-surgical hypoparathyroidism rates between 10% and 35% (Table 10.1).[9,31–44]

2. *Less than subtotal parathyroidectomy (LSPx)* consists of the removal of the elongated parathyroid glands. Usually, 2–2½ glands are removed, leaving in situ 1½–2 parathyroids. These remnant glands are marked with titanium clips or nonabsorbable sutures, to make it easier to identify in case of

reoperation. In the past, this technique was widely supported due to the high rates of permanent hypoparathyroidism in radical neck surgeries. Currently, it is generally recognized that LSPx in MEN1/HPT patients is associated with high rates of persistence and recurrence that reach 23%–61%; therefore, it is not recommended in these patients.[9,36,38–40,42,45]

Minimally invasive parathyroidectomy (MIP) corresponds to the standard of care in sHPT, although its applicability in MEN1/HPT is being evaluated in selected cases. Versnick et al. compared in 2013 the use of MIP ($n = 6$) and subtotal parathyroidectomy ($n = 46$), demonstrating zero incidence of recurrence, permanent hypoparathyroidism, and recurrent laryngeal nerve paralysis for the group subjected to MIP, with a clinical follow-up interval of 1.6 years for MIP and 8.8 years for subtotal parathyroidectomy ($P \leq .001$).[46] Recently, Kluijfhout et al. evaluated the clinical results between subtotal parathyroidectomy ($n = 16$) and unilateral clearance ($n = 8$), defined in patients with MEN1/HPT utilizing sestamibi and ultrasound concordant imaging in the detection of a single, enlarged parathyroid gland.

Patients undergoing subtotal parathyroidectomy were younger than those who had undergone unilateral clearance. In these patients subjected to subtotal parathyroidectomy, one developed persistent hyperparathyroidism, five experienced recurrence, and two had permanent hypoparathyroidism. In patients subjected to unilateral clearance, one had persistence, one had recurrence, and none developed permanent hypoparathyroidism. The mean of clinical follow-up was 47 and 68 months, respectively ($P = .62$).[47].

3. *Total parathyroidectomy (TPx)* consists of the total removal of the parathyroid glands with autotransplantation of fresh or cryopreserved parathyroid tissue. It has been widely reported in the literature that this surgical option has a wide range of recurrence rates, from 4% to 23%, with postsurgical hypoparathyroidism ranging from 22% to 66% (Table 10.2).[11,36,40,44,45,48–50] The autotransplant, usually located in a single pocket in the brachioradialis muscle of the nondominant forearm, could be beneficial in bypassing the need for postoperative vitamin D. Additionally, if hypercalcemia recurs, the autotransplant can be removed under local anesthesia.[11,51,52] Commonly, for the preparation of fresh or cryopreserved tissue, the fragments should be cut into the smallest sizes possible, ideally around 1 mm^3, to facilitate implantation.[51] The number of fragments to be implanted is still a matter of clinical debate, but generally 20–25 fragments are considered optimal. Other series did not exceed 12 parathyroid fragments and had a 20%–30% of

nonfunctioning parathyroid grafts.[33,53,54] Although it is uncertain what factors are associated with a successful autotransplantation, it generally depends on technical, local, and parathyroid histopathology factors.

It is recommended to perform a transcervical thymectomy (TCT) with MEN1-associated parathyroidectomy. This allows the removal of intrathymic parathyroid glands and may help prevent thymic carcinoid tumors that may develop in patients with MEN1 syndrome.[55] Nonetheless, it is estimated that TCT removes only 30%–40% of the thymus leading certain authors to question its prophylactic value[56]

SPx versus TPx

Our favored approach to PHPT in the MEN1 patient is subtotal parathyroidectomy. It avoids any period of time in which the patient is grossly hypocalcemic and dependent on calcium supplementation. We will however discuss the advantages and disadvantages of both surgical options in patients with MEN1-associated HPT. Older studies have shown similar rates of recurrence and of postoperative hypoparathyroidism although SPx is one of the therapeutic approaches of choice in specialized endocrine surgery centers. Two particular investigations attempted to address this question: one of them was randomized by Lairmore et al. in 2014, and the other was the meta-analysis by Schreinemakers et al. in 2011.[9,57]

In the randomized study by Lairmore et al., 33 cases with MEN1-HPT were analyzed between 1996 and

TABLE 10.2
Clinical Outcomes After Total Parathyroidectomy (TPx) in Multiple Endocrine Neoplasia Type 1-Hyperparathyroidism (MEN1-HPT).

Year	Period	Patients	Mean Follow-Up (years)	Persistent HPT %	Recurrent HPT %	Hypoparathy-roidism %	References
1986	1961–82	18	2	0	0	27.8	Malmaeus et al.[48]
1992	1982–91	23	8.9	0	22	30	Hellmann et al.[36]
1998	1969–96	15	11.3	0	20	47	Hellmann et al.[45]
2003	1960–2002	16	7	0	23	46	Elaraj et al.[40]
2007	1990–2006	45	6.7	0	11	22	Tonelli et al.[11]
2010	1987–2009	23	7	4	4	22	Waldmann et al.[49]
2012	1987–2011	45	N.A	N.A	14.3	40	Montenegro et al.[50]
2012	1990–2009	32	4.3	19		66	Pieterman et al.[44]

N.A., not applicable.

2012, of which 17 were randomized to SPx and 15 to TPx. The incidence of postoperative hypocalcemia was higher in the TPx group, reaching 47% compared with the SPx group with 35%. Permanent hypoparathyroidism was diagnosed in two (12%) patients in the SPx group and in one (7%) of the TPx (*P* = not significant). Only one patient from the SPx group had persistent PHPT; and later underwent a TCT for the resection of the ectopic mediastinal parathyroid gland. Four patients (24%) in the SPx group experienced recurrence during postoperative follow-up, and two patients (13%) in the TPx group showed no difference upon analysis. Therefore, there were no differences between both groups in regards to clinical outcomes such as persistent HPT, recurrent HPT, and permanent hypoparathyroidism.[57] The study however did not evaluate the time for which the patient had an altered quality of life because of copious oral calcium supplementation.

In a systematic review conducted by Schreinemakers et al. in 2011, 12 studies (52 patients) were selected with complete, original, and available information on different surgical treatments undergone by patients with MEN1/HPT. The studies were selected from Medline, Embase, and Cochrane. They were grouped according to type of surgical resection performed: LSPTx (29 patients), SPx (17 patients), and TPx (6 patients). The clinical results related to persistence and recurrence of PTH, and postoperative permanent hypoparathyroidism were analyzed. When the meta-analysis between SPx and TPx was performed, it showed that there was

no greater risk of recurrent HPT in SPx compared to TPx (OR = 2.15, 95% CI = 0.82−5.61, *P* = .12). Nor was there an increased risk of persistent HPT in the two groups (OR = 2.37, 95% CI = 0.54−10.44, *P* = .25). However, after SPx, patients had a lower risk of permanent hypoparathyroidism than patients in the TPx (OR = 0.25, 95% CI = 0.11−0.54, *P* = .0004).[9]

Intraoperative Parathyroid Hormone Monitoring as a Predictor of MultiGland Parathyroid Disease

The use of intraoperative parathyroid hormone (ioPTH) monitoring has become an essential tool in the surgical treatment of sporadic primary hyperparathyroidism due to its high sensitivity, which exceeds 95%.[58] However, it has not proven to be such a straightforward tool in patients with multiglandular disease. The removal of a single parathyroid adenoma normalizes ioPTH within 15 min in most cases, in multiglandular disease this decrease is progressive, and, rarely reaches normal levels within 15 min of the removal of all affected parathyroid glands.[59,60]

Various studies have tried to evaluate the reliability of using ioPTH in multiglandular or hyperplasic parathyroid disease, which are referenced in Table 10.3, with a percentage of false positives ranging between 9% and 75%.[32,39,54,61−63] Additionally, Thompson et al.[61] and Clerici et al.[63] demonstrated a reduction in the false positive rate using a cutoff for ioPTH ≥70% drop at 20 min after the parathyroid excision. The authors do not routinely use ioPTH in

TABLE 10.3
Different Intraoperative Parathyroid Hormone (ioPTH) Protocols in Multiglandular Parathyroid Disease After Parathyroidectomy.

Year	Patients	Time (minute) after Final Gland Removed	PTH Cut off	True Positive	False Negative	False Positive	True Negative	References
1999	11	10	≥50%	9	1	1	1	Thompson et al.[61]
2001	14[a]	10	≥50%	8	0	2	4	Kivlen et al.[54]
2002	7	10	≥50%	0	0	2	5	Jaskowiak et al.[62]
2002	20[b]	5	≥50%	18	1	0	1	Arnalsteen et al.[39]
2004	8	10	≥50%	0	0	6	2	Clerici et al.[63]
2005	14[b]	N.A	Decrease to ≤60 pg/mL	12	0	2	0	Lambert et al.[32]

N.A., not applicable.
[a] All reoperative MEN1/HPT patients.
[b] All patients with MEN1/HPT.

multiglandular disease as it will not guide the extent of the procedure—all four glands will be removed during the intervention, and using ioPTH will increase costs and operative time.

Identification of the Parathyroid Glands

One of the difficulties during bilateral cervical exploration in multiglandular parathyroid disease is being able to identify all four (or more) glands. We use an alphabetical nomenclature system to standardize our exploration.[64] Superior parathyroid glands will be located lateral to the recurrent laryngeal nerve and can be found posterior to the thyroid capsule (Type A), in the tracheoesophageal groove behind the thyroid lobe (Type B) or posterior in the tracheoesophageal groove and inferiorly toward the clavicle (Type C). Occasionally, the gland may course along the recurrent laryngeal nerve, usually within 1 cm of it at the level of its junction with the inferior thyroid artery (Type D). Inferior parathyroid glands can be found near the lateral edge of the inferior thyroid pole (Type E) or in the thyrothymic ligament or thymus (Type F). As mentioned previously, we use a neck ultrasound for our preoperative imaging, and this will aid in identifying an intrathyroidal gland (Type G). We believe that by using this systematic approach, all ectopic parathyroid glands should be identified.

Operative Technique

As described previously, we favor performing SPx in our MEN1 patients with PHPT. Following is a description of our technique for SPx in patients undergoing their first neck operation and how we process the remnant parathyroid.

Our patient is placed in a semi-Fowler position on the operating table with hyperextension of the neck. We do not use a nerve monitor in the initial surgery, as it has not been shown to decrease the risk of nerve injury. We start the operation on the patient's right side to ensure consistency with our surgical team. The skin is incised two fingerbreadths above the sternum and clavicles in the midline. We traverse the subcutaneous tissue and platysma. The strap muscles are retracted medially and the sternocleidomastoid muscle laterally. Two Kochers are then placed on the right thyroid lobe—both 1/3 away from either pole—and retract the gland toward the ceiling and away from the primary surgeon in an up and over fashion (Fig. 10.1). This exposes the recurrent laryngeal nerve and the right-sided parathyroid glands. Both glands are dissected with the bipolar device taking care not to disrupt the blood vessels laterally.

First of all, we start crafting our remnant. Most commonly we favor the right inferior parathyroid, as the inferior glands are easier to access in case of recurrence. Various factors are considered when choosing which gland to leave as a remnant such as size, nodularity, most normal appearing gland, and location relative to the recurrent laryngeal nerve and to the thymus. Once the remnant is chosen, we start crafting it by placing a large Hemoclip across the distal third of the gland. We hold the clip in place and sharply resect the distal end with the scalpel. The Hemoclip is left in place for easier future identification if needed. The specimen is sent for frozen section to confirm the presence of parathyroid tissue. The superior gland is then removed with the bipolar device.

We direct our attention to the patient's left neck and proceed with the thymic resection. The thymus is retracted with right-angled retractors in a delivering motion from the mediastinum into the neck. We grasp the most inferior portion of the thymus that has revealed itself and resect it with the electrocautery. The right thymus is then transected if it is anatomically separated from the left side. If we believe the remnant's viability will be jeopardized through the right-sided thymectomy, we may decide to skip this step. We then proceed toward the left thyroid and perform the up and over motion of the left thyroid gland. Once the other two parathyroids have been dissected, but before their resection, we reevaluate our remnant's viability. By this time, at least 20 min have passed, allowing us to appropriately evaluate the remnant's perfusion, and we should have results from our frozen section confirming parathyroid tissue. We then resect our last two parathyroid glands with the bipolar device. If we are concerned by

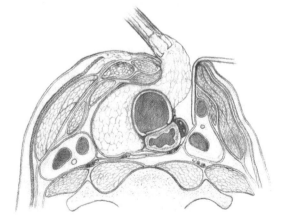

FIG. 10.1 "Up and over" motion during parathyroidectomy. Retraction of the thyroid for parathyroid exposure.

our remnant's viability at any time, we craft another remnant from one of the left parathyroid glands and remove the original one. All removed tissue is sent for pathology.

FOLLOW-UP

After undergoing surgery, patients should be followed regularly. In our practice, we survey our patients annually with intact PTH and calcium levels at 6 months and then annually. Additionally, they undergo a bone mineral density scan at 1 year postoperatively and then every 2 years.

RECURRENCES IN PATIENTS DIAGNOSED WITH MEN1/HPT AND PREVIOUSLY TREATED

Clinical outcomes of surgery are usually worse than those reported in sporadic primary hyperparathyroidism due to high rates of recurrence of the disease. This high rate of recurrence is due to various factors. First of all, in more than 10% of the cases, the parathyroid glands appear macroscopically normal intraoperatively in these patients.[11] This is due to the *MEN1* germline mutation that induces the parathyroid glands to be variably susceptible to expressing tumorigenesis only after another somatic mutation (second hit)[65–67] or epigenetics alteration[68] takes place, therefore favoring the regrowth of unrecognized parathyroid glands as a result of the inactivation of the *MEN1* gene. Additionally, up to 20% of the cases associated with ectopic parathyroid glands[11,45] remain unnoticed in the primary surgical intervention.

It is widely recognized that patients with MEN1/HPT are characterized histopathologically by the development of parathyroid hyperplasia, but also with the sequential formation of parathyroid adenomas.[4] Furthermore, the germline mutation MEN1 induces asymmetries in size, weight, and appearance, which are not necessarily synchronic, also adding the high incidence of ectopic parathyroid glands.[45,69] All these previously mentioned factors are related to one of the most significant factors in the development of recurrence in these patients, the extended clinical follow-up.[31,37,45] The surgical reexploration in a patient with MEN1/HPT corresponds to a challenge for any endocrine surgeon. The indications for reexploration are similar to those of the primary intervention; severe hypercalcemia, symptoms, or alterations in bone mineral density. For these cases, a thorough preoperative clinical, including primary operative protocols and pathological reports, and preoperative imaging study (neck ultrasound,

sestamibi parathyroid scintigraphy) are necessary to minimize the inherent risk of a neck reintervention such as recurrent laryngeal nerve injury, postoperative hypoparathyroidism, chylous fistula, and cervical hematoma.[26,44,54,70] Moreover, this reexploration could involve the resection of an ectopic parathyroid gland, the resection of one or more hyperplastic parathyroid glands, transcervical thymectomy, or resection of the parathyroid graft in the forearm.[43,71] All patients should undergo an evaluation of vocal cord function before undergoing a repeat cervical exploration as this could influence surgical planning. The use of ioPTH is less controversial in reoperative cervical exploration in MEN1-HPT patients. In their retrospective study, Keutgen et al. found that ioPTH in reoperative surgery in these patients had a positive predictive value of 92% for postoperative eucalcemia with persistent PHPT present in 13% of the patients.[71] The authors use ioPTH in reoperative parathyroidectomy in MEN1-HPT patients as this will guide them in the extent of their cervical exploration. Additionally, due to scaring and the high risk of nerve injury associated with these cases, they routinely use intraoperative nerve monitoring.

CONCLUSION/DISCUSSION

Parathyroid surgery for MEN1/HPT is in continuous development due to greater understanding of the pathophysiology of the disease, improved imaging modalities, and the introduction of new technologies. The fundamental objectives in the surgical management of patients with MEN1/HPT are as follows: obtain and maintain long-term normocalcemia, avoid postoperative hypoparathyroidism and all related surgical complications, and, finally, facilitate the surgical reexploration in cases of recurrent or persistent HPT. Therefore, the surgical treatment of choice should be intimately linked to the particularities of each case, but above all should consider the balance of risk and benefit to which the patient will be subjected.

Patients with MEN1/HPT are commonly subjected to SPx or TPx with immediate autotransplantation, due to the higher risk of permanent hypoparathyroidism after a TPx and the high rates of persistence/recurrence after LSPx in MEN1/HPT. Based on previously exposed evidence, we recommend subtotal parathyroidectomy in patients diagnosed with MEN1/HPT as the initial surgical treatment. In addition, transcervical thymectomy with the initial surgery should be performed for all patients with MEN1/HPT, mainly to control the frequent risk of ectopic parathyroid within the thymus but not as prevention of the development of neuroendocrine tumors in these patients.

Due to the limited evidence currently available regarding reoperation in MEN1/HPT patients, the recommended strategies to face this challenging surgical scenario are multiple. The first is the confirmation of the diagnosis of HPT before any surgical examination. Second, a detailed review of previous operative notes, and histopathological reports are required to obtain more information about the anatomy and potentially remaining glands. Third, preoperative imaging is used to rule out concomitant disease such as thyroid cancer. It should be obtained to determine the most precise location of the tumor. Last, cryopreservation should be considered in a reoperative case if removal of tissue is presumed to be the last functional tissue present. If this is the case, immediate autotransplant should be performed to prevent permanent hypoparathyroidism.

REFERENCES

1. Wermer P. Genetic aspects of adenomatosis of endocrine glands. *Am J Med.* 1954;16:363−371.
2. Perrier ND. From initial description by Wermer to present-day MEN1: what have we learned? *World J Surg.* 2018;42: 1031−1035.
3. Thakker RV. *Multiple Endocrine Neoplasia Type 1, Endocrinology: Adult and Pediatric.* Seventh). Elsevier Inc.; 2016: 2566−2593.e9.
4. Brandi ML, Gagel RF, Angeli A, et al. Guidelines for diagnosis and therapy of MEN type 1 and type 2. *J Clin Endocrinol Metab.* 2001;86:5658−5671.
5. Thakker RV, Newey PJ, Walls GV, et al. Clinical practice guidelines for multiple endocrine neoplasia type 1 (MEN1). *J Clin Endocrinol Metab.* 2012;97:2990−3011.
6. Kraimps JL, B A, Donatini G. Familial hyperparathyroidism in multiple endocrine neoplasia syndromes. In: Clark OHDQ-Y, Kebebew E, et al., eds. *Textbook of Endocrine Surgery.* Third. The health sciences publisher; 2016.
7. Romero Arenas MA, Morris LF, Rich TA, et al. Preoperative multiple endocrine neoplasia type 1 diagnosis improves the surgical outcomes of pediatric patients with primary hyperparathyroidism. *J Pediatr Surg.* 2014;49:546−550.
8. Kouvaraki MA, Greer M, Sharma S, et al. Indications for operative intervention in patients with asymptomatic primary hyperparathyroidism: practice patterns of endocrine surgery. *Surgery.* 2006;139:527−534.
9. Schreinemakers JM, Pieterman CR, Scholten A, et al. The optimal surgical treatment for primary hyperparathyroidism in MEN1 patients: a systematic review. *World J Surg.* 2011;35:1993−2005.
10. Giusti F, Tonelli F, Brandi ML. Primary hyperparathyroidism in multiple endocrine neoplasia type 1: when to perform surgery? *Clinics.* 2012;67(suppl 1):141−144.
11. Tonelli F, Marcucci T, Fratini G, et al. Is total parathyroidectomy the treatment of choice for hyperparathyroidism in multiple endocrine neoplasia type 1? *Ann Surg.* 2007;246: 1075−1082.
12. de Laat JM, Tham E, Pieterman CR, et al. Predicting the risk of multiple endocrine neoplasia type 1 for patients with commonly occurring endocrine tumors. *Eur J Endocrinol.* 2012;167:181−187.
13. Caldarella C, Treglia G, Pontecorvi A, et al. Diagnostic performance of planar scintigraphy using (9)(9)mTc-MIBI in patients with secondary hyperparathyroidism: a meta-analysis. *Ann Nucl Med.* 2012;26:794−803.
14. Alkhalili E, Tasci Y, Aksoy E, et al. The utility of neck ultrasound and sestamibi scans in patients with secondary and tertiary hyperparathyroidism. *World J Surg.* 2015;39: 701−705.
15. Nilubol N, Weinstein L, Simonds WF, et al. Preoperative localizing studies for initial parathyroidectomy in MEN1 syndrome: is there any benefit? *World J Surg.* 2012;36: 1368−1374.
16. Sugg SL, Krzywda EA, Demeure MJ, et al. Detection of multiple gland primary hyperparathyroidism in the era of minimally invasive parathyroidectomy. *Surgery.* 2004; 136:1303−1309.
17. Goudet P, Murat A, Cardot-Bauters C, et al. Thymic neuroendocrine tumors in multiple endocrine neoplasia type 1: a comparative study on 21 cases among a series of 761 MEN1 from the GTE (Groupe des Tumeurs Endocrines). *World J Surg.* 2009;33:1197−1207.
18. Ferolla P, Falchetti A, Filosso P, et al. Thymic neuroendocrine carcinoma (carcinoid) in multiple endocrine neoplasia type 1 syndrome: The Italian series. *J Clin Endocrinol Metab.* 2005;90:2603−2609.
19. Gibril F, Chen YJ, Schrump DS, et al. Prospective study of thymic carcinoids in patients with multiple endocrine neoplasia type 1. *J Clin Endocrinol Metab.* 2003;88: 1066−1081.
20. Wilhelm SM, Wang TS, Ruan DT, et al. The American association of endocrine surgeons guidelines for definitive management of primary hyperparathyroidism. *Jama Surgery.* 2016;151:959−968.
21. Thakker RV. Multiple endocrine neoplasia type 1 (MEN1) and type 4 (MEN4). *Mol Cell Endocrinol.* 2014; 386:2−15.
22. Burgess JR, David R, Greenaway TM, et al. Osteoporosis in multiple endocrine neoplasia type 1: severity, clinical significance, relationship to primary hyperparathyroidism, and response to parathyroidectomy. *Arch Surg.* 1999;134: 1119−1123.
23. Eller-Vainicher C, Chiodini I, Battista C, et al. Sporadic and MEN1-related primary hyperparathyroidism: differences in clinical expression and severity. *J Bone Miner Res.* 2009;24:1404−1410.
24. Silva AM, Vodopivec D, Christakis I, et al. Operative intervention for primary hyperparathyroidism offers greater bone recovery in patients with sporadic disease than in those with multiple endocrine neoplasia type 1-related hyperparathyroidism. *Surgery.* 2017;161:107−115.
25. Lourenco Jr DM, Coutinho FL, Toledo RA, et al. Biochemical, bone and renal patterns in hyperparathyroidism associated with multiple endocrine neoplasia type 1. *Clinics.* 2012;67(suppl 1):99−108.

26. Carling T, Udelsman R. Parathyroid surgery in familial hyperparathyroid disorders. *J Intern Med*. 2005;257:27–37.

27. Shih RY, Fackler S, Maturo S, et al. Parathyroid carcinoma in multiple endocrine neoplasia type 1 with a classic germline mutation. *Endocr Pract*. 2009;15:567–572.

28. del Pozo C, Garcia-Pascual L, Balsells M, et al. Parathyroid carcinoma in multiple endocrine neoplasia type 1. Case report and review of the literature. *Hormones (Athens)*. 2011;10:326–331.

29. Christakis I, Busaidy NL, Cote GJ, et al. Parathyroid carcinoma and atypical parathyroid neoplasms in MEN1 patients; A clinico-pathologic challenge. The MD Anderson case series and review of the literature. *Int J Surg*. 2016;31:10–16.

30. O'Riordain DS, O'Brien T, van Heerden JA, et al. Surgical management of insulinoma associated with multiple endocrine neoplasia type I. *World J Surg*. 1994;18:488–493; discussion 493-4.

31. Goudet P, Cougard P, Verges B, et al. Hyperparathyroidism in multiple endocrine neoplasia type I: surgical trends and results of a 256-patient series from Groupe D'etude des Neoplasies Endocriniennes Multiples Study Group. *World J Surg*. 2001;25:886–890.

32. Lambert LA, Shapiro SE, Lee JE, et al. Surgical treatment of hyperparathyroidism in patients with multiple endocrine neoplasia type 1. *Arch Surg*. 2005;140:374–382.

33. Edis AJ, van Heerden JA, Scholz DA. Results of subtotal parathyroidectomy for primary chief cell hyperplasia. *Surgery*. 1979;86:462–469.

34. van Heerden JA, Kent 3rd RB, Sizemore GW, et al. Primary hyperparathyroidism in patients with multiple endocrine neoplasia syndromes. Surgical experience. *Arch Surg*. 1983;118:533–536.

35. Goretzki PE, Dotzenrath C, Roeher HD. Management of primary hyperparathyroidism caused by multiple gland disease. *World J Surg*. 1991;15:693–697.

36. Hellman P, Skogseid B, Juhlin C, et al. Findings and long-term results of parathyroid surgery in multiple endocrine neoplasia type 1. *World J Surg*. 1992;16:718–722; discussion 722-3.

37. O'Riordain DS, O'Brien T, Grant CS, et al. Surgical management of primary hyperparathyroidism in multiple endocrine neoplasia types 1 and 2. *Surgery*. 1993;114:1031–1037; discussion 1037-9.

38. Dotzenrath C, Cupisti K, Goretzki PE, et al. Long-term biochemical results after operative treatment of primary hyperparathyroidism associated with multiple endocrine neoplasia types I and IIa: is a more or less extended operation essential? *Eur J Surg*. 2001;167:173–178.

39. Arnalsteen LC, Alesina PF, Quiereux JL, et al. Long-term results of less than total parathyroidectomy for hyperparathyroidism in multiple endocrine neoplasia type 1. *Surgery*. 2002;132:1119–1124; discussion 1124-5.

40. Elaraj DM, Skarulis MC, Libutti SK, et al. Results of initial operation for hyperparathyroidism in patients with multiple endocrine neoplasia type 1. *Surgery*. 2003;134:858–864; discussion 864-5.

41. Hubbard JG, Sebag F, Maweja S, et al. Subtotal parathyroidectomy as an adequate treatment for primary hyperparathyroidism in multiple endocrine neoplasia type 1. *Arch Surg*. 2006;141:235–239.

42. Norton JA, Venzon DJ, Berna MJ, et al. Prospective study of surgery for primary hyperparathyroidism (HPT) in multiple endocrine neoplasia-type 1 and Zollinger-Ellison syndrome: long-term outcome of a more virulent form of HPT. *Ann Surg*. 2008;247:501–510.

43. Salmeron MD, Gonzalez JM, Sancho Insenser J, et al. Causes and treatment of recurrent hyperparathyroidism after subtotal parathyroidectomy in the presence of multiple endocrine neoplasia 1. *World J Surg*. 2010;34:1325–1331.

44. Pieterman CR, van Hulsteijn LT, den Heijer M, et al. Primary hyperparathyroidism in MEN1 patients: a cohort study with longterm follow-up on preferred surgical procedure and the relation with genotype. *Ann Surg*. 2012;255:1171–1178.

45. Hellman P, Skogseid B, Oberg K, et al. Primary and reoperative parathyroid operations in hyperparathyroidism of multiple endocrine neoplasia type 1. *Surgery*. 1998;124:993–999.

46. Versnick M, Popadich A, Sidhu S, et al. Minimally invasive parathyroidectomy provides a conservative surgical option for multiple endocrine neoplasia type 1-primary hyperparathyroidism. *Surgery*. 2013;154:101–105.

47. Kluijfhout WP, Beninato T, Drake FT, et al. Unilateral clearance for primary hyperparathyroidism in selected patients with multiple endocrine neoplasia type 1. *World J Surg*. 2016;40:2964–2969.

48. Malmaeus J, Benson L, Johansson H, et al. Parathyroid surgery in the multiple endocrine neoplasia type I syndrome: choice of surgical procedure. *World J Surg*. 1986;10:668–672.

49. Waldmann J, Lopez CL, Langer P, et al. Surgery for multiple endocrine neoplasia type 1-associated primary hyperparathyroidism. *Br J Surg*. 2010;97:1528–1534.

50. Montenegro FL, Lourenco Jr DM, Tavares MR, et al. Total parathyroidectomy in a large cohort of cases with hyperparathyroidism associated with multiple endocrine neoplasia type 1: experience from a single academic center. *Clinics*. 2012;67(suppl 1):131–139.

51. Wagner PK, Seesko HG, Rothmund M. Replantation of cryopreserved human parathyroid tissue. *World J Surg*. 1991;15:751–755.

52. Wells Jr SA, Ellis GJ, Gunnells JC, et al. Parathyroid autotransplantation in primary parathyroid hyperplasia. *N Engl J Med*. 1976;295:57–62.

53. Feldman AL, Sharaf RN, Skarulis MC, et al. Results of heterotopic parathyroid autotransplantation: a 13-year experience. *Surgery*. 1999;126:1042–1048.

54. Kivlen MH, Bartlett DL, Libutti SK, et al. Reoperation for hyperparathyroidism in multiple endocrine neoplasia type 1. *Surgery*. 2001;130:991–998.

55. Lim LC, Tan MH, Eng C, et al. Thymic carcinoid in multiple endocrine neoplasia 1: genotype-phenotype correlation and prevention. *J Intern Med*. 2006;259:428–432.

56. Powell AC, Alexander HR, Pingpank JF, et al. The utility of routine transcervical thymectomy for multiple endocrine neoplasia 1-related hyperparathyroidism. *Surgery.* 2008; 144:878−883; discussion 883-4.

57. Lairmore TC, Govednik CM, Quinn CE, et al. A randomized, prospective trial of operative treatments for hyperparathyroidism in patients with multiple endocrine neoplasia type 1. *Surgery.* 2014;156:1326−1334; discussion 1334-5.

58. Barczynski M, Golkowski F, Nawrot I. The current status of intraoperative iPTH assay in surgery for primary hyperparathyroidism. *Gland Surg.* 2015;4:36−43.

59. Proye CA, Goropoulos A, Franz C, et al. Usefulness and limits of quick intraoperative measurements of intact (1-84) parathyroid hormone in the surgical management of hyperparathyroidism: sequential measurements in patients with multiglandular disease. *Surgery.* 1991;110: 1035−1042.

60. Richards ML, Thompson GB, Farley DR, et al. An optimal algorithm for intraoperative parathyroid hormone monitoring. *Arch Surg.* 2011;146:280−285.

61. Thompson GB, Grant CS, Perrier ND, et al. Reoperative parathyroid surgery in the era of sestamibi scanning and intraoperative parathyroid hormone monitoring. *Arch Surg.* 1999;134:699−704; discussion 704-5.

62. Jaskowiak NT, Sugg SL, Helke J, et al. Pitfalls of intraoperative quick parathyroid hormone monitoring and gamma probe localization in surgery for primary hyperparathyroidism. *Arch Surg.* 2002;137:659−668; discussion 668-9.

63. Clerici T, Brandle M, Lange J, et al. Impact of intraoperative parathyroid hormone monitoring on the prediction of multiglandular parathyroid disease. *World J Surg.* 2004; 28:187−192.

64. Perrier ND, Edeiken B, Nunez R, et al. A novel nomenclature to classify parathyroid adenomas. *World J Surg.* 2009; 33:412−416.

65. Friedman E, Sakaguchi K, Bale AE, et al. Clonality of parathyroid tumors in familial multiple endocrine neoplasia type 1. *N Engl J Med.* 1989;321:213−218.

66. Marx SJ, Simonds WF, Agarwal SK, et al. Hyperparathyroidism in hereditary syndromes: special expressions and special managements. *J Bone Miner Res.* 2002;17(suppl 2):N37−N43.

67. Carling T. Molecular pathology of parathyroid tumors. *Trends Endocrinol Metabol.* 2001;12:53−58.

68. Yang YJ, Song TY, Park J, et al. Menin mediates epigenetic regulation via histone H3 lysine 9 methylation. *Cell Death Dis.* 2013;4:e583.

69. Marx SJ, Menczel J, Campbell G, et al. Heterogeneous size of the parathyroid glands in familial multiple endocrine neoplasia type 1. *Clin Endocrinol.* 1991;35:521−526.

70. Hubbard JG, Sebag F, Maweja S, et al. Primary hyperparathyroidism in MEN 1–how radical should surgery be? *Langenbeck's Arch Surg.* 2002;386:553−557.

71. Keutgen XM, Nilubol N, Agarwal S, et al. Reoperative surgery in patients with multiple endocrine neoplasia type 1 associated primary hyperparathyroidism. *Ann Surg Oncol.* 2016;23:701−707.

CHAPTER 11

Advances in Diagnosis and Management of Primary Hyperparathyroidism due to Multiple Endocrine Neoplasia (MEN) Type 2 Syndrome

JAMES A. LEE, MD • SARAH S. PEARLSTEIN, MD

INTRODUCTION

Although the distinctive feature of the MEN2 syndromes is medullary thyroid cancer, primary hyperparathyroidism (PHP) is an associated disorder in MEN2A but not in familial medullary thyroid cancer or MEN 2B. PHP is defined as the autonomous overproduction of parathyroid hormone by one or more parathyroid glands. The relative risk of developing PHP in MEN 2A correlates with the specific codon mutation. Approximately 10%–35% of MEN2A patients with a C634R[1] mutation will develop PHP, while mutations in codons 609–620 are associated with a lower frequency of 2%–12%.[2] Over 80% of PHP in MEN 2A is caused by multigland disease.[3] Different from the often more aggressive form of PHP seen in MEN 1, PHP in MEN2A is often asymptomatic and mild.[4] Parathyroid carcinoma is rarely associated with MEN 2A.[5]

DIAGNOSIS

Diagnosis of Hyperparathyroidism in the General Population

As in sporadic cases of PHP, it is important to obtain a thorough history for possible signs and symptoms of PHP such as nephrolithiasis, fragility fractures, osteoporosis, gastrointestinal complaints, and neuropsychiatric disturbances. Although the well-known mnemonic of "stones, bones, groans, and psychic overtones" represents the classic presentation of PHP, with the addition of calcium in the standard basic metabolic profile, this classic presentation is becoming increasingly less common. Up to 68%–85% of patients are asymptomatic.[2,6] In addition to a detailed history and review of symptoms, a thorough family history is especially important. Patients with sporadic PHP who are younger than 40 years old should be considered for genetic evaluation.[4] Clearly, patients with a syndromic presentation or strong family history of inherited syndromes such as MEN 2A should undergo genetic testing. If a family member has a known codon mutation, the patient may be screened specifically for that mutation.

The diagnosis of PHP in patients with MEN 2A is made the same way as in sporadic cases—25-hydroxyvitamin D, total serum calcium, PTH, and creatinine and is covered in more detail in the corresponding chapter. A 24-h urine calcium measurement can be used to distinguish PHP from familial hypocalciuric hypercalcemia.[4] Given the propensity for developing PHP, a high index of suspicion should be maintained for patients with MEN2A and lifelong screening is necessary.

In addition to a thorough history, physical exam, and biochemical evaluation, patients should have a bone densitometry examination, survey for kidney stones, and screening for occult fractures, especially lumbar fractures.

Diagnosis of Hyperparathyroidism in Patients with Known MEN2A

The diagnosis of MEN2A is rarely made based on hyperparathyroidism as medullary thyroid carcinoma usually precedes it with a typical age of diagnosis between 25 and 35. There are case reports of hyperparathyroidism

Advances in Treatment and Management in Surgical Endocrinology. https://doi.org/10.1016/B978-0-323-66195-9.00011-X

being the first manifestation of MEN2A; however, they are rare and atypical.[7] In MEN2A, hyperparathyroidism is typically diagnosed at a median age of 33—37 years with a range of 12—70 years. However, with molecular testing procedures, the age of diagnosis has progressively decreased over time since the 1990s.[2] Diagnosis of MEN2A based on genetics or other manifestations will be discussed in another chapter. Briefly, the genetic diagnosis of MEN2A is typically made by RET sequencing.[8] Overall, for patients with MEN2A, the American Thyroid Association recommends beginning biochemical screening for hyperparathyroidism at age 8.[9] Biochemical screening involves annual calcium, parathyroid hormone, and albumin levels. In addition, before a planned thyroidectomy for medullary thyroid cancer, patients should be screened for PHP so that if present, both thyroidectomy and parathyroidectomy can be undertaken at the same time.

Localization

As there is a high rate of four-gland hyperplasia and multigland disease in PHP associated with MEN 2A, preoperative imaging is not strictly necessary. However, in many cases, preoperative imaging studies can be helpful to localize parathyroid glands for operative planning. The different types of studies are covered more extensively in another chapter. However, the most important recommendation from the American Association of Endocrine Surgeons Parathyroid Guidelines is that the surgeon should determine which imaging study/studies to order based on his/her knowledge of the results and expertise at his/her institution as the sensitivity and specificity of imaging vary from institution to institution.

Technetium 99m sestamibi scintigraphy (sestamibi scan) has traditionally been used for parathyroid gland imaging. Sestamibi is a monovalent cation that accumulates in mitochondria and has a particular affinity for the parathyroid gland. Increasingly, sestamibi scans are fused with SPECT imaging for better anatomic definition especially of small lesions. Unfortunately, sestamibi has lower sensitivity with multiglandular disease, a situation that is common in MEN2A.[10]

Ultrasound has been increasingly utilized in parathyroid disease given that it is inexpensive, noninvasive, readily available, and able to evaluate thyroid pathology. Ultrasound is highly operator dependent and cannot visualize the mediastinum and is less accurate for small lesions and lesions in the tracheoesophageal groove (because of air-interface issues with the trachea). However, when combined with sestamibi, the sensitivity for identifying a single parathyroid adenoma

increases from 80% to 95% when used in combination.[10] In the most recent American Association of Endocrine Surgeons Guidelines, cervical ultrasonography is recommended for operative planning for most patients as it also allows for assessment of thyroid disease.[4]

Parathyroid four-dimensional computed tomography (4D-CT) is an imaging modality that has emerged in the past 15 years that uses multidetector CT image acquisition during multiple contrast enhancement phases. 4D-CT provides both anatomic and functional data that help to determine a parathyroid gland's precise anatomic location. The fourth dimension in a 4D-CT is the characteristic contrast enhancement over time in different tissues. 4D-CT is able to localize lesions in atypical locations that are more difficult to visualize with ultrasound such as the mediastinum. In the setting of a negative sestamibi scan with patients with primary hyperparathyroidism, 4D-CT was 85% sensitive and 94% specific for lateralizing the side of the diseased gland and 66% sensitive and 89% specific for predicting the exact location.[11] When comparing initial localization study, 4D-CT was able to lateralize 93.9% of abnormal glands versus 71.2% for US and 61.5% for sestamibi.[12] In solitary adenomas, 4D-CT had a sensitivity of 85% and specificity of 92%; and with multigland disease had a sensitivity of 55%.[13] 4D-CT's high sensitivity and specificity allow it to be an excellent first- or second-line imaging choice for localizing parathyroid adenomas in the appropriate patient.

Parathyroid biopsy may create fibrosis in the adenomas that may make differentiation from parathyroid cancer difficult on final pathology and therefore should be avoided. However, parathyroid fine needle biopsy may be considered to confirm that a lesion in an uncommon location (ex. Undescended, intrathyroidal, etc.) is parathyroid tissue. When a parathyroid biopsy is performed, it is important to also send a sample for PTH washout as parathyroid cells on biopsy may look very similar to follicular thyroid cells.

Preoperative Treatment

A normal daily adult intake of calcium of 1000—1200 mg is recommended for patients preoperatively and they should not restrict calcium. Vitamin D repletion is recommended for patients who are deficient in Vitamin D.[4]

Preoperatively, patients should be evaluated for voice quality, and definitive objective evaluation should be carried out for any subjective voice changes, cervical trauma, or operations that would put the vagus nerve or recurrent laryngeal nerve at risk, which can be done with laryngoscopy.[4] Patients should also undergo preoperative evaluation of the thyroid, most preferentially by ultrasound.

THERAPY

In general, there are three surgical options: selective, subtotal parathyroidectomy (i.e., Three and a half gland excision), and total parathyroidectomy with autotransplantation. Total parathyroidectomy with autotransplantation was the traditional approach in MEN2A patients. However, recent guidelines suggest that this may be excessive in some patients that do not have enlargement of all four glands or high-risk mutations. The most recent ATA guidelines recommend subtotal parathyroidectomy only in patients with four glands enlargement or with those at high risk of hyperparathyroidism based on RET mutation.[9] Furthermore, the ATA recommends that if patients at low risk for hyperparathyroidism accidentally have normal parathyroid glands resected during thyroidectomy, they should undergo parathyroid autotransplantation into the sternocleidomastoid. Alternatively, patients with high-risk mutations should undergo subtotal parathyroidectomy or total parathyroidectomy with autotransplantation into a heterotopic muscle bed such as the forearm.[9] Although very rare, there have been cases reported of proliferation of autotransplanted parathyroid tissue, and so monitoring of this parathyroid tissue remains important.[6] In patients with less than four glands diseased and low-risk mutations, intraoperative PTH may guide how many glands should be removed.[4]

When comparing the three surgical options (selective, subtotal, and total parathyroidectomy) in a retrospective study of 119 patients, Herfath et al. found that the recurrence rate was 0% after no total parathyroidectomy with autotransplantation, 9% after selective, and 14% after subtotal resection.[14] There was an equivalent rate of permanent hypoparathyroidism after subtotal versus total parathyroidectomy with autotransplantation (29% vs. 20%). Given the lower rate of recurrence and hypoparathyroidism, this group recommended total parathyroidectomy with forearm autotransplantation. However, patients who have a total parathyroidectomy with autotransplantation typically have a period of temporary, but potentially severe, hypoparathyroidism while the autotransplanted tissue reestablishes a blood supply. The choice between techniques should be determined by the individual surgeon based on his/her comfort with the different techniques and the particular clinical factors for each individual patient.

One special consideration in MEN2A patients is that often these patients have had a prior thyroidectomy for medullary thyroid cancer. In reoperative cases, it is imperative to perform preoperative localization to try to determine which glands are diseased and their location so as limited of an operation as possible can be performed.

Complications

Complications from parathyroidectomy in MEN2A mirror complications of parathyroidectomy in the general population. Meticulous hemostasis must be achieved to avoid bleeding and hematoma in the neck. The recurrent laryngeal nerve must be identified throughout its course to be avoided, and care must be taken to avoid diathermy nearby the nerve as the area affected is often much larger than the point of diathermy. As there are many patients undergoing parathyroidectomy in MEN2A who have had previous neck dissections, special care must be taken to avoid injury to the recurrent laryngeal and superior laryngeal nerve as anatomy may be disturbed and planes may be less recognizable. The risk of hypoparathyroidism varies depending on the type of procedure performed and has been discussed earlier.

PROGNOSIS

Cure is defined as eucalcemia at more than 6 months.[4] However, in MEN 2A, patients should be followed for life with annual calcium labs. Different from PHP associated with MEN 1, PHP associated with MEN 2A has good outcomes with well-selected procedures and excellent rates of long-term eucalcemia.

REFERENCES

1. Valdes N, Navarro E, Mesa J, et al. RET Cys634Arg mutation confers a more aggressive multiple endocrine neoplasia type 2A phenotype than Cys634Tyr mutation. *Eur J Endocrinol.* 2015;172(3):301–307.
2. DeLellis D, Mangray S. Heritable forms of primary hyperparathyroidism: a current perspective. *Histopathology.* 2018;72:117–132.
3. Lairmore T, Moley J. The multiple endocrine neoplasia syndromes. In: Townsend C, Beauchamp R, Evers B, Mattox K, eds. *Sabiston Textbook of Surgery: The Biological Basis of Modern Surgical Practice.* 20th ed. Philadelphia, PA: Elsevier; 2017:996–1010.
4. Wilhelm SM, Wang TS, Ruan DT, et al. The American association of endocrine surgeons guidelines for definitive management of primary hyperparathyroidism. *JAMA Surg.* 2016;151(10):959–968.

5. Jenkins PJ, Satta MA, Simmgen M, et al. Metastatic parathyroid carcinoma in the MEN2A syndrome. *Clin Endocrinol.* 1997;47(6):747–751.

6. Hughes MS, Feliberti E, Perry RR, Vinik A. Multiple endocrine neoplasia type 2A (including familial medullary carcinoma) and type 2B. In: De Groot LJ, Chrousos G, Dungan K, et al., eds. *Endotext.* South Dartmouth (MA): MDText.com, Inc; 2000. NBK481898 [bookaccession].

7. Magalhaes PK, Antonini SR, de Paula FJ, de Freitas LC, Maciel LM. Primary hyperparathyroidism as the first clinical manifestation of multiple endocrine neoplasia type 2A in a 5-year-old child. *Thyroid.* 2011;21(5):547–550.

8. Taieb D, Kebebew E, Castinetti F, Chen CC, Henry JF, Pacak K. Diagnosis and preoperative imaging of multiple endocrine neoplasia type 2: current status and future directions. *Clin Endocrinol.* 2014;81(3):317–328.

9. Wells Jr SA, Asa SL, Dralle H, et al. Revised american thyroid association guidelines for the management of medullary thyroid carcinoma. *Thyroid.* 2015;25(6):567–610.

10. Quinn C, Udelsman R. The parathyroid glands. In: Townsend C, Beauchamp R, Evers B, Mattox K, eds. *Sabiston Textbook of Surgery: The Biological Basis of Modern Surgical Practice.* 20th ed. Philadelphia, PA: Elsevier; 2017:923–938.

11. Harari A, Zarnegar R, Lee J, Kazam E, Inabnet 3rd WB, Fahey 3rd TJ. Computed tomography can guide focused exploration in select patients with primary hyperparathyroidism and negative sestamibi scanning. *Surgery.* 2008; 144(6):970–976. discussion 976-9.

12. Starker LF, Mahajan A, Bjorklund P, Sze G, Udelsman R, Carling T. 4D parathyroid CT as the initial localization study for patients with de novo primary hyperparathyroidism. *Ann Surg Oncol.* 2011;18(6): 1723–1728.

13. Yeh R, Kwang Y, Donovan T, Tabacco G, Coronel E, Dercle L. Comparison of sestamibi SPECT/CT and parathyroid 4D CT with a 1-stop simultaneous imaging protocol. *J Nucl Med.* 2018;59:233.

14. Herfarth KK, Bartsch D, Doherty GM, Wells Jr SA, Lairmore TC. Surgical management of hyperparathyroidism in patients with multiple endocrine neoplasia type 2A. *Surgery.* 1996;120(6):966–973. discussion 973-4.

CHAPTER 12

Advances in Diagnosis and Management of Primary Hyperparathyroidism During Pregnancy

ALEXANDER SHIFRIN, MD, FACS, FACE, ECNU, FEBS (ENDOCRINE), FISS

Primary hyperparathyroidism (PHPT) may have serious consequences to the mother and to the fetus during pregnancy. Literature has limited data with single case reports or small case series described. Reason being the detection of PHPT during pregnancy is difficult due to physiological changes that mask this disease in earlier stages. Prevalence of PHPT during pregnancy was reported between 0.15% and 1.4%.[1-3] During pregnancy, maternal calcium homeostasis adapts to provide calcium for the fetus. Normal pregnancy is associated with the following maternal changes that contribute to physiological hypocalcemia: hemodilution related to intravascular fluid expansion, hypoalbuminaemia, increased glomerular filtration rate, and transplacental transfer of calcium. Nevertheless, the active, ionized calcium level remains unchanged.[3,4] Hypercalciuria occurs as the result of increased maternal glomerular filtration rate. PTH-related protein (PTHrp), secreted by placenta and fetus, mediates active calcium transport through the placenta. This process is independent of maternal PTH secretion.[5] The increased calcium demand during pregnancy is facilitated by the increased maternal intestinal calcium absorption that is facilitated by 1,25-dihydroxyvitamin D production. The placental delivery of calcium to the fetus is the highest during the third trimester and it is independent of maternal PTH level. Parathyroid hormone, 1,25-dihydroxyvitamin D3, and calcitonin do not cross the placenta. The previously mentioned physiological changes may mask gestational PHPT that remains undiagnosed in up to 80% of the cases. The causes of maternal PHPT are the same as in nonpregnancy-related PHPT.[2,3,6]

PRESENTATION AND SYMPTOMS

The clinical presentation of PHPT in pregnancy is directly related to the serum calcium level and cause significant fetal (up to 80%) and maternal (up to 67%) morbidity, with a mortality rate approaching 30%.[3,7-9] Being underdiagnosed in the past, gestational PHPT was most commonly presented with maternal nephrolithiasis and fetal complications, such as neonatal hypocalcemia with seizures, intrauterine growth retardation, low birth weight, premature birth, stillbirth, and miscarriages. Currently, hypercalcemia and the diagnosis of PHPT are established in earlier stages. This has resulted in significantly lower risk of maternal and fetal complications.[3,10] Clinical presentation of PHPT may range from hyperemesis, lethargy, hypertension, thirst, abdominal pain, depression, constipation, bone fracture, maternal heart rhythm disorders, maternal hypertension to preeclampsia, nephrolithiasis, pancreatitis, hyperemesis gravidarum, and hypercalcemic crisis. Despite presenting features of the condition, recent studies showed that PHPT during pregnancy has not been associated with an increased risk of spontaneous abortions, but might be associated with an increased risk of cesarean section.[2,3,5,11] Neonatal hypocalcemia was reported in up to 50% of newborns, it is usually transient, lasting up to 3-5 months and can be managed with calcium and vitamin D supplements.[12]

DIAGNOSIS

The same diagnostic approach should be applied to the pregnant female patient as to nonpregnant, with exception of some radiological studies. Routine blood work

Advances in Treatment and Management in Surgical Endocrinology. https://doi.org/10.1016/B978-0-323-66195-9.00012-1

would include serum calcium, PTH, Vitamin D, creatinine levels, **Glomerular filtration rate (GFR)**, and 24-h urine for calcium. It is important to understand that normal physiological changes will mask maternal PHPT and may result in lower serum total calcium level. When diagnosis of PHPT is suspected, it is therefore essential to measure not only ionized calcium level but albumin corrected calcium level as well, even when total serum calcium level is within normal ranges. PTH level, as well as ionized calcium level, remains unaffected during pregnancy. As with nonpregnancy-related PHPT, maternal PHPT is also most commonly caused by a single parathyroid adenoma. As pregnant patients are mostly younger age females, the testing for familial endocrine syndromes is advocated (multiple endocrine neoplasia (MEN) type 1 and 2 syndromes). In one study series, two of eight pregnant patients who have undergone parathyroidectomy were found to carry MEN 1 gene mutations, consistent with MEN 1 syndrome. Usual diagnostic tests, such as computerized tomography and 99 mTc-sestamibi scintigraphy, should be avoided due to the fetal risk of ionizing radiation. The only option for localization of parathyroid adenoma would be a dedicated ultrasonography of the neck[1-3,5]

MANAGEMENT OF PRIMARY HYPERPARATHYROIDISM DURING PREGNANCY

Management of PHPT during pregnancy should be individualized based on symptoms, the severity of the hypercalcemia, and gestational age. Mild form of PHPT causes low risk of maternal and obstetrical complications. If symptoms are limited and calcium level is mildly elevated, the patient can be managed with conservative therapy. These include intensive intravenous or oral hydration with or without forced diuresis, and low calcium intake. Bisphosphonates cannot be used during pregnancy because they cross the placenta and are embryotoxic at high doses.[13] Calcitonin does not cross the placenta and appears safe in pregnancy, but safety data are limited and its effectiveness is poor.[14] Cinacalcet has also been used in few cases with good results, but safety data are also limited.[15,16]

SURGERY

Surgery remains the standard of care approach in treatment of patients with PHPT, including PHPT during pregnancy, with minimally invasive approach remaining the gold standard.[2] The main questions would be when to perform the surgery, and can the surgery be postponed to after the delivery? Surgery is indicated in severe hypercalcemia when calcium level is above 11 mg/dL (2.75 mmol/L) and all symptomatic PHPT.[2,3,17] Surgery should be performed during the second trimester, to avoid consequences of anesthetic medications on incomplete organogenesis in the first trimester and the risk of inducing preterm labor in the third trimester. With severe hypercalcemia, some authors advocate that all pregnant patients should be offered surgical intervention independent of gestational age.[1] Small series of eight pregnant patients who underwent parathyroidectomy during the pregnancy, reported no maternal or fetal complications.[2] If hypercalcemia is severe during the pregnancy, some authors recommend performing cesarean section with concurrent parathyroidectomy.[19] If surgery is deferred to after the delivery, it should be performed as soon as possible to prevent a hypercalcemia crisis.[1] In our own experience, we have performed successful parathyroidectomies in several symptomatic pregnant patients with PHPT in the second trimester under the local anesthesia with a deep cervical block and mild sedation that helped to decrease the risk of general anesthesia. We also tend to follow patients with mild, asymptomatic PHPT, especially those patients diagnosed in the third trimester, and the parathyroidectomy was performed after delivery. Recent paper published by Rigg et al., retrospectively reviewed data of 28 pregnant patients with PHPT (22 managed medically and 6 surgically by elective parathyroidectomies), showed that 30% of those who were managed medically developed preeclampsia and 66% managed medically had preterm deliveries.[18]

REFERENCES

1. McMullen TP1, Learoyd DL, Williams DC, Sywak MS, Sidhu SB, Delbridge LW. Hyperparathyroidism in pregnancy: options for localization and surgical therapy. *World J Surg.* 2010;34(8):1811–1816.
2. Stringer K, Gough J, Gough I. Primary hyperparathyroidism during pregnancy: management by minimally invasive surgery based on ultrasound localization. *ANZ J Surg.* 2017;87(10):E134–E137.
3. Dochez V, Ducarme G. Primary hyperparathyroidism during pregnancy. *Arch Gynecol Obstet.* 2015;291(2):259–263.
4. Dahlman T, Sjoberg HE, Bucht E. Calcium homeostasis in normal pregnancy and puerperium. A longitudinal study. *Acta Obstet Gynecol Scand.* 1994;73(5):393–398.
5. Kamenický P, Lecoq AL, Chanson P. Primary hyperparathyroidism in pregnancy. *Ann Endocrinol.* 2016;77(2):169–171.
6. Hosking DJ. Calcium homeostasis in pregnancy. *Clin Endocrinol.* 1996;45(1):1–6.

7. Schnatz PF, Curry SL. Primary hyperparathyroidism in pregnancy: evidence-based management. *Obstet Gynecol Surv.* 2002;57(6):365–376.

8. Parks J, Coe F, Favus M. Hyperparathyroidism in nephrolithiasis. *Arch Intern Med.* 1980;140(11): 1479–1481.

9. Delmonico FL, Neer RM, Cosimi AB, Barnes AB, Russell PS. Hyperparathyroidism during pregnancy. *Am J Surg.* 1976;131(3):328–337.

10. Hirsch D, Kopel V, Nadler V, Levy S, Toledano Y, Tsvetov G. Pregnancy outcomes in women with primary hyperparathyroidism. *J Clin Endocrinol Metab.* 2015; 100(5):2115–2122.

11. Abood A, Vestergaard P. Pregnancy outcomes in women with primary hyperparathyroidism. *Eur J Endocrinol.* 2014;171(1):69–76.

12. Shangold MM, Dor N, Welt SI, Fleischman AR, Crenshaw MC. Hyperparathyroidism and pregnancy: a review. *Obstet Gynecol Surv.* 1982;37(4):217–228.

13. Djokanovic N, Klieger-Grossmann C, Koren G. Does treatment with bisphosphonates endanger the human pregnancy? *J Obstet Gynaecol Can.* 2008;30(12):1146–1148.

14. Krysiak R, Wilk M, Okopien B. Recurrent pancreatitis induced by hyperparathyroidism in pregnancy. *Arch Gynecol Obstet.* 2011;284(3):531–534.

15. Edling KL, Korenman SG, Janzen C, et al. A pregnant dilemma: primary hyperparathyroidism due to parathyromatosis in pregnancy. *Endocr Pract.* 2014;20(2):e14–e17.

16. Vera L, Oddo S, Di Iorgi N, Bentivoglio G, Giusti M. Primary hyperparathyroidism in pregnancy treated with cinacalcet: a case report and review of the literature. *J Med Case Rep.* 2016;10:361.

17. Kelly TR. Primary hyperparathyroidism during pregnancy. *Surgery.* 1991;110(6):1028–1033.

18. Rigg J, Gilbertson E, Barrett HL, Britten FL, Lust K. Primary hyperparathyroidism in pregnancy: maternofetal outcomes at a quaternary referral obstetric hospital, 2000 through 2015. *J Clin Endocrinol Metab.* 2019;104(3): 721–729.

19. Trebb C, Wallace S, Ishak F, Splinter KL. Concurrent parathyroidectomy and caesarean section in the third trimester. *J Obstet Gynaecol Can.* 2014;36(6):502–505.

CHAPTER 13

Update on the Diagnosis and Management of Primary Aldosteronism

MARI SUZUKI, MD • CONSTANTINE A. STRATAKIS, MD, PHD

INTRODUCTION

Primary aldosteronism was first described by Dr. Jerome Conn, at the University of Michigan in 1954. A patient with resistant hypertension and hypokalemia, after biochemical studies were performed concluding excess salt-retaining corticoid, was scheduled for bilateral adrenalectomy. She was intraoperatively found with a unilateral 13 g adrenal tumor.[1] Resection of this tumor cured the patient of hypertension and hypokalemia, opening-up the field of adrenal steroid studies.[2]

Initially thought to be a rare disorder, primary aldosteronism is now thought to constitute 6% of hypertensive patients, with reports of prevalence as high as 13%. The classic presentation of Conn's syndrome is described as difficult to control hypertension, on three antihypertensives or more, with the presence of hypokalemia. This stereotype has now been proven to be different from the status quo, by findings of normal serum potassium in more than 50% of primary aldosteronism patients.[3]

Patients recommended for screening include those with repeatedly elevated blood pressures above 150/100 mmHg, or resistant hypertension defined as being on three antihypertensive drugs but with blood pressure 140/90 mmHg, or patients on four antihypertensives to achieve blood pressure control, hypertension in the setting of hypokalemia that may be induced by a diuretic, finding of an adrenal incidentaloma, hypertension and obstructive sleep apnea, or strong family history of early cardiovascular disease (before age 40), and first-degree relatives of patients with primary aldosteronism.[4]

Primary aldosteronism has long been associated with chronic maladies. A number of cardiovascular studies comparing primary aldosteronism patients to those with essential hypertension found an increased risk of cardiovascular events,[5] with respect to myocardial infarction, stroke, and atrial fibrillation. A study following patients treated for primary aldosteronism compared to essential hypertension found that the former group had higher cardiovascular events before treatment, with no difference after 7 years follow-up.[6] The cardiovascular outcomes were similar in the adrenalectomy and mineralocorticoid antagonist groups, indicating the effect of reduction of high aldosterone levels, in reducing cardiac risk.

Echocardiographic studies of the heart have found remodeling, in left ventricular mass, septal wall thickness, and increased incidence of diastolic dysfunction in primary aldosteronism. This was independent of high blood pressure effects, as compared to patients with essential hypertension alone. Primary aldosteronism patients have been demonstrated to have an increased rate of carotid wall thickening, based on ultrasound study of carotid intima-media thickness.[7] A prospective study has found that cardiac remodeling changes are reversible though, either with adrenalectomy or mineralocorticoid antagonist treatment.[8]

A recently reported association, of a high frequency of primary aldosteronism with cortisol dysregulation in patients, may mire the view of a single steroid hormone effect on cardiac remodeling. The German Conn group followed echocardiograms of patients after primary aldosteronism treatment, and found that cardiac remodeling reversibility was not found in those who additionally had subclinical Cushing's.[9]

The increased risk for cardiovascular events and cardiac remodeling, seen with primary aldosteronism, is thought to be from aldosterone mediated inflammation, cell growth and vascular remodeling, and fibrosis

Advances in Treatment and Management in Surgical Endocrinology. https://doi.org/10.1016/B978-0-323-66195-9.00013-3

on cardiovascular and renal tissue leading to arterial stiffening and myocardial fibrosis.[10,11] This is an independent process from essential hypertension alone. As this is a treatable cause, there is impetus for diagnosis and treatment.

Renal insufficiency is often uncovered following unilateral adrenalectomy or spironolactone treatment, in primary aldosteronism patients. This has been established with comparison to hypertensive patients, at 1 year follow-up to adrenalectomy. This is attributed to the hyperfiltration effect of hyperaldosteronism, which overestimates the creatinine clearance in primary aldosteronism patients, before treatment.[12]

Metabolic syndrome correlations with dyslipidemia, diabetes, and obesity, are noted to be higher with hypertensive patients than those without hypertension.[13] This is putatively from target organ damage. With respect to primary aldosteronism patients, Jerome Conn reviewed 145 primary aldosteronism cases and found 39 patients to have impaired glucose tolerance (54%), in 1964. Subsequently, a high prevalence (10%–50%) of glucose intolerance or diabetes has been found, and the metabolic conditions alleviated after treatment for the primary aldosteronism with adrenalectomy.[14,15]

Insulin clamp studies found decreased metabolic clearance, lower glucose disposal, and insulin sensitivity in primary aldosteronism patients[16] compared to healthy controls. The primary aldosteronism group contained adrenal-producing adenomas and bilateral adrenal hyperplasia subjects. After adrenalectomy, there was improvement in insulin action; those on medical treatment with spironolactone did not show improvement, leading to the presumption that aldosterone had direct effects on insulin sensitivity.

Calcium and parathyroid hormone (PTH) level changes have been observed in primary aldosteronism patients, from higher serum PTH levels.[17] An analogy can be drawn to end stage and moderate severe heart failure patients, where reductions in bone mineral density, in the context of elevated PTH and PTH-related peptide, with consequent normocalcemic secondary hyperparathyroidism have been found. Lower bone mineral density and higher PTH, elevated urinary calcium was found in primary aldosteronism patients when compared to nonfunctional adrenal incidentaloma patients. Primary aldosteronism patients additionally had higher prevalence of osteoporosis and higher prevalence of vertebral fractures compared to control subjects.[18] Following treatment with either adrenalectomy or mineralocorticoid antagonist, there was reduction in urinary calcium excretion and improvement in bone mineral density.

Primary aldosteronism's relationship with obstructive sleep apnea is postulated to be bidirectional.[19] The severity of primary aldosteronism has been correlated with the severity of obstructive sleep apnea, with the premise that aldosterone promotes fluid accumulation, thereby worsening obstructive sleep apnea with increased upper airway resistance from fluid shift to the neck. This may contribute to resistant hypertension. The correlation is strong, such that primary aldosteronism patients are recommended for obstructive sleep apnea screening.

DIAGNOSIS

Primary aldosteronism is increasingly detected in the population, with the ease of screening with plasma aldosterone to plasma renin activity ratio (ARR). After this was first used in 1973 by Buhler, Dunn and Espiner applied the ratio to the diagnosis of primary aldosteronism in 1976. After establishment of its use in aldosterone-producing adenoma patients by Hiramitsu et al. in 1981,[20] showing prevalence of 2.6% in hypertensive patients, the ARR has been used. Although most blood pressure medications may affect the aldosterone renin ratio, precluding the usage of mineralocorticoid receptor antagonists, the screening labs may be drawn. If the aldosterone level is greater than 15 ng/dL and the renin level is below the lower limit of reference range or undetectable, this is considered a positive finding.[1]

With the ease of implementing ARR for screening, it was also found that 67% of aldosterone-producing adenoma subjects had normal potassium levels. With the advent of mass spectroscopy for laboratory testing, there has been increased reliability in the results. With increased detection, two main subtypes of primary aldosteronism became apparent:
- Aldosterone-producing adenomas
- Bilateral adrenal hyperplasia

A high aldosterone to renin ratio (ARR) is not diagnostic by itself, and a confirmatory test is recommended to evaluate for excess aldosterone secretion. There are four tests that may be used for confirmation: oral salt load test, normal saline suppression test, fludrocortisone suppression test, and captopril challenge test. The first two are most commonly used.

The oral salt load test involves excess salt intake for 3 days, greater than 6 g per day. This may be administered as sodium chloride tablets. On the third day, 24-h urine is collected for sodium and aldosterone levels. Urinary sodium equal to or greater than 200 mmol/L and urinary aldosterone greater than

12−14 mcg/24 h are diagnostic. This can be performed as outpatient and is frequently utilized. The saline suppression test is the comparable inpatient test, involving normal saline intravenous infusion over 4 h, at a rate of 500 mL/h. Hourly aldosterone levels are drawn, and a 4-h time point plasma aldosterone level greater than 10 ng/dL is considered diagnostic.

Less utilized tests are the fludrocortisone suppression test and captopril challenge test. The fludrocortisone suppression test involves administration of 100 mcg of fludrocortisone every 6 h for 4 days, additionally with sodium chloride 30 mmol tablets thrice daily with meals. Potassium chloride supplementation should be taken as needed. Daily 24-h urinary sodium levels are collected, and on day 4 morning plasma cortisol is drawn at 7:00 a.m. and 10:00 a.m., and renin is drawn at 7:00 a.m. For reliable interpretation of the urinary aldosterone, prerequisites of 24-h urinary sodium excretion greater than 3 mmol/kg/day, cortisol on day 4 lower at 10:00 a.m. than at 7:00 a.m., and renin less than 1 ng/mL/h are required. If the prerequisites are met, a urinary aldosterone level greater than 6 ng/dL is considered diagnostic.

The captopril challenge test involves administration of captopril 25 mg in the morning, and drawing plasma aldosterone and renin 1 h later. The test is considered positive if the aldosterone to renin ratio is greater than 20, and the aldosterone value is greater than 15 ng/dL. Tests are summarized in Table 13.1.

In addition to biochemical studies, imaging plays a role in the proper subtype diagnosis of primary aldosteronism. Since its advent in the 1970s, anatomical imaging with CT is helpful in localization of distinct aldosterone-producing adenomas, but it cannot distinguish between nonfunctional and functional adrenal nodules. As there is expected increased incidence of adrenal nodules with age, this is important to keep in mind. The practical application of CT adrenals is to map the vasculature surrounding the adrenal glands and to help rule out the likelihood of insidious processes, such as adrenocortical carcinoma.[21]

Because of the limitation in biochemical evaluation of adrenal adenomas with anatomical imaging alone, adrenal vein sampling has been considered to be the gold standard in differentiating between an aldosterone-producing adenoma and bilateral adrenal hyperplasia. There is a greater chance of successful cannulation of the proper veins with an experienced interventional radiologist. Comparison between different centers performing the procedure has been limited, due to variations in the protocol. There may be adrenal vein sampling alone, or with cosyntropin stimulation, with the purpose of trying to overcome situations where there may be cortisol cosecretion.[21]

Due to the limited centers that offer adrenal vein sampling, and the cost and invasiveness of the procedure, alternatives to simplify the diagnostic algorithm for aldosterone-producing adenoma have been studied. The SPARTACUS trial was a multicenter, randomized study of treatment based either on CT and adrenal vein sampling or CT adrenals alone with anatomical characterization. CT adrenals were used to prognosticate for adrenalectomy if one side was enlarged. If the adrenal glands had normal appearance or bilateral enlargement was seen, mineralocorticoid therapy was selected. Adrenal vein sampling with lateralization

TABLE 13.1
Confirmatory Testing for Primary Aldosteronism.

Test	Protocol	Positive Result Interpretation
Oral salt load test	Salt intake of >6 g/day for 3 days Third day, collect 24-h urine and 24-h aldosterone	Urinary sodium ≥200 mmol/L Urinary aldosterone >12−14 mcg/24 h
Saline suppression test	Normal saline infusion at 500 mL/h for 4 h. Collect plasma aldosterone levels hourly	Plasma aldosterone >10 ng/dL at 4 h
Fludrocortisone suppression test	Fludrocortisone 100 mcg every 6 h, for 4 days, NaCl 30 mmol tablets thrice daily with meals and potassium chloride supplementation as needed. Measure 24 h urinary sodium daily. Day 4, 7 a.m.: Measure cortisol and renin.	Prerequisites: 24-h U sodium excretion > 3 mmol/kg/day cortisol on day 4 is lower at 10 a.m. than at 7 a.m. Renin <1 ng/mL/h positive if: aldosterone >6 ng/dL
Captopril challenge test	Captopril 25 mg in the morning. Check aldosterone to renin ratio 1 h later	Positive if ARR> 20 and aldosterone >15 ng/dL

ratio >4 led to adrenalectomy; in instances of failed adrenal vein sampling with cannulation, the CT adrenals were used to prognosticate. The endpoints studied were number of antihypertensives used at follow-up, blood pressure, and quality of life.

The SPARTACUS trial did not have a large enough sample size to prove noninferiority of CT adrenals to adrenal vein sampling. The argument against adrenal vein sampling was that it involved 60% higher cost compared to CT adrenals alone, and based on select endpoints, comparable outcomes.

The limits to the study were that the study sample was different from other precedents, with a higher predominance of males, constituting over three quarters, and more patients with severe primary aldosteronism, give the higher incidence of hypokalemia at 60%. The low hypertension cure rate of 15% also is consistent with the subjects having more severe disease.[22]

It is important to keep in mind that a higher proportion of patients undergoing sequential CT then adrenal vein sampling, end up having discordant results between the two procedures, as high as 50%. This brings into consideration the possibility of selecting the wrong adrenal gland for removal.

Alternative imaging modalities have been explored for subtyping primary aldosteronism[21] but barriers to implementation exist, such as long half-lives of the radioactive steroids, such as with (6-β-131I)-iodomethyl-19-norcholesterol or NP-59[23], approved for use in Europe and Japan, but not used in the United States. Others imaging modalities are pending proof of concept, such as with metomidate. Radiolabeled metomidate binds to adrenal cortex specific enzymes, including CYP11B1 and CYP11B2, involved in cortisol and aldosterone synthesis. Given that metomidate cannot differentiate between the different enzymes, its potential utility in subtyping primary aldosteronism is low.

Steroid profiling is another area where proof of concept is pending. With the advent of more reliable laboratory results with liquid chromatography and mass spectrometry, identification of aldosterone-producing adenoma specific or bilateral hyperplasia specific steroid profiles may help with proper diagnosis. 18-hydroxycortisol and 18-oxocortisol are potential steroids under investigation. Early work by Biglieri, in 1979, showed that 18-hydroxycorticosterone level of >100 ng/dL was highly predictive of an aldosterone-producing adenoma.[21]

Steroid profiling with adrenal vein sampling is another area of investigation. A study has shown three-fold increase in 18-hydroxycorticosterone in adrenal veins draining from aldosterone-producing adenomas compared to bilateral adrenal hyperplasia.[21] The utility of this steroid in the selectivity index (when corrected with a ratio with cortisol) did not show more usefulness than aldosterone to cortisol ratio. Other steroids that may have clinical utility are 18-oxocortisol and 18-hydroxycortisol, which were higher in adrenal venous samples from aldosterone-producing adenomas than bilateral adrenal hyperplasia. Higher urinary excretion of 18-hydroxycortisol and 18-oxocortisol in aldosterone-producing adenoma subtypes of primary aldosteronism patients was a phenomenon observed as far back as 1992 by Ulrick et al. Particularly, with urinary 18-hydroxycortisol, values greater than 510 µg/day were indicative of aldosterone-producing adenoma, though the sensitivity was 30%. Additionally, with the advent of mass spectroscopy, alternative steroids to aldosterone and cortisol have been studied in adrenal vein sampling lateralization studies, including 11-deoxycortisol.[24]

Steroid profiles have been studied in peripheral blood alone, with 18-hydroxycortisol and 18-oxocortisol using liquid chromatography and mass spectroscopy. These steroids were found in higher concentrations with aldosterone-producing adenomas compared to bilateral adrenal hyperplasia, with 18-oxocortisol found 12.5-fold higher, and 18-hydroxycortisol 2.5-fold higher.[21] In 80% of patients, classification of primary aldosteronism subtype was correct, using 12 steroids. The most common genetic mutation for aldosterone-producing adenoma, KCNJ5, has been found with a distinct steroid profile, with the highest peripheral plasma of 18-oxocortisol.

GENETICS

Important insight into the genetics of aldosterone-producing adenomas came about from sequencing of somatic mutations in these adrenal tumors, after observation of subcapsular aldosterone-producing tumors. KCNJ5 was discovered by Robert Lifton and colleagues, after sequencing distinct adrenal tumors in primary aldosteronism patients. Most aldosterone-producing adenomas have KCNJ5 gene mutation, shown to be present in 35%–70% of aldosterone-producing adenomas. The KCNJ5 gene codes for the selectivity filter of G protein activated inward rectifier potassium channel GIRK4. This mutation tends to be in the zona fasciculata and is prevalent in east Asians.

Additional mutations in aldosterone-producing adenomas have been identified as ATP1A1 gene, which encodes the sodium-potassium ATPase, ATP2B3 gene for membrane calcium ATPase, and CACNA1D gene, which encodes the calcium channel subunit Cav1.3, tend to be of the zona glomerulosa phenotype. Along with *KCNJ5*, these are the dominant aldosterone-producing adenoma-causing genes, accounting for over half of the cases.

CACNA1D is found in 10% of aldosterone-producing adenomas, encoding for a voltage-gated calcium channel. Mutation in *CACNA1D* cause direct increased calcium influx through the channel. *ATP1A1* mutations are found in 5% of aldosterone-producing adenomas. *ATP2B3* mutations are found in 2% of mutations, this leads to abnormal permeability to sodium/proton ions, leading to increased depolarization, much like in *KCNJ5* mutations. *CTNNB1* mutations are found in 2%–5% of aldosterone-producing adenomas; this encodes for β-catenin. *CTNNB1* may have additional regulatory pathways. Based on studies, it is postulated that *CTNNB1* may cause adrenal proliferation by Wnt signaling activation. Cortisol-producing adenomas with *CTNNB1* mutations have been found to additionally have GNAS variants.

Fig. 13.1 depicts an aldosterone-producing adenoma, with a list of commonly known underlying mutations and their frequency of occurrence.

A study of macronodular adrenal hyperplasia, at the National Institutes of Health found mutations in *ARMC5*, a tumor-suppressor gene[25] commonly associated with hypercortisolemia, to have a subset of patients additionally with primary aldosteronism. This mutation was particularly deleterious in African American patients.

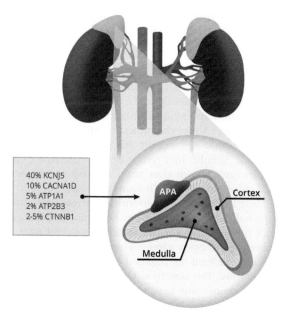

FIG. 13.1 Frequency of commonly known somatic mutations in aldosterone producing adenomas.

Despite discoveries of aldosterone-producing adenomas, 40% of them do not have identified mutations. Reasons for this may include limitations in sample size, narrowing of tissue to study with immunohistologic staining, and biopsies containing normal adrenal tissue that may dilute the variants below detection in Sanger sequencing. Small sample size evading exome sequencing is another possibility. Copy number variations of undetermined significance and single nucleotide variants in the germline may be areas for further study. Additional consideration is that large genes, such as *CACNA1D* are difficult to sequence in entirety, where only partial mutations may have been found so far.

Histologic staining of adrenal glands has shown either adrenocortical micronodules or diffuse zona glomerulosa hyperplasia. The micronodules were found with somatic mutations to known mutations (*KCNJ5*, *CACNA1D*, *ATP1A1*, and *ATP2B3*). Additionally, there has been speculation that zona glomerulosa cells in aldosterone-producing cell clusters with *KCNJ5* mutations morph into zona fasciculata cells, thereby creating aldosterone-producing adenomas. Hyperplasia regions without nodules were not found with known mutations.[26]

Immunohistologic staining for CYP11B2 has allowed for elucidation of putative subtypes in primary aldosteronism. There is either uniform expression of the enzyme in the zona glomerulosa, or aldosterone-producing cell clusters. Aldosterone-producing adenomas themselves have variation in CYP11B2 staining, which vary from uniform to homogeneous. Moreover, 30% of unilateral primary aldosteronism patients have zona glomerulosa hyperplasia or CYP11B2-expressing micronodules, rather than distinct aldosterone-producing adenomas. This raises the possibility that the pathophysiology of primary aldosteronism is bilateral hyperplasia, with nodules that develop into aldosterone-producing adenomas. As potentially likely underlying genetic mutations, it has been pointed out that aldosterone-producing cell clusters in normal adrenal gland tissue found somatic variants in *CACNA1D* and *ATP1A1* genes.[27]

Phenotypic characterization has shed light on biochemical activity in relation to aldosterone-secreting adenoma size. Larger aldosterone-producing adenomas tend to secrete higher amounts of aldosterone than smaller adenomas. However, this is not a linear relationship. Larger adenomas, despite being 9 times larger than smaller adenomas, only had plasma aldosterone concentrations 2–2.5 times greater. This indicated the potency of smaller aldosterone-producing adenomas.

Familial Primary Aldosteronism

Although most primary aldosteronism patients present with a sporadic aldosterone-producing adenomas or bilateral adrenal hyperplasia, 1%−6% cases have a familial presentation.[28] The importance of the familial subtypes is that identification leads to appropriate diagnosis and treatment, forgoing the need for adrenal vein sampling.

Familial studies from 1966 have elucidated glucocorticoid-remediable aldosteronism,[28] with familial hyperaldosteronism type I shown to be caused by a chimera of *CYP11B1*, encoding 11 β-hydroxylase, which produces cortisol, and *CYP11B2*, which encodes aldosterone synthase. This was shown in 1992 by Richard Lifton and colleagues to occur on chromosome 8. This family's hypertension and hypokalemia were found to be treated with dexamethasone. This particular chimeric enzyme also produces 18-OH-cortisol and 18-oxo cortisol, which were initially used as pathogenic markers for this disease.[28] This accounts for less than 1% of primary aldosteronism cases.[1]

Type II is the most common form, with prevalence of 5% in primary aldosteronism patients, but the genetic basis has not been well established.[28] This is diagnosed when two first-degree family members are diagnosed with primary aldosteronism. Presently, there are no distinct genetic mutations that would distinguish this from sporadic presentations. This has been linked to chromosome 7p22 in some families. Due to the frequency of this familial form of hyperaldosteronism, Endocrine Society guidelines recommend screening for primary aldosteronism in first-degree family members.

Type III is a particularly aggressive form of primary aldosteronism, due to mutations in the *KCNJ5* gene, located on chromosome 11, which changes the selectivity of the GIRK4 potassium channel.

De novo germline variants, have also been found in association with seizures and neurologic abnormalities, now known as PASNA syndrome (primary aldosteronism, seizures, neurologic abnormalities), which is associated with *CACNA1D* mutations.[28] In one pediatric patient with PASNA, treatment with amlodipine, a dihydropyridine calcium channel blocker, treated hypertension, and thus suggested that this class of drugs may be effective against aldosterone-producing adenomas with this mutation.

Type IV is from mutations in *CACNA1H* gene, on chromosome 16, where a voltage-gated calcium channel subunit is mutated. The familial hyperaldosteronism types are summarized in Table 13.2.

TABLE 13.2
Familial Hyperaldosteronism Types.

Familial Hyperaldosteronism Type	Description
I	Glucocorticoid-remediable aldosteronism Chimera of *CYP11B1* with *CYP11B2* on chromosome 8
II	Nonglucocorticoid-remediable aldosteronism Childhood onset cases Underlying genetics unknown
III	De novo germline variants *KCNJ5* mutations
IV	Germline mutants in *CACNA1H*, gain of function of calcium channel

Although most mutations responsible for primary aldosteronism involve either aldosterone production or calcium channel regulation, *CTNNB1* mutations, on chromosome 3, encoding β-catenin, are associated with adherens junctions proteins.[28] This is thought to play a role in adrenal gland phenotype. Other regulatory genes of WNT/β-catenin, such as *SFRP2*, which is a WNT inhibitor, has shown increased aldosterone production, suggesting an alternative pathogenic mechanism for primary aldosteronism.

THERAPY

Unilateral subtypes of primary aldosteronism are candidates for adrenalectomy, which would alleviate hypertension and hypokalemia associated with excess aldosterone. Although mineralocorticoid antagonist therapy would still benefit this particular subtype of patients, should they elect against adrenalectomy, studies have shown over years that the requirement for antihypertensive medications increases.

Adrenalectomy is performed increasingly with minimally invasive surgery—either laparoscopically or with robotic surgery. Complication rates and rates of conversion to open adrenalectomy are low, such that this is considered the standard of care for benign adrenal tumors. The operative time and recovery period may be shorter with smaller incisions.

Complications requiring conversion to open adrenalectomy include intraoperative bleeding.[29]

Aldosterone to renin ratio may be obtained 1–2 days postoperatively, to evaluate for cure. Postoperatively, the diet may be liberalized in salt intake.

Bilateral adrenal hyperplasia would be best managed with mineralocorticoid receptor antagonist therapy, either spironolactone at doses of 12.5–25 mg daily (up to 50 mg daily), in combination with other antihypertensives. Although higher doses are prescriptible, the low dose of spironolactone is recommended, to avoid unwanted side effects and foster medication compliance. The addition of amiloride is used in practice, in some circumstances. Efficacy against hypokalemia is relatively immediate, but blood pressure response may take 1–2 months. Side effects of spironolactone include gynecomastia, erectile dysfunction, and decreased libido for males. Menstrual irregularity may occur in women.[1]

Alternatively, there is off-label use of eplerenone. This may be started at a dosage of 25 mg twice daily,[1] and titrated up to a minimum of 50 mg twice daily (100 mg daily is minimum for efficacy). Patient should be counseled regarding potential side effects, including dizziness, headache, elevated liver enzymes, fatigue, and diarrhea.[1] Eplerenone may be preferred in instances where there is concern for gynecomastia with spironolactone.

Additional lifestyle factors that contribute to successful control of blood pressure include sodium restriction, avoiding weight gain, exercise, and smoking avoidance.

PROGNOSIS

Remission of hypertension, following unilateral adrenalectomy, is dependent on several variables, the most commonly defined being duration of hypertension, number of antihypertensives, age, gender, and pathologic findings. Male gender, age, and number of years with hypertension have been noted to be predictors of lack of complete remission.[30] The expected rate of complete resolution of hypertension is 33%–35%,[30] based on past studies that evaluated blood pressure at 6 months. Patient requiring continuous need for antihypertensive medications or with blood pressure greater than 140/90 mmHg were considered to have persisting hypertension. Taking fewer than three antihypertensive mediations, shorter duration of hypertension, younger age, and female gender were predictors of resolution.

The aldosteronoma reduction score was created based on these predictive factors. This is a four-item resolution score, based on a study of 100 patients who had undergone unilateral adrenalectomy for primary aldosteronism, with validation performed on

TABLE 13.3 Aldosteronoma Resolution Score. Best Predictors for Complete Resolution of Hypertension After Adrenalectomy.	
2 or Fewer Antihypertensive Medications	Low (0–1)
Hypertension ≤6 years	Medium (2–3)
Female gender BMI ≤25 Kg/m²	High (4–5)

Zarnegar et al., The aldosteronoma resolution score: predicting complete resolution of hypertension after adrenalectomy for aldosteronoma, Ann Surg 247 (3) (2008) 511–8.

the cases of 67 patients who had undergone adrenalectomy at another institution. The aldosteronoma resolution score is summarized in Table 13.3.

Predictive factors were defined as follows: two or fewer antihypertensive medications, hypertension greater than or equal to 6 years, female gender, body mass index less than or equal to 25 kg/m². Stratification of likelihood of hypertension remission was devised as follows: low (0–1), medium (2–3), and high (4–5).

Following unilateral adrenalectomy, low to normal aldosterone levels are expected. This is thought to be from suppression of the contralateral adrenal gland. Patients without hypertensive cure were studied. They were characterized as having higher preoperative systolic blood pressure 159.7 mmHg (compared to 147.5 mmHg), worsening serum creatinine 1.32 (compared to 0.94), and higher body mass index 32.7 (compared to 27.4), duration of hypertension 14.9 years (compared to 9.1), and number of antihypertensive medications 3.7 (compared to 2.1).[31]

Reasons for partial success in hypertension remission after unilateral adrenalectomy for aldosterone-producing adenoma include vascular damage sustained during the course of hypertensive state, and coexisting essential hypertension.

Cortisol cosecretory status is another factor for consideration for prognosis, especially with cardiac remodeling recovery. "Connshing syndrome," described as primary aldosteronism and subclinical Cushing's syndrome is a phenomenon increasingly described. This has been demonstrated recently by mass spectroscopy of 24-h urinary steroids, with establishment of mild glucocorticoid excess. A proportion of these patients—approximately 30%—had postoperative partial adrenal insufficiency. In reported studies, adrenalectomy resolved aldosterone and cortisol excess.

Histologic studies of the adrenal glands showed intratumor expression of CYP11B1 (cortisol synthesis enzyme). Additionally, study of metabolic risk parameters were studied, and were found to correlate with glucocorticoid production, rather than mineralocorticoid. Although adrenalectomy would remove excess of aldosterone and cortisol, those on medical therapy with mineralocorticoid antagonist may have metabolic risk that remains, given glucocorticoid excess goes unchecked.

This is supported by studies performed in areas with a nationalized health service, where risk of osteoporotic fracture in women with primary aldosteronism, on mineralocorticoid receptor antagonist treatment, compared to those who underwent adrenalectomy, remained elevated. Hypercortisolism, even in mild forms, may increase the risk for osteoporosis and diabetes mellitus.[32,33]

SUMMARY

With the establishment of reliable laboratory testing and the aldosterone renin ratio as a screening test for primary aldosteronism, there is capability for increased detection. With elucidation of the various subtypes of primary aldosteronism, as spontaneous mutations or familial conditions, this has helped with setting up appropriate guidelines for screening. Presently, in addition to resistant hypertension, requiring multiple antihypertensive agents, with or without the absence of hypokalemia, family history of early cardiovascular events, screening guidelines also include first-degree relatives of primary aldosteronism patients. Confirmatory testing is predominantly with salt loading and evaluation for an inappropriate response in aldosterone with persistent elevation.

Reliable subtyping of primary aldosteronism into unilateral disease versus bilateral adrenal hyperplasia remains a challenge. Anatomical imaging with CT adrenals may discern adenomas that may be biochemically active; however, adrenal vein sampling has proven that anatomy alone is not always accurate. Based on immunohistochemical staining of adrenalectomies, it is evident that not all culprit adrenal glands will have a discernible aldosteronoma or adenoma. Some adrenal glands were noted to be hyperplastic, in some cases with aldosterone-producing cell clusters. Based on the difference in appearance, it is postulated that the underlying pathologic development of the aldosterone-secreting cells may be different.

Performing adrenal vein sampling successfully depends on the experience of the interventional radiologist and may not be offered at all centers. Arguments have been made for mineralocorticoid antagonist

therapy, as noninferior to unilateral adrenalectomy, but emerging studies have found other steroids factor into prognosis, such as cortisol cosecretion, where cardiac remodeling may persist, and risk for osteopenia and fracture risk may remain elevated. Less invasive diagnostic methods have been proposed, such as steroid profiling, but presently lack proof of concept to implement in practice.

Mineralocorticoid receptor antagonist (MRA) therapy, with spironolactone or eplerenone, is well established in efficacy at treatment of the underlying process. Limitations may be if there are additional steroids such as glucocorticoids involved in the pathologic disease process, which would not be blocked by the mineralocorticoid antagonist. Despite its address of the underlying pathologic process, long-term hypertension treatment on MRA would be expected to require a higher degree of antihypertensive agents.

With advances in elucidating genetic mutations underlying aldosterone-producing adenomas, identification of the best medical therapies is certainly a possibility. De novo aldosterone-producing adenoma sequencing has unveiled dominant mutations: *KCNJ5*, *CACNA1D*, *ATP1A1*, and *ATP2B3*. Additionally, regulatory pathways such as Wnt/β-catenin are now under investigation for their role in adrenal gland hyperplasia, and consequent hyperaldosteronism.

Familial aldosteronism conditions, which may have been described in the literature from the 1960s, now increasingly have more known underlying genetic mutations.

Additionally investigations into best therapeutic modalities continue to be underway. Prior study of index patients has found efficacy of calcium channel blockers in treatment. Recently, Lifton et al. have shown macrolides to be effective in *KCNJ5* mutations.[34] Further elucidation of underlying genetic mutations is expected to help with identification of the best medical treatment methods.

Additional consideration would be the steroid profile of the aldosterone-producing adenomas or bilateral adrenal hyperplasia. Should there be glucocorticoid excess secretion, we will not be dealing with one pathologic process alone, and there would be the considerations for mitigating the effects of excess glucocorticoid hormone.

ACKNOWLEDGMENTS

This work was supported by the NICHD, NIH intramural research program.

REFERENCES

1. Melmed S, et al. *Williams Textbook of Endocrinology.* 2016.
2. Buffolo F, et al. Is primary aldosteronism still largely unrecognized? *Horm Metab Res.* 2017;49(12):908–914.
3. Gordon RD, et al. Primary aldosteronism: hypertension with a genetic basis. *Lancet.* 1992;340(8812):159–161.
4. Funder JW, et al. The management of primary aldosteronism: case detection, diagnosis, and treatment: an endocrine society clinical practice guideline. *J Clin Endocrinol Metab.* 2016;101(5):1889–1916.
5. Milliez P, et al. Evidence for an increased rate of cardiovascular events in patients with primary aldosteronism. *J Am Coll Cardiol.* 2005;45(8):1243–1248.
6. Catena C, et al. Cardiovascular outcomes in patients with primary aldosteronism after treatment. *Arch Intern Med.* 2008;168(1):80–85.
7. Holaj R, et al. Increased intima-media thickness of the common carotid artery in primary aldosteronism in comparison with essential hypertension. *J Hypertens.* 2007;25(7):1451–1457.
8. Giacchetti G, et al. Aldosterone as a key mediator of the cardiometabolic syndrome in primary aldosteronism: an observational study. *J Hypertens.* 2007;25(1):177–186.
9. Adolf C, et al. Cortisol excess in patients with primary aldosteronism impacts left ventricular hypertrophy. *J Clin Endocrinol Metab.* 2018;103(12):4543–4552.
10. Weber KT, Brilla CG. Pathological hypertrophy and cardiac interstitium. Fibrosis and renin-angiotensin-aldosterone system. *Circulation.* 1991;83(6):1849–1865.
11. Choi EY, et al. Increased plasma aldosterone-to-renin ratio is associated with impaired left ventricular longitudinal functional reserve in patients with uncomplicated hypertension. *J Am Soc Echocardiogr.* 2008;21(3):251–256.
12. Sechi LA, et al. Intrarenal hemodynamics in primary aldosteronism before and after treatment. *J Clin Endocrinol Metab.* 2009;94(4):1191–1197.
13. Schillaci G, et al. Prognostic value of the metabolic syndrome in essential hypertension. *J Am Coll Cardiol.* 2004;43(10):1817–1822.
14. Corry DB, Tuck ML. The effect of aldosterone on glucose metabolism. *Curr Hypertens Rep.* 2003;5(2):106–109.
15. Shimamoto K, et al. Does insulin resistance participate in an impaired glucose tolerance in primary aldosteronism? *J Hum Hypertens.* 1994;8(10):755–759.
16. Sindelka G, et al. Insulin action in primary hyperaldosteronism before and after surgical or pharmacological treatment. *Exp Clin Endocrinol Diabetes.* 2000;108(1):21–25.
17. Rossi E, et al. Alterations of calcium metabolism and of parathyroid function in primary aldosteronism, and their reversal by spironolactone or by surgical removal of aldosterone-producing adenomas. *Am J Hypertens.* 1995;8(9):884–893.
18. Salcuni AS, et al. Bone involvement in aldosteronism. *J Bone Miner Res.* 2012;27(10):2217–2222.
19. Prejbisz A, et al. Primary aldosteronism and obstructive sleep apnea: is this a bidirectional relationship? *Horm Metab Res.* 2017;49(12):969–976.
20. Hiramatsu K, et al. A screening test to identify aldosterone-producing adenoma by measuring plasma renin activity. Results in hypertensive patients. *Arch Intern Med.* 1981;141(12):1589–1593.
21. Lenders JWM, Eisenhofer G, Reincke M. Subtyping of patients with primary aldosteronism: an update. *Horm Metab Res.* 2017;49(12):922–928.
22. Beuschlein F, et al. The SPARTACUS trial: controversies and unresolved issues. *Horm Metab Res.* 2017;49(12):936–942.
23. Naruse M, et al. The latest developments of functional molecular imaging in the diagnosis of primary aldosteronism. *Horm Metab Res.* 2017;49(12):929–935.
24. Nilubol N, et al. 11-Deoxycortisol may be superior to cortisol in confirming a successful adrenal vein catheterization without cosyntropin: a pilot study. *Int J Endocr Oncol.* 2017;4(2):75–83.
25. Zilbermint M, et al. Primary aldosteronism and ARMC5 variants. *J Clin Endocrinol Metab.* 2015;100(6):E900–E909.
26. Gomez-Sanchez CE, et al. Disordered CYP11B2 expression in primary aldosteronism. *Horm Metab Res.* 2017;49(12):957–962.
27. Scholl UI. Unanswered questions in the genetic basis of primary aldosteronism. *Horm Metab Res.* 2017;49(12):963–968.
28. Monticone S, et al. Genetics in endocrinology: the expanding genetic horizon of primary aldosteronism. *Eur J Endocrinol.* 2018;178(3):R101–r111.
29. Sommerey S, et al. Laparoscopic adrenalectomy–10-year experience at a teaching hospital. *Langenbeck's Arch Surg.* 2015;400(3):341–347.
30. Zarnegar R, et al. The aldosteronoma resolution score: predicting complete resolution of hypertension after adrenalectomy for aldosteronoma. *Ann Surg.* 2008;247(3):511–518.
31. Worth PJ, et al. Characteristics predicting clinical improvement and cure following laparoscopic adrenalectomy for primary aldosteronism in a large cohort. *Am J Surg.* 2015;210(4):702–709.
32. Wu VC, et al. Risk of new-onset diabetes mellitus in primary aldosteronism: a population study over 5 years. *J Hypertens.* 2017;35(8):1698–1708.
33. Beuschlein F, Reincke M, Arlt W. The impact of Connshing's syndrome – mild cortisol excess in primary aldosteronism drives diabetes risk. *J Hypertens.* 2017;35(12):2548.
34. Scholl UI, et al. Macrolides selectively inhibit mutant KCNJ5 potassium channels that cause aldosterone-producing adenoma. *J Clin Investig.* 2017;127(7):2739–2750.

CHAPTER 14

Update on Diagnosis and Management of Pheochromocytoma

YUFEI CHEN, MD • QUAN-YANG DUH, MD

INTRODUCTION

Pheochromocytomas are rare catecholamine-secreting tumors that arise from the chromaffin cells of the adrenal medulla. Similar tumors that arise from the sympathetic ganglia, or paragangliomas, are often termed "extraadrenal pheochromocytomas," although there are important clinical distinctions between the two.

History

The first description of pheochromocytoma is credited to Felix Fraenkel in 1886. He reported the discovery of bilateral adrenal tumors on autopsy of a young woman who presented with palpitations, anxiety, and headaches, and subsequently collapsed and died.[1] The term pheochromocytoma was not coined until 1912 and was based on the tumor's response of turning dark brown upon exposure to chromium salts described by Ludwig Pick.[2] The first surgical removal of pheochromocytoma was performed in 1926 by César Roux in Europe and 1927 by Charles Mayo in the United States.[3] Since then, there have been numerous advances in the diagnosis, treatment, and management of pheochromocytomas and paragangliomas.

Incidence

The incidence of pheochromocytomas is estimated to be approximately 2–8 per million persons per year.[4,5] The peak incidence occurs in the 4th to 5th decades of life with no gender predisposition. In autopsy series, the prevalence rate varies between 0.05% and 0.3%, suggesting that a significant number of pheochromocytomas remain clinically silent or underdiagnosed.[6] It accounts for approximately 5% of patients with incidentally discovered adrenal masses, and may be a contributing factor in 0.1%–1% of patients with hypertension.[7]

DIAGNOSIS

Signs and Symptoms

Symptoms of pheochromocytoma are associated with the tumor's excess secretion of catecholamines. The classic presentation is that of a patient with episodic headaches, diaphoresis, and tachycardia. The majority will also have hypertension, either paroxysmal or sustained. Symptoms can be precipitated during times of stress such as exercise, trauma, or general anesthesia. Foods rich in tyramine such as aged cheeses and cured meats as well as certain medications, particularly monoamine oxidase inhibitors, have also been associated as pheochromocytoma triggers. However, most patients do not present with this classic triad and the clinical presentation can be so variable that it is sometimes termed "the great masquerader." Other signs and symptoms associated with pheochromocytoma include postural hypotension, abdominal pain, bowel obstruction, fever, and new onset diabetes.[8] Some pheochromocytomas present incidentally on abdominal imaging and signs and symptoms may only be obvious in retrospect.

A small portion of patients, who make up a disproportionate number of case reports, also present with pheochromocytoma crisis. This can lead to myocardial infarction, cardiomyopathy, heart failure, stroke, pulmonary edema, and even sudden death.

Genetics

The historic "rule of 10s" for pheochromocytoma has since been debunked with more recent studies suggesting that 30%–40% of patients have the disease as part of a hereditary syndrome.[9] Patients with familial pheochromocytoma and paraganglioma usually present at a younger age than their sporadic counterparts, often with bilateral or more advanced disease. Our evolving knowledge of the genetics of pheochromocytoma and paraganglioma has led us to routinely refer our patients

Advances in Treatment and Management in Surgical Endocrinology. https://doi.org/10.1016/B978-0-323-66195-9.00014-5

for genetic counseling and testing, as a positive result has implications for therapy, follow-up, and screening.

Multiple endocrine neoplasia type 2

Probably, the most well-known familial association with pheochromocytoma is multiple endocrine neoplasia (MEN) type 2. These patients have mutations in the RET proto-oncogene, which encodes a transmembrane receptor tyrosine kinase. It is inherited in an autosomal dominant fashion and is divided into two main phenotypes, MEN2A and MEN2B. Approximately 90% of patients will have the MEN2A subtype, with the most common mutation being found in codon 634.[9] Patients with MEN2A have an almost 100% incidence of medullary thyroid carcinoma, 50% incidence of pheochromocytoma and 20% will develop primary hyperparathyroidism. MEN2B patients usually carry a mutation in codon 918 and are similarly characterized by an almost 100% incidence of medullary thyroid carcinoma and 50% incidence of pheochromocytoma but develop distinctive phenotypical features with a "marfanoid" body habitus, mucocutaneous neuromas (usually on the tongue and lips), skeletal deformities, chronic constipation, and a lack of lacrimation during childhood.

Patients with MEN2-related pheochromocytoma are more likely to have bilateral although rarely malignant tumors. They also tend to have a biochemical profile that is higher in epinephrine (and metanephrine), due to a higher expression of phenylethanolamine N-methyltransferase (PNMT) that converts norepinephrine to epinephrine, and consequently can be more symptomatic.[10]

von Hippel-Lindau syndrome

von Hippel-Lindau (VHL) is an autosomal-dominant syndrome caused by a germline mutation in the VHL tumor suppressor gene. Similar to MEN, it has several subtypes and only patients with VHL type II are at increased risk for developing pheochromocytoma. Pheochromocytomas are seen in approximately 10%–20% of patients with VHL, and may be extraadrenal, often bilateral and rarely malignant.[10] The syndrome is associated with a variety of other tumors, most commonly renal cell carcinoma and central nervous system hemangioblastoma. Pheochromocytomas in VHL tend to have a very low expression of PNMT, and biochemically these patients typically have isolated elevations in normetanephrines with normal metanephrine levels.

Neurofibromatosis type 1

Neurofibromatosis type 1 (NF-1) is another autosomal-dominant tumor syndrome associated with pheochromocytoma. It is caused by mutations in the NF1 tumor suppressor gene, and pheochromocytomas can develop in approximately 3% of the affected individuals. It is a disorder that is distinguished and clinically diagnosed by its phenotypical appearance with multiple café au lait spots, neurofibromas, inguinal and axillary freckling, iris harmatomas (Lisch nodules), and central nervous system gliomas. Patients with NF-1 typically have pheochromocytomas that are unilateral and have a similar rate of malignancy (12%) as patients with sporadic disease.[11]

Paraganglioma syndromes

Familial paragangliomas are another group of autosomal-dominant disorders characterized by mutations in the succinate dehydrogenase gene. There are several different subunit genes affected, with the most common being SDHD (54%) followed by SDHB (40%), SDHC (6%), and the rarer SHDA and SDHAF2 subtypes.[12] These patients develop paragangliomas that are located throughout the body, including the skull base, neck, mediastinum, abdomen, and pelvis and can be associated with the development of gastrointestinal stromal tumors and renal cell carcinomas. Patients with paragangliomas located below the diaphragm are more likely to be biochemically active. The particular subunit affected in the familial paraganglioma syndrome has important prognostic information, with SDHB-associated tumors often being larger and having a higher risk of malignancy.[10]

Other genes

As our knowledge behind the genetics of pheochromocytomas and paragangliomas continues to expand, it is likely that an even larger proportion of patients will be found to have a hereditary mutation in the future. Other mutations that have been reported in recent years include TMEM127, MYC-associated factor X (MAX), fumarate hydratase (FH), and KIF1B genes.[13] Although the clinical and genetic implications of some of these mutations are yet to be fully elucidated, all patients with a young age at presentation (<45 years), multiple tumors, extraadrenal tumors, metastatic disease, positive family history, or clinical features suggestive of a known syndromic disorder should be referred for genetic counseling and testing.

Biochemical Diagnosis

Confirming the diagnosis of pheochromocytoma requires both detecting the presence of catecholamine hypersecretion as well as identifying the tumor on imaging. A number of biochemical tests have been utilized in the diagnosis of pheochromocytoma, including the measurement of chromogranin A and dopamine. Historically, the clonidine suppression test and provocative tests with glucagon were used to confirm a borderline case of pheochromocytoma. However, these tests have largely been supplanted by the measurement of fractionated catecholamines and their metabolites, metanephrines, both in the plasma and 24-h urine collections. The sensitivity and specificity of various biochemical tests vary among institutions and laboratories, so it is important to understand the local environment when ordering tests. In general, plasma free metanephrines are more sensitive and 24-h urinary metanephrines are more specific for diagnosis of pheochromocytoma.[14]

A number of medications can alter the interpretation of results, including tricyclic antidepressants, most psychoactive agents, prochlorperazine, ethanol, and common decongestants. These should ideally be discontinued for 2 weeks before biochemical testing. In times of illness or physical stress, catecholamines can be appropriately increased, so results should be interpreted with caution in hospitalized patients.

Patients with small "preclinical" tumors and those being screened for hereditary pheochromocytoma will often tend to have lower or even normal levels of catecholamine secretion. Biochemical tests performed in these populations may have lower sensitivity such that an individualized interpretation is required, which may include serial imaging and repeat biochemical testing.

In patients where there is suspicion for pheochromocytoma, we prefer to start with measuring plasma free metanephrines. In most centers, it has a sensitivity of 96%–100% and a specificity of 85%–100%.[14,15] This should ideally be drawn with the patient supine and having rested for 30 min. Although not as specific as a 24-h urine collection, its simplicity increases patient compliance and it is an effective "rule-out" test when the results are negative, and we find it particularly useful in the workup of adrenal incidentaloma. We consider it a positive test when the result is over two times the upper limit of normal in the absence of any confounding medications. Patients with intermediate results, between one and two times the upper limit of normal, should have their tests repeated under ideal circumstances or proceed to 24-h urine collection.

The current gold standard biochemical test for diagnosing pheochromocytoma is a 24-h urinary fractionated metanephrines and catecholamines with a reported sensitivity and specificity of 98%–100%.[15] A 24-h urine creatinine should be measured concurrently to confirm adequate collection. Positive results typically have metanephrine and catecholamine levels over twofold the upper limit of normal. In patients who experience paroxysms of hyperadrenergic symptoms highly suggestive of pheochromocytoma but with negative biochemical testing, they can be instructed to repeat their 24-h urinary collection immediately after experiencing an attack.

Screening for pheochromocytoma should be done selectively, especially among hypertensive patients as the disease contributes to elevated blood pressure in only 0.1% of patients. Appropriate populations in whom screening should take place include any patients with a known or suspected familial syndrome that includes pheochromocytoma, young patients with new onset or resistant hypertension, hypertensive crisis during stressful situations such as induction of anesthesia and paradoxical hypertension with commencement of β-blockers.

Imaging

In modern practice, localization of pheochromocytoma often precedes biochemical diagnosis. Indeed, in patients with symptoms suggestive of pheochromocytoma, negative imaging effectively rules out pheochromocytoma as extremely small tumors are unlikely to produce sufficient catecholamines to cause symptoms. Most symptomatic patients have tumors at least 2 cm in size or larger. An increasing proportion of patients with pheochromocytomas are incidentally diagnosed, usually with a computed tomography (CT) scan of the abdomen or chest for another indication. In retrospect, some of these patients describe symptoms that can be attributed to their pheochromocytoma but in most cases, they are asymptomatic.

First-line imaging for pheochromocytoma can be either with CT (Fig. 14.1) or magnetic resonance imaging (MRI) (Fig. 14.2). In our practice, an adrenal protocol CT of the abdomen and pelvis is the most commonly ordered test, with MRI reserved for younger patients, during pregnancy or patients with renal insufficiency. An adrenal protocol CT is easily accessible, cheap, and provides sufficient anatomic detail of the tumor and its relationship with surrounding structures, and is the modality most surgeons are comfortable with interpreting. CT and MRI both have a sensitivity exceeding 98% but specificity of only around 70%.[16]

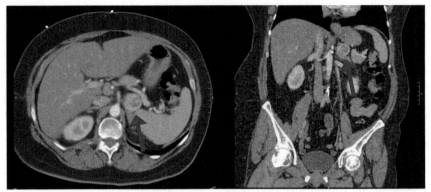

FIG. 14.1 Adrenal protocol CT scan demonstrating 3 × 3 cm heterogeneous pheochromocytoma in the anterior and superior aspect of the left adrenal gland. It has central hypoattenuation representing tumor necrosis and had delayed contrast washout at 10 min.

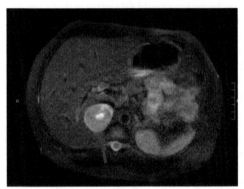

FIG. 14.2 Abdominal MRI showing a high intensity 4.6 cm right adrenal pheochromocytoma on T2-weighted images.

Despite earlier concern of precipitating a crisis, using contrast for imaging studies appear to be safe.

Classical imaging characteristics of pheochromocytoma and paraganglioma include elevated Hounsfield units (>20) on noncontrast CT, delayed contrast washout <50% at 10 min, increased mass vascularity, and high signal intensity on T2-weighted MRI, although the absence of these features does not preclude pheochromocytoma.[16] Patients with cystic or hemorrhagic pheochromocytomas have also been described. If there is suspicion for paraganglioma syndromes or extraadrenal lesions, the imaging can be extended to include the chest and neck.

In most patients, a localized CT or MRI with confirmatory biochemical diagnosis is sufficient to proceed with surgical resection. Additional functional imaging can be obtained in patients with bilateral disease, tumors larger than 10 cm, suspicion for malignant pheochromocytoma or in patients with symptoms and highly suggestive biochemical testing but negative CT/MRI.

The most commonly used functional imaging test is metaiodobenzylguanidine scintigraphy (MIBG) (Fig. 14.3). Metaiodobenzylguanidine is a structural analog of epinephrine that is taken up by the adrenal gland and other neuroendocrine tissues and is usually tagged with a radioisotope of ^{131}I or ^{123}I so it can be detected via scintigraphy. It has a high sensitivity and specificity of 88%−100% when an adrenal tumor is present.[17] The sensitivity decreases to 67%−85% for extraadrenal and metastatic pheochromocytoma/paraganglioma. Disadvantages of MIBG are that it is not widely available, requires up to 48−72 h for imaging acquisition, and needs CT/MRI for anatomic correlation. It is mainly used to predict whether the tumor may be responsive to ^{131}I-MIBG treatment if it is not resectable.

Positron-emission tomography (PET) fused with CT has emerged as an alternative to MIBG for identifying pheochromocytomas. Several isotopes have been described including fludeoxyglucose (^{18}F-FDG PET/CT) that has been shown to have excellent sensitivity for the detection of metastatic disease. The discovery of somatostatin receptor expression in pheochromocytomas and paragangliomas has led to the utilization of octreotide-based functional imaging. Gallium 68 coupled to octreotate (^{68}Ga-DOTATATE PET/CT) (Fig. 14.4), although less readily available, has in some studies been shown to have the highest sensitivity and accuracy for detecting disease compared with other functional imaging modalities and has led some to recommend it to be the first-line study for mapping metastatic pheochromocytoma and paraganglioma.[18]

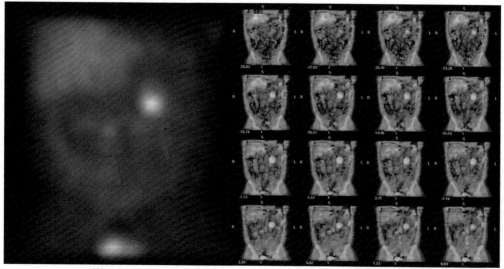

FIG. 14.3 ^{123}I-MIBG in a patient with SDHB mutation demonstrating bilateral paraganglioma.

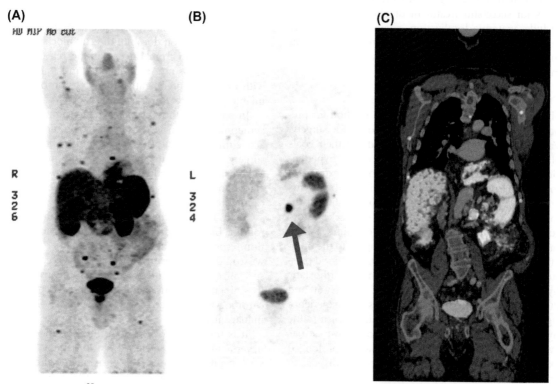

FIG. 14.4 ^{68}Ga-DOTATATE PET/CT in patient with recurrent pheochromocytoma in the left adrenal bed and widespread metastatic disease. **(A)** demonstrates initial followed by **(B)** subtraction PET images. **(C)** shows radiotracer uptake overlaid on fusion PET/CT.

Selective venous sampling for catecholamine levels is rarely performed or indicated. Fine-needle aspiration biopsy has a diagnostic accuracy of 80%–90%. It is almost never indicated in the workup of adrenal pheochromocytoma as it carries the risk of precipitating a dangerous hypertensive crisis and increases the risk of tumor spillage and recurrence.[19]

THERAPY

Surgical resection remains the only curative option for patients with pheochromocytoma and paraganglioma.[20] An experienced multidisciplinary team incorporating surgeons, endocrinologists, and anesthesiologists is required as the perioperative management of pheochromocytoma can be challenging. Nonsurgical active surveillance of pheochromocytoma, outside of select patients with asymptomatic, biochemically inert familial disease, is rarely indicated. Untreated pheochromocytoma can lead to hypertensive crises, arrhythmias, heart failure, and even death especially in times of stress such as undergoing surgical procedures.[21] The key goals for successful treatment of pheochromocytoma include anatomic localization, adequate preoperative medical treatment, complete surgical resection without tumor spillage, and close perioperative hemodynamic monitoring.

Preoperative Medical Treatment

There is no universally recommended method for preparing patients with pheochromocytoma for surgery. Various regimens have been described but their goals all include sympathetic blockade to control hypertension and tachycardia and adequate volume expansion to overcome the prolonged vasoconstriction that occurs with catecholamine excess. Preoperative medical treatment should take place for at least 1–2 weeks before surgery. Patients are encouraged to consume a high salt diet with liberal fluid intake leading up to the operation with an objective of achieving a target blood pressure of less than 130/80 mmHg, minimal orthostatic hypotension, and resting heart rate of between 60 and 80 beats per minute (bpm).[20] Patients who experience significant orthostasis can be preadmitted for a saline infusion the day before surgery. Preoperative cardiac evaluation should also be considered as the prolonged exposure to elevated catecholamines can predispose to arrhythmias, coronary ischemia, and cardiomyopathy.

The first choice agent at most centers is an α-adrenergic receptor blocker. Although clinical trials have suggested that there is no overall difference regarding the use of nonselective α-versus selective α1-adrenergic receptor blockers, in our experience we find that patients who use nonselective α-adrenergic blockers experience less intraoperative hemodynamic variability.[22] As such, we typically start our patients on phenoxybenzamine at 10 mg b.i.d and uptitrate as necessary. Side effects can include orthostasis, nasal congestion, and fatigue. In circumstances where phenoxybenzamine is not available or if cost is prohibitive, we utilize a selective α1-adrenergic blocker such as doxazosin starting at 2 mg/day.

Once adequate α-blockade is obtained, patients who experience tachycardia are commenced on β-adrenergic blockers until a goal heart rate of 60–80 bpm is reached. An agent such as propranolol or atenolol is started at low doses and increased as necessary. Care must be taken in patients with concomitant cardiomyopathy. Initiation of β-blockade should never precede α-blockade as unopposed α-adrenergic stimulation can lead to hypertensive crises.

An alternative regimen for preparing patients with pheochromocytoma is with the use of calcium channel blockers.[23] This can be used alone or in conjunction with α-blockade to assist with blood pressure control, with the most commonly used agents being nifedipine or amlodipine. As it does not directly block the adrenergic stimulation from catecholamine release, its use as a solo agent is not recommended unless in patients with only mild preoperative hypertension or who are unable to tolerate α-blockade.

In patients with refractory hypertension, which can sometimes be seen in those with large, biochemically active tumors, metyrosine can be added shortly before surgery to help with blood pressure management. Metyrosine, a competitive inhibitor of tyrosine hydroxylase, directly inhibits catecholamine synthesis and thus can deplete catecholamine levels.

There have also been centers that report not using routine blockade prior to pheochromocytoma resection, especially in normotensive patients.[24] However, we would caution against this approach except in highly specialized centers with experienced surgeons and anesthesiologists as the risks of treating an unblocked pheochromocytoma exceeds the side effects of medical management.

It is important to note that pheochromocytoma is never a surgical emergency. Even in patients who present in pheochromocytoma crisis, taking them to the operating room immediately would result in high morbidity and mortality.[25] Patients should have their hemodynamics supported acutely and then be commenced on appropriate adrenergic blockade. Medical management and optimization can continue for weeks to months, often as an outpatient, until the patient has fully stabilized. In patients with cardiomyopathy, cardiac function can recover during this time although patients need to be careful not to have excessive salt loading as it can precipitate congestive cardiac failure.

Surgical Resection

A number of surgical approaches have been described for the resection of pheochromocytoma. Generally, minimally invasive adrenalectomy is recommended as these patients have been shown to experience fewer complications, shorter length of stay and faster postoperative recovery.[26] Open resection is reserved for larger tumors (>8 cm) or where there is concern for adjacent tissue invasion. Conversion to an open procedure should also occur when there are uncertainties as to completeness of tumor resection or concern for tumor rupture. The technique and approach for paraganglioma resection should be based on tumor size, location, and surgeon expertise.

Minimally invasive adrenalectomy—anterior approach

The anterior, or lateral transabdominal laparoscopic approach, is performed with the patient in the lateral decubitus position with the tumor side elevated.[27] The operative bed is flexed, expanding the space between the lower ribs and iliac crest. Pneumoperitoneum is established. Four trocars are placed underneath the ipsilateral costal margin. On the left, the colon, spleen, and tail of pancreas are mobilized and retracted anteromedially, thereby exposing the adrenal gland and the tumor. On the right, the triangular ligament of the liver is divided, and the liver is retracted medially and superiorly. The tumor is identified and in most patients, a complete adrenalectomy is performed. The adrenal with a rim of periadrenal fat is dissected circumferentially, with hemostasis of small adrenal vessels with a vessel-sealing device. The adrenal vein draining into the renal vein on the left and inferior vena cava on the right is identified and divided. Division of adrenal vein is a critical time; following division, the blood pressure can fall precipitously as the source of excess catecholamines is abruptly ceased so the anesthesiologist needs to be forewarned. Early division of the vein can however lead to venous congestion of the tumor that causes increased bleeding and friability. Once the adrenalectomy is complete, the specimen is placed into an endocatch bag and removed.

Minimally invasive adrenalectomy—posterior approach

The posterior retroperitoneoscopic approach is ideally suited for patients who have had previous abdominal surgery or who require bilateral adrenalectomy as no patient repositioning is required.[28] The patient is placed a prone half-jackknife position with the hips and knees bent at 90 degrees. An initial incision is made just below the tip of the 12th rib and the retroperitoneal space is bluntly dissected. Two additional ports are placed and insufflation of the retroperitoneal space is commenced, typically at a higher pressure of 20−25 mmHg to assist with dissection and hemostasis. The adrenal gland is identified and mobilized starting medially and the adrenal vein is located and divided at the inferior medial border. The dissection is then continued laterally and cranially, dissecting the adrenal gland off the superior pole of the kidney. The specimen is then retrieved via an endocatch bag.

Special Considerations
Children

Approximately 10% of pheochromocytomas and paragangliomas present in the pediatric population, although it still remains a rare condition. Pediatric patients have a male preponderance and are more likely to present with sustained hypertension. Compared with adults, their tumors are more likely to be familial, bilateral and located in extraadrenal locations. Treatment goals of adequate medical optimization followed by complete surgical resection are identical to their adult counterparts. All children who present with pheochromocytoma or paraganglioma should be referred for genetic counseling and testing and all require close lifelong monitoring as recurrence and malignancy rates are elevated.

Pregnancy

Much has been written about pheochromocytoma in pregnancy although this is an extremely rare situation. However, it should be considered if severe or uncontrolled hypertension develops as undiagnosed and untreated during pregnancy is associated with maternal and fetal mortality rates exceeding 50%.[29] Biochemical testing is the same as in nonpregnant patients but MRI is the localizing study of choice as CT and MIBG are contraindicated due to radiation. Once diagnosed, phenoxybenzamine remains a safe drug for α-adrenergic blockade as it does not cross the placenta. Surgical resection can be performed laparoscopically during the second trimester. Otherwise, blockade is continued and an elective cesarean section can be performed in the third trimester with careful monitoring, followed by laparoscopic adrenalectomy 4 weeks postpartum. Spontaneous labor and normal vaginal delivery increases the risk of hypertensive crisis and subsequent maternal and fetal morbidity. Needless to say, a specialized team is needed for both maternal and fetal monitoring.

Bilateral pheochromocytoma

Cortical sparing (partial) adrenalectomy can be considered in patients who undergo bilateral adrenalectomy or those with familial syndromes such as MEN2 to prevent permanent steroid dependency. However, these patients will need to be counseled on the possible increased risk of tumor recurrence and the need for reoperation.[30] Complete bilateral adrenalectomy with autotransplantation of cortical adrenal tissue has been described but there is insufficient evidence to recommend this approach currently.

Perioperative Monitoring

The operative management of pheochromocytoma requires close communication between the surgeon and anesthesiologist. The surgery is performed under general anesthesia with endotracheal intubation. In addition to standard monitoring, adequate large bore intravenous access as well as an arterial catheter is necessary for real-time hemodynamic monitoring. Central venous and pulmonary artery catheterization are used selectively. A foley catheter is routinely placed. An epidural catheter is inserted for open procedures but is ideally not utilized intraoperatively as the resulting sympathectomy can result in more exaggerated hypotension.

In most well-blocked patients, the operative course of pheochromocytoma resection is relatively smooth. However, the anesthesiologist needs to be well prepared to manage labile blood pressures. With intubation, peritoneal insufflation and with any tumor manipulation, the patient can become hypertensive due to surge of catecholamine release that is often managed with short acting vasodilators such as sodium nitroprusside.[31] Additional agents that can be utilized include phentolamine, nicardipine, and esmolol. In patients with particularly labile hypertension, magnesium sulfate, a vasodilator that inhibits catecholamine release while also having cardiac stabilizing properties, can be added. Cardiac arrhythmias that develop can usually resolve with cessation of tumor manipulation and with the addition of lidocaine, amiodarone, or a short acting β-blocker.

After ligation of the draining adrenal veins, profound hypotension can occur as the source of catecholamine excess is abruptly ceased. Vasodilators should be stopped and intravenous fluids and vasopressors should be administered. Phenylephrine and norepinephrine are first line agents that can be titrated rapidly to effect. In patients who experience resistant hypotension, vasopressin infusion at 0.02–0.04 units/min can be added as an adjunct. Both the surgeon and anesthesiologist need to keep in mind the presence of additional adrenal veins in patients who develop rebound hypertension after ligation of the initial adrenal vein, and will need to be prepared to rapidly switch between vasodilators and vasopressors.

Postoperative monitoring of patients after pheochromocytoma resection can usually occur in a regular postanesthesia care unit (PACU) although some patients with prolonged hemodynamic instability may require intensive care admission. In our practice, we observe patients for 4 h in the PACU before making the decision of sending them to the hospital floor or intensive care. Postoperative hypotension is common due to a combination of downregulation of adrenergic receptors, residual antihypertensives, or hypovolemia. Blood glucose should be monitored perioperatively as rebound hyperinsulinemia can lead to hypoglycemia.[32] We monitor blood glucose hourly in the PACU and then every 6 h subsequently until eating and all patients receive dextrose containing maintenance fluids. Patients with underlying cardiomyopathy can be particularly susceptible to the fluid shifts that occur perioperatively, so fluid resuscitation needs to be used judiciously to avoid pulmonary edema. Patients who undergo bilateral adrenalectomy or who have previously had their contralateral adrenal removed will need stress dose perioperative glucocorticoids followed by a postoperative taper.

Metastatic Pheochromocytoma/Paraganglioma

Approximately 10% of pheochromocytomas and up to a quarter of patients with paraganglioma can have malignant disease. Malignancy is defined by the presence of metastases, either regional or distant, and as such is difficult to diagnose on initial pathology. Various tumor features have been identified that are associated with increased risk of malignancy. The Pheochromocytoma of the Adrenal gland Scaled Score (PASS) (Table 14.1) is most commonly utilized with a PASS ≥ 4 associated with more biologically aggressive tumors that may require closer monitoring.[33]

Treatment options for patients with metastatic disease depend on extent and location of tumor burden, with the goal of decreasing tumor bulk and slowing

TABLE 14.1
Pheochromocytoma of the Adrenal Gland Scaled Score (PASS).

Histological Feature	Score
Vascular invasion	1
Capsular invasion	1
Periadrenal adipose tissue invasion	2
Large nests or diffuse growth	2
Focal or confluent necrosis	2
High cellularity	2
Tumor cell spindling	2
Cellular monotony	2
Increased mitotic figures (>3/10 high power fields)	2
Atypical mitotic figures	2
Profound nuclear pleomorphism	1
Hyperchromasia	1

tumor progression. Symptoms from catecholamine excess should be controlled with medical therapy, like in patients with benign disease. Combined α- and β-adrenergic blockades are most commonly used, with selective α1-adrenergic blockers such as prazosin or doxazosin preferred over phenoxybenzamine for long-term administration.

In patients with isolated, resectable metastatic disease, complete removal of tumor can result in long-term remission. Even when an R0 resection cannot be obtained or in patients with widespread disease, surgical tumor debulking can lead to a significant decrease in catecholamine secretion and improve efficacy of adjuvant therapies.[34] Other local therapies that can offer debulking benefits or slow disease progression in patients not amenable to surgical intervention include cryoablation, radiofrequency ablation, stereotactic radiation especially for bony metastases, ethanol injection, and tumor embolization for liver metastases.

Several systemic therapies can be utilized in the treatment of metastatic pheochromocytoma/paraganglioma.[11] Conventional cytotoxic chemotherapy, with the most common regimens utilizing cyclophosphamide, vincristine, doxorubicin, and dacarbazine, has been shown to slow disease progression and control symptoms but has limited effect on overall survival.[35] Radionucleotide therapy has emerged as a more targeted form of systemic therapy and is based on the tumors uptake of MIBG or somatostatin analogs that

can be determined on pretreatment scans.[36] Radioactive iodine coupled to MIBG (^{131}I-MIBG) is effective in approximately 60%–70% of tumors and can be repeated, with the most common toxicity being myelosuppression. Tumors that uptake on ^{68}Ga-DOTATATE PET may benefit from peptide receptor radioligand therapy with radiolabeled somatostatin analogs such as ^{177}Lu-DOTATATE, and although early results are promising, our experience with these agents is still evolving.

PROGNOSIS

Following successful surgical resection of pheochromocytoma, approximately 80% of patients are expected to become normotensive. Most patients with persistent elevated blood pressure will likely have a component of essential hypertension although their blood pressure will usually be more easily controlled. Those with persistent symptoms of catecholamine excess or episodic episode of hypertension should raise suspicion for persistent or metastatic pheochromocytoma.

Approximately 10%–15% of patients will develop disease recurrence after initial surgical therapy, and as recurrence can occur decades later, surveillance for pheochromocytoma and paraganglioma is lifelong. Follow-up needs to be individualized, and those with familial disease, multiple tumors, or aggressive histological features are at higher risk of recurrence and need more stringent follow-up. All patients should be offered genetic testing and counseling, if not done already preoperatively. Biochemical testing should occur as early as 2–4 weeks after surgery to document successful tumor removal, every 3–6 months for the first year and then annually for life.[20] Elevations in metanephrines should prompt imaging with high resolution CT or functional imaging especially if there was preoperative uptake. A baseline whole body functional imaging test is often performed postoperatively in those with high-risk pathologic features. In patients with nonfunctional tumors (often seen in head and neck paragangliomas in patients with SDHx or VHL mutations), surveillance should be with serial imaging such as MRI.

Patients who are detected to have recurrence in the surgical resection bed should raise suspicion for pheochromocytomatosis, where tumor cells seed the surrounding tissue, often from rupture of the tumor capsule during the initial operation.[37] Treatment involves a combination of surgical resection of tumor implants, adjuvant systemic therapy, and/or stereotactic radiation, and although the clinical course is generally benign, local recurrence rates are high.

Long-term survival rates in patients with pheochromocytoma or paraganglioma are highly variable. Patients who have apparently "benign" disease that never develop disease recurrence should have an overall survival that approaches age-matched individuals. In patients with metastatic disease, 5-year survival is approximately 50%–80% with appropriate therapy although this differs depending on location of the primary tumor, extent of metastases, and response to adjuvant therapies.

SUMMARY

Pheochromocytoma and paraganglioma are rare diseases that require an experienced multidisciplinary team to manage effectively. Although our patients are now presenting increasingly with adrenal incidentalomas rather than clinical features of pheochromocytoma, the principles of treatment remain the same. Confirming the biochemical diagnosis and accurate anatomic localization followed by preoperative medical optimization are all essential for patients to undergo successful surgical resection of the tumor, the only form of cure. Clinicians need to remain informed of ongoing developments in the field, as our knowledge of tumor genetics and adjuvant therapies continues to evolve and influence the management of these complicated patients.

REFERENCES

1. Fraenkel F. Classics in oncology. A case of bilateral completely latent adrenal tumor and concurrent nephritis with changes in the circulatory system and retinitis: Felix Fränkel, 1886. *CA Cancer J Clin.* 1984;34(2):93–106.
2. Bausch B, Tischler AS, Schmid KW, Leijon H, Eng C, Neumann HPH. Max schottelius: pioneer in pheochromocytoma. *J Endocr Soc.* 2017;1(7):957–964.
3. Goldstein RE, O'Neill JA, Holcomb GW, et al. Clinical experience over 48 years with pheochromocytoma. *Ann Surg.* 1999;229(6):755–764; discussion 764-6.
4. Beard CM, Sheps SG, Kurland LT, Carney JA, Lie JT. Occurrence of pheochromocytoma in Rochester, Minnesota, 1950 through 1979. *Mayo Clin Proc.* 1983;58(12):802–804.
5. Berends AMA, Buitenwerf E, de Krijger RR, et al. Incidence of pheochromocytoma and sympathetic paraganglioma in The Netherlands: a nationwide study and systematic review. *Eur J Intern Med.* 2018;51:68–73.
6. Sutton MG, Sheps SG, Lie JT. Prevalence of clinically unsuspected pheochromocytoma. Review of a 50-year autopsy series. *Mayo Clin Proc.* 1981;56(6):354–360.
7. Young WF. The incidentally discovered adrenal mass. *N Engl J Med.* 2007;356(6):601–610.
8. Soltani A, Pourian M, Davani BM. Does this patient have Pheochromocytoma? a systematic review of clinical signs and symptoms. *J Diabetes Metab Disord.* 2015;15:6.
9. Martucci VL, Pacak K. Pheochromocytoma and paraganglioma: diagnosis, genetics, management, and treatment. *Curr Probl Cancer.* 2014;38(1):7–41.
10. King KS, Pacak K. Familial pheochromocytomas and paragangliomas. *Mol Cell Endocrinol.* 2014;386(1–2):92–100.
11. Angelousi A, Kassi E, Zografos G, Kaltsas G. Metastatic pheochromocytoma and paraganglioma. *Eur J Clin Investig.* 2015;45(9):986–997.
12. Lefebvre M, Foulkes WD. Pheochromocytoma and paraganglioma syndromes: genetics and management update. *Curr Oncol.* 2014;21(1):e8–e17.
13. Casey RT, Warren AY, Martin JE, et al. Clinical and molecular features of renal and pheochromocytoma/paraganglioma tumor association syndrome (RAPTAS): case series and literature review. *J Clin Endocrinol Metab.* 2017;102(11):4013–4022.
14. Sawka AM, Jaeschke R, Singh RJ, Young WF. A comparison of biochemical tests for pheochromocytoma: measurement of fractionated plasma metanephrines compared with the combination of 24-hour urinary metanephrines and catecholamines. *J Clin Endocrinol Metab.* 2003;88(2):553–558.
15. Lenders JWM, Pacak K, Walther MM, et al. Biochemical diagnosis of pheochromocytoma. *J Am Med Assoc.* 2002;287(11):1427–1434.
16. Blake MA, Kalra MK, Maher MM, et al. Pheochromocytoma: an imaging chameleon. *Radiographics.* 2004;24(suppl 1):S87–S99.
17. Havekes B, King K, Lai EW, Romijn JA, Corssmit EPM, Pacak K. New imaging approaches to phaeochromocytomas and paragangliomas. *Clin Endocrinol.* 2010;72(2):137–145.
18. Maurice JB, Troke R, Win Z, et al. A comparison of the performance of 68Ga-DOTATATE PET/CT and 123I-MIBG SPECT in the diagnosis and follow-up of phaeochromocytoma and paraganglioma. *Eur J Nucl Med Mol Imaging.* 2012;39(8):1266–1270.
19. Cheah WK, Clark OH, Horn JK, Siperstein AE, Duh Q-Y. Laparoscopic adrenalectomy for pheochromocytoma. *World J Surg.* 2002;26(8):1048–1051.
20. Lenders JWM, Duh Q-Y, Eisenhofer G, et al. Pheochromocytoma and paraganglioma: an endocrine society clinical practice guideline. *J Clin Endocrinol Metab.* 2014;99(6):1915–1942.
21. Lenders JWM, Eisenhofer G, Mannelli M, Pacak K. Phaeochromocytoma. *Lancet.* 2005;366(9486):665–675.
22. Randle RW, Balentine CJ, Pitt SC, Schneider DF, Sippel RS. Selective versus non-selective α-blockade prior to laparoscopic adrenalectomy for pheochromocytoma. *Ann Surg Oncol.* 2017;24(1):244–250.
23. Brunaud L, Boutami M, Nguyen-Thi P-L, et al. Both preoperative alpha and calcium channel blockade impact intraoperative hemodynamic stability similarly in the

management of pheochromocytoma. *Surgery.* 2014; 156(6):1410–1418.

24. Shao Y, Chen R, Shen Z, et al. Preoperative alpha blockade for normotensive pheochromocytoma. *J Hypertens.* 2011; 29(12):2429–2432.

25. Scholten A, Cisco RM, Vriens MR, et al. Pheochromocytoma crisis is not a surgical emergency. *J Clin Endocrinol Metab.* 2013;98(2):581–591.

26. Shen WT, Grogan R, Vriens M, Clark OH, Duh Q-Y. One hundred two patients with pheochromocytoma treated at a single institution since the introduction of laparoscopic adrenalectomy. *Arch Surg.* 2010;145(9):893.

27. Lal G, Duh Q-Y. Laparoscopic adrenalectomy—indications and technique. *Surg Oncol.* 2003;12:105–123.

28. Walz MK, Alesina PF, Wenger FA, et al. Posterior retroperitoneoscopic adrenalectomy—results of 560 procedures in 520 patients. *Surgery.* 2006;140(6):943–950.

29. Lenders JWM. Endocrine disorders in pregnancy: pheochromocytoma and pregnancy: a deceptive connection. *Eur J Endocrinol.* 2012;166(2):143–150.

30. Castinetti F, Qi X-P, Walz MK, et al. Outcomes of adrenal-sparing surgery or total adrenalectomy in phaeochromocytoma associated with multiple endocrine neoplasia type 2: an international retrospective population-based study. *Lancet Oncol.* 2014;15(6):648–655.

31. O'Riordan JA. Pheochromocytomas and anesthesia. *Int Anesthesiol Clin.* 1997;35(4):99–127.

32. Chen Y, Hodin RA, Pandolfi C, Ruan DT, McKenzie TJ. Hypoglycemia after resection of pheochromocytoma. *Surgeon.* 2014;156(6):1404–1408.

33. Thompson LDR. Pheochromocytoma of the Adrenal gland Scaled Score (PASS) to separate benign from malignant neoplasms: a clinicopathologic and immunophenotypic study of 100 cases. *Am J Surg Pathol.* 2002;26(5):551–566.

34. Hamidi O, Young WF, Iñiguez-Ariza NM, et al. Malignant pheochromocytoma and paraganglioma: 272 patients over 55 years. *J Clin Endocrinol Metab.* 2017;102(9): 3296–3305.

35. Gonias S, Goldsby R, Matthay KK, et al. Phase II study of high-dose [131I]metaiodobenzylguanidine therapy for patients with metastatic pheochromocytoma and paraganglioma. *J Clin Oncol.* 2009;27(25):4162–4168.

36. Kong G, Grozinsky-Glasberg S, Hofman MS, et al. Efficacy of peptide receptor radionuclide therapy for functional metastatic paraganglioma and pheochromocytoma. *J Clin Endocrinol Metab.* 2017;102(9):3278–3287.

37. Li ML, Fitzgerald PA, Price DC, Norton JA. Iatrogenic pheochromocytomatosis: a previously unreported result of laparoscopic adrenalectomy. *Surgery.* 2001;130(6): 1072–1077.

CHAPTER 15

Advances in the Diagnosis and Medical Management of Cushing's Syndrome

DANAE A. DELIVANIS, MD, PHD • ANU SHARMA, MBBS • OKSANA HAMIDI, DO • MEERA SHAH, MD • IRINA BANCOS, MD

INTRODUCTION

The clinical constellation of signs and symptoms consistent with glucocorticoid excess is termed Cushing syndrome (CS). By far, the most common etiology for CS is the administration of exogenous glucocorticoids. However, this chapter will mainly focus on endogenous forms of overt cortisol excess.

Endogenous CS affects 0.2−5 people/million per year, with an estimated annual incidence of pituitary Cushing disease (CD) of 1.2−2.4 cases/million, CS due to adrenal adenoma—0.6 cases/million, and CS due to adrenocortical carcinoma—0.2 cases/million.[1−4] Although endogenous CS is thought to be rare based on available population-based studies, its incidence may be grossly underestimated.[5−7] For instance, in a prospective study of 200 overweight patients with type 2 diabetes mellitus, CS was diagnosed in four (2%) patients: three with CD and one with adrenal CS.[7] In another retrospective analysis of obese patients with poorly controlled diabetes mellitus, the prevalence of preclinical CS was 3.3%, higher than previously reported.[5] However, these findings were not confirmed in follow-up studies.[8,9] Therefore, routine screening for CS is not recommended. Instead, a case-finding approach is recommended in patients with features predictive of CS, children with decreasing height and increasing weight percentile, and patients with incidental adrenal adenoma.[10]

Patients with CS can have a wide range of clinical presentations. Cortisol excess may lead to development of hypertension, weight gain, skin thinning, menstrual irregularity, and mood changes. However, no one single symptom or sign is specific enough to make a diagnosis of CS. The "classic" phenotype of prominent dorsal, supraclavicular and temporal fat pads, bruising, abdominal striae, proximal myopathy, and hypertension is observed in patients with severe CS. However, less severe presentations are more commonly encountered in clinical practice. The tissue-specific action of cortisol at the glucocorticoid receptor is what seems to determine the resulting phenotype, which in turn is driven by the rate of production of cortisol, activity of the glucocorticoid receptor, and rate of cortisol metabolism, all of which show variability between individuals.[11] In addition to classic phenotype of CS, endogenous cortisol excess should be suspected in patients who present with unusual clinical features, such as rapid weight gain or severe bone loss. CS should also be suspected in those who have had a significant change in a previously stable comorbidity, such as rapidly worsening hypertension or type 2 diabetes.

DIAGNOSIS OF CUSHING SYNDROME
General Remarks

Making the diagnosis of CS can be challenging and should be performed by an experienced endocrinologist. When CS is suspected based on typical or atypical clinical presentation, biochemical confirmation is required through a combination of several tests assessing the hypothalamic−pituitary−adrenal (HPA) axis (Table 15.1), each presenting with its own limitations and pitfalls (Table 15.2). As recommended by the clinical practice guideline from the Endocrine Society, at least two of three different screening tests should indicate abnormal HPA axis functioning to confirm CS. These tests include assessment of free cortisol in the 24-h urine collection (UFC), measurement of late-night salivary cortisol (LNSC) concentrations, and the 1-mg overnight dexamethasone suppression test (DST) or alternatively the 2-day 2-mg DST.[10] These tests are complimentary to each other, and the results should generally be concordant.

Advances in Treatment and Management in Surgical Endocrinology. https://doi.org/10.1016/B978-0-323-66195-9.00015-7

TABLE 15.1
Tests Used in Diagnosis and Differential Diagnosis of Cushing Syndrome.
FIRST-LINE TESTING—ESTABLISHING DIAGNOSIS
24-h urinary free cortisol (UFC) excretion (2 measurements) Late-night salivary cortisol (2 measurements) 1-mg overnight dexamethasone suppression test (DST) Two-day low-dose DST (2 mg/d for 48 h)
ADDITIONAL TESTS FOR DIAGNOSIS AND SUBTYPE OF CUSHING SYNDROME
Plasma ACTH High dose (8mgDST) dexamethasone suppression test Corticotropin-releasing hormone stimulation test Desmopressin stimulation test Inferior petrosal sinus sampling Cross-sectional imaging of adrenal glands or MRI of pituitary gland Somatostatin receptor scintigraphy

ACTH, Adrenocorticotropic hormone; *CT*, Computed tomography; *MRI*, Magnetic resonance imaging.

Cortisol may be measured by an immunoassay (such as radioimmunoassay) or a structurally based assay (such as high performance liquid chromatography mass spectrometry). Assays differ in their accuracy. Antibody-based immunoassays such as radioimmunoassay can be affected by cross-reactivity with cortisol metabolites and synthetic glucocorticoids. In contrast, structurally based assays such as liquid chromatography mass spectrometry do not pose this issue and are being used with increasing frequency. Each test has important caveats and pitfalls that need to be carefully considered during interpretation (Table 15.2).

After confirming biochemical cortisol excess, the next step is to determine whether the hypercortisolism is adrenocorticotropic hormone (ACTH)-dependent (due to a pituitary or ectopic ACTH-secreting tumor) or ACTH-independent (due to an adrenal source) by measuring 8 AM plasma ACTH (Fig. 15.1). Additional radiological investigations should be undertaken only after biochemical confirmation of cortisol excess and its subtype.

Diagnostic Algorithm

Cortisol excess is confirmed when at least two different first-line diagnostic tests are abnormal as proposed by the 2008 Endocrine Society guidelines (Fig. 15.1).[10]

If initial testing is normal in an individual with low suspicion for CS, it is unlikely that the patient has CS unless the disease is very mild or cyclical. Further testing is not recommended in these situations unless symptoms progress or cyclical CS is suspected.

If initial testing is normal in an individual with high suspicion of CS (based on history and clinical exam), excluding physiologic causes of cortisol excess, repeating first-line tests, or performing additional testing might be warranted. Exclusion of exogenous glucocorticoid exposure is key in these situations.

If initial testing is abnormal (at least one abnormal test) then additional evaluation is recommended to determine whether a patient had a false-positive result, mild CS or physiological cause of cortisol excess (pseudo-Cushing syndrome).

FIRST-LINE DIAGNOSTIC TESTS

24-Hour Urinary Free Cortisol Excretion

Measurement of UFC excretion provides a direct measurement of circulating biologically active cortisol.[12] The advantage of UFC is that unlike serum cortisol, UFC is unaffected by medications and conditions that alter cortisol-binding globulin (CBG) (e.g., estrogen containing oral contraceptives). The disadvantage is that the 24-h urine collection can be cumbersome and clinicians need to confirm appropriateness of the sample collection (Table 15.2).

UFC is considered the gold standard test for detection of hypercortisolism with several studies reporting a sensitivity and specificity of 95%–100% and 98%, respectively.[12,13] However, other studies showed lower specificity with up to 24% of surgically proven CS demonstrating normal UFC.[14] A systematic review and meta-analysis of studies on diagnostic tests for CS concluded that UFC diagnosed CS with a high

TABLE 15.2
Tests Used in Diagnosis and Differential Diagnosis of Cushing Syndrome.

Test	Advantages	Pitfalls
24-h urinary free cortisol excretion	• high sensitivity • not affected by conditions that alter CBG • No cross-reactivity with other steroids or cortisol metabolites • not affected by circadian secretion of cortisol • performed in the outpatient setting • inexpensive test	• low specificity • cumbersome test and requires evaluation of appropriateness of the collection • false-positive with high fluid intake >5 L/day • false-positive in pseudo-Cushing cases • false-positive if HPLC method is used and individual is taking fibrate and carbamazepine • false-negative in mild and cyclic CS • false-negative in the setting of renal impairment
Late-night salivary cortisol	• noninvasive and easy to collect	• falsely abnormal in patients with erratic sleep schedule (e.g., shift workers) • false-positive in pseudo-Cushing syndrome • false-positive due to gingivitis and steroid containing oral gels • false-positive in patients who chew tobacco or eat licorice limited availability outside USA
Low DST tests	• 1-mg DST easy to perform	• false-positive in pseudo-Cushing syndrome • false-positive with elevated CBG (e.g., due to oral estrogen) • false-positive with poor absorption of tdexamethasone • false abnormal with medications that alter CYP3A4 activity • false-negative with slow dexamethasone metabolism (e.g., liver failure, drugs) • false-positive with chronic renal failure (creatinine clearance<15 mL/min)
Late-night serum cortisol		• false-positive by stress before blood collection • false-positive with pseudo-Cushing syndrome
Two-day 2-mg DST with CRH		• same as low dose DSTs • requires hospitalization
Desmopressin stimulation test		• requires hospitalization • lack of large validating studies

CBG, Cortisol-binding globulin; *CRH*, corticotropin-releasing hormone; *CS*, Cushing syndrome; *DST*, dexamethasone suppression test; *HPLC*, High-performance liquid chromatography.

sensitivity but a low specificity.[15] Although values more than fourfold the upper limit of normal are virtually diagnostic for CS, false-positive results may be seen in patients with physiological cortisol excess, individuals who drink large volumes of liquid (>5 L per day), in patients treated with carbamazepine or fenofibrate when UFC is measured by high performance liquid chromatography, or when there is contamination with hydrocortisone preparations (Table 15.3).[16–20] Conversely, false-negative results may be seen in patients with mild or cyclic CS[10,21–23] and in patients with moderate-to-severe renal impairment and/or incomplete urine collection.[24]

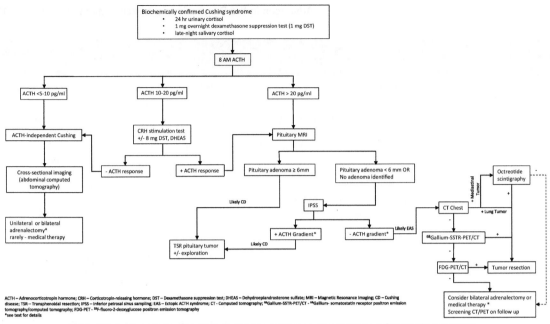

FIG. 15.1 Diagnostic algorithm for testing patients with suspected Cushing's syndrome.

ACTH – Adrenocorticotropin hormone; CRH – Corticotropin-releasing hormone; DST – Dexamethasone suppression test; DHEAS – Dehydroepiandrosterone sulfate; MRI – Magnetic Resonance Imaging; CD – Cushing disease; TSR – Transphenoidal resection; IPSS – Inferior petrosal sinus sampling; EAS – Ectopic ACTH syndrome; CT - Computed tomography; 68Gallium-SSTR-PET/CT - 68Gallium- somatostatin receptor positron emission tomography/computed tomography; FDG-PET – 18F-fluoro-2-deoxyglucose positron emission tomography
*see text for details

TABLE 15.3
Drugs that Interfere With the Screening Tests for Cushing Syndrome.

DRUGS THAT DECREASE DEXAMETHASONE METABOLISM BY INHIBITING CYP3A4

Itraconazole
Ritonavir
Fluoxetine
Diltiazem
Cimetidine
Aprepitant/fosaprepitant

DRUGS THAT INCREASE DEXAMETHASONE METABOLISM BY INDUCING CYP3A4

Phenobarbital
phenytoin
carbamazepine
primidone
Rifampin
Topiramate
Nifedipine
Rifapentine
St. John's wort
Ethosuximide
Pioglitazone Bicalutamide Enzalutamide

DRUGS THAT INCREASE CBG

Estrogens
Mitotane

DRUGS THAT INCREASE UFC

Carbamazepine
Fenofibrate
Some synthetic glucocorticoids (hydrocortisone)
Drugs that inhibit 11β-hydroxysteroid dehydrogenase type 2 (e.g., licorice)

CBG, Cortisol-binding globulin; UFC, Urinary free cortisol.

Late-Night Salivary Cortisol

Measurement of salivary cortisol takes advantage of the fact that patients with CS lose the normal circadian cortisol secretion, which leads to inappropriate elevation of the late-night cortisol concentrations.[25] The sample is collected at home between 2300 and 2400 h, ideally on two separate evenings. Healthy individuals and patients with physiological cortisol excess usually have normal circadian cortisol secretion; therefore, LNSC can be used in conjunction with other first-line tests to establish the diagnosis of CS.[26–28] Overall, LNSC diagnoses CS with 92%−100% sensitivity and 93%−100% specificity.[27,29,30] The accuracy of LNSC is similar to that of UFC.[15] Advantages of LNSC is that salivary cortisol is a noninvasive easy to collect test, and patients can collect many samples over a period of time making it an attractive option for patients with suspected cyclical CS (Table 15.2).

Potential disadvantages of LNSC are that it is not always readily available outside of the United States and that the diagnostic performance depends on the method used to measure salivary cortisol. Normal reference ranges are assay-dependent, necessitating to be validated for each laboratory, thus comparing diagnostic accuracy of LNSC in different studies is challenging.[31–33]

False-positive results may be seen in individuals with physiological causes of cortisol excess,[34,35] in shift workers[36] in whom the circadian rhythm may be blunted, and with direct contamination from blood (gingivitis)[33,37] or hydrocortisone-containing oral gels.[38] Licorice or tobacco chewing can have a falsely elevated LNSC as both contain glycyrrhizic acid that deactivates 11β-hydroxysteroid dehydrogenase type 2.[39,40] The use of mass spectrometry instead of a radioimmunoassay technique was reported to increase the specificity of the LNSC[41].

Low-Dose Dexamethasone Suppression Tests

In normal subjects, the administration of a supraphysiological dose of a glucocorticoid results in suppression of ACTH, and in turn decreased endogenous cortisol secretion. In endogenous CS of any cause, a failure to suppress cortisol with administration of dexamethasone is indicative of a positive result.[42,43]

The two tests commonly used in clinical practice are the 1-mg overnight DST and the 2-day 2-mg DST. The 1-mg overnight DST consists of administration of 1 mg of dexamethasone at 11 p.m., followed by measurement of serum cortisol at 8 a.m. the next morning. In contrast, in the 2-day 2-mg DST, dexamethasone is administered at a dose of 0.5 mg every 6 h for eight doses, followed by measurement of serum cortisol during 2−6 h after the last dexamethasone dose. Cortisol of <1.8 mcg/dL (<50 nmol/L) is considered normal suppression in both tests[10]

The reported specificities for the 1-mg overnight DST and the 2-day 2-mg DST are 87.5% and 97%−100%, respectively,[42,44] whereas sensitivity for both tests varies between 98% and 100%. DST has several limitations. Dexamethasone absorption is variable and can be affected in individuals with hepatic or renal disease or in those who take medications that alter CYP3A4 activity and dexamethasone clearance (Table 15.3).[45] Therefore, measurement of dexamethasone concentrations, when available, may be needed to clarify otherwise confusing results caused by noncompliance and individual variability in dexamethasone metabolism and drug−drug interactions.[46] On the other hand, false-positive results are seen in pregnant women or those receiving oral estrogen treatment that increase CBG levels[47] (Tables 15.2 and 15.3). Free cortisol measurement may aid in diagnosis in these situations, but is not widely available.[48]

Diagnosis of Subtype of Cushing Syndrome

Once CS is confirmed with initial tests, the next step is to measure plasma ACTH to determine the cause of CS. In adrenal CS, plasma ACTH concentration is usually low (<10 pg/mL or <2.2 pmol/L), Fig. 15.1. Plasma ACTH concentration between 10 pg/mL and 20 pg/mL (2.2 pmol/L and 4.4 pmol/L, respectively) is equivocal, and could indicate an ACTH-dependent CS, especially in patients with moderate or severe CS.[49] Patients with mild adrenal CS may not have suppressed ACTH and demonstrate ACTH in this range. An inappropriately normal or elevated ACTH level (>20 pg/mL, 4.4 pmol/L) is consistent with an ACTH-dependent CS. Dehydroepiandrosterone sulfate measurement is helpful to distinguish between ACTH-dependent (normal to elevated) and ACTH-independent CS (low to undetectable in benign adrenal disease).[50] Corticotropin-releasing hormone (CRH) stimulation and high-dose dexamethasone suppression tests (8 mgDST) may further aid in diagnosis of adrenal versus ACTH-dependent forms of CS when ACTH concentrations are equivocal (10−20 pg/mL, 2.2−4.4 pmol/L)[2] Fig. 15.1.

ACTH-DEPENDENT CUSHING SYNDROME

Epidemiology and Clinical Presentation

After exclusion of iatrogenic causes, CD is the most common cause of CS accounting for 60% of cases with a female preponderance (female:male ratio of 3−15:1).[1,4] Incidence rates of CD differ by region studied and the year the study was undertaken likely due to differing diagnostic accuracies and thresholds. Higher rates were reported in the United States compared with Spain and Denmark (8 cases per million vs. 2.4 cases per million vs. 1.2−1.7 cases per million).[1,3,4]

Ectopic ACTH syndrome (EAS) accounts for 10% of all causes of CS[1] with the most common etiology being a bronchial carcinoid tumor (25%−38%).[51−53] Reported female to male ratios vary between 1 and 1.5:1 with the mean age at presentation 35−60 years.[51−53] EAS has been traditionally described in the setting of small cell lung cancer (SCLC) at which time it represents paraneoplastic progression of the tumor.[54] This often portends poor prognosis with goals of treatment focused on palliation rather than curative intent.

A very rare entity is ectopic CRH syndrome (<1%). These tumors can secrete purely CRH[55] or cosecrete CRH and ACTH.[56]

EAS is more likely to have a rapid and dramatic presentation (e.g., in SCLC); however, bronchial carcinoids can have a more indolent, progressive course similar to CD.[54]

Diagnostic Testing

Once hypercortisolism is established (see first-line tests earlier), the next step is to determine the source. An inappropriately normal or elevated ACTH concentration confirms ACTH-dependent CS (Fig. 15.1). Generally, ACTH concentrations and the degree of hypercortisolism are significantly higher in EAS compared to CD, however there is overlap. Once ACTH-dependent CS is established, the next step is to determine whether hypercortisolism is due to CD or EAS. Diagnostic tests used to differentiate these two entities are described later.

High-Dose Dexamethasone Suppression Tests

This test is based on the assumption that ACTH secretion due to a pituitary adenoma demonstrates negative feedback with high-dose dexamethasone (8 mg/day for 48 h or 8 mg overnight) and that nonpituitary tumors do not.[57,58] A morning cortisol concentration after the 8 mgDST of less than 5 mcg/dL (140 nmol/L) indicates a pituitary source. The caveat to this, however, is EAS due to bronchial carcinoid tumors may demonstrate similar ACTH suppression as found in CD.[59] Due to a specificity of less than 100% and a sensitivity lower that the pretest probability for CD, the 8mgDST is no longer recommended to be used alone.[60] In addition, in ectopic CRH syndrome, pituitary ACTH can also be suppressed by dexamethasone.[55,56,61]

Corticotropin-Releasing Hormone Stimulation Test

The basis of this test is that ACTH-secreting pituitary tumors generally respond to corticotropin-releasing hormone (CRH), whereas ectopic ACTH-secreting tumors do not. CRH is expensive and not widely available at most centers. In addition, response to CRH is dependent on the type of CRH injected (ovine vs. human). Human CRH has a higher metabolic clearance rate compared with ovine CRH resulting in a longer duration of action in the latter.[62]

The test is performed after 4-h fasting. CRH is injected at a dose of 1 mcg/kg body weight (maximum 100 mcg) as an intravenous bolus. Blood samples are drawn for ACTH and cortisol at time points −15, 0, 5, 10, 15, 30, 45, 60, 90, and 120 min in relation to administration of CRH. Compared with human CRH, ovine CRH has superior diagnostic accuracy based on cortisol response but is similar with respect to ACTH response.[63] Using ovine CRH, a ≥35%−50% increase in ACTH concentrations had a sensitivity of 86%−93% and a specificity of 90%−100%[64,65] to diagnose CD, while a ≥20% increase in cortisol had a sensitivity of 91%[64] to diagnose CD.

If CRH is combined with desmopressin, the ACTH response is exaggerated with a 218%−350% increase in ACTH concentrations in CD compared with EAS.[66,67] Despite this, diagnostic accuracy still does not reach 100%, as 8% of patients with CD do not exhibit a significant increase in ACTH in response to CRH.[65] Moreover, an ACTH response can be occasionally detected in EAS.[65]

Pituitary Magnetic Resonance Imaging

In the setting of biochemically proven ACTH-dependent CS, it is reasonable to proceed with pituitary magnetic resonance imaging (MRI) given the high probability of CD (80%), Fig. 15.1.[68] In CD, up to 50% of pituitary tumors are <5 mm in size[68] with standard pituitary MRI failing to detect an adenoma in up to 40% of cases.[69] Conversely, pituitary incidentalomas can occur in up to 10% of healthy individuals[70] and in up to 23% of EAS cases.[71]

The standard protocol for pituitary MRI includes coronal T1 spin echo sequences with 2−3 mm slices before and after gadolinium intravenous contrast administration with dynamic imaging. This technique increases the sensitivity to detect pituitary microadenomas (67% with dynamic imaging vs. 52% without dynamic imaging) at the downfall of lower specificity (80% vs. 100%).[72]

Advancement in imaging technology may lead to improvement in imaging diagnostic accuracy in CD. The 7.0 T MRI was able to detect three out of five microadenomas in CD when the 1.5 T MRI failed to do so.[73] The combination of methionine-PET (positron emission tomography) with 3.0 T MRI increases diagnostic accuracy to 100%.[74] The addition of the 3D volumetric interpolated breath-hold examination, a spoiled-gradient echo 3D T1 sequence, to dynamic MRI was able to detect three additional adenomas that increased sensitivity to 54% from 47% with dynamic imaging only.[75]

Inferior Petrosal Sinus Sampling

The pituitary gland is drained by the cavernous sinus that flows into the petrosal venous sinus. Under fluoroscopic guidance, catheters are inserted into either the femoral or jugular veins (both right and left) and advanced into the inferior petrosal sinuses bilaterally. The position of the catheters is confirmed radiologically with contrast. Samples are drawn simultaneously from both inferior petrosal sinuses and peripheral veins for ACTH at time intervals −5, 0, 5, 10, and 15 min with time 0 signifying the time at administration of a 100 µg bolus of CRH.[76]

A central to peripheral ACTH ratio of ≥3.0 after CRH stimulation is diagnostic for CD with both sensitivity and specificity as high as 100%. A ratio of ≥2.0 has been used without CRH stimulation however, sensitivity is lower.[76] An ACTH concentration lateralization ratio of ≥1.4 between the two inferior petrosal sinuses accurately predicted the location in 68% of cases.[77] Lower sensitivities and specificities have been reported in more recent reports due to differing protocols, lack of CRH stimulation, use of ovine versus human CRH, use of desmopressin stimulation with CRH, and varying technical expertise.[78–82]

False-positive results are rare but have been reported in EAS.[53,83] False-negative results occur in 0.8%−11% of cases,[79,84] and are more commonly due to incorrect catheter placement or anomalous venous drainage. It has been suggested that low ACTH concentrations (<400 pg/mL) after CRH stimulation should raise suspicion for a false-negative study.[85] This, however, has not been investigated in other centers. Simultaneous measurement of prolactin allows normalization of petrosal to peripheral ACTH ratios to petrosal to peripheral prolactin ratios. Much like measuring cortisol in adrenal vein sampling for aldosterone-producing adrenal adenomas, prolactin is used to validate accurate placement and increase diagnostic accuracy when the ACTH gradient does not meet diagnostic criteria. The cut-off for a prolactin-normalized ACTH petrosal-to-peripheral ratio however has not been standardized.[86–89]

Inferior petrosal sinus sampling (IPSS) is an invasive procedure and therefore carries risk of complications. Reported complications include groin hematoma (4%),[90] cerebrovascular accident/brain stem injury (1/508),[91] transient cranial nerve palsy (1/166),[92] subarachnoid hemorrhage (1/94),[93] deep vein thrombosis (2/34),[94] and pulmonary embolism (1/34).[94]

Jugular Vein Sampling

Jugular vein sampling is less invasive than IPSS and has been suggested as an alternative to IPSS when expertise for IPSS is not available. Catheters are placed in the internal jugular veins and positioned at the angle of the mandible where the inferior petrosal sinus drains and mixes with the internal jugular effluent. Samples are drawn for ACTH measurement at time points −5, 0, 3, 5, and 10 min in relation to CRH administration as with IPSS. A central to peripheral ratio is then calculated to determine the presence of CD. Reported sensitivities for jugular vein sampling in diagnosing CD range from 80% to 83%.[95–97] Although these are lower than IPSS, jugular vein sampling can improve diagnostic accuracy in ACTH-dependent CS when IPSS is not available.

Diagnostic Imaging in EAS

A standardized imaging protocol has not been agreed upon for tumor localization in EAS. Nuclear imaging increases the sensitivity when added to conventional radiology. Indeed, tumor localization can prove to be difficult with no tumor being identified in 9%−27% of patients with biochemical EAS during long term follow-up.[51–53] Given 55% of tumors are located in the lung,[98] the logical first step would be CT chest (overall sensitivity 53%−66%; sensitivity for lung tumor 79.4%).[98,99] Small bronchial carcinoids, however, can be missed. In a systematic review including 231 patients, after CT chest, [68]Gallium-SSTR-PET/CT ([68]Gallium-somatostatin receptor positron emission tomography/computed tomography including the use of DOTATATE, DOTATOC, or DOTANOC) had the highest sensitivity for tumor localization in the lung (overall 81.8%; lung 77.8%) followed by [8]F-fluorodopa (F-DOPA)-PET (overall 57.1%, lung 71.4%), and then MRI (overall 51.5%, lung 66.7%).[98]

After lung, the most common sites are mediastinum, pancreas, adrenal glands, and gastrointestinal tract, in order of decreasing frequency. For mediastinal/thymic tumors, scintigraphy utilizing 111-In-octreotide or one of its analogues (octreotide scan) would be the best modality (sensitivity 85.7%).[98] For pancreatic and gastrointestinal lesions both ^{18}F-fluoro-2-deoxyglucose (FDG)-PET and [68]Gallium-SSTR-PET/CT had 100% sensitivities for tumor localization.[98] Adrenal gland tumors were localized with 100% sensitivity using CT abdomen, MRI abdomen, FDG-PET, or F-DOPA-PET.[98] The accuracy of octreotide scanning in nonmediastinal tumors is inconsistent likely due to variable somatostatin receptor expression on tumors.[99,100]

Treatment of ACTH-Dependent Cushing Syndrome

Urgency and type of treatment should be dictated by the type of disease (CD vs. EAS), degree of cortisol excess, possibility of surgical cure, and local expertise/availability of treatment options.

FIRST-LINE THERAPIES
Transphenoidal Selective Adenomectomy

Endoscopic transphenoidal selective adenomectomy (TSS) is the first-line treatment for CD.[101] Remission has been defined as a postoperative morning serum cortisol <5 µg/dL (<138 nmol/L) or 24-h urinary free cortisol <56 nmol/day (<20 µg/day) within the first week of resection.[101] In the hands of a high volume surgeon, remission rates of 73%–76% for microadenomas and 43% for macroadenomas have been reported.[102–104] With IPSS-directed hemihypophysectomy, remission was achieved in only 56%–69% of cases.[85,105] In mild CD or cyclic CD, midnight salivary cortisol more accurately detects remission or persistent disease.[103]

Postoperative hypopituitarism including diabetes insipidus (DI) is more frequent in CD compared to other functioning adenomas likely due to the need for more aggressive surgery. In the immediate postoperative period, serum sodium should be monitored due to the possibility of both transient syndrome of inappropriate antidiuretic hormone secretion (SIADH) and transient DI (triphasic response). Free thyroxine levels should be checked 1–2 weeks after surgery and replaced if low.[101]

Other possible postoperative complications are rare (<5%) and include epistaxis, mucocele, aseptic meningitis, permanent DI (more likely in repeat TSS), and carotid artery injury.[106]

Recurrence in CD is high, ranging from 15% to 66% and is dependent on the adenoma size (macroadenomas are more likely to recur), age at diagnosis, postoperative cortisol (>3 µg/dL, more likely to recur), early recovery of the hypothalamic–pituitary axis (<6 months), surgical expertise, and underlying adenoma molecular alterations (e.g., *USP8* mutation more likely to recur).[102,104,107–109] Midnight salivary cortisol is the first detectable abnormal test to document recurrence. Screening for recurrence should occur once there is recovery from postoperative adrenal insufficiency and annually thereafter.[101] Once recurrence is documented, repeat TSS (if there is incomplete resection with persistent tumor noted on imaging), radiation, medical therapy, or bilateral adrenalectomy can be employed.

EAS Tumor Resection

Once a single primary tumor has been localized, radical resection results in 83% cure rate in EAS.[51] Overall cure rates, however, are lower (30%–47%)[51,53] and multiple surgical excisions are often required. In the setting of metastases or inability to localize the tumor, medical therapy to reduce cortisol production or bilateral adrenalectomy are the treatment options.

SECOND-LINE THERAPIES
Medical Treatment

Medical treatment can be divided into steroidogenesis inhibitors, pituitary directed or glucocorticoid receptor antagonists.[101] Steroidogenesis inhibitors include ketoconazole (oral, quick onset of action with multiple daily dosing),[110] metyrapone (oral, quick onset of action, multiple daily dosing),[111] mitotane (oral, slow onset of action, once to twice daily dosing),[112] and etomidate (intravenous, quick onset of action, requires intensive care unit monitoring).[113] Pituitary-directed therapies include cabergoline (oral, twice weekly dosing)[114] and pasireotide (subcutaneous injection, twice daily dosing).[115] Monitoring on medical therapy includes clinical response and measuring UFC and morning cortisol, in most cases. There is an increased risk of adrenal insufficiency and steroid replacement may be necessary especially in the setting of acute physical stress.[112]

Ketoconazole

Ketoconazole, an imidazole derivative with antifungal activity, is commonly the first choice of medical therapy for cortisol excess in the United States, Table 15.4. It impairs adrenal and gonadal steroidogenesis by inhibiting side-chain cleavage, 17,20-lyase, and 11-β-hydroxylase enzymes.[110] Ketoconazole has a rapid onset of

TABLE 15.4
Medical Therapy for Adrenal Cushing's Syndrome.

Drug	Dose	Efficacy	Advantages	Disadvantages
Ketoconazole	400–1600 mg/d; every 6–8 h dosing; requires acid for biological activity	∼70% (25%–93% in individual studies)	Fast onset of action	Gastrointestinal side effects, hepatotoxicity, male hypogonadism, gynecomastia, drug–drug interactions
Metyrapone	500 mg/d to 6 g/day; every 6–8 h dosing	50%–75%	Fast onset of action	Gastrointestinal side effects, hirsutism, hypertension, hypokalemia; accessibility variable across countries
Mitotane	Starting dose, 250 mg; 500 mg to 8 g/day	72%–82% of patients while awaiting the effects of radiation therapy or when surgery was not possible	Adrenolytic, approved for adrenal cancer	Slow onset of action; lipophilic/long half-life, teratogenic; gastrointestinal side effects, gynecomastia, hepatotoxicity, adrenal insufficiency, dyslipidemia, low free thyroxine, drug–drug interactions
Etomidate	Bolus and titrate, 0.1–0.3 mg/kg/h intravenously		Intravenous, quick onset of action	Requires monitoring in ICU, gastrointestinal side effects, myoclonus, pain at injection site
Mifepristone	300–1200 mg/d	38% and 60% of patients with improvement in hypertension and/or diabetes, respectively		Difficult to titrate (no biomarker), adrenal insufficiency, endometrial hyperplasia, edema, abortifacient, fatigue, nausea, vomiting, arthralgias, headache, hypertension, hypokalemia

action within 24—48 h, which can be monitored by measuring serum cortisol or UFC. Ketoconazole is usually initiated at a dose of 200 mg two or three times daily and is increased promptly to 400 mg three times daily. Higher doses are infrequently more effective. Proton pump inhibitors may reduce the bioavailability of ketoconazole by 50% and therefore should be discontinued or avoided.[116] A summary of available data from case series, ketoconazole monotherapy (daily doses of 400—1200 mg) restored normal UFC in 57 of 82 patients with CS at a rate of 25%—93% in individual studies, regardless of the dose or duration of treatment.[117–119] Ketoconazole is relatively safe, except for its potential to induce hepatotoxicity, which can affect 1 in 15,000 exposed individuals.[120] Thus, monitoring liver enzymes is recommended at the initiation of therapy or at the dose increase. If liver enzymes increase by more than three times the upper limit of normal, the medication should be either reduced or discontinued.

Metyrapone

Metyrapone is an inhibitor of 11-β hydroxylase, which in turn blocks conversion of 11-deoxycortisol to cortisol, Table 15.4. Starting dose is 250 mg two or three times a day. The dose can be increased rapidly to a maximum of 6 g/day, based on serum cortisol or UFC values.[116] The goal of treatment is either normalization of UFC or mean serum cortisol concentration between 5.4 and 10.8 mcg/dL (150—300 nmol/L) throughout the day.[101] Near-maximal responses are commonly seen at a dose of 2 g/day in most patients. Metarypone achieves eucortisolemia in 50%—75% of patients with CS.[111,121] Although none of the medical therapies are approved for use in pregnancy, metyrapone was not associated with apparent adverse effects to mother or offspring when given in pregnant women with CS.[122] Metyrapone side effects are mostly gastrointestinal but can be alleviated by taking the drug with food or milk. With long-term use, metyrapone can worsen hirsutism and acne pertaining to the accumulation of androgen precursors. Additionally, blockade of cortisol synthesis can lead to accumulation of mineralocorticoid precursors, which in turn can lead to hypokalemia, hypertension, and edema.

Mitotane

Mitotane is a highly effective adjunctive therapy in the long-term management of CS, Table 15.4. It can be added to ketoconazole or metyrapone as a second/third agent but its onset of action is slow and can take several months to normalize UFC.[112] It is primarily used for treatment of adrenal carcinoma and can also be used to achieve medical adrenalectomy in patients with CS by inhibiting CYP11A1 (P450 side-chain cleavage) and direct cytotoxic action on the adrenal cortex.[112] Mitotane should be initiated at a dose of 0.5 g at bedtime, with slow dose increase as tolerated by 0.5 g/week taken with fatty food, to reach a maximum dose of 2—3 g/day. The median dose and concentration of mitotane required to control hypercortisolism in CD was 2.7 g/day and 8.5 mg/L, respectively.[112] Mitotane has a long half-life and gets stored in adipose tissue, thus maintaining sustained effects. In patients with pituitary CD after unsuccessful transsphenoidal surgery, mitotane led to normalization of cortisol in 72%—82% of patients while awaiting the effects of radiation therapy or when surgery was not possible.[112]

Etomidate

Similar to ketoconazole, etomidate is a member of the imidazole family that inhibits 11-β hydroxylation of deoxycortisol to produce cortisol, Table 15.4. It is an anesthetic drug that has been proposed as a fast-acting anticortisol agent, which can be useful in an emergency setting with acute life-threatening symptoms such as respiratory failure or severe psychosis.[123,124] It can be also used as a bridge to other medical or surgical therapies in hospitalized patients. In a summary of available data, etomidate was effective and safe for rapid control of hypercortisolemia in patients requiring parenteral therapy who cannot take oral medications or who are not immediate surgical candidates, with cortisol levels falling within 12—24 h.[125] Etomidate is administered intravenously with a loading dose of 3—5 mg, followed by continuous infusion of 0.03—0.10 mg/kg/h (2.5—3.0 mg/h), with dose adjustment based on serum cortisol concentration. Although sedation has not been reported at these doses, the dose should be reduced in patients with renal failure due to potential drug hypofiltration.[101]

Etomidate requires a multidisciplinary approach and an intensive care for close patient monitoring and frequent cortisol measurements (every 4—6 h) to achieve either complete or partial blockade and to prevent adrenal insufficiency. The target serum cortisol based on mean 24-h cortisol levels in patients in an intensive care setting is 10—20 mcg/dL (280—560 nmol/L).[101] If "block and replace" complete cortisol blockade method is elected, intravenous hydrocortisone at a dose of 0.5—1 mg/h is required.[36]

Mifepristone

Mifepristone (oral, once daily dosing) is the only currently available drug falling under the glucocorticoid receptor antagonist category, Table 15.4.[126] Mifepristone is a glucocorticoid (and progestin) antagonist, which is approved in the United States for treatment of glucose intolerance in patients with CS with nonresectable tumors or who are not surgical candidates.[126] Mifeprisone has high clinical efficacy in patients with CS and can also be used in severe CS. Because of its rapid onset of action and potent glucocorticoid receptor inhibition, mifepristone can be useful in life-threatening hypercortisolism though data are lacking. In one study of 34 patients, mifepristone (administered at doses of 300–1200 mg daily) resulted in improvement in hypertension, diabetes, and overall clinical status.[126] Mifepristone is difficult to monitor directly because of the persistently elevated urinary free cortisol excretion during treatment. Monitoring requires resolution of clinical symptoms of CS (glucose control, weight loss and blood pressure improvement). Given that it is an antagonist, ACTH levels usually rise and cortisol concentrations are either normal or increased. It should be started at a dose 300 mg/day and titrated slowly based on secondary clinical parameters, primarily glucose and weight reduction. Common adverse events include symptoms of adrenal insufficiency, increased mineralocorticoid, and antiprogestin action such as fatigue, nausea, headache, arthralgia, vomiting, hypokalemia, edema, and endometrial thickening in women.[126] It is an abortifacient and therefore contraception is required with its use. Hypoadrenalism can also occur; therefore, steroid replacement may be necessary. Suspected adrenal insufficiency can be treated with drug discontinuation or dexamethasone 2–8 mg/day.[126]

Combination therapy

If medical monotherapy is ineffective in controlling hypercortisolism or when immediate treatment of severe SC is not feasible, combination therapy can be considered as an alternative to emergent bilateral adrenalectomy. Combination therapy may also be useful during palliative care of patients with diffuse disease. Using a combination of medical therapy allows the drugs to work synergistically at the lower starting doses, thus optimizing therapeutic benefits while lowering the incidence of side effects.

Other therapy

As some pituitary and ectopic ACTH-producing tumors express somatostatin receptors (somatostatin type 2 and dopamine 2 receptors), several reports reported therapy with octreotide, pasireotide, and cabergoline in CD and EAS.[127]

Radiation

Pituitary radiation can be a first-line option if the patient is not a surgical candidate or if the tumor is not amenable to resection. It is recommended, however, as second-line therapy in most cases if surgery fails. The onset of therapeutic action is months to years; therefore, medical management should be initiation first and once cortisol concentrations are controlled, radiation can then be administered. Radiation is recommended especially in situations when the pituitary tumor is invasive or atypical with aggressive histopathology. Conventional radiation induces remission in 83% of patients within 2 years.[128] Stereotactic radiosurgery results in 80% cumulative control at 10 years.[129] Hypopituitarism can occur in up to 25% of cases.[129]

Bilateral Adrenalectomy

If TSS is not successful and CD is severe, or, in EAS with rapid onset and severity, bilateral adrenalectomy can be lifesaving. It results in immediate cure of the hypercortisolism state but requires glucocorticoid and mineralocorticoid replacement, and monitoring for Nelson's syndrome in the case of CD, and occult tumor growth in EAS.[130,131] Rarely, hypercortisolism can recur due to stimulation of cortisol-producing cells left in the surgical bed or present in the gonads.[101]

ACTH-INDEPENDENT CUSHING SYNDROME

Epidemiology

ACTH-independent CS represents around 20%–30% of endogenous CS cases and is caused by primary adrenal disorders, of which at least 90% are due to unilateral adrenal tumors (Table 15.5).[1] Rare adrenal causes of CS include bilateral macronodular adrenal hyperplasia (BMAH), primary pigmented nodular adrenocortical disease (PPNAD) (sporadic or as part of Carney's complex), its nonpigmented variant, isolated micronodular adrenocortical disease, and McCune–Albright syndrome. Overall, the causes of endogenous CS in children and adolescents are similar to those in adults, albeit with some variations. In infancy, CS is usually associated with McCune–Albright syndrome, while in children less than 5–7 years of age, adrenocortical tumors are the most common cause, and CD is the commonest cause beyond 7 years of age, while ectopic CS is extremely rare in the pediatric population.[132]

TABLE 15.5
Etiology of ACTH-independent Cushing's Syndrome.

Etiology	Proportion	Age	Female:male	Features
Adrenal adenoma (unilateral or bilateral)	80%–90%	4th–5th decades	4–8:1	Most pure cortisol secretion
Adrenal carcinoma (unilateral)	5%–7%	1st, 5th–6th decades	1.5–3:1	Commonly cortisol and androgen cosecretion
Bilateral macronodular adrenal hyperplasia • aberrant G-protein-coupled receptors • autocrine and paracrine ACTH production • sporadic or familial (*ARMC5*)	<2%	5th–6th decades	2–3:1	Modest cortisol secretion compared with size; raised steroid precursors; might have combined androgen and mineralocorticoid cosecretion
Bilateral micronodular adrenal hyperplasia • primary pigmented nodular adrenocortical disease • isolated or familial with Carney complex • isolated micronodular adrenocortical disease • primary bimorphic adrenocortical disease	Rare	1st–3rd decades	0.5:1 < 12 years 2:1 > 12 years	Adrenal size often normal Paradoxical increase of urine free cortisol with Liddle's oral dexamethasone suppression test Nonpigmented adrenal micronodules
McCune–Albright syndrome	Rare	Infants (<6 months)	1:1	Internodular adrenal atrophy

ACTH, adrenocorticotropic hormone; *ARMC5*, armadillo repeat containing five.

Increased use of CT and MRI led to an increasing number of incidentally discovered adrenal masses without associated symptomatic disease (incidentalomas). The prevalence of adrenal masses discovered on radiographic studies is 1.3%–8.7% among adults, with prevalence up to 10% with increasing age. Albeit mild, clinically important CS has been reported in 5%–10% of these patients.[133]

The incidence of CS is dependent on gender and age. Women are approximately three times more likely than men to develop either benign or malignant adrenal tumors, and approximately four to five times more likely to have CS associated with an adrenal tumor.[134] After puberty, PPNAD is more common among females than males.[135]

Adrenal tumors have a bimodal distribution by age, with small peak at approximately 50 years for adenomas and 40 years for carcinomas.[134,136,137] Adrenal carcinoma is the cause of one-half of all cases of childhood CS, and adenomas account for another one-sixth.[134,138] CS due to PPNAD manifests at a young age, typically before 30 years old and before 15 years old in 50% of cases.[139]

Cortisol-Secreting Adrenal Cortical Adenoma

Adrenal adenomas have been linked to mutations or activation of the cAMP-dependent pathway, including ACTH-receptor (*MC2R* gene), *PRKAR1A* and *PDE11A*.[140] Somatic-activating mutations of *GNAS* (encoding Gsα) are reported in 5%–17% of cortisol-secreting adenomas and β-catenin gene (*CTNNB1*) mutations in 16%–20% of sporadic cortisol-secreting adenomas.[141,142] Somatic *PRKAR1A* mutations are present in 20% of adrenal adenomas and deletions at *PRKAR1A* locus in 23% of adenomas.[143] Somatic mutations in the gene encoding the catalytic subunit of protein kinase A (*PRKACA*) were identified in 35%–65% of adrenal adenomas with overt Cushing's syndrome.[144] Defects in the phosphodiesterase 11A (*PDE11A*) or phosphodiesterase 8B (*PDE8B*) genes can lead to adrenocortical tumorigenesis, including adrenal adenomas, carcinomas, and bilateral macronodular adrenal hyperplasia.[145,146] Although more common in bilateral adrenal macronodular hyperplasia, cortisol secretion in adrenal adenomas can be regulated by hormones other than ACTH via aberrant expression and function of various membrane-bound hormone G-protein-coupled receptors.[147]

Bilateral Macronodular Adrenal Hyperplasia

BMAH is characterized by multiple bilateral adrenal nodules with diameter $\geq$1 cm. BMAH ultimately affects both adrenal glands, although it may initially present as a unilateral nodule.[148] Familial forms of BMAH appear to have autosomal dominant transmission. Inactivating mutations of armadillo repeat containing five genes (*ARMC5*) were identified in large families with BMAH and in up to 50% of patients with apparently sporadic BMAH. Similarly, nearly half of first-degree relatives of patients with apparently sporadic cases of CS carried the same *ARMC5* mutation and had autonomous cortisol secretion.[149] In addition to somatic *ARMC5* mutations, BMAH is occasionally associated with multiple endocrine neoplasia type 1, familial adenomatous polyposis, and fumarate hydratase gene mutations.[150]

Primary Pigmented Nodular Adrenal Disease

PPNAD is a micronodular bilateral adrenal disease that represents a rare cause of CS. Most cases of PPNAD are associated with Carney complex. Carney complex is inherited as an autosomal dominant condition, which can manifest with a variety of other abnormalities, including cardiac myxomas, myxomatous masses of skin or breast, blue nevi or lentigines, Other endocrinopathies associated with Carney complex include precocious puberty, Sertoli or Leydig cell tumors, adrenal rest tumors, acromegaly ($\sim$10%) and CS ($\sim$30%). Approximately half of the patients with Carney complex have a mutation in the tumor suppressor gene *PRKAR1A*, encoding for the type 1A regulatory subunit of protein kinase A. Mutations in this gene and also in the phosphodiesterase 11A (*PDE11A*) gene have been shown to be associated with an isolated distinct form of PPNAD.[151]

Adrenocortical Carcinoma

About 45%–70% of adrenocortical carcinomas are associated with autonomous hormone production. Among hormone-secreting adrenocortical carcinomas, hypercortisolemia alone is present in 50%–80% of cases or with androgen excess in 25%.[152,153] The vast majority of adrenocortical carcinomas in adults appear to be sporadic. Occasionally, however, they occur as part of hereditary syndromes such as Li–Fraumeni syndrome, Lynch syndrome, Beckwith–Wiedemann syndrome, multiple endocrine neoplasia type 1, and

familial adenomatous polyposis.[154] Adrenal cortical carcinomas are usually large, heterogeneous tumors (usually > 6 cm). Although many are discovered based on symptoms of hormone excess and adrenal mass effect, almost half are discovered incidentally.[137]

Diagnosis

Once ACTH-independent cortisol excess is confirmed (Fig. 15.1), cross-sectional adrenal imaging should be obtained to identify the cause of CS. Noncontrast CT is an acceptable initial imaging modality, which is sufficiently reliable in ruling out adrenocortical cancer when the adrenal lesion is homogeneous and has low nonenhance CT density $\leq$10 HU. If adrenocortical carcinoma is suspected based on a suspicious imaging phenotype, large tumor size, androgen excess, acute onset of symptoms, or young age, additional imaging (such as 18F-fluorodeoxyglucose PET scan) might be indicated before adrenalectomy, particularly to evaluate for distant metastases.[153]

Some uncertainty exists on optimal diagnostic workup of patients with adrenal CS due to bilateral disease. Adrenal venous sampling (AVS) to identify the site with dominant cortisol secretion could be considered in patients with bilateral adenomas of similar size.[155,156] In one study of 10 patients with bilateral nodules and cortisol excess, AVS was successful in all cases to identify the source of cortisol excess and guide adrenalectomy.[155] In a more recent study of 32 patients with mild cortisol excess (14 patients with bilateral disease), AVS accurately diagnosed the source of cortisol excess, and imaging findings were not always concordant with AVS.[156]

In micronodular adrenal hyperplasia, adrenal glands are generally not enlarged and may appear normal on the cross-sectional imaging[151] Diagnostic workup in these situations should include evaluation for exogenous glucocorticoid use, evaluation for other features of Carney complex, and possibly genetic testing for *PRKAR1A* mutations.[135] A paradoxical rise in urinary free cortisol after dexamethasone administration (0.5 mg every 6 h for 2 days and 2 mg every 6 h for another 2 days) has been reported in PPNAD.[157]

TREATMENT OF ADRENAL CUSHING SYNDROME
Adrenalectomy

Minimally invasive laparoscopic transabdominal or retroperitoneal unilateral adrenalectomy is the standard of care for the removal of nonmalignant cortisol-secreting unilateral adrenal tumors.

Laparoscopic surgical techniques are safe, effective, and less expensive than open adrenalectomy. Other recent developments include robotic retroperitoneal adrenalectomy, single-incision laparoendoscopic surgery, and ambulatory adrenalectomy. Generally, open adrenalectomy is recommended if adrenocortical carcinoma is suspected, although for tumors <6 cm without evidence of local invasion laparoscopic approach is reasonable, provided sufficient experience of the surgeon.[158]

In patients with bilateral adrenal adenomas unequal in size, proceeding directly to unilateral adrenalectomy of the larger adrenal mass has been reported effective.[159] In patients with bilateral adrenal adenomas of equal size, AVS may indicate the dominant lesion guiding toward a curative unilateral adrenalectomy.[155,156]

In patients with BMAH (detected as bilateral macronodular adrenal disease on imaging), the mainstay of therapy used to be bilateral adrenalectomy. However, in patients with BMAH and mild CS, unilateral adrenalectomy of the larger adrenal gland has been reported to lead to long-term remission of cortisol excess, along with sustained improvement of several cardiovascular risk factors such as hypertension, DM2, and obesity.[160–162] Postoperative adrenal insufficiency is a common occurrence even in these cases, thus a careful postoperative evaluation of the HPA axis is needed. As BMAH is a progressive disease, contralateral cortisol secretion may eventually increase, which may necessitate a complete adrenalectomy.

In children with BMAH due to McCune–Albright syndrome, hypercortisolism can be severe and life threatening, and bilateral adrenalectomy is usually indicated.[163] In contrast, spontaneous remission with medical therapy has been reported, suggesting that medical treatment to control hypercortisolemia may be considered in milder cases.

In PPNAD, laparoscopic bilateral adrenalectomy is the definitive treatment of choice, which leads to remission of CS in most cases.[164] In some pediatric patients, unilateral adrenalectomy significantly reduced clinical and biochemical features of hypercortisolism, although a subsequent relapse has been reported requiring resection of the second gland.[165] In patients with suspected or confirmed PPNAD, it is important to screen for features of Carney complex, particularly for atrial myxoma.[164] Importantly, family members of patients with Carney complex should undergo appropriate testing.[101]

In rare cases, remnant adrenocortical tissue, either in the surgical bed or sometimes in the gonads, can lead to residual or recurrent cortisol secretion. If patients develop features of cortisol excess after bilateral adrenalectomy, endogenous cortisol secretion should be evaluated by withholding glucocorticoids for 24 h and testing for cortisol excess.

When adrenalectomy is indicated, it is important to plan appropriately for postoperative adrenal insufficiency, a consequence of chronic HPA axis suppression and atrophy of the contralateral normal adrenal gland. Glucocorticoid replacement therapy is indicated until the hypothalamic–pituitary–adrenal axis recovery is established.[166] Recovery of HPA axis after adrenalectomy has been reported to range between 2 months and several years.[166]

Medical Therapy

Medical therapy may be elected in select patients, particularly in patients with BMAH or PPNAD, in patients who are poor surgical candidates, and in patients with CS due to metastatic adrenal cortical carcinoma.[101] The choice of medical therapy should be guided by patient-related factors, efficacy, and cost. Combination medical therapy may be necessary in patients with moderate-to-severe hypercortisolism, in which case using a combination of medications at lower effective doses may be attempted to reduce medication-related adverse events (see Medical therapy section).

PROGNOSIS

Patients with CS present with high prevalence of obesity, hypertension, hyperglycemia, depression, and osteoporosis.[167] In addition, patients with CS demonstrate an increased cardiovascular risk and mortality, but also increased risk of infections and suicide.[168] Although remission is associated with significant improvement in quality of life and reduction in both morbidity and mortality, patients remain at higher risk of morbidity and mortality when compared to the general population.

Initial morbidity experienced postoperatively is hypoadrenalism during recovery of the HPA axis. Recovery can take up to 6–12 months (or longer) after resection.[169] Many patients suffer with glucocorticoid withdrawal symptoms including anorexia, nausea, fatigue, and myalgias.[166] There is also increased risk to develop/unmask or have worsening of underlying autoimmune diseases.[170]

With cure, patients demonstrate improvement in metabolic parameters including hypertension, obesity, and glycemic control; however, overall prevalence rates of these comorbidities continue to be higher than the general population (up to 25%).[171,172] Depression, anxiety, and cognitive impairment also continue to persist despite cure.[167] This leads to significant impairment in health-related quality of life.[173] On the other hand, osteoporosis significantly improves with evidence of normalization of bone mineral density within 2–5 years after remission.[101,174]

CYCLIC CUSHING SYNDROME

Cyclic CS is rare. It is characterized by intermittent episodes of cortisol excess interspersed by normalcy. It has been referred to as periodic, intermittent, or cyclic CS due to its episodic nature. Frequency of hypercortisolism phases can range from days to months.[21] Interestingly, in most cases of CS, there is day-to-day variation in cortisol production more so in CD as compared to EAS and adrenal CS.[175] In cyclic CS, however, the trough cortisol is normal. Suggested criteria for diagnosis has been three peak cortisol concentrations (abnormal high) and two trough concentrations (normal) in the setting of a high pretest probability for CS.[176] Its prevalence has been suggested to be as high as 15%.[177] Moreover, 54% of cases with cyclic CS are due to CD, 26% from EAS, and 11% from an adrenal tumor.[21] Confirmation of CS should rely on the midnight salivary cortisol or 24-h urine cortisol concentrations as the 1-mg overnight dexamethasone suppression test can often be inaccurate in cyclic CS.[176,178] Testing should be done when the pretest probability is highest, that is, when the patient is most symptomatic. Several tests and follow-up would be required to confirm the diagnosis.

PSEUDO-CUSHING SYNDROME

The term pseudo-Cushing syndrome is used to describe physiologic hypercortisolism (Table 15.6). This can be very difficult to differentiate from pathologic CS because of a significant overlap in clinical and biochemical features due to the shared etiology of HPA-axis stimulation. Some evidence also suggests that individuals with Pseudo-Cushing exhibit heightened sensitivity to glucocorticoid-negative feedback, which in turn leads to mild elevations in cortisol. Over time, longitudinal exposure to glucocorticoids results in similar clinical features.[179]

Some physiologic conditions are more likely to result in physical features of Cushing syndrome. This includes depression and other psychiatric conditions, alcohol dependence, obesity, poorly controlled type 2 diabetes, and stage 5 chronic kidney disease. Rarely, cases of glucocorticoid resistance may present with mineralocorticoid excess without features of cortisol excess (Table 15.6).

TABLE 15.6
Conditions Associated With Physiologic Hypercortisolism not Caused by Cushing Syndrome.

Pregnancy, usually in late second and third trimester
Severe obesity
Psychological stress
Psychiatric disorders
Physical stress (illness, hospitalization/surgery, pain)
Uncontrolled diabetes mellitus
Chronic alcoholism
Untreated sleep apnea
Malnutrition, anorexia nervosa
Intense chronic exercise
Hypothalamic amenorrhea
Glucocorticoid resistance

Alcohol-induced hypercortisolism is mediated through increased CRH secretion into the portal veins supplying the anterior pituitary gland and can biochemically mimic ACTH-dependent CD. Additionally, liver dysfunction can lead to decreased clearance of cortisol, leading to hypercortisolism. Typically, late-night salivary cortisol, overnight dexamethasone suppression testing, and urinary cortisol excretion are abnormal, although alcohol abstinence for 4 weeks has been reported to resolve these abnormalities.[180] In a small study comparing patients with Cushing disease with alcoholic patients, desmopressin administration resulted in abnormally elevated ACTH concentrations in the former, but not the latter.[181] However, this protocol is not widely used in clinical practice and is limited by the lack of normative data for ACTH and cortisol after desmopressin stimulation in normal nonobese subjects.[182,183] Ultimately, history and surrogate markers may be a better way to make the diagnosis of chronic alcoholism, while repeat testing after a period of abstinence may be a better differentiator between physiologic and pathologic hypercortisolism when alcohol is a confounder.

Several forms of depression or other neuropsychiatric disorders have been associated with hypercortisolism as a result of increased HPA axis activity and resistance to cortisol-negative feedback.[184] What makes this particularly difficult to differentiate from pathologic ACTH-dependent hypercortisolism is the high prevalence (about 65%) of neuropsychiatric illness in patients with pathologic CS.[49] The use of the dexamethasone-CRH test (see below) has been used by psychiatrists to monitor response to antidepressant therapy with the idea that persistent elevations in cortisol suggest inadequate treatment. Additionally, in a pooled cohort of patients with CS and pseudo-Cushing, the rate of false-positive testing after dexamethasone-CRH testing was reported as 8%–50%; and 8%–10% after desmopressin stimulation.[185] Thus, the dexamethasone-CRH test may not be useful to differentiate between physiologic and pathologic disease, and there are limitations to the desmopressin stimulation as outlined earlier. As with chronic alcoholism, improvements in the underlying mood disorder are associated with improvements in biochemical hypercortisolism[186] although in clinical practice this is not an easy assessment to make. Unfortunately, distinguishing between physiological and pathological hypercortisolism in this patient population remains one of the most diagnostically challenging clinical scenarios that an endocrinologist faces.

Obesity results in a clinical phenotype that overlaps significantly with hypercortisolism, both in terms of associated comorbidities and physical changes. There is a general consensus that patients with simple obesity have normal basal salivary, plasma, and urinary cortisol levels no matter their body fat distribution.[187,188] However, there may be subtle differences in the central and peripheral mechanisms involved in cortisol metabolism that may affect the interpretation of cortisol following dexamethasone suppression (Table 15.3). As with other conditions that can result in physiologic hypercortisolism, the clinical suspicion for pathological hypercortisolism should drive how extensively a diagnostic workup should be pursued.

Chronic kidney disease and uncontrolled type 2 diabetes mellitus may result in a physical phenotype that is suggestive of hypercortisolism. The mechanism for the increase in cortisol in both these conditions is activation of the HPA axis, as plasma ACTH is typically increased in these patients. As with other causes of physiologic hypercortisolism discussed earlier, there should be caution when interpreting subtle abnormalities in HPA-axis testing.

Glucocorticoid resistance is a rare, familial, receptor-mediated disorder that typically manifests with either signs of excess androgens or mineralocorticoids.[189,190] Patients may have elevated ACTH and cortisol levels but do not exhibit catabolic features of excess cortisol. Some patients may have bilateral adrenal enlargement. This condition should be suspected in patients with biochemical ACTH-dependent hypercortisolism, but no physical features consistent with cortisol excess.

Apart from the conditions discussed earlier, there are certain conditions associated with physiologic hypercortisolism that do not result in a clinical phenotype similar to CS. These include physical stress brought on by acute illness, pain or surgery, anorexia or starvation, pregnancy, and intense chronic exercise. Studies on amenorrheic women with anorexia nervosa show a negative association between serum concentrations of cortisol and degree of bone loss; however, it is unclear if cortisol excess is the cause or the consequence of the underlying psychiatric pathology.[191] Despite higher evening basal cortisol concentrations, highly trained runners have an attenuated cortisol response to exercise when compared to sedentary or moderately trained runners.[192]

In summary, making the diagnosis of physiologic hypercortisolism or pseudo-Cushing is particularly challenging because of the great overlap in clinical presentation and lack of definitive diagnostic testing to discriminate it from pathologic hypercortisolism. The history and physical examination still are the best tools for a clinician trying to make that distinction in a patient with multiple confounders. Repeat biochemical testing after several months is reasonable and most useful particularly when there is an expectation that the process that may be contributing to physiologic hypercortisolism may improve.

DIAGNOSTIC TESTS IN PSEUDO-CUSHING SYNDROME
Low-Dose Dexamethasone Suppression-CRH Stimulation Test
In an effort to distinguish patients with CD from those with pseudo-Cushing syndrome, Yanovski et al. developed the low-dose dexamethasone suppression-CRH stimulation test.[193]

Dexamethasone fails to suppress serum cortisol concentrations in individuals with CD as well as in a small number of patients with pseudo-Cushing syndrome. However, if given CRH, patients with pseudo-Cushing syndrome demonstrate a blunted serum cortisol in comparison to patients with CD. The test is performed by administering dexamethasone over 2 days (2 mg), followed by administration of CRH (1 g/kg, intravenous) 2 h after the last dose of dexamethasone; cortisol is then measured 15 min later.

The initial studies of this strategy reported high diagnostic accuracy.[21,194] A plasma cortisol concentration greater than 38 nmol/L (1.4 g/dL) measured 15 min after the administration of CRH correctly identified all cases of CD and all cases of pseudo-Cushing syndrome (100% specificity, sensitivity, and diagnostic accuracy).[193] Subsequent studies, however, reported a lower diagnostic accuracy.[195–197] Large variability in interpersonal metabolism of dexamethasone, differences in testing protocols, diagnostic thresholds, and cortisol assays used in each study most likely account for these noted differences.

Desmopressin Test

The desmopressin stimulation test involves measurement of plasma ACTH and cortisol at baseline and 10, 20, and 30 min after intravenous administration of 10-g 1-desamino-8-D-arginine vasopressin. The rationale behind this test is that desmopressin stimulates ACTH release in patients with CD but not in most normal individuals and those with pseudo-Cushing syndrome. Diagnostic accuracy of the test varies across different studies; the sensitivity to diagnose CD ranges from 63% to 75% and the specificity from 85% to 91%.[198–200]

In a study comparing the low-dose dexamethasone suppression-CRH stimulation test with the desmopressin test in patients with CD and pseudo-Cushing tests demonstrated sensitivities of 100% and 90% and specificities of 62.5% and 81.5, respectively.

Iatrogenic Cushing Syndrome

It is estimated that 1% of population uses exogenous glucocorticoids. Iatrogenic CS is caused by administration of synthetic glucocorticoids for a prolonged period of time and/or in excessive amounts. It is the most common cause of CS seen in clinical practice and therefore exclusion of iatrogenic CS is of great importance before entering the diagnostic cascade of testing for endogenous CS.

The most common cause of hypercortisolism is ingestion of prescribed oral steroid (such as prednisone or dexamethasone) for treatment of a nonendocrine disease. However, CS can also be caused by other injected, topical, and inhaled glucocorticoids,[201–203] and by megestrol acetate and other progestins with intrinsic glucocorticoid activity.[204] The clearance of some inhaled steroids may be delayed by ritonavir leading to CS.[205,206] Several over-the-counter herbal preparations have been implicated in the development of CS, likely due to contamination with steroids.

Development of CS features depends on the dose, duration, and potency of the corticosteroids use. Several clinical features are more commonly seen in iatrogenic rather than endogenous CS, such as increase in intraocular pressure, cataracts, benign intracranial hypertension, aseptic necrosis of the femoral head, osteoporosis, and pancreatitis.

Clinical evaluation, physical exam, and history or current synthetic glucocorticoid exposure are usually sufficient to make the diagnosis of iatrogenic CS. In rare situations when history of glucocorticoid exposure is unclear, patients with iatrogenic CS can demonstrate undetectable ACTH and low serum and urine cortisol concentrations.

Supraphysiological glucocorticoid use also suppresses HPA axis with ensuing adrenal atrophy (and consequent adrenal insufficiency), thus abrupt cessation of glucocorticoids should never be attempted, and a glucocorticoid taper with physiologic replacement is required until HPA axis recovers.[207]

CONCLUSION

In conclusion, CS presents with a spectrum of clinical manifestations ranging from metabolic abnormalities to classical features of CS. Clinical presentation depends on the severity and duration of cortisol excess, and individual susceptibility. CS presents with high morbidity and mortality, especially if unrecognized or diagnosis is delayed. After excluding iatrogenic CS through a careful history and exam, biochemical and imaging workup guide the most appropriate therapy. Postoperative adrenal insufficiency and glucocorticoid withdrawal syndrome should be appropriately treated with glucocorticoid supplementation therapy and monitoring.

REFERENCES

1. Lindholm J, et al. Incidence and late prognosis of cushing's syndrome: a population-based study. *J Clin Endocrinol Metab*. 2001;86(1):117–123.
2. Sharma ST, Nieman LK, Feelders RA. Cushing's syndrome: epidemiology and developments in disease management. *Clin Epidemiol*. 2015;7:281–293.
3. Broder MS, et al. Incidence of Cushing's syndrome and Cushing's disease in commercially-insured patients <65 years old in the United States. *Pituitary*. 2015;18(3):283–289.
4. Etxabe J, Vazquez JA. Morbidity and mortality in Cushing's disease: an epidemiological approach. *Clin Endocrinol*. 1994;40(4):479–484.
5. Leibowitz G, et al. Pre-clinical Cushing's syndrome: an unexpected frequent cause of poor glycaemic control in obese diabetic patients. *Clin Endocrinol*. 1996;44(6):717–722.
6. Terzolo M, et al. Screening of Cushing's syndrome in outpatients with type 2 diabetes: results of a prospective multicentric study in Italy. *J Clin Endocrinol Metab*. 2012;97(10):3467–3475.
7. Catargi B, et al. Occult Cushing's syndrome in type-2 diabetes. *J Clin Endocrinol Metab*. 2003;88(12):5808–5813.

8. Reimondo G, et al. Screening of Cushing's syndrome in adult patients with newly diagnosed diabetes mellitus. *Clin Endocrinol.* 2007;67(2):225–229.

9. Gagliardi L, et al. Screening for subclinical Cushing's syndrome in type 2 diabetes mellitus: low false-positive rates with nocturnal salivary cortisol. *Horm Metab Res.* 2010;42(4):280–284.

10. Nieman LK, et al. The diagnosis of cushing's syndrome: an endocrine society clinical practice guideline. *J Clin Endocrinol Metab.* 2008;93(5):1526–1540.

11. Tomlinson JW, et al. Absence of Cushingoid phenotype in a patient with Cushing's disease due to defective cortisone to cortisol conversion. *J Clin Endocrinol Metab.* 2002;87(1):57–62.

12. Mengden T, et al. Urinary free cortisol versus 17-hydroxycorticosteroids: a comparative study of their diagnostic value in Cushing's syndrome. *Clin Investig.* 1992;70(7):545–548.

13. Nieman LK. Diagnostic tests for Cushing's syndrome. *Ann N Y Acad Sci.* 2002;970:112–118.

14. Lin CL, et al. Urinary free cortisol and cortisone determined by high performance liquid chromatography in the diagnosis of Cushing's syndrome. *J Clin Endocrinol Metab.* 1997;82(1):151–155.

15. Elamin MB, et al. Accuracy of diagnostic tests for Cushing's syndrome: a systematic review and metaanalyses. *J Clin Endocrinol Metab.* 2008;93(5):1553–1562.

16. Cizza G, et al. Factitious cushing syndrome. *J Clin Endocrinol Metab.* 1996;81(10):3573–3577.

17. Carroll BJ, et al. Urinary free cortisol excretion in depression. *Psychol Med.* 1976;6(1):43–50.

18. Mericq MV, Cutler Jr GB. High fluid intake increases urine free cortisol excretion in normal subjects. *J Clin Endocrinol Metab.* 1998;83(2):682–684.

19. Findling JW, et al. Pseudohypercortisoluria: spurious elevation of urinary cortisol due to carbamazepine. *Endocrinololgist.* 1998;8(2):51–54.

20. Meikle AW, et al. Pseudo-Cushing syndrome caused by fenofibrate interference with urinary cortisol assayed by high-performance liquid chromatography. *J Clin Endocrinol Metab.* 2003;88(8):3521–3524.

21. Meinardi JR, Wolffenbuttel BH, Dullaart RP. Cyclic Cushing's syndrome: a clinical challenge. *Eur J Endocrinol.* 2007;157(3):245–254.

22. Leeflang MM, et al. Use of methodological search filters to identify diagnostic accuracy studies can lead to the omission of relevant studies. *J Clin Epidemiol.* 2006;59(3):234–240.

23. Montori VM, Guyatt GH. Summarizing studies of diagnostic test performance. *Clin Chem.* 2003;49(11):1783–1784.

24. Chan KC, et al. Diminished urinary free cortisol excretion in patients with moderate and severe renal impairment. *Clin Chem.* 2004;50(4):757–759.

25. Glass AR, et al. Circadian rhythm of serum cortisol in Cushing's disease. *J Clin Endocrinol Metab.* 1984;59(1):161–165.

26. Viardot A, et al. Reproducibility of nighttime salivary cortisol and its use in the diagnosis of hypercortisolism compared with urinary free cortisol and overnight dexamethasone suppression test. *J Clin Endocrinol Metab.* 2005;90(10):5730–5736.

27. Papanicolaou DA, et al. Nighttime salivary cortisol: a useful test for the diagnosis of Cushing's syndrome. *J Clin Endocrinol Metab.* 2002;87(10):4515–4521.

28. Putignano P, et al. Midnight salivary cortisol versus urinary free and midnight serum cortisol as screening tests for Cushing's syndrome. *J Clin Endocrinol Metab.* 2003;88(9):4153–4157.

29. Luthold WW, Marcondes JA, Wajchenberg BL. Salivary cortisol for the evaluation of Cushing's syndrome. *Clin Chim Acta.* 1985;151(1):33–39.

30. Laudat MH, et al. Salivary cortisol measurement: a practical approach to assess pituitary-adrenal function. *J Clin Endocrinol Metab.* 1988;66(2):343–348.

31. Raff H, Homar PJ, Burns EA. Comparison of two methods for measuring salivary cortisol. *Clin Chem.* 2002;48(1):207–208.

32. Trilck M, et al. Salivary cortisol measurement–a reliable method for the diagnosis of Cushing's syndrome. *Exp Clin Endocrinol Diabetes.* 2005;113(4):225–230.

33. Yaneva M, et al. Midnight salivary cortisol for the initial diagnosis of Cushing's syndrome of various causes. *J Clin Endocrinol Metab.* 2004;89(7):3345–3351.

34. Butler PW, Besser GM. Pituitary-adrenal function in severe depressive illness. *Lancet.* 1968;1(7554):1234–1236.

35. Liu H, et al. Elevated late-night salivary cortisol levels in elderly male type 2 diabetic veterans. *Clin Endocrinol.* 2005;63(6):642–649.

36. Ross RJ, et al. Levels of GH binding activity, IGFBP-1, insulin, blood glucose and cortisol in intensive care patients. *Clin Endocrinol.* 1991;35(4):361–367.

37. Raff H, Raff JL, Findling JW. Late-night salivary cortisol as a screening test for Cushing's syndrome. *J Clin Endocrinol Metab.* 1998;83(8):2681–2686.

38. Kivlighan KT, et al. Quantifying blood leakage into the oral mucosa and its effects on the measurement of cortisol, dehydroepiandrosterone, and testosterone in saliva. *Horm Behav.* 2004;46(1):39–46.

39. Smith RE, et al. Localization of 11 beta-hydroxysteroid dehydrogenase type II in human epithelial tissues. *J Clin Endocrinol Metab.* 1996;81(9):3244–3248.

40. Badrick E, Kirschbaum C, Kumari M. The relationship between smoking status and cortisol secretion. *J Clin Endocrinol Metab.* 2007;92(3):819–824.

41. Baid SK, et al. Radioimmunoassay and tandem mass spectrometry measurement of bedtime salivary cortisol levels: a comparison of assays to establish hypercortisolism. *J Clin Endocrinol Metab.* 2007;92(8):3102–3107.

42. Newell-Price J, et al. The diagnosis and differential diagnosis of Cushing's syndrome and pseudo-Cushing's states. *Endocr Rev.* 1998;19(5):647–672.

43. Crapo L. Cushing's syndrome: a review of diagnostic tests. *Metabolism.* 1979;28(9):955–977.

44. Wood PJ, et al. Evidence for the low dose dexamethasone suppression test to screen for Cushing's syndrome–recommendations for a protocol for biochemistry laboratories. *Ann Clin Biochem.* 1997;34(Pt 3):222–229.

45. Luo G, et al. CYP3A4 induction by xenobiotics: biochemistry, experimental methods and impact on drug discovery and development. *Curr Drug Metabol.* 2004;5(6):483–505.

46. Meikle AW. Dexamethasone suppression tests: usefulness of simultaneous measurement of plasma cortisol and dexamethasone. *Clin Endocrinol.* 1982;16(4):401–408.

47. Nickelsen T, Lissner W, Schoffling K. The dexamethasone suppression test and long-term contraceptive treatment: measurement of ACTH or salivary cortisol does not improve the reliability of the test. *Exp Clin Endocrinol.* 1989;94(3):275–280.

48. Bancos I, et al. Performance of free versus total cortisol following cosyntropin stimulation testing in an outpatient setting. *Endocr Pract.* 2015;21(12):1353–1363.

49. Lacroix A, et al. Cushing's syndrome. *Lancet.* 2015;386(9996):913–927.

50. Dennedy MC, et al. Low DHEAS: a sensitive and specific test for the detection of subclinical hypercortisolism in adrenal incidentalomas. *J Clin Endocrinol Metab.* 2017;102(3):786–792.

51. Isidori AM, et al. The ectopic adrenocorticotropin syndrome: clinical features, diagnosis, management, and long-term follow-up. *J Clin Endocrinol Metab.* 2006;91(2):371–377.

52. Aniszewski JP, et al. Cushing syndrome due to ectopic adrenocorticotropic hormone secretion. *World J Surg.* 2001;25(7):934–940.

53. Ilias I, et al. Cushing's syndrome due to ectopic corticotropin secretion: twenty years' experience at the National Institutes of Health. *J Clin Endocrinol Metab.* 2005;90(8):4955–4962.

54. Alexandraki KI, Grossman AB. The ectopic ACTH syndrome. *Rev Endocr Metab Disord.* 2010;11(2):117–126.

55. Carey RM, et al. Ectopic secretion of corticotropin-releasing factor as a cause of Cushing's syndrome. A clinical, morphologic, and biochemical study. *N Engl J Med.* 1984;311(1):13–20.

56. O'Brien T, et al. Cushing's syndrome associated with ectopic production of corticotrophin-releasing hormone, corticotrophin and vasopressin by a phaeochromocytoma. *Clin Endocrinol.* 1992;37(5):460–467.

57. Liddle GW. Tests of pituitary-adrenal suppressibility in the diagnosis of Cushing's syndrome. *J Clin Endocrinol Metab.* 1960;20:1539–1560.

58. Liddle GW, et al. Clinical and laboratory studies of ectopic humoral syndromes. *Recent Prog Horm Res.* 1969;25:283–314.

59. Malchoff CD, et al. Ectopic ACTH syndrome caused by a bronchial carcinoid tumor responsive to dexamethasone, metyrapone, and corticotropin-releasing factor. *Am J Med.* 1988;84(4):760–764.

60. Daniel E, Newell-Price JDC. Diagnosis of Cushing's disease. *Pituitary.* 2015;18(2):206–210.

61. Schteingart DE, et al. Cushing's syndrome secondary to ectopic corticotropin-releasing hormone-adrenocorticotropin secretion. *J Clin Endocrinol Metab.* 1986;63(3):770–775.

62. Schurmeyer TH, et al. Human corticotropin-releasing factor in man: pharmacokinetic properties and dose-response of plasma adrenocorticotropin and cortisol secretion. *J Clin Endocrinol Metab.* 1984;59(6):1103–1108.

63. Pecori Giraldi F, Invitti C, Cavagnini F. The corticotropin-releasing hormone test in the diagnosis of ACTH-dependent Cushing's syndrome: a reappraisal. *Clin Endocrinol.* 2001;54(5):601–607.

64. Nieman LK, et al. A simplified morning ovine corticotropin-releasing hormone stimulation test for the differential diagnosis of adrenocorticotropin-dependent Cushing's syndrome. *J Clin Endocrinol Metab.* 1993;77(5):1308–1312.

65. Reimondo G, et al. The corticotrophin-releasing hormone test is the most reliable noninvasive method to differentiate pituitary from ectopic ACTH secretion in Cushing's syndrome. *Clin Endocrinol.* 2003;58(6):718–724.

66. Tsagarakis S, et al. The desmopressin and combined CRH-desmopressin tests in the differential diagnosis of ACTH-dependent Cushing's syndrome: constraints imposed by the expression of V2 vasopressin receptors in tumors with ectopic ACTH secretion. *J Clin Endocrinol Metab.* 2002;87(4):1646–1653.

67. Newell-Price J, et al. A combined test using desmopressin and corticotropin-releasing hormone in the differential diagnosis of Cushing's syndrome. *J Clin Endocrinol Metab.* 1997;82(1):176–181.

68. Invitti C, et al. Diagnosis and management of cushing's syndrome: results of an Italian multicentre study. Study group of the Italian society of endocrinology on the pathophysiology of the hypothalamic-pituitary-adrenal Axis. *J Clin Endocrinol Metab.* 1999;84(2):440–448.

69. Chowdhury IN, et al. A change in pituitary magnetic resonance imaging protocol detects ACTH-secreting tumours in patients with previously negative results. *Clin Endocrinol.* 2010;72(4):502–506.

70. Hall WA, et al. Pituitary magnetic resonance imaging in normal human volunteers: occult adenomas in the general population. *Ann Intern Med.* 1994;120(10):817–820.

71. Yogi-Morren D, et al. Pituitary MRI findings in patients with pituitary and ectopic acth-dependent Cushing syndrome: Does a 6-mm pituitary tumor size cut-off value exclude ectopic acth syndrome? *Endocr Pract.* 2015;21(10):1098–1103.

72. Tabarin A, et al. Comparative evaluation of conventional and dynamic magnetic resonance imaging of the pituitary gland for the diagnosis of Cushing's disease. *Clin Endocrinol.* 1998;49(3):293–300.

73. de Rotte AA, et al. High resolution pituitary gland MRI at 7.0 tesla: a clinical evaluation in Cushing's disease. *Eur Radiol.* 2016;26(1):271–277.

74. Ikeda H, Abe T, Watanabe K. Usefulness of composite methionine-positron emission tomography/3.0-tesla magnetic resonance imaging to detect the localization and extent of early-stage Cushing adenoma. *J Neurosurg.* 2010;112(4):750–755.

75. Grober Y, et al. Comparison of MRI techniques for detecting microadenomas in Cushing's disease. *J Neurosurg.* 2018;128(4):1051–1057.

76. Kaltsas GA, et al. A critical analysis of the value of simultaneous inferior petrosal sinus sampling in Cushing's disease and the occult ectopic adrenocorticotropin syndrome. *J Clin Endocrinol Metab.* 1999;84(2):487–492.

77. Oldfield EH, et al. Petrosal sinus sampling with and without corticotropin-releasing hormone for the differential diagnosis of Cushing's syndrome. *N Engl J Med.* 1991;325(13):897–905.

78. Findling J, et al. Routine inferior petrosal sinus sampling in the differential diagnosis of adrenocorticotropin (ACTH)-dependent Cushing's syndrome: early recognition of the occult ectopic ACTH syndrome. *J Clin Endocrinol Metab.* 1991;73:408–413.

79. Swearingen B, et al. Diagnostic errors after inferior petrosal sinus sampling. *J Clin Endocrinol Metab.* 2004;89:3752–3763.

80. Colao A, et al. Inferior petrosal sinus sampling in the differential diagnosis of Cushing's syndrome: results of an Italian multicenter study. *Eur J Endocrinol.* 2001;144:499–507.

81. Tsagarakis S, et al. The application of the combined corticotropin-releasing hormone plus desmopressin stimulation during petrosal sinus sampling is both sensitive and specific in differentiating patients with Cushing's disease from patients with the occult ectopic adrenocorticotropin syndrome. *J Clin Endocrinol Metab.* 2007;92:2080–2086.

82. Machado M, et al. The role of desmopressin in bilateral and simultaneous inferior petrosal sinus sampling for differential diagnosis of ACTH-dependent Cushing's syndrome. *Clin Endocrinol (Oxf).* 2007;66:136–142.

83. Yamamoto Y, et al. False-positive inferior petrosal sinus sampling in the diagnosis of Cushing's disease. Report of two cases. *J Neurosurg.* 1995;83(6):1087–1091.

84. Doppman JL, et al. The hypoplastic inferior petrosal sinus: a potential source of false-negative results in petrosal sampling for Cushing's disease. *J Clin Endocrinol Metab.* 1999;84(2):533–540.

85. Wind JJ, et al. The lateralization accuracy of inferior petrosal sinus sampling in 501 patients with Cushing's disease. *J Clin Endocrinol Metab.* 2013;98(6):2285–2293.

86. Findling JW, Raff H, Aron DC. The low-dose dexamethasone suppression test: a reevaluation in patients with Cushing's syndrome. *J Clin Endocrinol Metab.* 2004;89(3):1222–1226.

87. Sharma ST, Raff H, Nieman LK. Prolactin as a marker of successful catheterization during IPSS in patients with ACTH-dependent Cushing's syndrome. *J Clin Endocrinol Metab.* 2011;96(12):3687–3694.

88. Mulligan GB, et al. Prolactin measurement during inferior petrosal sinus sampling improves the localization of pituitary adenomas in Cushing's disease. *Clin Endocrinol.* 2012;77(2):268–274.

89. Grant P, Dworakowska D, Carroll P. Maximizing the accuracy of inferior petrosal sinus sampling: validation of the use of Prolactin as a marker of pituitary venous effluent in the diagnosis of Cushing's disease. *Clin Endocrinol.* 2012;76(4):555–559.

90. Zampetti B, et al. Bilateral inferior petrosal sinus sampling. *Endocr Connect.* 2016;5(4):R12.

91. Miller DL, et al. Neurologic complications of petrosal sinus sampling. *Radiology.* 1992;185(1):143–147.

92. Lefournier V, et al. One transient neurological complication (sixth nerve palsy) in 166 consecutive inferior petrosal sinus samplings for the etiological diagnosis of Cushing's syndrome. *J Clin Endocrinol Metab.* 1999;84(9):3401–3402.

93. Bonelli F, et al. Venous subarachnoid hemorrhage after inferior petrosal sinus sampling for adrenocorticotropic hormone. *AJNR Am J Neuroradiol.* 1999;20:306–307.

94. Blevins Jr LS, Clark RV, Owens DS. Thromboembolic complications after inferior petrosal sinus sampling in patients with cushing's syndrome. *Endocr Pract.* 1998;4(6):365–367.

95. Ilias I, et al. Jugular venous sampling: an alternative to petrosal sinus sampling for the diagnostic evaluation of adrenocorticotropic hormone-dependent Cushing's syndrome. *J Clin Endocrinol Metab.* 2004;89(8):3795–3800.

96. Erickson D, et al. Internal jugular vein sampling in adrenocorticotropic hormone-dependent Cushing's syndrome: a comparison with inferior petrosal sinus sampling. *Clin Endocrinol (Oxf).* 2004;60(4):413–419.

97. Doppman JL, Oldfield EH, Nieman LK. Bilateral sampling of the internal jugular vein to distinguish between mechanisms of adrenocorticotropic hormone-dependent cushing syndrome. *Ann Intern Med.* 1998;128(1):33–36.

98. Isidori AM, et al. Conventional and nuclear medicine imaging in ectopic cushing's syndrome: a systematic review. *J Clin Endocrinol Metab.* 2015;100(9):3231–3244.

99. Pacak K, et al. The role of [(18)F]fluorodeoxyglucose positron emission tomography and [(111)In]-diethylenetriaminepentaacetate-D-Phe-pentetreotide scintigraphy in the localization of ectopic adrenocorticotropin-secreting tumors causing Cushing's syndrome. *J Clin Endocrinol Metab.* 2004;89(5):2214–2221.

100. Tabarin A, et al. Usefulness of somatostatin receptor scintigraphy in patients with occult ectopic adrenocorticotropin syndrome. *J Clin Endocrinol Metab.* 1999;84(4):1193–1202.

101. Nieman LK, et al. Treatment of cushing's syndrome: an endocrine society clinical practice guideline. *J Clin Endocrinol Metab.* 2015;100(8):2807–2831.

102. Alexandraki KI, et al. Long-term remission and recurrence rates in Cushing's disease: predictive factors in a single-centre study. *Eur J Endocrinol.* 2013;168(4):639−648.

103. Valassi E, et al. Delayed remission after transsphenoidal surgery in patients with Cushing's disease. *J Clin Endocrinol Metab.* 2010;95(2):601−610.

104. Hofmann BM, et al. Long-term results after microsurgery for Cushing disease: experience with 426 primary operations over 35 years. *J Neurosurg.* 2008;108(1):9−18.

105. Liu C, et al. Cavernous and inferior petrosal sinus sampling in the evaluation of ACTH-dependent Cushing's syndrome. *Clin Endocrinol.* 2004;61(4):478−486.

106. Smith TR, et al. Complications after transsphenoidal surgery for patients with Cushing's disease and silent corticotroph adenomas. *Neurosurg Focus.* 2015;38(2):E12.

107. Aranda G, et al. Long-term remission and recurrence rate in a cohort of Cushing's disease: the need for long-term follow-up. *Pituitary.* 2015;18(1):142−149.

108. Atkinson AB, et al. Long-term remission rates after pituitary surgery for Cushing's disease: the need for long-term surveillance. *Clin Endocrinol.* 2005;63(5):549−559.

109. Albani A, et al. The USP8 mutational status may predict long-term remission in patients with Cushing's disease. *Clin Endocrinol.* 2018.

110. Castinetti F, et al. Ketoconazole in Cushing's disease: is it worth a try? *J Clin Endocrinol Metab.* 2014;99(5):1623−1630.

111. Daniel E, et al. Effectiveness of metyrapone in treating cushing's syndrome: a retrospective multicenter study in 195 patients. *J Clin Endocrinol Metab.* 2015;100(11):4146−4154.

112. Baudry C, et al. Efficiency and tolerance of mitotane in Cushing's disease in 76 patients from a single center. *Eur J Endocrinol.* 2012;167(4):473−481.

113. Schulte HM, et al. Infusion of low dose etomidate: correction of hypercortisolemia in patients with Cushing's syndrome and dose-response relationship in normal subjects. *J Clin Endocrinol Metab.* 1990;70(5):1426−1430.

114. Pivonello R, et al. The medical treatment of Cushing's disease: effectiveness of chronic treatment with the dopamine agonist cabergoline in patients unsuccessfully treated by surgery. *J Clin Endocrinol Metab.* 2009;94(1):223−230.

115. Colao A, et al. A 12-month phase 3 study of pasireotide in Cushing's disease. *N Engl J Med.* 2012;366(10):914−924.

116. Ogawa R, Echizen H. Drug-drug interaction profiles of proton pump inhibitors. *Clin Pharmacokinet.* 2010;49(8):509−533.

117. Pascal V, et al. Value of ketoconazole in the treatment of Cushing disease. *Rev Med Interne.* 1993;14(1):58−61.

118. Vong CH, Forest M, Nicolino M. Ketoconazole treatment for Cushing syndrome in McCune-Albright syndrome. *J Pediatr.* 2009;154(3):467−468. author reply 468-9.

119. Loli P, Berselli ME, Tagliaferri M. Use of ketoconazole in the treatment of Cushing's syndrome. *J Clin Endocrinol Metab.* 1986;63(6):1365−1371.

120. Greenblatt HK, Greenblatt DJ. Liver injury associated with ketoconazole: review of the published evidence. *J Clin Pharmacol.* 2014;54(12):1321−1329.

121. Verhelst JA, et al. Short and long-term responses to metyrapone in the medical management of 91 patients with Cushing's syndrome. *Clin Endocrinol.* 1991;35(2):169−178.

122. Blanco C, et al. Cushing's syndrome during pregnancy secondary to adrenal adenoma: metyrapone treatment and laparoscopic adrenalectomy. *J Endocrinol Investig.* 2006;29(2):164−167.

123. Chan LF, et al. Use of intravenous etomidate to control acute psychosis induced by the hypercortisolaemia in severe paediatric Cushing's disease. *Horm Res Paediatr.* 2011;75(6):441−446.

124. Drake WM, et al. Emergency and prolonged use of intravenous etomidate to control hypercortisolemia in a patient with Cushing's syndrome and peritonitis. *J Clin Endocrinol Metab.* 1998;83(10):3542−3544.

125. Preda VA, et al. Etomidate in the management of hypercortisolaemia in Cushing's syndrome: a review. *Eur J Endocrinol.* 2012;167(2):137−143.

126. Fleseriu M, et al. Mifepristone, a glucocorticoid receptor antagonist, produces clinical and metabolic benefits in patients with Cushing's syndrome. *J Clin Endocrinol Metab.* 2012;97(6):2039−2049.

127. Pivonello R, et al. Cabergoline plus lanreotide for ectopic Cushing's syndrome. *N Engl J Med.* 2005;352(23):2457−2458.

128. Estrada J, et al. The long-term outcome of pituitary irradiation after unsuccessful transsphenoidal surgery in Cushing's disease. *N Engl J Med.* 1997;336(3):172−177.

129. Mehta GU, et al. Stereotactic radiosurgery for cushing disease: results of an international, multicenter study. *J Clin Endocrinol Metab.* 2017;102(11):4284−4291.

130. Assie G, et al. Corticotroph tumor progression after adrenalectomy in Cushing's Disease: a reappraisal of Nelson's Syndrome. *J Clin Endocrinol Metab.* 2007;92(1):172−179.

131. Osswald A, et al. Favorable long-term outcomes of bilateral adrenalectomy in Cushing's disease. *Eur J Endocrinol.* 2014;171(2):209−215.

132. Storr HL, et al. Paediatric Cushing's syndrome: epidemiology, investigation and therapeutic advances. *Trends Endocrinol Metabol.* 2007;18(4):167−174.

133. Mantero F, et al. A survey on adrenal incidentaloma in Italy. Study group on adrenal tumors of the Italian society of endocrinology. *J Clin Endocrinol Metab.* 2000;85(2):637−644.

134. Luton JP, et al. Clinical features of adrenocortical carcinoma, prognostic factors, and the effect of mitotane therapy. *N Engl J Med.* 1990;322(17):1195−1201.

135. Bertherat J, et al. Mutations in regulatory subunit type 1A of cyclic adenosine 5'-monophosphate-dependent protein kinase (PRKAR1A): phenotype analysis in 353 patients and 80 different genotypes. *J Clin Endocrinol Metab.* 2009;94(6):2085−2091.

136. Bertagna C, Orth DN. Clinical and laboratory findings and results of therapy in 58 patients with adrenocortical tumors admitted to a single medical center (1951 to 1978). *Am J Med.* 1981;71(5):855–875.

137. Iniguez-Ariza NM, et al. Clinical, biochemical, and radiological characteristics of a single-center retrospective cohort of 705 large adrenal tumors. *Mayo Clin Proc Innov Qual Outcomes.* 2018;2(1):30–39.

138. Neville AM, Symington T. Bilateral adrenocortical hyperplasia in children with Cushing's syndrome. *J Pathol.* 1972;107(2):95–106.

139. Carney JA, et al. Primary pigmented nodular adrenocortical disease: the original 4 cases revisited after 30 years for follow-up, new investigations, and molecular genetic findings. *Am J Surg Pathol.* 2014;38(9):1266–1273.

140. Mazzuco TL, et al. Genetic aspects of adrenocortical tumours and hyperplasias. *Clin Endocrinol.* 2012;77(1):1–10.

141. Kobayashi H, et al. Mutation analysis of Gsalpha, adrenocorticotropin receptor and p53 genes in Japanese patients with adrenocortical neoplasms: including a case of Gsalpha mutation. *Endocr J.* 2000;47(4):461–466.

142. Beuschlein F, et al. Constitutive activation of PKA catalytic subunit in adrenal Cushing's syndrome. *N Engl J Med.* 2014;370(11):1019–1028.

143. Bertherat J, et al. Molecular and functional analysis of PRKAR1A and its locus (17q22-24) in sporadic adrenocortical tumors: 17q losses, somatic mutations, and protein kinase A expression and activity. *Cancer Res.* 2003;63(17):5308–5319.

144. Goh G, et al. Recurrent activating mutation in PRKACA in cortisol-producing adrenal tumors. *Nat Genet.* 2014;46(6):613–617.

145. Libe R, et al. Phosphodiesterase 11A (PDE11A) and genetic predisposition to adrenocortical tumors. *Clin Cancer Res.* 2008;14(12):4016–4024.

146. Rothenbuhler A, et al. Identification of novel genetic variants in phosphodiesterase 8B (PDE8B), a cAMP-specific phosphodiesterase highly expressed in the adrenal cortex, in a cohort of patients with adrenal tumours. *Clin Endocrinol.* 2012;77(2):195–199.

147. Reznik Y, et al. Aberrant adrenal sensitivity to multiple ligands in unilateral incidentaloma with subclinical autonomous cortisol hypersecretion: a prospective clinical study. *Clin Endocrinol.* 2004;61(3):311–319.

148. Lacroix A. Heredity and cortisol regulation in bilateral macronodular adrenal hyperplasia. *N Engl J Med.* 2013;369(22):2147–2149.

149. Assie G, et al. ARMC5 mutations in macronodular adrenal hyperplasia with Cushing's syndrome. *N Engl J Med.* 2013;369(22):2105–2114.

150. Lacroix A. ACTH-independent macronodular adrenal hyperplasia. *Best Pract Res Clin Endocrinol Metab.* 2009;23(2):245–259.

151. Stratakis CA, Boikos SA. Genetics of adrenal tumors associated with Cushing's syndrome: a new classification for bilateral adrenocortical hyperplasias. *Nat Clin Pract Endocrinol Metab.* 2007;3(11):748–757.

152. Else T, et al. Adrenocortical carcinoma. *Endocr Rev.* 2014;35(2):282–326.

153. Fassnacht M, et al. European society of endocrinology clinical practice guidelines on the management of adrenocortical carcinoma in adults, in collaboration with the european network for the study of adrenal tumors. *Eur J Endocrinol.* 2018;179(4):G1–G46.

154. Petr EJ, Else T. Adrenocortical carcinoma (ACC): when and why should we consider germline testing? *Presse Med.* 2018;47(7–8 Pt 2):e119–e125.

155. Young Jr WF, et al. The clinical conundrum of corticotropin-independent autonomous cortisol secretion in patients with bilateral adrenal masses. *World J Surg.* 2008;32(5):856–862.

156. Ueland GA, et al. Adrenal venous sampling for assessment of autonomous cortisol secretion. *J Clin Endocrinol Metab.* 2018;103(12):4553–4560.

157. Stratakis CA, et al. Paradoxical response to dexamethasone in the diagnosis of primary pigmented nodular adrenocortical disease. *Ann Intern Med.* 1999;131(8):585–591.

158. Fassnacht M, et al. Management of adrenal incidentalomas: european society of endocrinology clinical practice guideline in collaboration with the european network for the study of adrenal tumors. *Eur J Endocrinol.* 2016;175(2):G1–G34.

159. Perogamvros I, et al. Biochemical and clinical benefits of unilateral adrenalectomy in patients with subclinical hypercortisolism and bilateral adrenal incidentalomas. *Eur J Endocrinol.* 2015;173(6):719–725.

160. Debillon E, et al. Unilateral adrenalectomy as a first-line treatment of cushing's syndrome in patients with primary bilateral macronodular adrenal hyperplasia. *J Clin Endocrinol Metab.* 2015;100(12):4417–4424.

161. Lamas C, et al. Is unilateral adrenalectomy an alternative treatment for ACTH-independent macronodular adrenal hyperplasia?: long-term follow-up of four cases. *Eur J Endocrinol.* 2002;146(2):237–240.

162. Iacobone M, et al. The role of unilateral adrenalectomy in ACTH-independent macronodular adrenal hyperplasia (AIMAH). *World J Surg.* 2008;32(5):882–889.

163. Collins MT, Singer FR, Eugster E. McCune-Albright syndrome and the extraskeletal manifestations of fibrous dysplasia. *Orphanet J Rare Dis.* 2012;7(suppl 1):S4.

164. Powell AC, et al. Operative management of Cushing syndrome secondary to micronodular adrenal hyperplasia. *Surgery.* 2008;143(6):750–758.

165. Guana R, et al. Laparoscopic unilateral adrenalectomy in children for isolated primary pigmented nodular adrenocortical disease (PPNAD): case report and literature review. *Eur J Pediatr Surg.* 2010;20(4):273–275.

166. Hurtado MD, et al. Extensive clinical experience: hypothalamic-pituitary-adrenal axis recovery after adrenalectomy for corticotropin-independent cortisol excess. *Clin Endocrinol.* 2018;89(6):721–733.

167. Feelders RA, et al. The burden of Cushing's disease: clinical and health-related quality of life aspects. *Eur J Endocrinol.* 2012;167(3):311–326.

168. Graversen D, et al. Mortality in Cushing's syndrome: a systematic review and meta-analysis. *Eur J Intern Med.* 2012;23(3):278–282.

169. Avgerinos PC, et al. The corticotropin-releasing hormone test in the postoperative evaluation of patients with cushing's syndrome. *J Clin Endocrinol Metab.* 1987;65(5):906–913.

170. da Mota F, Murray C, Ezzat S. Overt immune dysfunction after Cushing's syndrome remission: a consecutive case series and review of the literature. *J Clin Endocrinol Metab.* 2011;96(10):E1670–E1674.

171. Giordano R, et al. Metabolic and cardiovascular outcomes in patients with Cushing's syndrome of different aetiologies during active disease and 1 year after remission. *Clin Endocrinol.* 2011;75(3):354–360.

172. Geer EB, et al. Body composition and cardiovascular risk markers after remission of Cushing's disease: a prospective study using whole-body MRI. *J Clin Endocrinol Metab.* 2012;97(5):1702–1711.

173. van Aken MO, et al. Quality of life in patients after long-term biochemical cure of Cushing's disease. *J Clin Endocrinol Metab.* 2005;90(6):3279–3286.

174. Kristo C, et al. Restoration of the coupling process and normalization of bone mass following successful treatment of endogenous Cushing's syndrome: a prospective, long-term study. *Eur J Endocrinol.* 2006;154(1):109–118.

175. Sederberg-Olsen P, et al. Episodic variation in plasma corticosteroids in subjects with Cushing's syndrome of differing etiology. *J Clin Endocrinol Metab.* 1973;36(5):906–910.

176. Carmichael JD, Zada G, Selman WR. Making the diagnosis of cyclic Cushing's syndrome: a position statement from the topic editors. *Neurosurg Focus.* 2015;38(2):E8.

177. Alexandraki KI, et al. The prevalence and characteristic features of cyclicity and variability in Cushing's disease. *Eur J Endocrinol.* 2009;160(6):1011–1018.

178. Alexandraki KI, Grossman AB. Is urinary free cortisol of value in the diagnosis of Cushing's syndrome? *Curr Opin Endocrinol Diabetes Obes.* 2011;18(4):259–263.

179. Keller-Wood M. Hypothalamic-Pituitary–Adrenal axis-feedback control. *Comp Physiol.* 2015;5(3):1161–1182.

180. Lambers SW, de Jong FH, Birkenhager JC. Biochemical characteristics of alcohol-induced Pseudo-Cushing's syndrome [proceedings]. *J Endocrinol.* 1979;80(2):62P–63P.

181. Coiro V, et al. Desmopressin and hexarelin tests in alcohol-induced Pseudo-Cushing's syndrome. *J Intern Med.* 2000;247(6):667–673.

182. Pecori Giraldi F. PseudoCushing: why a clinical challenge? *J Endocrinol Investig.* 2015;38(10):1137–1139.

183. Pecori Giraldi F, Ambrogio AG. Variability in laboratory parameters used for management of Cushing's syndrome. *Endocrine.* 2015;50(3):580–589.

184. Ising M, et al. The combined dexamethasone/CRH test as a potential surrogate marker in depression. *Prog Neuro-Psychopharmacol Biol Psychiatry.* 2005;29(6):1085–1093.

185. Findling JW, Raff H. Diagnosis of Endocrine Disease: differentiation of pathologic/neoplastic hypercortisolism (Cushing's syndrome) from physiologic/non-neoplastic hypercortisolism (formerly known as pseudo-Cushing's syndrome). *Eur J Endocrinol.* 2017;176(5):R205–R216.

186. Amsterdam JD, et al. The oCRH stimulation test before and after clinical recovery from depression. *J Affect Disord.* 1988;14(3):213–222.

187. Duclos M, et al. Abdominal obesity increases overnight cortisol excretion. *J Endocrinol Investig.* 1999;22(6):465–471.

188. Boushaki FZ, Rasio E, Serri O. Hypothalamic-pituitary-adrenal axis in abdominal obesity: effects of dexfenfluramine. *Clin Endocrinol.* 1997;46(4):461–466.

189. Malchoff CD, Malchoff DM. Glucocorticoid resistance and hypersensitivity. *Endocrinol Metab Clin N Am.* 2005;34(2):315–326. viii.

190. Bronnegard M, Werner S, Gustafsson JA. Primary cortisol resistance associated with a thermolabile glucocorticoid receptor in a patient with fatigue as the only symptom. *J Clin Investig.* 1986;78(5):1270–1278.

191. Lawson EA, et al. Adrenal glucocorticoid and androgen precursor dissociation in anorexia nervosa. *J Clin Endocrinol Metab.* 2009;94(4):1367–1371.

192. Luger A, et al. Acute hypothalamic-pituitary-adrenal responses to the stress of treadmill exercise. Physiologic adaptions to physical training. *N Engl J Med.* 1987;316(21):1309–1315.

193. Yanovski JA, et al. Corticotropin-releasing hormone stimulation following low-dose dexamethasone administration. A new test to distinguish Cushing's syndrome from Pseudo-Cushing's states. *Jama.* 1993;269(17):2232–2238.

194. Yanovski JA, et al. The dexamethasone-suppressed corticotropin-releasing hormone stimulation test differentiates mild Cushing's disease from normal physiology. *J Clin Endocrinol Metab.* 1998;83(2):348–352.

195. Martin NM, et al. Comparison of the dexamethasone-suppressed corticotropin-releasing hormone test and low-dose dexamethasone suppression test in the diagnosis of Cushing's syndrome. *J Clin Endocrinol Metab.* 2006;91(7):2582–2586.

196. Erickson D, et al. Dexamethasone-suppressed corticotropin-releasing hormone stimulation test for diagnosis of mild hypercortisolism. *J Clin Endocrinol Metab.* 2007;92(8):2972–2976.

197. Gatta B, et al. Reevaluation of the combined dexamethasone suppression-corticotropin-releasing hormone test for differentiation of mild cushing's disease from pseudo-Cushing's syndrome. *J Clin Endocrinol Metab.* 2007;92(11):4290–4293.

198. Moro M, et al. The desmopressin test in the differential diagnosis between Cushing's disease and pseudo-Cushing states. *J Clin Endocrinol Metab.* 2000;85(10):3569–3574.

199. Tsagarakis S, Vassiliadi D, Thalassinos N. Endogenous subclinical hypercortisolism: diagnostic uncertainties and clinical implications. *J Endocrinol Investig.* 2006; 29(5):471−482.

200. Pecori Giraldi F, et al. The dexamethasone-suppressed corticotropin-releasing hormone stimulation test and the desmopressin test to distinguish Cushing's syndrome from pseudo-Cushing's states. *Clin Endocrinol.* 2007; 66(2):251−257.

201. Hughes JM, et al. Cushing's syndrome from the therapeutic use of intramuscular dexamethasone acetate. *Arch Intern Med.* 1986;146(9):1848−1849.

202. Decani S, et al. Iatrogenic Cushing's syndrome and topical steroid therapy: case series and review of the literature. *J Dermatol Treat.* 2014;25(6):495−500.

203. Nutting CM, Page SR. Iatrogenic Cushing's syndrome due to nasal betamethasone: a problem not to be sniffed at!. *Postgrad Med.* 1995;71(834):231−232.

204. Steer KA, Kurtz AB, Honour JW. Megestrol-induced Cushing's syndrome. *Clin Endocrinol.* 1995;42(1):91−93.

205. Colpitts L, et al. Iatrogenic cushing syndrome in a 47-year-old HIV-positive woman on ritonavir and inhaled budesonide. *J Int Assoc Phys AIDS Care.* 2017;16(6): 531−534.

206. Mann M, et al. Glucocorticoidlike activity of megestrol. A summary of Food and Drug Administration experience and a review of the literature. *Arch Intern Med.* 1997; 157(15):1651−1656.

207. Paragliola RM, et al. Treatment with synthetic glucocorticoids and the hypothalamus-pituitary-adrenal Axis. *Int J Mol Sci.* 2017;18(10).

CHAPTER 16

Advances in the Diagnosis and Management of Adrenocortical Carcinoma

SARAH B. FISHER, MD, MS • ELLIOT A. ASARE, MD, MS •
MOUHAMMED AMIR HABRA, MD • NANCY D. PERRIER, MD, FACS

INTRODUCTION

Adrenocortical carcinoma (ACC) is rare, with an estimated annual incidence of 0.7—2.0 cases per million individuals worldwide.[1-3] It is an aggressive malignancy that often presents in advanced stages and portends a poor prognosis. Surgical resection offers the best opportunity for cure, but 5-year overall survival (OS) remains a disappointing 39%—55% after curative intent resection,[4] and survival for patients with progressive metastatic disease is often less than a year. Age at presentation is bimodal, peaking at age 5 in childhood and again in the 4th—6th decades of life, with a slight female predominance.[1,3] When possible, patients with ACC should be treated in a multidisciplinary setting with providers experienced in the management of this rare disease, and enrollment in clinical trials should be encouraged.[5]

CLINICAL PRESENTATION AND EVALUATION

Patients with ACC typically present in one of three ways: symptoms related to adrenal hormone excess, abdominal or back pain related to mass effect, or as an incidental finding on imaging studies performed for other reasons. Among the 50%—60% of patients who present with hormone excess, 50%—70% will demonstrate symptoms of cortisol excess (Cushing syndrome), 20%—30% virilization (in females), 5% feminization (in males), and an additional 2%—3% will demonstrate other symptoms of mineralocorticoid excess.[5] The classic presentation of Cushing syndrome with ACC involves significant proximal muscle weakness, noticeable striae, and weight gain with disproportionate distribution in the abdominal and dorsocervical

regions, although the total weight gained may be less pronounced as these symptoms present rapidly (Fig. 16.1). Severe hypertension and hypokalemia may be mediated by mineralocorticoid excess or

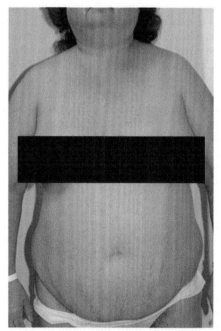

FIG. 16.1 **Clinical characteristics of Cushing's associated with adrenocortical carcinoma.** Marked abdominal striae, increased abdominal and dorsocervical fat deposition, and proximal muscle weakness are among the many signs and symptoms that patients with Cushing's experience. The severity of signs and symptoms, as well as the rapidity of the onset, are factors that suggest malignancy.

Advances in Treatment and Management in Surgical Endocrinology. https://doi.org/10.1016/B978-0-323-66195-9.00016-9

glucocorticoid excess. Many patients exhibit signs and symptoms of multiple hormonal excesses, pathognomonic for ACC. Particular attention should be paid to the timeline and severity of the symptoms related to hormone excess, with rapid-onset and severe electrolyte disturbances more concerning for underlying malignancy. Diagnostic workup should include serum cortisol and adrenocorticotropic hormone, with low-dose dexamethasone suppression test, late-night salivary cortisol, or 24-h urinary free cortisol as confirmatory tests to evaluate for Cushing syndrome. To evaluate for sex hormone, excess dehydroepiandrosterone sulfate, 17-hydroxy progesterone, androstenedione, testosterone (in women), and 17-β-estradiol (in men and postmenopausal women) should be obtained. Finally, plasma aldosterone concentration and plasma renin activity should be checked to evaluate for mineralocorticoid excess.

The identification of subclinical or clinical hormone hypersecretion provides information regarding diagnosis and has therapeutic and prognostic implications. For indeterminate adrenal lesions, hormone functionality involving more than one line of adrenal steroids is suggestive of malignancy.[6] Electrolyte disturbances related to mineralocorticoid excess should be corrected preoperatively. Deconditioning due to hypercortisolism may be severe, limiting performance status. Even in the setting of metastatic disease, resection may be appropriate to palliate symptoms of hypercortisolism. Recognition and appropriate perioperative management of hypercortisolism with postoperative stress dose steroids is important to minimize the risk of subsequent adrenal insufficiency.[7,8] Functional tumors appear to have a more aggressive phenotype. Clinical hypercortisolism has been associated with poorer recurrence free (RFS) and OS, even after adjusting for gender, age, tumor stage, and mitotane therapy in a multinational retrospective series of patients undergoing curative intent resection (RFS hazard ratio [HR] 1.3, 95% confidence interval [CI] 1.04–2.62, $P = .02$; OS HR 1.55, 95% CI 1.15–2.09, $P = .004$).[9] It is unclear whether the poor outcome is driven by the morbidity associated with cortisol overproduction, including the possibility of immunosuppression leading to micrometastases early on, or if the poor prognosis is linked to tumor-related factors. In another study that included 330 patients, (n=138 with functional excess: 55% cortisol, 10.1% aldosterone, 15.2% androgen, 19.6% multiple hormone excess) tumor functionality remained a negative prognostic factor for OS after accounting for age and stage (HR 1.4, 95% CI 1.06–1.86, $P = .02$)[10]

In the absence of hormone production, ACCs may present with abdominal or back pain due to mass effect,

often at advanced stages. The median size of most ACCs is greater than 10–11 cm, while most adenomas are less than 5 cm.[1,6,11] In surgical series, the risk of malignancy increases with tumor size, with ACC identified in 2% of tumors smaller than or equal to 4 cm, 6% of tumors between 4.1 and 6 cm, and 25% of tumors larger than 6 cm.[8]

Finally, ACC may be identified as an incidental finding on cross-sectional imaging performed for other reasons. Societal demand for imaging is increasing, and with it the incidence of the "incidentaloma."[12] Adrenocortical carcinoma comprises 5%–14% of surgically resected adrenal incidentalomas.[8,13] In theory, incidental diagnosis should correlate with identification of ACC at an earlier stage, and allow curative intent treatment of ACC with potentially better outcomes. This is not supported by two recent large database analyses. One National Cancer Database analysis showed that the median tumor size, proportion of patients presenting with metastatic or nodal disease, and OS were unchanged between 1985 and 2000.[3] A surveillance, epidemiology, and end results (SEER) analysis that examined patients with ACC treated between 1973 and 2000 also showed no differences in age at diagnosis, gender, race/ethnicity, tumor size or grade, stage, and frequency of distant metastasis either by quartile or annually, but in contrast to the NCDB study showed that diagnosis in a more recent time period was associated with improved cause-specific mortality.[13] The possibility of malignancy should be considered in patients with adrenal masses presenting with rapid-onset and/or severe symptoms of hormone excess, radiographic evidence of local invasion or tumor thrombus, nodal or distant metastases, size > 6 cm, or positron emission tomography avid tumors (Fig. 16.2).[6]

Imaging

Computed tomography (CT) is the most common imaging modality for evaluating adrenal tumors. When performed with an initial unenhanced (noncontrasted) phase, tumors with Hounsfield units (HU) less than 10 are safely classified as lipid-rich adenomas. Absolute washout and relative washout can also be calculated if the precontrast density is greater than 10 HU, suggestive of a lipid poor mass. The relative washout is particularly useful in circumstances in which noncontrast phase images are not available (Fig. 16.3A–C). Absolute washout greater than or equal to 60%, or relative washout greater than or equal to 40% is associated with a high sensitivity (88%–96%) and specificity (96% –100%) for an adrenal adenoma.[14] Other techniques

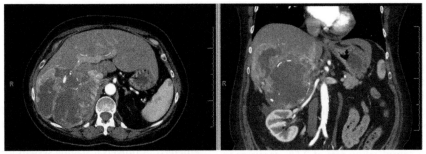

FIG. 16.2 **Radiographic characteristics of adrenocortical carcinoma.** Characteristics suggestive of adrenocortical carcinoma include tumor size greater than 6 cm, invasion into adjacent soft tissues and organs, and radiographic heterogeneity as pictured here.

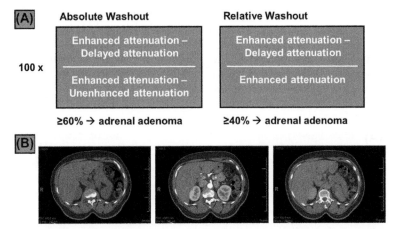

FIG. 16.3 **Radiographic characteristics of an adrenal mass.** When the initial Hounsfield units on an adrenal mass are > 10, or if a noncontrast CT is unavailable absolute washout and relative washout **(A)** can be calculated to assist in discerning the origin of an adrenal mass, as shown in **(B)**, representative unenhanced, enhanced, and delayed computed tomography images of an adrenal mass. In this scenario, the Hounsfield units on unenhanced imaging = 37, enhanced = 108, and delayed = 72, with absolute washout = 50% and the relative washout = 33%, is not clearly consistent with an adenoma. Although an atypical adenoma remains possible, further evaluation is merited.

involving CT have been evaluated, with variable but generally lower sensitivity and specificity for adenomas using dual-energy CT (near simultaneous image acquisition at two different tube voltages) or CT perfusion imaging (quantification of perfusion parameters).[14] In contrast to adenomas, ACCs are generally larger (>6 cm in 90% of cases) with ill-defined margins often with a thin enhancing rim, heterogeneous internal appearance often with a central area of low attenuation, and slow washout of intravenous contrast.[11] Adjacent organ or vascular invasion, regional lymphadenopathy, and distant metastases are highly suggestive of malignancy. Magnetic resonance imaging, either with gadolinium enhancement or chemical-shift

assessment, may aid in characterization of the ACC itself as well as discernment of venous thrombus or invasion and/or hepatic metastases.

Baseline staging for all patients with suspected or confirmed ACC should include cross-sectional imaging of the chest, abdomen, and pelvis. Of patients presenting with metastatic disease, the most common sites are regional or para-aortic/paracaval lymph nodes (25%–46%), lung (45%–97%), liver (48%–96%), and bone (11%–33%).[6] Positron emission tomography (often combined with CT) may be appropriate as part of an initial evaluation and is particularly useful for whole body imaging, but has the drawback of cost, radiation exposure, and test availability.[5]

Biopsy

Once characterized biochemically and radiographically, percutaneous image-guided biopsy is rarely indicated for the patient suspected of having ACC. Biopsy should only be performed in situations in which management would be directly altered such as nonfunctioning tumors that might require systemic therapy. Concerns of tumor seeding along the biopsy tract, risk of capsular rupture, the possibility of misdiagnosis on biopsy, a demonstrable nondiagnostic rate (8.7% in one meta-analysis), and a complication rate of 2.5% converge to discourage the practice.[5]

Genetic Testing

Although most cases of ACC are sporadic, up to 10% of all patients with ACC will have an identifiable genetic predisposition.[15] Adrenocortical carcinoma is most commonly associated with Li–Fraumeni syndrome, Lynch syndrome, and rarely in multiple endocrine neoplasia type 1, although ACC is also reported in patients with Beckwith–Wiedemann syndrome (pediatric patients), congenital adrenal hyperplasia, familial adenomatous polyposis, and Carney complex.[5,15] Genetic testing for germline mutations is recommended in all patients presenting with ACC.[5]

STAGING

A tumor, node, metastasis (TNM) staging system for ACC was first proposed by MacFarlane in 1958.[16] Since then, several competing staging systems for ACC have emerged. A universal staging system for ACC is important for a number of reasons: (1) allows for communication among clinicians/pathologists across the world, (2) facilitates the collection and pooling of data from different institutions to support research for a rare cancer, (3) utilization as selection criteria for enrollment in clinical trials, and (4) tool for prognostication.[17]

The American Joint Committee on Cancer (AJCC) first published a TNM staging system for ACC in the seventh edition of the Cancer Staging System (2010–17, Fig. 16.4A–B).[18] This staging system was adopted

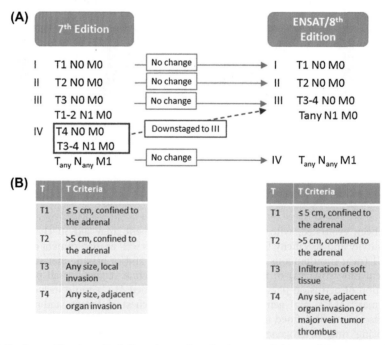

FIG. 16.4 **Radiographic characteristics of an adrenal adenoma.** Schema of the changes between the American Joint Committee on Cancer 7th edition and the European Network for the Study of Adrenal Tumors/AJCC 8th edition staging systems for adrenocortical carcinoma (A) with the corresponding T category definitions (B) representative unenhanced, enhanced, and delayed computed tomography images of an adrenal mass. In this scenario, the Hounsfield units on unenhanced imaging = 37, enhanced = 108, and delayed = 72, with absolute washout = 50% and the relative washout = 33%, not clearly consistent with an adenoma. Although an atypical adenoma remains possible, further evaluation is merited.

from the publication in 2004 by the International Union against Cancer (UICC) and the World Health Organization (WHO). Studies that attempted to validate the TNM staging system for ACC in the seventh edition of the AJCC found significant limitations.[17,19,20] Fassnacht et al.[19] examined 416 patients with ACC treated between 1986 and 2003 in the German ACC registry. They reported a disease-specific survival of 82%, 58%, 55%, and 18% for stages I, II, III, and IV, respectively, although the differences in survival between stages I, II, and III were not statistically significant. Additionally, there were no differences in survival between patients with stage IV disease without distant metastases (T3N1M0, T4N0M0) and those with stage III disease. The presence of nodal disease (HR 2.5, 95% CI: 1.2–5.7), infiltration of surrounding tissue (HR 1.9, 95% CI: 1.2–3), and tumor thrombus in a large vein (HR 2.7, 95% CI: 1.2–6) were poor prognostic factors for disease-specific survival. The authors proposed the European Network for the Study of Adrenal Tumors (ENSAT) staging system in which patients with nodal disease, infiltration of surrounding tissue, or venous tumor thrombus were considered stage III, while stage IV was restricted to patients with distant metastases (Fig. 16.4A–B). Disease-specific 5-year survival based on the ENSAT proposal was 82%, 61%, 50%, and 13%, respectively.[19]

An external validation of the ENSAT staging using the National Cancer Database demonstrated statistically significant differences in OS between stages II/III and III/IV, but not between stages I and II. In this study of 1579 patients treated between 1985 and 2006, multivariable analysis identified positive resection margin status, higher grade, and age >55 years as negative prognostic factors; the authors proposed incorporating age >55 years as an automatic upgrade to stage II for patients with early (T1/2 N0M0) disease. Using age in addition to the ENSAT staging resulted in 5-year OS of 70%, 53%, 37%, and 10% for stages I, II, III, and IV, respectively.[21]

Alternatively, the United States Adrenocortical Carcinoma Group proposed incorporating the presence or absence of lymphovascular invasion (LVI) into the TNM seventh edition staging system, based on their findings that LVI remained a significant poor prognostic factor (HR 2.81, 95% CI: 1.46–5.41) even after accounting for T category and extraadrenal invasion (Table 16.1).[4]

The ENSAT staging system was adopted by the eighth edition of the AJCC Cancer Staging System in January 2018.[22] Factors such as age and LVI should be further evaluated and potentially incorporated in future

TABLE 16.1 Proposed Changes to T-Category for Adrenocortical Carcinoma Staging by the United States Adrenocortical Carcinoma Group.	
T-Category	**Definition**
T1	≤5 cm, (−) local invasion, ±LVI
T2	>5 cm, (−) local invasion, −LVI
	Any size, (+) local invasion, −LVI
T3	>5 cm, (−) local invasion, +LVI
	Any size, (+) local invasion, +LVI
T4	Any size, (+) adjacent organ invasion, ±LVI

LVI, Lymphovascular invasion.

renditions of the AJCC TNM staging system. In addition, the AJCC has recommended that the following variables be collected in cancer registries: tumor weight (g), vascular invasion, mitotic count, Ki-67 proliferative index, and Weiss score. Robust prognostic models that incorporate other factors in addition to T, N, and M could be developed in the future once high-quality data with pertinent variables is accrued.

SURGICAL THERAPY

Operative Approach

Complete surgical resection without tumor rupture at the time of the initial operation offers the best opportunity for cure, although locoregional and distant recurrence rates remain high.[6,23] When suspicion for malignancy is low and size is less than 6 cm, a minimally invasive approach (laparoscopic transabdominal or retroperitoneoscopic) to adrenalectomy is associated with shorter hospital stays, less postoperative pain, and lower costs and is preferred over an open approach.[24] For a suspected malignancy, concern over tumor capsule rupture, spillage, and tumor seeding with later development of peritoneal carcinomatosis and poorer long-term outcomes has historically precluded the minimally invasive approach.[25,26] In one tertiary referral center series of 170 patients, the laparoscopic approach was more frequently associated with development of peritoneal carcinomatosis than an open approach (83% vs. 8%, $P = .0001$).[25] Recently, retrospective series of well-selected patients with smaller ACC undergoing minimally invasive resection at referral institutions have demonstrated equivalent long-term outcomes as compared to the open approach.[27-29] In one recent multiinstitutional series of 201 patients, 47 of whom underwent a minimally invasive approach, there was no difference between the groups with regards to intraoperative tumor rupture, R0 resection, morbidity, recurrence rates, disease free, and OS ($P > .05$); however, the patients in the minimally invasive arm had significantly smaller tumors (5.5 vs. 10.9 cm, $P < .001$). The authors note that stringent patient selection, smaller tumor size, and increased proficiency of minimally invasive surgeons at the included institutions likely attributed to the overall low rate of tumor rupture, and suggest that the ability to achieve a complete and appropriate oncologic resection should guide the choice of surgical approach.[30] Retrospective comparisons are plagued by selection bias, and randomized clinical trials assessing operative approach are unlikely to be feasible. The European Society of Endocrinology Clinical Practice Guidelines suggest that for adrenal tumors <6 cm, a laparoscopic approach may be considered reasonable in the absence of local invasion provided adequate surgical expertise; in situations in which malignancy is suspected, an open approach remains the standard of care.[5] It is the authors' preference to approach suspected or known malignancy with an open approach.

Lymphadenectomy

Although lymph node metastases are accepted as a negative prognostic factor,[1,3] regional lymphadenectomy is inconsistently performed (8%–32.5% of modern series).[3,31-33] A SEER analysis showed that lymphadenectomy was performed in only 67 (8%) of 802 patients undergoing resection for ACC between 1973 and 2011. Although the presence of lymph node metastases was a negative prognostic factor, there was no survival benefit associated with lymphadenectomy in the study group. However, the authors noted that lymphadenectomy was more likely to be performed in patients with locally advanced tumors and distant metastases, and encouraged the consideration of lymphadenectomy in patients with T3 or T4 tumors.[32] In contrast, data from the German ACC registry and a recent United States multiinstitutional cohort support lymphadenectomy as both a prognostic and therapeutic tool, with a survival advantage observed for those undergoing lymphadenectomy.[33,34] After controlling for age, tumor stage, multivisceral resection, and receipt of adjuvant therapy, the German series of 283 patients concluded that patients who underwent lymphadenectomy (defined arbitrarily as >5 lymph nodes resected) had a reduced risk of tumor recurrence (HR 0.65, 95% CI 0.43–0.98, $P = .042$) and/or disease-related death

(HR 0.54, 95% CI 0.29–0.99, $P = .049$) as compared to those who did not undergo lymphadenectomy.[33] The United States series of 120 patients demonstrated that although patients who underwent lymphadenectomy more often had larger tumors, a palpable mass at presentation, suspicious lymph nodes on preoperative imaging, and required multivisceral resection, 5-year OS was better than patients who did not undergo lymphadenectomy (76% vs. 59%, $P = .041$, with lymphadenectomy defined from operative notes).[34] It is the authors' practice to resect ipsilateral periadrenal and renal hilar nodes, with selective inclusion of the ipsilateral celiac, para-aortic, and paracaval lymph nodes from the level of the aortic hiatus on the left or the inferior aspect of the liver on the right to the renal vein inferiorly, as guided by preoperative imaging.

Locally Advanced, Recurrent, or Oligometastatic Disease

When local invasion is suspected en bloc resection of adjacent organs is appropriate. The kidney (56%), liver (28%), spleen (24%), and pancreas (16%) were the most common extraadrenal organs resected in one multiinstitutional study of 26 patients undergoing multivisceral resection for ACC.[35] Although some have suggested planned ipsilateral nephrectomy at the time of resection to avoid renal capsular disruption, this does not appear to confer a survival benefit in the absence of direct invasion.[6,35]

Tumor thrombus or direct invasion of the adrenal vein, renal vein, or inferior vena cava is noted in 15%–25% of patients and is not considered a contraindication to operation if a margin negative resection can be achieved.[6] Although perioperative mortality is high at 13%, 3 year survival has been reported to be between 25% and 29% for such patients.[36,37] Major venous resections should only be performed in high volume centers well versed in techniques to prevent tumor embolus with the ability to accomplish suprahepatic control of the inferior vena cava and/or consideration for cardiopulmonary bypass. Stringent patient selection, surgical and critical care expertise, and frank discussion of the risks, benefits, and alternatives of resection in the setting of localized disease with major vascular involvement are warranted.

Recurrence rates after resection of ACC range from 37% to 80%, with one multiinstitutional study recently demonstrating recurrence in 116 of 180 patients (64.4%) treated with curative intent resection at a median time of 18.8 months. In this study, distant metastases were the most common pattern of recurrence (45.1%) and most commonly occurred in the lung or liver. Patients with locoregional recurrence alone experienced a longer RFS than those with distant metastases (16.1 vs. 9.8 months), and those with both distant metastases and locoregional disease had the worst RFS (7.9 months).[38]

In well-selected patients resection, and sometimes repeat resection, of hepatic and/or pulmonary metastases or locoregional recurrence has conferred a survival advantage as compared to patients with recurrent disease treated medically.[39–44] Longer disease-free interval (>6–12 months) and ability to obtain a complete margin negative resection correlate with improved OS (29%–41% 5-year OS).[39,41,45,46] It is important to counsel patients that resection in the metastatic setting is unlikely to cure, as disease-free survival remains low (7–9 months).[42,47] Other prognostic factors associated with longer OS after metastasectomy include a lower Ki-67 proliferation index,[44] response to neoadjuvant chemotherapy,[47] and unifocal disease.[46] In addition to surgical therapy, locoregional approaches such as radiation therapy, ablation, or chemoembolization may be considered under the guidance of a multidisciplinary team experienced in managing ACC.[5]

MEDICAL THERAPY

The adrenolytic agent, mitotane, is a synthetic derivative of the insecticide dichlorodiphenyltrichloroethane and was approved in the United States in 1970 for the treatment of advanced ACC. Thought to block 11β-hydroxylase, mitotane reduces adrenal steroid production in the adrenal cortex and increases peripheral glucocorticoid clearance.[48] Adverse effects of mitotane therapy include gastrointestinal upset, adrenal insufficiency, neurologic complaints (lethargy, somnolence, dizziness, confusion, and impaired memory), hepatotoxicity, alterations in thyroid hormone levels, and hypercholesterolemia.[49] In addition to these effects, mitotane is a potent CYP3A4 inducer, resulting in the increased clearance of medications often used to correct the adverse effects, including calcium channel blockers, HGM-CoA reductase inhibitors, benzodiazepines, oral contraceptives, some macrolide antibiotics, and some opioids, as well as select anti-ACC drugs.[1] The upregulation of hepatic metabolism associated with mitotane requires close attention and often increasing the glucocorticosteroid dose to ensure adequate steroid replacement in patients with mitotane induced adrenal insufficiency.

With an objective response rate between 20% and 24%, effective systemic therapy for ACC is lacking.[1,5] As a result, mitotane is often combined with cytotoxic therapy. The combination of etoposide, doxorubicin, cisplatin, and mitotane (EDP-M) is the only therapy

for ACC successfully evaluated in a randomized controlled trial to date (FIRM-ACT). In 304 patients, combination therapy with EDP-M had better objective response rate (23.2% vs. 9.2%, $P < .001$) and progression-free survival (5.0 vs. 2.1 months, $P < .001$) as compared to therapy with streptozotocin and mitotane (Sz-M), although OS between the two groups was similar (14.8 vs. 12.0 months, $P = .07$).[50] It is possible the crossover design of the trial contributed to the lack of a significant difference in survival. Currently, EDP-M is recommended for patients with unresectable disease and aggressive disease parameters (high tumor burden, uncontrolled symptoms, high Ki-67 proliferation index, or clinical evidence of a fast-growing tumor) when performance status allows. Mitotane monotherapy may be considered with the understanding that titration to therapeutic serum level (levels > 14 mg/L) may require weeks to months.[5] In cases of progression on EDP-M, Sz-M may be offered (9% response rate) or the combination of gemcitabine and capecitabine; single agent cisplatin or carboplatin has also been proposed.[48,49] Case reports have demonstrated response to therapy with the targeted agents, with one phase 2 study demonstrating progression-free survival ranging between 5.6 and 11.2 months in patients using sunitinib after progression on mitotane and multiple cytotoxic therapies.[48] Unfortunately small trials in heavily pretreated populations have failed to show response with other targeted agents (epidermal growth factor receptor, mammalian target of rapamycin, insulin-like growth factor one receptor, fibroblast growth factor receptor, and vascular endothelial growth factor). Recently, the activation of cMET receptors has been suggested as potential mechanism associated with ACC resistance to therapy, and preclinical data suggested that silencing cMET signaling could be a potential therapeutic target.[51] A phase II clinical trial is ongoing to evaluate the effect of simultaneous targeting of tumor vasculature (VEGFR) and cMET in ACC using cabozantinib, a multitarget oral tyrosine kinase inhibitor (NCT03370718).[52] The role of immunotherapy in ACC management is evolving, and a recent study found a response rate of 6% to programmed death-ligand 1 (PDL1) inhibitor (avelumab) though half of the study participants received simultaneous mitotane therapy. Although rare, surgery or other locoregional therapy may be considered in the patient demonstrating disease stability on systemic therapy.[1]

Adjuvant Therapy

Data for adjuvant therapy are limited to retrospective reviews, with the strongest evidence for adjuvant mitotane stemming from the comparison of 47 Italian patients treated at centers who routinely recommended adjuvant mitotane, compared to 55 Italian patients treated at centers that did not, with an additional comparison to 75 patients from the German ACC Registry treated with surgery alone. Recurrence-free survival for patients treated with mitotane (42 months) was higher than the Italian surgery-only group (10 months, $P < .001$) or the German surgery-only group (25 months, $P = .005$). Similarly, OS was longest for patients treated with mitotane (110 months) as compared to the Italian surgery-only group (52 months, $P = .01$) or the German surgery-only group (67 months, $P = .10$). After accounting for age, gender, and tumor stage, the lack of adjuvant mitotane therapy remained a negative prognostic factor for RFS (HR 2.93, CI 1.74–4.94, German group; HR 3.79, 95% CI 2.27–6.32 Italian group, $P < .001$).[53] Despite this, others have failed to identify a benefit for adjuvant mitotane.[31,54] A recent study from multiple institutions in the United States retrospectively examined 207 patients, 88 of whom received adjuvant mitotane between 1993 and 2014. After accounting for margin status, stage, and receipt of cytotoxic chemotherapy, mitotane was not associated with RFS or OS, but the impact of selection bias treated at multiple centers over a large time period must be considered.[55] Another retrospective single-institution study of 218 patients demonstrated improved disease-free survival (DFS) for patients who received adjuvant mitotane (30 vs. 12 months for surgery alone, $P = .05$), but noted similar recurrence rates between patients treated initially at a tertiary referral center, the majority of whom had grossly complete resections and did not receive adjuvant mitotane, as compared to patients undergoing resection before referral, many of whom had incomplete resections and were more likely to receive mitotane. They hypothesized that completeness of initial resection was a more powerful driving factor of survival than receipt of adjuvant mitotane.[56] It is the authors' practice, in concordance with the European Society of Endocrinology Clinical Practice Guidelines, to consider adjuvant mitotane for patients perceived to be at higher risk for recurrence (stage III, R1 resection, or Ki-67 proliferation index greater than 10%). The ADIUVO phase III trial (NCT00777244), which randomizes low-risk patients to postoperative mitotane versus observation after curative intent resection, is ongoing. For patients with high risk ACC (Ki-67 greater than 10%), the ADIUVO-2 phase III trial compares 2 years of mitotane therapy versus 2 years of mitotane with 3 months of adjuvant cisplatin and etoposide (NCT03583710).[57,58]

Neoadjuvant Therapy

Combination chemotherapy may be beneficial preoperatively for patients with borderline resectable disease. Defined as a concern for technical resectability such that a margin negative resection, even with concomitant multiorgan resection, is not assured, the borderline resectable nomenclature may also apply to the patient with radiographically indeterminate or suspicious distant metastases or marginal performance status. Although randomized data are lacking, a retrospective review of clinical practice at a tertiary referral center demonstrated similar if not better survival (DFS 27.6 vs. 12.6 months, $P = .48$; OS median not reached vs. 110 months, $P = .75$) between patients with borderline resectable disease treated with neoadjuvant therapy compared to those undergoing immediate resection, despite larger tumors and more advanced stage disease in the neoadjuvant group.[59] Future studies examining the utility of a neoadjuvant approach should also evaluate the potential for downstaging the planned operation—salvage of organs at risk (i.e., the ipsilateral kidney) will directly impact ability to tolerate later (nephrotoxic) systemic therapy.

Radiation Therapy

Adjuvant radiation therapy to the operative field is particularly attractive in situations in which there is a higher theoretical risk of recurrence (i.e., tumor capsule rupture or spillage, or close or positive margins), yet there is conflicting data on its utility. One retrospective comparison of 16 patients who received adjuvant radiation after curative intent surgery compared to 32 patients who did not failed to demonstrate a difference in local recurrence rate (44% vs. 31%, respectively).[60] In contrast, a retrospective cohort of 20 patients undergoing adjuvant radiation after curative intent resection compared to 20 controls undergoing surgery alone matched on stage, margin status, grade, and adjuvant mitotane use showed local recurrence was less in the radiation arm.[61] There were no difference in RFS or OS in either study, a finding that may be explained by the high propensity of ACC to recur distantly. Further study of patient and disease factors associated with locoregional recurrence and thus identifying who may benefit from radiation is necessary. In the advanced setting, palliative radiation is a useful adjunct for symptom control and may be particularly effective for pain related to bony metastases.[48]

FOLLOW-UP

Despite curative intent resection, most patients with ACC will experience recurrence. In the absence of published studies that address timing of surveillance imaging, expert consensus suggests cross-sectional imaging every 3 months for the first 2 years and then every 3−6 months for an additional 3 years.[5] Biochemical evaluation focused on the steroid hormones or metabolites present at the initial diagnosis should also be performed at regular intervals and as indicated by new or recurrent symptoms.

CONCLUSION

Adrenocortical carcinoma is a rare and aggressive disease. Complete surgical resection without tumor rupture offers the best chance for survival, yet many patients experience locoregional and distant recurrence. Tenets of therapy include en bloc resection, routine lymphadenectomy, and treatment in high volume centers with multidisciplinary care teams. Resection of locoregional and oligometastatic distant disease is appropriate for well-selected patients with favorable disease biology. Systemic therapies include the adrenolytic agent mitotane and cytotoxic drugs, although response rates are low and effective regimens are lacking.

DISCLOSURES

This work is not supported by a specific funding source. The authors have no financial disclosures or competing interests.

CONTRIBUTIONS

All authors have made substantial contributions to conception and design, have participated in drafting and revising the chapter for important intellectual content, and have given final approval of the submitted version.

REFERENCES

1. Fassnacht M, Kroiss M, Allolio B. Update in adrenocortical carcinoma. *J Clin Endocrinol Metab*. 2013;98:4551−4564.
2. Schteingart DE, Doherty GM, Gauger PG, et al. Management of patients with adrenal cancer: recommendations of an international consensus conference. *Endocr Relat Cancer*. 2005;12:667−680.
3. Bilimoria KY, Shen WT, Elaraj D, et al. Adrenocortical carcinoma in the United States: treatment utilization and prognostic factors. *Cancer*. 2008;113:3130−3136.
4. Poorman CE, Ethun CG, Postlewait LM, et al. A novel T-stage classification system for adrenocortical carcinoma: proposal from the US adrenocortical carcinoma study group. *Ann Surg Oncol*. 2018;25:520−527.
5. Fassnacht M, Dekkers O, Else T, et al. European society of Endocrinology clinical practice guidelines on the management of adrenocortical carcinoma in adults, in collaboration with the European Network for the study of adrenal tumors. *Eur J Endocrinol*. 2018.
6. Gaujoux S, Mihai R. European society of endocrine surgeons (ESES) and European Network for the study of adrenal Tumours (ENSAT) recommendations for the surgical management of adrenocortical carcinoma. *Br J Surg*. 2017;104:358−376.
7. Shen WT, Lee J, Kebebew E, Clark OH, Duh QY. Selective use of steroid replacement after adrenalectomy: lessons from 331 consecutive cases (Chicago, Ill: 1960) *Arch Surg*. 2006;141:771−774. discussion 4-6.
8. Zeiger MA, Thompson GB, Duh QY, et al. The American association of clinical Endocrinologists and American association of endocrine surgeons medical guidelines for the management of adrenal incidentalomas. *Endocr Pract*. 2009;15(Suppl 1):1−20.
9. Berruti A, Fassnacht M, Haak H, et al. Prognostic role of overt hypercortisolism in completely operated patients with adrenocortical cancer. *Eur Urol*. 2014;65:832−838.
10. Ayala-Ramirez M, Jasim S, Feng L, et al. Adrenocortical carcinoma: clinical outcomes and prognosis of 330 patients at a tertiary care center. *Eur J Endocrinol*. 2013;169:891−899.
11. Zhang HM, Perrier ND, Grubbs EG, et al. CT features and quantification of the characteristics of adrenocortical carcinomas on unenhanced and contrast-enhanced studies. *Clin Radiol*. 2012;67:38−46.
12. Wagner J, Aron DC. Incidentalomas: a "disease" of modern imaging technology. *Best Pract Res Clin Endocrinol Metab*. 2012;26:3−8.
13. Kebebew E, Reiff E, Duh QY, Clark OH, McMillan A. Extent of disease at presentation and outcome for adrenocortical carcinoma: have we made progress? *World J Surg*. 2006;30:872−878.
14. Elsayes KM, Emad-Eldin S, Morani AC, Jensen CT. Practical approach to adrenal imaging. *Urol Clin*. 2018;45:365−387.
15. Petr EJ, Else T. Genetic predisposition to endocrine tumors: diagnosis, surveillance and challenges in care. *Semin Oncol*. 2016;43:582−590.
16. Macfarlane DA. Cancer of the adrenal cortex; the natural history, prognosis and treatment in a study of fifty-five cases. *Ann R Coll Surg Engl*. 1958;23:155−186.
17. Asare EA, Washington MK, Gress DM, Gershenwald JE, Greene FL. Improving the quality of cancer staging. *CA A Cancer J Clin*. 2015;65:261−263.
18. Edge SB, CCC, Fritz AG, Greene FL, Trotti III A, Byrd D, eds. *AJCC Cancer Staging Manual*. 7th ed. New York, NY: Springer; 2011.
19. Fassnacht M, Johanssen S, Quinkler M, et al. Limited prognostic value of the 2004 International union against cancer staging classification for adrenocortical carcinoma: proposal for a revised TNM classification. *Cancer*. 2009;115:243−250.

20. Lughezzani G, Sun M, Perrotte P, et al. The European network for the study of adrenal tumors staging system is prognostically superior to the international union against cancer-staging system: a North American validation. *Eur J Cancer.* 2010;46:713–719 (Oxford, England : 1990).

21. Asare EA, Wang TS, Winchester DP, Mallin K, Kebebew E, Sturgeon C. A novel staging system for adrenocortical carcinoma better predicts survival in patients with stage I/II disease. *Surgery.* 2014;156:1378–1385. discussion 85-6.

22. Amin MB, Edge SB, Greene FL, et al., eds. *AJCC Cancer Staging Manual.* 8th. Springer; 2017.

23. Margonis GA, Kim Y, Prescott JD, et al. Adrenocortical carcinoma: impact of surgical margin status on long-term outcomes. *Ann Surg Oncol.* 2016;23:134–141.

24. Brunt LM, Doherty GM, Norton JA, Soper NJ, Quasebarth MA, Moley JF. Laparoscopic adrenalectomy compared to open adrenalectomy for benign adrenal neoplasms. *J Am Coll Surg.* 1996;183:1–10.

25. Gonzalez RJ, Shapiro S, Sarlis N, et al. Laparoscopic resection of adrenal cortical carcinoma: a cautionary note. *Surgery.* 2005;138:1078–1085. discussion 85-6.

26. Miller BS, Gauger PG, Hammer GD, Doherty GM. Resection of adrenocortical carcinoma is less complete and local recurrence occurs sooner and more often after laparoscopic adrenalectomy than after open adrenalectomy. *Surgery.* 2012;152:1150–1157.

27. Donatini G, Caiazzo R, Do Cao C, et al. Long-term survival after adrenalectomy for stage I/II adrenocortical carcinoma (ACC): a retrospective comparative cohort study of laparoscopic versus open approach. *Ann Surg Oncol.* 2014;21: 284–291.

28. Lombardi CP, Raffaelli M, De Crea C, et al. Open versus endoscopic adrenalectomy in the treatment of localized (stage I/II) adrenocortical carcinoma: results of a multiinstitutional Italian survey. *Surgery.* 2012;152:1158–1164.

29. Porpiglia F, Fiori C, Daffara F, et al. Retrospective evaluation of the outcome of open versus laparoscopic adrenalectomy for stage I and II adrenocortical cancer. *Eur Urol.* 2010;57:873–878.

30. Lee CW, Salem AI, Schneider DF, et al. Minimally invasive resection of adrenocortical carcinoma: a multiinstitutional study of 201 patients. *J Gastrointest Surg.* 2017;21:352–362.

31. Icard P, Goudet P, Charpenay C, et al. Adrenocortical carcinomas: surgical trends and results of a 253-patient series from the French Association of Endocrine Surgeons study group. *World J Surg.* 2001;25:891–897.

32. Nilubol N, Patel D, Kebebew E. Does lymphadenectomy improve survival in patients with adrenocortical carcinoma? A population-based study. *World J Surg.* 2016;40: 697–705.

33. Reibetanz J, Jurowich C, Erdogan I, et al. Impact of lymphadenectomy on the oncologic outcome of patients with adrenocortical carcinoma. *Ann Surg.* 2012;255: 363–369.

34. Gerry JM, Tran TB, Postlewait LM, et al. Lymphadenectomy for adrenocortical carcinoma: is there a therapeutic benefit? *Ann Surg Oncol.* 2016;23:708–713.

35. Marincola Smith P, Kiernan CM, Tran TB, et al. Role of additional organ resection in adrenocortical carcinoma: analysis of 167 patients from the U.S. Adrenocortical carcinoma database. *Ann Surg Oncol.* 2018;25:2308–2315.

36. Chiche L, Dousset B, Kieffer E, Chapuis Y. Adrenocortical carcinoma extending into the inferior vena cava: presentation of a 15-patient series and review of the literature. *Surgery.* 2006;139:15–27.

37. Mihai R, Iacobone M, Makay O, et al. Outcome of operation in patients with adrenocortical cancer invading the inferior vena cava–a European Society of Endocrine Surgeons (ESES) survey. *Langenbeck's Arch Surg.* 2012;397: 225–231.

38. Amini N, Margonis GA, Kim Y, et al. Curative resection of adrenocortical carcinoma: rates and patterns of postoperative recurrence. *Ann Surg Oncol.* 2016;23:126–133.

39. Datrice NM, Langan RC, Ripley RT, et al. Operative management for recurrent and metastatic adrenocortical carcinoma. *J Surg Oncol.* 2012;105:709–713.

40. Dy BM, Strajina V, Cayo AK, et al. Surgical resection of synchronously metastatic adrenocortical cancer. *Ann Surg Oncol.* 2015;22:146–151.

41. Dy BM, Wise KB, Richards ML, et al. Operative intervention for recurrent adrenocortical cancer. *Surgery.* 2013; 154:1292–1299. discussion 9.

42. Gaujoux S, Al-Ahmadie H, Allen PJ, et al. Resection of adrenocortical carcinoma liver metastasis: is it justified? *Ann Surg Oncol.* 2012;19:2643–2651.

43. Kemp CD, Ripley RT, Mathur A, et al. Pulmonary resection for metastatic adrenocortical carcinoma: the National Cancer Institute experience. *Ann Thorac Surg.* 2011;92:1195–1200.

44. op den Winkel J, Pfannschmidt J, Muley T, et al. Metastatic adrenocortical carcinoma: results of 56 pulmonary metastasectomies in 24 patients. *Ann Thorac Surg.* 2011;92: 1965–1970.

45. Ripley RT, Kemp CD, Davis JL, et al. Liver resection and ablation for metastatic adrenocortical carcinoma. *Ann Surg Oncol.* 2011;18:1972–1979.

46. Tran TB, Maithel SK, Pawlik TM, et al. Clinical score predicting long-term survival after repeat resection for recurrent adrenocortical carcinoma. *J Am Coll Surg.* 2016;223: 794–803.

47. Baur J, Buntemeyer TO, Megerle F, et al. Outcome after resection of Adrenocortical Carcinoma liver metastases: a retrospective study. *BMC Cancer.* 2017;17:522.

48. Varghese J, Habra MA. Update on adrenocortical carcinoma management and future directions. *Curr Opin Endocrinol Diabetes Obes.* 2017;24:208–214.

49. Puglisi S, Perotti P, Cosentini D, et al. Decision-making for adrenocortical carcinoma: surgical, systemic, and endocrine management options. *Expert Rev Anticancer Ther.* 2018:1–9.

50. Fassnacht M, Terzolo M, Allolio B, et al. Combination chemotherapy in advanced adrenocortical carcinoma. *N Engl J Med.* 2012;366:2189–2197.

51. Phan LM, Fuentes-Mattei E, Wu W, et al. Hepatocyte growth factor/cMET pathway activation Enhances cancer hallmarks in adrenocortical carcinoma. *Cancer Research.* 2015;75:4131–4142.

52. Cabozantinib in Unresectable/Metastatic Adrenocortical Carcinoma. https://clinicaltrialsgov/ct2/show/NCT0337 0718.NCT03370718.

53. Terzolo M, Angeli A, Fassnacht M, et al. Adjuvant mitotane treatment for adrenocortical carcinoma. *N Engl J Med.* 2007;356:2372–2380.

54. Schulick RD, Brennan MF. Long-term survival after complete resection and repeat resection in patients with adrenocortical carcinoma. *Ann Surg Oncol.* 1999;6: 719–726.

55. Postlewait LM, Ethun CG, Tran TB, et al. Outcomes of adjuvant mitotane after resection of adrenocortical carcinoma: a 13-institution study by the US adrenocortical carcinoma group. *J Am Coll Surg.* 2016;222: 480–490.

56. Grubbs EG, Callender GG, Xing Y, et al. Recurrence of adrenal cortical carcinoma following resection: surgery alone can achieve results equal to surgery plus mitotane. *Ann Surg Oncol.* 2010;17:263–270.

57. Efficacy of Adjuvant Mitotane Treatment (ADIUVO). https://clinicaltrialsgov/ct2/show/NCT00777244.NCT00 777244.

58. Mitotane With or Without Cisplatin and Etoposide After Surgery in Treating Participants With Stage I-III Adrenocortical Cancer With High Risk of Recurrence (ADIUVO-2). https://clinicaltrialsgov/ct2/show/NCT03583710.NCT035 83710.

59. Bednarski BK, Habra MA, Phan A, et al. Borderline resectable adrenal cortical carcinoma: a potential role for preoperative chemotherapy. *World J Surg.* 2014;38:1318–1327.

60. Habra MA, Ejaz S, Feng L, et al. A retrospective cohort analysis of the efficacy of adjuvant radiotherapy after primary surgical resection in patients with adrenocortical carcinoma. *J Clin Endocrinol Metab.* 2013;98:192–197.

61. Sabolch A, Else T, Griffith KA, et al. Adjuvant radiation therapy improves local control after surgical resection in patients with localized adrenocortical carcinoma. *Int J Radiat Oncol Biol Phys.* 2015;92:252–259.

CHAPTER 17

Adrenal Vein Sampling

HARRISON X. BAI, MD • SCOTT O. TREROTOLA, MD

PRIMARY ALDOSTERONISM

Primary aldosteronism (PA) was first described by Jerome Conn in 1945, the same year that the chemical structure of aldosterone was identified.[1] Conn postulated that a female patient's hypertension and hypokalemia were due to an adrenal tumor that produced aldosterone autonomously. In the 1950s, imaging and biochemical studies were rudimentary, so Conn persuaded urologist Dr. William Baum to perform a laparotomy and search for an adrenal tumor. Dr. Baum found and removed the responsible adrenal adenoma, which established Conn's syndrome as a secondary cause of hypertension.[2] Today, PA is the most common cause of secondary hypertension, accounting for approximately 5%–13% of hypertensive patients, predominantly those with severe hypertension.[3–5] As patients with unilateral adrenal hypersecretion of aldosterone may be cured by unilateral adrenalectomy, while bilateral adrenal hypersecretion of aldosterone is most often treated by medical therapy such as mineralocorticoid-receptor antagonists, differentiating between unilateral (most often from an adenoma) from bilateral (most often bilateral hyperplasia) aldosterone hypersecretion is critical. Adrenal vein sampling (AVS) plays a critical role in the management of PA, serving as the final determinant between surgical and medical management.[6] The 2016 Endocrine Society Guidelines state that AVS is the gold standard test to distinguish between unilateral and bilateral aldosterone overproduction and, therefore, to decide which patients with PA can be safely referred to surgery.[7]

DIAGNOSIS OF PRIMARY ALDOSTERONISM WITH OTHER IMAGING MODALITIES

Efforts have been devoted in the past few years to creating and identifying alternative tests to replace or to reduce the number of AVS performed. Nevertheless, no other test has demonstrated adequate accuracy to replace AVS in a significant number of patients. Conventional cross-sectional imaging with computed tomography (CT) and magnetic resonance imaging (MRI) can be as sensitive as 90% in the detection of adrenal adenomas. However, the high prevalence of nonfunctional adrenal adenomas (around 85% among incidentally detected adrenal masses) makes CT and MRI nonspecific for the diagnosis of aldosteronoma.[8,9] Furthermore, CT does not provide information about the secretory activity of a detected nodule, and densitometry parameters (Hounsfield units) and contrast washout have proven to be inadequate to distinguish aldosterone-producing adenoma (APA) from nonsecretory nodules.[10] MRI is a second-choice imaging modality after CT due to its lower spatial resolution.[11] A review of 38 studies that compared localization by CT/MRI versus AVS showed that 37.8% ($n = 950$) of the CT/MRI results disagreed with AVS results.[12] Based on CT/MRI alone, 14.6% of the patients would have had received adrenalectomy inappropriately (where AVS showed bilateral hypersecretion), 19.1% of the patients would have been inappropriately excluded from adrenalectomy (where AVS showed unilateral hypersecretion), and 3.9% of the patients would have received adrenalectomy on the wrong side (where AVS showed aldosterone secretion on the opposite side).[12] In a study of 367 patients who underwent AVS at our institution, AVS changed management in 43% of the patients ($n = 158$) in whom imaging and AVS results were discordant.[13] Discordant imaging and AVS results would have resulted in wrong-side adrenalectomy in 3% of patients where AVS lateralized to the contralateral side of the imaged mass and in unnecessary surgery in 25% of patients where AVS was nonlateralizing despite a unilateral adrenal mass on imaging.[13] Sixteen percent of patients would have been incorrectly excluded from surgery or potentially not referred for surgery where AVS was lateralizing despite negative cross-sectional imaging.[13] Despite this compelling evidence, it is important to note that AVS is not universally accepted as the gold standard. The SPARTACUS (Subtyping Primary Aldosteronism: A Randomized Trial Comparing Adrenal Vein Sampling and Computed

Advances in Treatment and Management in Surgical Endocrinology. https://doi.org/10.1016/B978-0-323-66195-9.00017-0

Tomography Scan) trial, in which 184 patients with follow-up (among 200 recruited) were randomized to receive CT-based versus AVS-based (post-CT) treatment, no significant difference in intensity of antihypertensive medication or clinical benefits was demonstrated after 1 year of follow-up.[14] However, the study has been criticized for its substantial referral bias, suboptimal outcome measure, and insufficient power.[15]

Imaging increases financial costs and poses health risks to patients. From 2000 to 2008, the use of cross-sectional imaging has risen dramatically in the United States, with increased spending on cross-sectional imaging by 80% and more than doubling the volume of non-brain CTs and MRIs.[16] In addition to the burden of time and cost, CT accounts for most radiation in medical imaging and the corresponding known risks associated with radiation exposure to patients and environmental pollution.[17] In a retrospective analysis of 337 AVS procedures done for PA at our institution from 2001 to 2013, Asmar et al. demonstrated that performing AVS before imaging could have avoided CT/MRI in 43% of patients.[18]

Efficacy of [131]I-6β-iodomethyl-19-norcholesterol adrenal scintigraphy has been suggested in lateralizing aldosterone-secreting adenomas. However, with an accuracy of only 77%, it has not been widely used in the workup of PA.[19] ^{11}C-metomidate positron emission tomography-CT has been assessed for PA-subtype diagnosis, but its sensitivity (76%) and specificity (87%) rendering is not comparable to AVS performed by an experienced operator.[20] Steroid profiling using liquid chromatography coupled to tandem mass spectrometry is currently being investigated for subtype diagnosis.

PATIENT SELECTION

Selection for AVS includes elevated aldosterone, elevated aldosterone-to-renin ratio, and suppressed renin.[21] A flowchart of the algorithm for patient selection is shown in Fig. 17.1. AVS is the only reliable way to correctly diagnose the subtype of PA according to Endocrine Society guidelines, and AVS is recommended to be performed in all patients who have a diagnosis of PA and want to pursue surgical treatment according to the US Endocrine Society guidelines and the Japanese Endocrine Society guidelines.[22,23] However, practice varies among institutions. For example, in the Adrenal Vein Sampling International Study (AVIS) for identifying major subtypes of PA, only 77% of PA patients underwent AVS.[24] The rate of patients undergoing AVS ranged from 19% to nearly 100% between institutions.[24] AVS is not indicated when the patient

prefers lifelong medical treatment or the risks of surgery outweigh the benefits (e.g., multiple comorbidities in elderly patients). AVS is also not required if surgery is already mandated for the patient due to the size of the adenoma or other radiological features suspicious for adrenocortical carcinoma. Before undertaking AVS, familial hyperaldosteronism types I and III should be considered and excluded, at least in young patients with PA and/or patients with a suggestive family history.[25]

Some experts suggest that patients under the age of 40, in whom the likelihood of adrenal incidentaloma is small, may potentially bypass AVS and proceed directly to adrenalectomy if a unilateral mass >10 mm is identified with clear visualization of a normal contralateral adrenal.[21] However, patients who meet these criteria constitute less than 10% of those who might undergo AVS.[26] Furthermore, in a study of 367 patients who underwent AVS at our institution, AVS changed management in 30% ($n = 15$) of patients ≤40 years old and in 16% ($n = 4$) of young patients with clearly identified adrenal masses on imaging.[13] Thus, we recommend AVS in patients under the age of 40.

PREPARATION FOR AVS

At our institution, all patients referred for AVS are screened using a standard intake procedure. This procedure includes obtaining values for aldosterone and renin, calculation of an aldosterone-to-renin ratio, obtaining the results of any imaging (however, based on the study cited above,[18] we do not require imaging before AVS), determining any potentially problematic medications, and obtaining other relevant laboratory data, such as potassium, creatinine, and coagulation parameters. The patient is scheduled for AVS after a diagnosis of PA is confirmed with available laboratory data. Careful adjustment of the antihypertensive agents before AVS is important. Renin-stimulating hypertensive agents, including amiloride, spironolactone, eplerenone, and aliskiren can increase aldosterone secretion from a normally functioning contralateral adrenal gland.[27] This effect may decrease lateralization in AVS resulting in a false-negative study.[28] For this reason, an expert consensus panel recommended that mineralocorticoid receptor antagonists and amiloride be stopped for 4–6 weeks before AVS.[22] Suspending these medications can be problematic as alternative antihypertensives often cannot adequately control patients' hypertension and may result in severe hypokalemia that requires potassium supplementation. In addition, alternatives are often poorly tolerated.[29] Data from

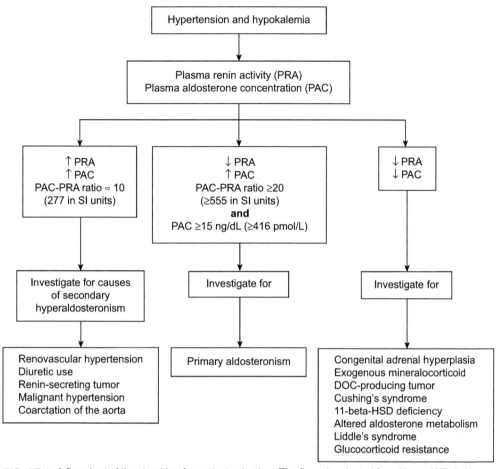

FIG. 17.1 A flowchart of the algorithm for patient selection. (The figure is adapted from Young WF, Jr, Hogan MJ. Renin-Independent hypermineralocorticoidism. *Trends Endocrinol Metab.* 1994;5 (3):97–106)

Ching et al. suggest that patients taking mineralocorticoid receptor (MR) antagonists and/or amiloride may withdraw these antihypertensives using the 2-week protocol without affecting the results of AVS.[30] When doing so, it is prudent to ensure that renin is suppressed on the day of the procedure, because a small percentage of patients will not have their renin suppressed. $\alpha 1$-adrenergic receptor blockers and long-acting calcium channel blockers (preferably nondihydropyridine, such as verapamil or diltiazem) which have no or minimum effects on renin secretion are the preferred drugs to manage blood pressure before AVS.[31] β-blockers and centrally acting antihypertensive agents inhibit renin secretion and should therefore not interfere with AVS results in patients with PA. AVS should be performed after an hour of supine rest if it is performed without

cosyntropin stimulation,[32] because aldosterone secretion by normal adrenal glands approximately doubles in the standing position and may blunt lateralization of aldosterone hypersecretion.

ADRENAL VEIN ANATOMY

A central vein in each adrenal gland constitutes the main venous system of the glands. The right adrenal vein (RAV), formed from three tributaries, arises from the anterior margin of the gland just below the apex and drains directly into the inferior vena cava (IVC) on its midposterior wall, just above the right renal vein. It usually arises from the IVC between T11 and L1 with a mean diameter of 2–5 mm.[33,34] The normal course is posteroinferiorly to the right. In 23% of patients, however, the vein courses posteriorly to the left, and in 11%–38% of patients, the vein runs cranially.[33,34] High-quality CT examination has been advocated in planning AVS; on a modern multislice scanner with reconstruction at 2 or 3 mm, the RAV can be visualized in more than half of patients.[27] However, cross-sectional imaging increases cost, exposes patients to additional radiation, and delays care. Although this approach may be useful for less-experienced operators, we use it very rarely and only after failed AVS.

The RAV and the inferior accessory hepatic vein (IAHV) can have a double-barrel common origin.[27] The IAHV is the most common variation in the hepatic venous system and is present in up to 51% of the population.[35] Previous studies reported that the RAV and IAHV shared and "almost" shared a common trunk in 8% (6 of 79) and 9% of patients, respectively.[27] In 58% of patients whose IAHV was identified on imaging, 12 of 42 (29%) RAVs were immediately adjacent to the IAHV (i.e., distance of 0 mm), and 20 of 42 (48%) or 30 of 42 (71%) RAVs were "almost" common depending on whether one defines "almost" as within 2 mm or 5 mm. The mean distance between the RAV and the IAVH was slightly more than 4 mm, and they were always within 2 cm of each other. Therefore, detection of an IAHV may be a very useful adjunct to all physicians looking to increase their RAV diagnostic yield.[36]

The left adrenal vein (LAV) arises inferiorly along the anterior surface of the adrenal gland and courses inferiorly to join the left inferior phrenic vein before draining into the superior aspect of the left renal vein. The LAV is typically lateral to the inferior phrenic vein. It is approximately 4–5 mm in diameter and extends 1–4 cm in length toward the inferior phrenic vein confluence. The confluence lies 1–3 cm from the left renal vein.[37] Rarely, likely in less than 1% of patients, the left adrenal and inferior phrenic veins enter the left renal vein separately.[38]

ADRENAL VEIN SAMPLING TECHNIQUE

AVS is optimally performed in the morning while the patient is in a fasting state.[39] However, this is likely applicable only when stimulation is not used. AVS is routinely performed with moderate sedation, though local anesthesia alone is an acceptable alternative in patients in whom sedation is not desired or contraindicated. A percutaneous femoral vein approach is typically taken with sequential or simultaneous catheterization of the adrenal veins (see discussion later). The correct position of the catheter is verified by gentle injection of a small volume (no more than 0.1–0.2 mL) of contrast, and blood is then collected by slow aspiration. Although some have advocated "dripping" the blood by gravity, this is not necessary for effective and diagnostic AVS.

LAV cannulation is relatively easy to perform, because it generally merges with the inferior phrenic vein to form a common trunk draining directly into the left renal vein.[40] For left AVS, the tip of the catheter can be placed either in the left inferior phrenic vein or in the adrenal-phrenic trunk.[41] The RAV inserts directly into the IVC in the vicinity of other veins of similar caliber such as the inferior accessory hepatic vein. It is shorter in length and, once cannulated, the catheter may fall out with the motion of breathing. The RAV also tends to collapse under aspiration. Therefore, it is more common to cannulate and sample effluent from an incorrect vein on the right and, even when successfully identified, the RAV is more challenging to sample. At our institution, we use the renal double curve (RDC) catheter to catheterize the RAV first. If catheterization with the RDC catheter is unsuccessful, the following catheters are used generally in the following order: Mikaelsson (Beacon Tip, Cook, Bloomington, IN), Multipurpose (Cook), Cobra (Imager, Boston Scientific, Natick, Massachusetts), HS2 (Cook), and Simmons 1 (Cordis, Miami Lakes, FL) catheters. The order of catheters may change to match the orientation of the RAV if it is identified with the RDC (or another catheter) but cannot be sampled with that catheter. For example, a vein entering the IVC at a right angle would be best sampled with a Mikaelsson. We have fairly recently introduced the multipurpose shape early in the rotation when no RAV is identified, because as noted earlier, the RAV has a cephalad orientation in a sizable percentage of patients. After successful sampling of the RAV, the LAV is catheterized and sampled. The LAV is almost always sampled with a Simmons 3 (Glidecath, Terumo, Somerset, NJ) catheter. Rarely, an exchange for a Berenstein or multipurpose shape is necessary to catheterize the LAV. All catheters have a single 0.025-inch side hole punched approximately 1 mm from the tip (Surgical punch, Syneo, Angleton, TX); for right-sided catheters, this is on the cephalad aspect, and for the left-sided catheter, it is on the inside of the curve (i.e., facing laterally when selective in the adrenal-phrenic trunk or left adrenal vein). The purpose of the holes was originally described to facilitate aspiration if the tip of the catheter is against the vein wall and to capture RAV blood at the origin of the vein if not fully catheterized. The latter remains important, however, when the position of the hole in the right-sided catheter might also help to avoid the "double down' phenomenon (see below) in which too-deep sampling gives a non-diagnostic AVS. If a standard hole punch is not available (Cook no longer sells the punch, however it can be obtained from Syneo as above), cutting a small "V" in the catheter tip has been described.[42] At most two side holes should be made (we make only one) because doing so may dilute the right adrenal sample with IVC blood, resulting in falsely low aldosterone and cortisol levels.[40] If considered necessary by the operator, a high flow microcatheter (e.g., Renegade Hi-Flo; Boston Scientific) can be used through the 5-F catheter. While using a microcatheter results in higher concentrations of hormones, these higher concentrations do not change the management.[43] Thus, microcatheters should only be used when needed to reach an elongated LAV or for superselective sampling prompted by the "double down" phenomenon. In our practice, we use microcatheters less than 5% of the time.

During the search for the RAV in particular, the catheter may engage other veins, including accessory hepatic, retroperitoneal, and phrenic veins.[40] Recognition of their venographic appearance is essential to avoid sampling error. Caution must be taken when using a reverse curve catheter on the right because they are more prone to deeper engagement of the vessel, which may result in overly selective sampling (i.e., beyond the draining vein of the adenoma, see "double down" phenomenon below) or vessel occlusion.[40] Ultimately, as is the case with many interventional procedures, the optimal catheter depends on operator experience, availability, and relevant anatomy.

One of the greatest pitfalls when catheterizing the RAV relates to the inadvertent catheterization of an accessory hepatic vein. Although gentle injection of contrast often delineates the two, appreciating their subtle difference on venography is important. A hepatic radicle may be identified by denser parenchymal staining and absence of discomfort with injection, which conversely may be experienced when the RAV is injected. In addition, communication of the vein with another hepatic vein effectively excludes it as the RAV since hepatic veins never communicate with the RAV, though they can have an origin immediately adjacent to them. In the authors' experience, only once in over 800 AVS procedures has the RAV communicated with a liver vein, and it was the portal vein. Multiple methods have been suggested to improve the results of RAV sampling (see later) and these are particularly useful for less-experienced operators. One of the most helpful of these is identifying an inferior emissary vein, which is 86% sensitive and 100% specific for successful RAV catheterization.[44]

After successful AVS, the patient is recovered; we use 2 h of bedrest for recovery. Once sampling is determined to be successful (see "rapid cortisol assay" later), patients can immediately resume mineralocorticoid receptor antagonists or other medications that were previously withheld, while pending the final aldosterone results.[45] Illustrative cases are shown in Figs. 17.2 and 17.3.

COSYNTROPIN STIMULATION
Cosyntropin is a synthetic derivative of the adrenocorticotropic hormone (ACTH), and infusion of this agent during the AVS procedure was introduced in 1967.[46] Cosyntropin stimulation enhances the plasma cortisol concentration gradient between the adrenal vein and the IVC, reduces stress-induced and diurnal fluctuations in cortisol and aldosterone secretion during sequential AVS, and increases aldosterone secretion from unilateral APA.[6,47,48] No randomized study has yet investigated the effect of using cosyntropin stimulation during AVS on the remission of hypertension and hypokalemia after adrenalectomy. Cosyntropin infusion improves selectivity but may theoretically compromise lateralization[49,50] because it can potentially increase aldosterone production within the normal suppressed gland rather than the one containing the adenoma.[51] Nonetheless, in the AVIS study, 55% of centers used stimulation.[24] Baseline (prestimulation) sampling does not contribute unique diagnostic information and may provide contradictory or confounding information in simultaneous AVS from our experience.[52]

Two main protocols of cosyntropin administration are currently used: (1) continuous infusion (50 μg/h, starting 60 min before the first sampling), and (2) bolus (250 μg [10 IU]). There is no gold standard protocol for method (bolus vs. infusion) or dosage of cosyntropin administration, and varying protocols may contribute to the conflicting data in the literature. A multicenter study compared the roles of continuous cosyntropin infusion and bolus on AVS.[53] Both infusion and bolus increased the selectivity index significantly, but did not affect the lateralization index. In most patients, the diagnosis made with AVS was the same with continuous infusion, bolus or without stimulation.[53] At our institution, 1 h before AVS, continuous infusion of cosyntropin (Amphastar, Rancho Cucamonga, CA) 0.25 mg/500 mL normal saline is initiated and

(A)   **(B)**   **(C)**

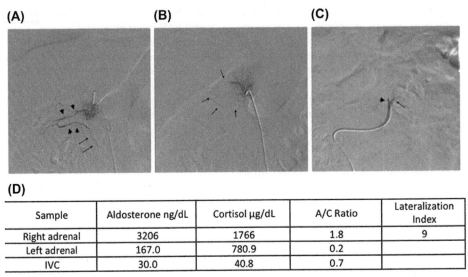

(D)

Sample	Aldosterone ng/dL	Cortisol µg/dL	A/C Ratio	Lateralization Index
Right adrenal	3206	1766	1.8	9
Left adrenal	167.0	780.9	0.2	
IVC	30.0	40.8	0.7	

FIG. 17.2 Illustrative case #1. A 63-year-old man presented with hypertension and hypokalemia. MRI of the abdomen demonstrated a 1.3 × 1.0 cm right adrenal adenoma. The plasma renin activity was 0.2 and aldosterone level 17. The patient underwent AVS. Initial right adrenal venogram **(A)** shows a classic delta sign (arrowheads) as well as an inferior emissary vein (arrows) confirming right adrenal catheterization. Note however that no upper pole adrenal vein is seen. Sampling in this location risks the "double down" phenomenon (see text). In **(B)** the catheter has been retracted slightly and now shows all of the right adrenal vein tributaries; note also the mass effect due to the adenoma (arrows). Sampling was done from this location. Venography on the left shows the catheter to be in the adrenal-phrenic trunk **(C)**. Note the Y-shaped confluence of the phrenic (arrowhead) and left adrenal vein (arrow). Sampling was done in this location. In the results table **(D)**, note a selectivity index (see text) of 43 on the right and 19 on the left, indicating a diagnostic study. The lateralization index (see text) of nine shows that the aldosteronism is due to the right adrenal adenoma; contralateral suppression is also present. The patient underwent right adrenalectomy. At 6-month follow-up, he was able to cease potassium supplementation and some of his antihypertensives with excellent blood pressure control.

maintained until the end of the procedure. If cosyntropin is not used, AVS is best performed in the morning to avoid false-negative results attributable to diurnal fluctuation in ACTH.

SIMULTANEOUS VERSUS SEQUENTIAL CANNULATION

Two techniques of AVS, simultaneous and sequential, are currently being practiced. Simultaneous AVS measures aldosterone and cortisol levels from the right and left adrenal veins and inferior vena cava via two accesses.[54] Sequential catheterization uses a single puncture site to sample both adrenal veins and the IVC.[48] Controversy remains regarding sequential versus simultaneous AVS.[27] In the AVIS study, 13 of the 20 centers used sequential catheterization, and 7 used bilateral simultaneous catheterization.[24]

Simultaneous bilateral catheterization was first introduced in 1980 to minimize differences between sides due to timing,[54] and catheters with different shapes were used on each side to further improve the technique.[50] The main proposed advantage of simultaneous cannulation of the adrenal veins is to avoid the gradient of aldosterone production between the two adrenals being artificially modified due to the oscillations of aldosterone and cortisol secretion, if the procedure is performed under basal conditions.[55] However, simultaneous AVS is more invasive (requiring the insertion of two catheters) and technically demanding than sequential technique. The sequential technique was described by Young et al.[48] in which patients underwent catheterization of the right adrenal vein followed by the left adrenal vein via a single access. Cosyntropin stimulation is used more often in the sequential technique than the simultaneous technique

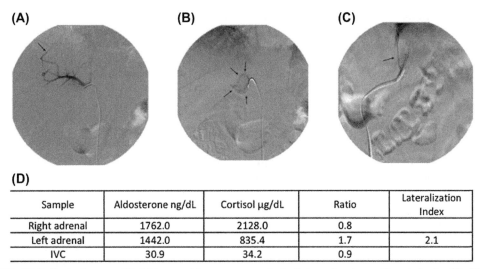

(D)

Sample	Aldosterone ng/dL	Cortisol µg/dL	Ratio	Lateralization Index
Right adrenal	1762.0	2128.0	0.8	
Left adrenal	1442.0	835.4	1.7	2.1
IVC	30.9	34.2	0.9	

FIG. 17.3 Illustrative case #2. A 64-year-old woman presented with hypertension and hypokalemia. CT of the abdomen and pelvis demonstrated a 2.5 × 2.9 cm right adrenal adenoma. The plasma renin activity was 0.3 and aldosterone level 19. The patient was referred for AVS. Initial catheterization on the right **(A)** is an inferior accessory hepatic vein; note the communication with another hepatic vein (arrow), which never occurs with the right adrenal vein. Finding this vein is helpful, as the right adrenal vein will generally be within 1 cm of it and usually much closer. **(B)** shows successful catheterization of the RAV; note that although there are no distinguishing features such as an inferior emissary vein or delta sign, the right adrenal mass is seen (arrows), which confirms RAV catheterization. Nonetheless, only biochemical confirmation can ultimately determine a successful AVS. **(C)** Venography on the left shows relatively deep catheterization of the LAV (arrowhead); the catheter was retracted somewhat before sampling. Note the left phrenic vein (arrow). In the results table **(D)**, note a selectivity index (see text) of 62 on the right and 24 on the left, indicating a diagnostic study. The LI of 2.1 and lack of contralateral suppression indicates that the excess aldosterone secretion is bilateral and the mass is likely nonfunctional. Thus, the patient did not undergo surgery and continued medical management. In this patient, operating on the basis of the CT alone would have resulted in unnecessary and ineffective surgery.

to stabilize hormonal variation.[56] In a study comparing sequential versus simultaneous AVS, mean elapsed time between acquisition of right and left samples was similar between the two techniques.[52]

IMPROVING THE SUCCESS RATE OF AVS

AVS is considered the gold standard in the preoperative localization of aldosterone-secreting adenomas in patients with PA, with high diagnostic rates ranging from 92% to 100%.[6,57–59] However, the utility of AVS has been limited in the past by failure rates as high as 70%,[27,60] which was likely because AVS is technically demanding.[39,40,60] Interventional radiologists' experience and dedication are fundamental to successful procedures. Some centers are fortunate to assign all AVS to one or a few interventional radiologists who are highly skilled in the procedure,[39] and this circumstance is ideal due to the infrequency of AVS in most practices. The

technical success rate of AVS at our institution is over 95%.[45] In a study of 343 AVS procedures performed over a 10-year period, AVS was nondiagnostic in 12 of 343 (3.5%) primary procedures and 2 secondary procedures.[45] Failure occurred via the following mechanisms: sample from the correctly identified vein was diluted ($n = 7$ [50%]; three right and four left); other vessel misidentified as adrenal vein ($n = 3$ [21%]; all right); adrenal vein could not be located ($n = 2$ [14%]; both right); cosyntropin stimulation failure ($n = 1$ [7%]; diagnostic by nonstimulated criteria); laboratory error ($n = 1$ [7%]; specimen loss). Recent innovations include the use of cone beam CT,[61] rapid cortisol assay,[62,63] and intraprocedural imaging adjuncts such as visualization of the inferior accessory hepatic vein[36] and the inferior emissary vein,[44] and the ultimate effect of these innovations in aggregate on AVS success at the global level is yet to be determined.

INTRAPROCEDURAL CORTISOL ANALYSIS

Hormonal data are normally not available until well after AVS is completed, and judgment of selectivity can only be achieved retrospectively. The so-called "rapid cortisol assay" enables the interventional radiologist to be confident that both adrenal veins are sampled adequately either during the procedure or while the patient is recovering.[64,65] Cortisol is measured immediately after sampling from each site, and results are available in a short time (less than 30 min), enabling almost immediate feedback on the success of the procedure. The rapid cortisol assay has been shown to be helpful in several studies.[60,63,65,66] In one center, intraprocedural cortisol measurement increased the success rate of AVS from 50% to 89%.[67] Cortisol can be measured in the central laboratory of the hospital[60,63,68] or in the interventional radiology (IR) suite using a benchtop analyzer.[65] The latter method, performed with a reliable cortisol immunofluorimetric assay[65] or with immunochromatography and gold nanoparticles,[69] more rapidly provides information to the interventional radiologist on the position of the catheter tip. Rapid cortisol measurements enable the operator to attempt cannulating the adrenal veins again if the sample is inadequate, and allow them to progressively improve their success rate.[60] In our practice, we only rarely use the rapid cortisol assay intraprocedurally because the 30-min delay inherent in the assay unnecessarily prolongs the procedure in experienced hands. However, the ability to tell the patient that the procedure was successful before they leave and to allow them to resume any medications they suspended makes it a patient-friendly addition to AVS.

CONE-BEAM CT AND CT VENOGRAPHY

C-arm cone-beam CT (CBCT) performed during AVS allows near perfect catheter placement according to small series.[61,70] The reader is reminded that simply identifying catheter placement in the RAV does not equate with successful AVS-only the biochemical result defines AVS success (see later). CBCT may be a useful tool for inexperienced operators; in our practice, we use it very rarely (<<5% of AVS) and as a problem-solving tool only. It is possible that high-resolution CT scanning with late venous-phase images and/or three-dimensional reconstruction will help to define the RAV anatomy before the procedure and improve success rates for difficult cases. However, using a modality with significant radiation exposure and cost can be challenging to justify for a small diagnostic yield gain when it is unnecessary in >95% of patients. For repeat

procedures, using CT venography might be the ideal way to maximize yield at the subsequent AVS attempt(s). In our published institutional experience, CT venography helped to successfully localize the right adrenal vein in two patients who were subjected to CT venography for repeat AVS.[45] Unfortunately, even when the vein's location was known and catheterization was successful, one of these samples proved to be diluted below our diagnostic threshold. Thus, merely knowing where the vein is, or even successful catheterization, does not guarantee successful sampling.

SEGMENTAL AVS

"Super-selective" adrenal venous sampling (ssAVS), where tributaries of each adrenal vein (superior, lateral, and inferior) are sampled with a microcatheter, has been recently described.[71-74] Segmental adrenal lesions can be detected by ssAVS, which allows for partial bilateral adrenalectomies that spare normal adrenal tissue. Theoretically, ssAVS could help to identify patients with bilateral focal lesions who are surgical candidates who otherwise would have been diagnosed with bilateral adrenal hyperplasia. However, segmental AVS is technically more demanding, time consuming, and expensive.[74] Furthermore, in two case series, contrast extravasation occurred in 12.6%[74] and 16%[73] of patients undergoing segmental AVS, a higher complication rate than in central AVS.[74] In addition, partial adrenalectomy is not widely practiced. Superselective AVS is probably most useful in repeat AVS following a "double down" result, see later.

AVS INTERPRETATION CRITERIA

Although there are accepted criteria to define selectivity of adrenal vein catheterization and lateralization of aldosterone, evidence for optimal diagnostic accuracy of selectivity and lateralization cutoffs ideally should come from prospective studies in patients undergoing unilateral adrenalectomy regardless of AVS results. The hormonal outcome of adrenalectomy would indicate whether the PA was truly lateralized or not, which would determine the selectivity and lateralization thresholds to achieve the best sensitivity and specificity. Unfortunately, no such prospective randomized study exists.

The selectivity index (SI), the ratio of cortisol in each adrenal vein to that in the infrarenal IVC, is used to assess the selectivity of adrenal catheterization based on the differential of plasma cortisol between the two vessels. The SI is the gold standard as it is biochemical proof (rather than imaging) of selectivity. To account for dilution, the raw aldosterone levels are not compared side to side. Rather, the aldosterone-to-cortisol ratio is determined and the A/C ratio is compared. The lateralization index (LI), which consists of the higher A/C ratio divided by the lower A/C ratio, is used to establish whether a lateralized aldosterone excess exists. The contralateral suppression index, determined by dividing the A/C ratio of each side by that of the IVC, is used to determine whether the aldosterone concentration in the adrenal vein blood is higher or lower than expected based on the peripheral venous level of the hormone. Simply put, unilateral hyperfunction should result in suppression of the contralateral gland, so the A/C ratio on that side should be below that of the IVC. The criteria for adequate SIs and localization by LIs are disturbingly empiric and historical. The late John Doppman was probably the first to propose a standard set of criteria, which have been adopted at most major centers that use cosyntropin infusion: SIs of >3−5:1 for adequacy and LI of >4:1 for lateralization.[54,75] When cosyntropin is not infused, the criteria must be adjusted to compensate for a lower rate of cortisol (and aldosterone) production. Typical SIs are much lower without cosyntropin, and a value of 2:1 is considered adequate,[76] although values as low as 1.1:1 have been suggested,[50] which is close to the inherent error of the cortisol assay. An LI as low as 2:1 in the absence of cosyntropin may be sufficient for lateralization.[50,51] A study by Tagawa et al. demonstrated that LI but not contralateral suppression at AVS predicts improvement in blood pressure after adrenalectomy for PA.[77]

REPEAT AVS

When repeating AVS in a high-volume practice, adjuncts such as CT venography, cone-beam CT, and rapid cortisol assay may be most helpful. Bouhanick et al. published a series of patients in whom repeat AVS was performed for various reasons, including initial failure in four of these patients, and all second procedures were diagnostic.[78] In addition, Betz et al. supported that imaging or cortisol assay adjuncts are more helpful in centers with lower diagnostic yield.[63]

In the 12 nondiagnostic AVS cases from our published experience of 343 AVS procedures, a second AVS procedure was diagnostic in three of five cases (60%), and a third AVS procedure was diagnostic in one of one case (100%).[45] Among the eight patients in whom AVS ultimately was not diagnostic, four underwent adrenalectomy based on diluted AVS samples, and one underwent adrenalectomy based on imaging; aldosteronism improved in all five.

THE "DOUBLE DOWN" PHENOMENON

If both adrenal vein A/C ratios are lower than that of the IVC, the differential diagnosis includes extraadrenal secretion (very rare), accessory adrenal veins not sampled, and too-deep sampling.[79] When preparing for a repeat AVS in this setting, a high-quality CT venogram may help determine anatomic variants; however, superselective sampling is still important (paradoxically) to exclude too-deep sampling. Unfortunately, the rapid cortisol assay is not helpful here, as this phenomenon is observed even though the SI shows successful catheterization of the adrenal veins.

COMPLICATIONS

AVS is a safe procedure with less than 1% reported complication rates. For example, in the AVIS study, the overall rate of adrenal vein rupture was only 0.61%.[24] Complications are more common in the right compared to the left adrenal vein, likely due to the anatomic diversity and complexity. The most common complication, as with any transvenous procedure, is femoral hematoma. Other rare complications, such as adrenal vein and gland hemorrhage, can result from strong adrenal vein injections, and present as pain that may persist for 1−2 days. Adrenal vein rupture clinically manifests as persistent pain during or after catheterization, which intensifies and requires large doses of analgesics for 24−48 h.[40] Major complications, such as adrenal insufficiency, hypertensive crisis, and thrombosis, are rare and inversely correlated to operator experience. There is a significant inverse correlation between the number of procedures performed and the rate of complications.[24] In the AVIS study, the average number of AVS performed annually for each center was generally below 40 and ranged between 16 in 2005 and 34 in 2010.[24] Thus, the ideal situation would be if all procedures should be assigned to one interventional radiologist in most centers where the limited number of AVS performed yearly makes it possible.

QUALITY IN AVS

To achieve optimal AVS results, in addition to developing operator expertise, all members of the team must be committed to maximizing diagnostic yield and minimizing errors. Redundancy protocols for specimens (e.g., time of specimen plus location) will allow problem solving when results seem erroneous. Handoff protocols will ensure specimens are not misplaced or lost. Keeping a backup sample allows repeat testing in the event of concerns about a result. A core team of nurses, IR techs, and laboratory techs should be fully educated on the indications for AVS and the implications of error to the patient. Operators should be fully cognizant in real time of their diagnostic yield and provide this to the patient during the informed consent process; educating patients that everyone fails in AVS is critical to setting expectations in the event of a nondiagnostic study. Operators should take responsibility for AVS interpretation and delivery of results to patients as soon as they are available.

SUMMARY

AVS is a challenging, interesting, and rewarding part of Interventional Radiology. While purely diagnostic in most centers, some IRs are pushing the envelope with adrenal ablation in highly selected cases instead of surgery.[80,81] It remains to be seen if this will open a new avenue for management of localized PA. Meanwhile, newer techniques for improving outcomes of AVS can help even beginners achieve acceptable outcomes in a relatively short period of time, which in turn should help further increase the acceptance of AVS as the gold standard worldwide.

REFERENCES

1. Conn JW, Louis LH. Primary aldosteronism, a new clinical entity. *Ann Intern Med.* 1956;44(1):1–15.
2. Conn JW. Presidential address. I. Painting background. II. Primary aldosteronism, a new clinical syndrome. *J Lab Clin Med.* 1955;45(1):3–17.
3. Rossi GP, Bernini G, Caliumi C, et al. A prospective study of the prevalence of primary aldosteronism in 1,125 hypertensive patients. *J Am Coll Cardiol.* 2006;48(11): 2293–2300.
4. Fardella CE, Mosso L, Gomez-Sanchez C, et al. Primary hyperaldosteronism in essential hypertensives: prevalence, biochemical profile, and molecular biology. *J Clin Endocrinol Metab.* 2000;85(5):1863–1867.
5. Gordon RD, Ziesak MD, Tunny TJ, et al. Evidence that primary aldosteronism may not be uncommon: 12% incidence among antihypertensive drug trial volunteers. *Clin Exp Pharmacol Physiol.* 1993;20(5):296–298.
6. Young WF, Stanson AW, Thompson GB, et al. Role for adrenal venous sampling in primary aldosteronism. *Surgery.* 2004;136(6):1227–1235.
7. Buffolo F, Monticone S, Williams TA, et al. Subtype diagnosis of primary aldosteronism: is adrenal vein sampling always necessary? *Int J Mol Sci.* 2017;18(4).
8. Mantero F, Terzolo M, Arnaldi G, et al. A survey on adrenal incidentaloma in Italy. Study group on adrenal tumors of the Italian society of endocrinology. *J Clin Endocrinol Metab.* 2000;85(2):637–644.
9. McAlister FA, Lewanczuk RZ. Primary hyperaldosteronism and adrenal incidentaloma: an argument for physiologic testing before adrenalectomy. *Can J Surg.* 1998;41(4): 299–305.
10. Blake MA, Cronin CG, Boland GW. Adrenal imaging. *AJR.* 2010;194(6):1450–1460.
11. Schieda N, Siegelman ES. Update on CT and MRI of adrenal nodules. *AJR.* 2017;208(6):1206–1217.
12. Kempers MJ, Lenders JW, van Outheusden L, et al. Systematic review: diagnostic procedures to differentiate unilateral from bilateral adrenal abnormality in primary aldosteronism. *Ann Intern Med.* 2009;151(5):329–337.
13. Wachtel H, Zaheer S, Shah PK, et al. Role of adrenal vein sampling in primary aldosteronism: impact of imaging, localization, and age. *J Surg Oncol.* 2016;113(5):532–537.
14. Dekkers T, Prejbisz A, Kool LJS, et al. Adrenal vein sampling versus CT scan to determine treatment in primary aldosteronism: an outcome-based randomised diagnostic trial. *Lancet Diabetes Endocrinol.* 2016;4(9):739–746.
15. Rossi GP, Funder JW. Adrenal venous sampling versus computed tomographic scan to determine treatment in primary aldosteronism (the SPARTACUS trial): a critique. *Hypertension.* 2017;69(3):396–397.
16. A Data Book: Healthcare Spending and the Medicare Program, Medicare Payment Advisory Commission.
17. Mettler Jr FA, Bhargavan M, Faulkner K, et al. Radiologic and nuclear medicine studies in the United States and worldwide: frequency, radiation dose, and comparison with other radiation sources–1950–2007. *Radiology.* 2009;253(2):520–531.
18. Asmar M, Wachtel H, Yan Y, et al. Reversing the established order: should adrenal venous sampling precede cross-sectional imaging in the evaluation of primary aldosteronism? *J Surg Oncol.* 2015;112(2):144–148.
19. Yen RF, Wu VC, Liu KL, et al. 131I-6beta-iodomethyl-19-norcholesterol SPECT/CT for primary aldosteronism patients with inconclusive adrenal venous sampling and CT results. *J Nucl Med.* 2009;50(10):1631–1637.
20. Burton TJ, Mackenzie IS, Balan K, et al. Evaluation of the sensitivity and specificity of (11)C-metomidate positron emission tomography (PET)-CT for lateralizing aldosterone secretion by Conn's adenomas. *J Clin Endocrinol Metab.* 2012;97(1):100–109.
21. Young Jr WF, Hogan MJ. Renin-Independent hypermineralocorticoidism. *Trends Endocrinol Metabol.* 1994;5(3):97–106.
22. Funder JW, Carey RM, Mantero F, et al. The management of primary aldosteronism: case detection, diagnosis, and treatment: an endocrine society clinical practice guideline. *J Clin Endocrinol Metab.* 2016;101(5):1889–1916.
23. Nishikawa T, Omura M, Satoh F, et al. Guidelines for the diagnosis and treatment of primary aldosteronism–the Japan Endocrine Society 2009. *Endocr J.* 2011;58(9): 711–721.

24. Rossi GP, Barisa M, Allolio B, et al. The Adrenal Vein Sampling International Study (AVIS) for identifying the major subtypes of primary aldosteronism. *J Clin Endocrinol Metab*. 2012;97(5):1606–1614.

25. Korah HE, Scholl UI. An update on familial hyperaldosteronism. *Horm Metab Res*. 2015;47(13): 941–946.

26. Kupers EM, Amar L, Raynaud A, et al. A clinical prediction score to diagnose unilateral primary aldosteronism. *J Clin Endocrinol Metab*. 2012;97(10):3530–3537.

27. Rossi GP, Auchus RJ, Brown M, et al. An expert consensus statement on use of adrenal vein sampling for the subtyping of primary aldosteronism. *Hypertension*. 2014;63(1): 151–160.

28. Rossi GP. A comprehensive review of the clinical aspects of primary aldosteronism. *Nat Rev Endocrinol*. 2011;7(8): 485–495.

29. Haase M, Riester A, Kropil P, et al. Outcome of adrenal vein sampling performed during concurrent mineralocorticoid receptor antagonist therapy. *J Clin Endocrinol Metab*. 2014;99(12):4397–4402.

30. Ching KC, Cohen DL, Fraker DL, et al. Adrenal vein sampling for primary aldosteronism: a 2-week protocol for withdrawal of renin-stimulating antihypertensives. *Cardiovasc Interv Radiol*. 2017;40(9):1367–1371.

31. Mulatero P, Rabbia F, Milan A, et al. Drug effects on aldosterone/plasma renin activity ratio in primary aldosteronism. *Hypertension*. 2002;40(6):897–902.

32. Rossi GP. New concepts in adrenal vein sampling for aldosterone in the diagnosis of primary aldosteronism. *Curr Hypertens Rep*. 2007;9(2):90–97.

33. Matsuura T, Takase K, Ota H, et al. Radiologic anatomy of the right adrenal vein: preliminary experience with MDCT. *AJR*. 2008;191(2):402–408.

34. Monkhouse WS, Khalique A. The adrenal and renal veins of man and their connections with azygos and lumbar veins. *J Anat*. 1986;146:105–115.

35. Radtke A, Sotiropoulos GC, Molmenti EP, et al. The influence of accessory right inferior hepatic veins on the venous drainage in right graft living donor liver transplantation. *Hepatogastroenterology*. 2006;53(70):479–483.

36. Trerotola SO, Smoger DL, Cohen DL, et al. The inferior accessory hepatic vein: an anatomic landmark in adrenal vein sampling. *J Vasc Interv Radiol*. 2011;22(9): 1306–1311.

37. Cesmebasi A, Du Plessis M, Iannatuono M, et al. A review of the anatomy and clinical significance of adrenal veins. *Clin Anat*. 2014;27(8):1253–1263.

38. Scholten A, Cisco RM, Vriens MR, et al. Variant adrenal venous anatomy in 546 laparoscopic adrenalectomies. *JAMA Surg*. 2013;148(4):378–383.

39. Young WF, Stanson AW. What are the keys to successful adrenal venous sampling (AVS) in patients with primary aldosteronism? *Clin Endocrinol*. 2009;70(1):14–17.

40. Daunt N. Adrenal vein sampling: how to make it quick, easy, and successful. *Radiographics*. 2005;25(suppl 1): S143–S158.

41. Takada A, Suzuki K, Mori Y, et al. Comparison of the central adrenal vein and the common trunk of the left adrenal vein for adrenal venous sampling. *J Vasc Interv Radiol*. 2013;24(4):550–557.

42. Thompson KR, Given MF, et al. Adrenal venous sampling. In: Mauro M, ed. *Image Guided Interventions*. Philadelphia: Elsevier; 2008:1147–1150.

43. Kishino M, Yoshimoto T, Nakadate M, et al. Optimization of left adrenal vein sampling in primary aldosteronism: coping with asymmetrical cortisol secretion. *Endocr J*. 2017;64(3):347–355.

44. Kohi MP, Agarwal VK, Naeger DM, et al. The inferior emissary vein: a reliable landmark for right adrenal vein sampling. *Acta Radiol*. 2015;56(4):454–457.

45. Trerotola SO, Asmar M, Yan Y, et al. Failure mode analysis in adrenal vein sampling: a single-center experience. *J Vasc Interv Radiol*. 2014;25(10):1611–1619.

46. Melby JC, Spark RF, Dale SL, et al. Diagnosis and localization of aldosterone-producing adenomas by adrenal-vein cateterization. *N Engl J Med*. 1967;277(20):1050–1056.

47. Weinberger MH, Grim CE, Hollifield JW, et al. Primary aldosteronism: diagnosis, localization, and treatment. *Ann Intern Med*. 1979;90(3):386–395.

48. Young Jr WF, Stanson AW, Grant CS, et al. Primary aldosteronism: adrenal venous sampling. *Surgery*. 1996;120(6): 913–919; discussion 9-20.

49. Rossi GP, Pitter G, Bernante P, et al. Adrenal vein sampling for primary aldosteronism: the assessment of selectivity and lateralization of aldosterone excess baseline and after adrenocorticotropic hormone (ACTH) stimulation. *J Hypertens*. 2008;26(5):989–997.

50. Rossi GP, Ganzaroli C, Miotto D, et al. Dynamic testing with high-dose adrenocorticotrophic hormone does not improve lateralization of aldosterone oversecretion in primary aldosteronism patients. *J Hypertens*. 2006;24(2): 371–379.

51. Seccia TM, Miotto D, De Toni R, et al. Adrenocorticotropic hormone stimulation during adrenal vein sampling for identifying surgically curable subtypes of primary aldosteronism: comparison of 3 different protocols. *Hypertension*. 2009;53(5):761–766.

52. Carr CE, Cope C, Cohen DL, et al. Comparison of sequential versus simultaneous methods of adrenal venous sampling. *J Vasc Interv Radiol*. 2004;15(11):1245–1250.

53. Monticone S, Satoh F, Giacchetti G, et al. Effect of adrenocorticotropic hormone stimulation during adrenal vein sampling in primary aldosteronism. *Hypertension*. 2012; 59(4):840–846.

54. Doppman JL, Gill Jr JR. Hyperaldosteronism: sampling the adrenal veins. *Radiology*. 1996;198(2):309–312.

55. Seccia TM, Miotto D, Battistel M, et al. A stress reaction affects assessment of selectivity of adrenal venous sampling and of lateralization of aldosterone excess in primary aldosteronism. *Eur J Endocrinol*. 2012;166(5):869–875.

56. Rossi GP, Sacchetto A, Chiesura-Corona M, et al. Identification of the etiology of primary aldosteronism with adrenal vein sampling in patients with equivocal computed

tomography and magnetic resonance findings: results in 104 consecutive cases. *J Clin Endocrinol Metab.* 2001; 86(3):1083–1090.

57. White ML, Gauger PG, Doherty GM, et al. The role of radiologic studies in the evaluation and management of primary hyperaldosteronism. *Surgery.* 2008;144: 926–933; discussion 933.

58. Espiner EA, Ross DG, Yandle TG, et al. Predicting surgically remedial primary aldosteronism: role of adrenal scanning, posture testing, and adrenal vein sampling. *J Clin Endocrinol Metab.* 2003;88(8):3637–3644.

59. heaves R, Goldin J, Reznek RH, et al. Relative value of computed tomography scanning and venous sampling in establishing the cause of primary hyperaldosteronism. *Eur J Endocrinol.* 1996;134(3):308–313.

60. Vonend O, Ockenfels N, Gao X, et al. Adrenal venous sampling: evaluation of the German Conn's registry. *Hypertension.* 2011;57:990–995.

61. eorgiades CS, Hong K, Geschwind JF, et al. Adjunctive use of C-arm CT may eliminate technical failure in adrenal vein sampling. *J Vasc Interv Radiol.* 2007;18(9): 1102–1105.

62. Reardon MA, Angle JF, Abi-Jaoudeh N, et al. Intraprocedural cortisol levels in the evaluation of proper catheter placement in adrenal venous sampling. *J Vasc Interv Radiol.* 2011;22(11):1575–1580.

63. Betz MJ, Degenhart C, Fischer E, et al. Adrenal vein sampling using rapid cortisol assays in primary aldosteronism is useful in centers with low success rates. *Eur J Endocrinol.* 2011;165(2):301–306.

64. Woods JJ, Sampson ML, Ruddel ME, et al. Rapid intraoperative cortisol assay: design and utility for localizing adrenal tumors by venous sampling. *Clin Biochem.* 2000;33(6): 501–503.

65. Mengozzi G, Rossato D, Bertello C, et al. Rapid cortisol assay during adrenal vein sampling in patients with primary aldosteronism. *Clin Chem.* 2007;53(11):1968–1971.

66. Rossi E, Regolisti G, Perazzoli F, et al. Intraprocedural cortisol measurement increases adrenal vein sampling success rate in primary aldosteronism. *Am J Hypertens.* 2011; 24(12):1280–1285.

67. Hayden JA, Kwan SW, Valji K. Implementation of rapid cortisol during adrenal vein sampling. *Hypertension.* 2014;63:e88.

68. Auchus RJ, Michaelis C, Wians Jr FH, et al. Rapid cortisol assays improve the success rate of adrenal vein sampling for primary aldosteronism. *Ann Surg.* 2009;249(2): 318–321.

69. Yoneda T, Karashima S, Kometani M, et al. Impact of new quick gold nanoparticle-based cortisol assay during adrenal vein sampling for primary aldosteronism. *J Clin Endocrinol Metab.* 2016;101(6):2554–2561.

70. Park SI, Rhee Y, Lim JS, et al. Right adrenal venography findings correlated with C-arm CT for selection during C-arm CT-assisted adrenal vein sampling in primary

aldosteronism. *Cardiovasc Interv Radiol.* 2014;37: 1469–1475.

71. Makita K, Nishimoto K, Kiriyama-Kitamoto K, et al. A novel method: super-selective adrenal venous sampling. *JoVE.* 2017;(127).

72. Omura M, Saito J, Matsuzawa Y, et al. Supper-selective ACTH-stimulated adrenal vein sampling is necessary for detecting precisely functional state of various lesions in unilateral and bilateral adrenal disorders, inducing primary aldosteronism with subclinical Cushing's syndrome. *Endocr J.* 2011;58(10):919–920.

73. Satani N, Ota H, Seiji K, et al. Intra-adrenal aldosterone secretion: segmental adrenal venous sampling for localization. *Radiology.* 2016;278(1):265–274.

74. Satoh F, Morimoto R, Seiji K, et al. Is there a role for segmental adrenal venous sampling and adrenal sparing surgery in patients with primary aldosteronism? *Eur J Endocrinol.* 2015;173(4):465–477.

75. Steichen O, Amar L. Diagnostic criteria for adrenal venous sampling. *Curr Opin Endocrinol Diabetes Obes.* 2016;23(3): 218–224.

76. Mailhot JP, Traistaru M, Soulez G, et al. Adrenal vein sampling in primary aldosteronism: sensitivity and specificity of basal adrenal vein to peripheral vein cortisol and aldosterone ratios to confirm catheterization of the adrenal vein. *Radiology.* 2015;277(3):887–894.

77. Tagawa M, Ghosn M, Wachtel H, et al. Lateralization index but not contralateral suppression at adrenal vein sampling predicts improvement in blood pressure after adrenalectomy for primary aldosteronism. *J Hum Hypertens.* 2017; 31(7):444–449.

78. Bouhanick B, Delchier MC, Fauvel J, et al. Is it useful to repeat an adrenal venous sampling in patients with primary hyperaldosteronism? *Ann Cardiol Angiol.* 2014; 63(1):23–27.

79. Shibayama Y, Wada N, Umakoshi H, et al. Bilateral aldosterone suppression and its resolution in adrenal vein sampling of patients with primary aldosteronism: analysis of data from the WAVES-J study. *Clin Endocrinol.* 2016;85(5):696–702.

80. Minowada S, Fujimura T, Takahashi N, et al. Computed tomography-guided percutaneous acetic acid injection therapy for functioning adrenocortical adenoma. *J Clin Endocrinol Metab.* 2003;88(12):5814–5817.

81. Munver R, Del Pizzo JJ, Sosa RE. Adrenal-preserving minimally invasive surgery: the role of laparoscopic partial adrenalectomy, cryosurgery, and radiofrequency ablation of the adrenal gland. *Curr Urol Rep.* 2003;4(1):87–92.

FURTHER READING

1. Monticone S, Viola A, Rossato D, et al. Adrenal vein sampling in primary aldosteronism: towards a standardised protocol. *The lancet Diabetes & Endocrinology.* 2015;3(4): 296–303.

CHAPTER 18

Advances in the Diagnosis and Management of Insulinoma

IRENE LOU, MD • WILLIAM B. INABNET III, MD, MHA

INTRODUCTION

Insulinomas are the most common of the functional pancreatic neuroendocrine tumors.[1] These tumors are typically small (<2 cm), well circumscribed and benign. Insulinomas occur in 1−4 people per million and represent 1%−2% of all pancreatic neoplasms.[2] Less than 10% are malignant or multiple, and they are equally distributed throughout the pancreas.[3] Most insulinoma are located within the pancreas and evenly distributed between the head, body, and tail; however, ectopic insulinoma can occur outside the pancreas within the duodenal wall.[2]

Pancreatic islet cells were first described in 1869 by Paul Langerhans.[4] It was not until 1922 that Frederick Banting and Charles Best discovered insulin itself, from a solution extract of canine pancreas.[5]

PRESENTATION

Patients typically present between 40 and 45 years old, with symptoms of hypoglycemia as a result of fasting. Typically, symptoms are due to hypoglycemia of the central nervous system resulting in headaches, confusion, and visual disturbances or because of an excess of catecholamines secondary to hypoglycemia resulting in symptoms such as palpitations, sweating, and tremors. The original description of Whipple's triad consists of symptoms of hypoglycemia, plasma glucose less than 40 mg/dL, and relief of symptoms with the administration of glucose.[4] Approximately 10% of insulinomas are associated with a hereditary syndrome, most commonly multiple endocrine neoplasia type 1 (MEN1) followed by von Hippel−Lindau disease.[6,7]

PATHOPHYSIOLOGY

Insulinoma can occur sporadically, or as part of MEN-1 syndrome. MEN-1 is an autosomal dominant disorder associated with mutations in the MEN1 gene, which maps to chromosome 11q13.[8] Somatic mutations and loss of heterozygosity in MEN1 have also been shown in nonhereditary endocrine tumors such as insulinoma.[9] A recent study specifically examining 38 human insulinomas revealed that many of these tumors display mutations and dysregulation of epigenetic modifying genes that are coupled with factors associated with cell proliferation. This work reveals potential candidates for inducing β-cell regeneration.[10]

DIAGNOSIS

Clinically, patients must demonstrate elevated insulin-to-glucose ratio during fasting with associated elevated levels of c-peptide. If factitious hypoglycemia is suspected, levels of urine or plasma sulfonylurea metabolites can also be measured. The gold standard for diagnosis is a 72-h fast during which plasma c-peptide, glucagon, proinsulin, insulin, and glucose levels are closely monitored. The patient has baseline insulin and glucose levels measured, and undergoes a fast for 72 h or until symptoms develop. Glucose is measured every 2 h, and insulin is checked at the onset of hypoglycemic symptoms or when the blood glucose falls below 50 mg/dL.[1,11] Failure of insulin suppression in the setting of hypoglycemia supports a diagnosis of an insulinoma. Symptoms appear in 75% of patients within the first 24 h of fasting, and 95% of patients after 48 h of fasting if an insulinoma is present. With currently available assays however, a 48 h fast has also

Advances in Treatment and Management in Surgical Endocrinology. https://doi.org/10.1016/B978-0-323-66195-9.00018-2

been found to have great success in making a diagnosis.[12]

Several provocative tests can also be administered if the diagnosis of insulinoma remains unclear. Patients with suspected insulinoma can be given an infusion of insulin until hypoglycemia develops, with c-peptide levels drawn at baseline and during infusion. Patients with insulinoma will show no suppression of c-peptide levels. Tolbutamide, a sulfonylurea oral hypoglycemia medication, stimulates the synthesis and release of endogenous insulin. Patients with insulinoma

when given the medication will have persistent hypoglycemia and elevated serum insulin levels. This boasts an 80% sensitivity. Glucagon, which stimulates liver glycogenolysis, when given to insulinoma patients will reveal a rapid rise in glucose with subsequent severe hypoglycemia and persistent elevated insulin levels, and can make the diagnosis in 70% of patients.[13] A diagnostic algorithm is shown in Table 18.1.

In tumors that are multiple, there should be a high clinical suspicion of MEN-1. While not the most common neuroendocrine tumor associated with MEN-1,

TABLE 18.1
Diagnostic Algorithm for Suspected Insulinoma.

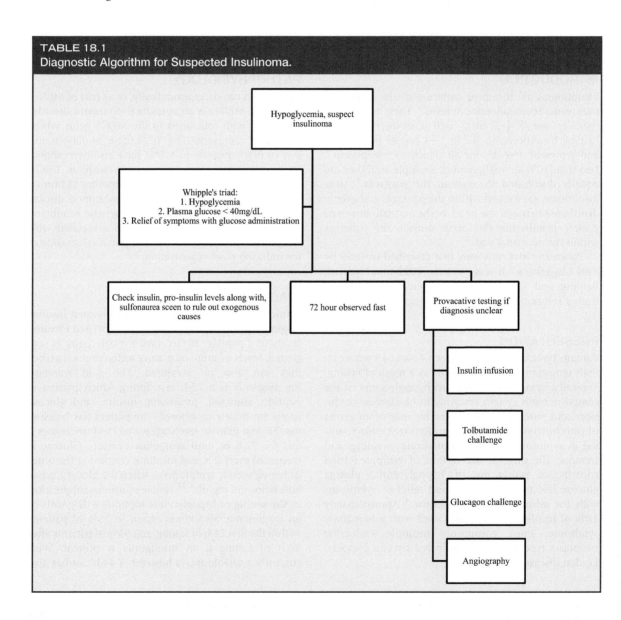

patients below 40 years old with MEN-1 more frequently have insulinomas.[14]

IMAGING

Insulinomas usually occur within the pancreas, but due to their small size with greater than 80% of tumors <2 cm, they can be difficult to localize. Thin section CT, and MRI are easily available and the initial imaging modality of choice. With improvements in advance imaging, a dual-phase thin section multidetector CT can detect insulinoma in 94%, 57% for dual-phase multidetector CT without thin sections.[15] (Fig. 18.1) A fat-saturated T1 weighted spin echosequence has improved MRI detection of insulinoma up to 94%.[16] Endoscopic ultrasound (EUS) has been shown to be positive in 70%–95% of cases, and is the procedures of choice if other noninvasive studies are negative. Some groups promote routine EUS, however, the success of this imaging modality is linked to the experience of the EUS team. EUS is particularly helpful in identifying small pancreatic lesions, especially when they are located in the head and body.[17] Pancreatic islet cell tumors can also be biopsied by EUS to assist with the diagnosis if the diagnosis has not been unequivocally confirmed. Visceral arteriography alone can be used to localize a suspected insulinoma, with localization rates reported as high as 84%.[18] Selective angiography can also be performed, and combined with hepatic venous sampling for insulin levels after calcium stimulation has reported high rates of successful localization.[19,20] This technique is based on the idea that the insulin response from tumor cells differ than normal β-cells when stimulated by calcium injection.[21,22] When given IV calcium, patients with insulinoma will have a rise in insulin levels, whereas normal patients will show no significant change in insulin or glucose levels.

Neuroendocrine tumors (NET) in general have a particularly high density of somatostatin receptors, which allows the use of radiolabeled somatostatin analogs for imaging. Somatostatin-receptor scans can sometimes be useful, however have a sensitivity of only 14% of insulinoma cases due to either the low density or lack of somatostatin receptors compared to other PNETs.[23]

The newest technique for localization of neuroendocrine tumor is the ^{68}Ga-DOTATATE PET/CT. DOTA-DPhe^1,Tyr^3-octreotate (DOTATATE) is a somatostatin-2 receptor (SSR-2) analog, which is radiolabeled with ^{68}Ga, a positron emitter.[24] The ^{68}Ga-DOTATATE molecule has high affinity for the SSR-2 receptor with rapid washout of nonreceptor sites allowing improved identification of NET. Combined with ^{18}F-fluorodeoxyglucose (^{18}F-FDG) positron emission tomography (PET)/CT, this boasts an accuracy of 87%, with an 81% positive predictive value and a 90% negative predictive value.[25] Comparing ^{68}Ga-DOTATATE PET/CT with the most commonly used type of octreotide scan for neuroendocrine tumors, the DOTATATE scan identified significantly more lesions as well as changed management in 70.6% of cases.[26] In insulinomas, ^{68}Ga-DOTATATE PET/CT is able to identify 90% of insulinomas, making this a useful adjunct when there is any question of localization, or when all other imaging studies have been negative.[27]

SURGICAL MANAGEMENT

William Mayo performed the first operative exploration for insulinoma in 1926 in a physician with a history of severe and unpredictable hypoglycemic attacks.[28] Since then, surgery has played an important role in the management of insulinomas. Insulinomas differ from other PNETs due to their low malignant potential. Less than 10% are malignant; therefore, over 90% of patients can achieve cure with resection. Localization is a cornerstone in insulinoma management with multiple invasive and noninvasive imaging modalities available. Localization also allows for a minimally invasive approach for resection. Exploratory laparotomy using bimanual palpation and intraoperative ultrasound can identify insulinomas with great sensitivity.[29] If exploration is unable to identify the tumor however, blind pancreatic resection is not advised.

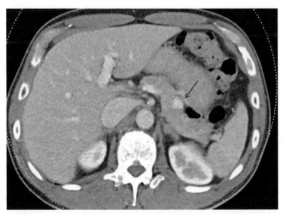

FIG. 18.1 Thin slice axial contrasted CT scan section of a well-localized insulinoma in the pancreatic body (arrow). The patient was able to undergo a minimally invasive pancreatic enucleation.

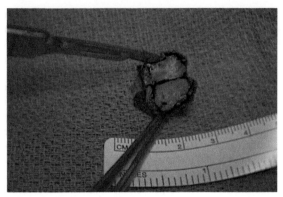

FIG. 18.2 Classic gross appearance of insulinoma postenucleation.

Insulinomas are located uniformly throughout the pancreas, with 1/3 in the head, 1/3 in the body, and 1/3 in the tail and generally small (Fig. 18.2). Most patients found to have an insulinoma undergo pancreatic enucleation, less commonly pancreatic resection with cure rates of 85%–95%. Enucleation is increasingly being performed laparoscopically and can be safely done if the tumor is farther than 2–3 mm away from the pancreatic duct. Otherwise, a partial pancreatic resection is warranted. In most cases, lymphadenectomy is not required, except in the rare exception when a malignant insulinoma is suspected. Reoperations if required for insulinomas can provide successful cure at experienced centers, though there is an increase in operative morbidity and postoperative diabetes.[30]

PREOPERATIVE

Control of hypoglycemia preoperatively is paramount. This can be done with lifestyle changes such as eating frequent mixed-carbohydrate meals, and reducing exercise that will increase overall metabolic requirements. Additionally, medications such as steroids and diazoxide may be used to aid in preventing hypoglycemia. The patient should be admitted the day before surgery and placed on an intravenous dextrose infusion so as to not develop hypoglycemia while fasting (Table 18.2).

There are multiple minimally invasive approaches to insulinoma resection. Early experiences with laparoscopy showed successful rates of pancreatic enucleation and distal pancreatectomy.[31] More recent studies on the safety and efficacy of minimally invasive pancreatic surgery demonstrated that laparoscopic distal pancreatectomy and enucleation of insulinoma is safe and reduces hospital length of stay compared to conventional open surgery.[32,33]

Robotic surgery has been widely applied to different specialties, including pancreatic surgery. The robotic approach is safe, with comparable short-term oncologic outcomes.[34] When compared to laparoscopy, the robotic approach reports lower rates of conversion to open and higher rates of splenic preservation, but with higher cost and longer operative times.[35] Both minimally invasive approaches report comparable outcomes including length of stay.

INTRAOPERATIVE

If the patient is preoperatively localized, enucleation or pancreatic resection may be performed in a minimally invasive way. In a nonlocalized patient with sporadic insulinoma, surgical exploration is indicated. When the insulinoma cannot be localized preoperatively or intraoperatively, blind distal resection is not recommended due to low likelihood of cure and high complication rates.[36] Close communication with the anesthesia team is paramount. Blood sugars should be monitored closely throughout the case, in 15-min intervals to detect intraoperative hypoglycemia. The IV dextrose infusion can be stopped once the tumor is removed, and blood sugars continue to be carefully monitored (Table 18.2).

As most of these tumors are intrapancreatic, intraoperative ultrasound (IOUS) is mandatory. Full mobilization of the pancreas is required to perform IOUS adequately. IOUS alone has been shown to identify up to 90% of insulinomas even without palpation.[37] IOUS also allows identification of the relationship of the tumor to vital structures, including the pancreatic duct, splenic vessels, common bile duct, and superior mesenteric vessels. Manual palpation alone also has an approximately 90% sensitivity in localization, with tumors in the tail and body easier to palpate than those located in the head of the pancreas or uncinate process. However, when manual palpation and IOUS are using in conjunction, this combination can virtually identify 100% of insulinomas.[38]

Frozen section of any removed tissue may also be helpful in identifying if neuroendocrine tissue was removed. Patients should be taken off any exogenous glucose after insulinoma resection. Intraoperative insulin sampling is another adjunctive measure. Blood from the exposed portal vein and a peripheral vein is simultaneously drawn before any manipulation or resection of the tumor. Twenty minutes after resection, simultaneous systemic and portal blood samples are again drawn. Resection is considered completed when a patient who had elevated insulin levels before resection

TABLE 18.2
Management for Patients With Insulinoma Preparing for Resection.

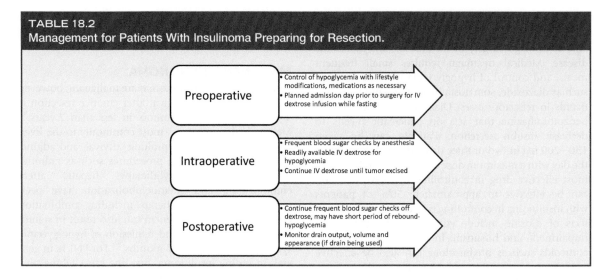

Preoperative
• Control of hypoglycemia with lifestyle modifications, medications as necessary
• Planned admission day prior to surgery for IV dextrose infusion while fasting

Intraoperative
• Frequent blood sugar checks by anesthesia
• Readily available IV dextrose for hypoglycemia
• Continue IV dextrose until tumor excised

Postoperative
• Continue frequent blood sugar checks off dextrose, may have short period of rebound-hypoglycemia
• Monitor drain output, volume and appearance (if drain being used)

achieves decreased levels to the normal range at 20 min after resection. In patients who demonstrate elevated insulin level before resection, the specificity and positive predictive value of complete resection if post-resection value normalized were 100%. In patients with MEN-1 or multiple tumors, this method may be useful to determine if additional operative exploration is warranted.[39] At the conclusion of the case, drain placement is recommended, though not required around the area of the dissection, to facilitate evaluation for possible pancreatic fistula.

Patients with known or suspected MEN-1 typically develop symptoms earlier, and these tumors are frequently multiple and have higher recurrence rates than sporadic cases.[40] Therefore, simple enucleation or local resection is less likely to be curative and subtotal pancreatectomy in addition to enucleation of tumors in the head of the pancreas may be required.[40–42] Genetic testing can be offered if the diagnosis has not been made, or is unclear. Despite a failure to detect the MEN1 mutation in 10%–25% of cases, genetic testing is important in the workup of patients with high clinical suspicious as it would allow other affected family members to be tested.[43]

POSTOPERATIVE

Initially, blood sugar should still be checked frequently to closely monitor for any hypoglycemia. Often, patients will experience a short period of rebound hyperglycemia, which can often be observed and managed without additional administration of insulin. Postoperative complications from the actual pancreatic surgery include formation of pseudocyst, pancreatitis, intraabdominal abscess, development of diabetes, and pancreatic fistula (Table 18.2).

Pancreatic fistula is a frequent complication encountered after pancreatic surgery. What constitutes a pancreatic fistula was previously unclear.[44] Therefore, the International Study Group of Pancreatic Fistula has developed a more universally accepted definition. The quality and quantity of fluid from the intraoperatively placed drain is important in the evaluation of possible pancreatic fistula, as the drain fluid can be subjectively tested for fluid amylase. Pancreatic fistula is defined by a grading system of severity; however, a drain output of any measureable volume with an amylase greater than three times the upper limit of institution normal in association with clinical correlation can confirm the diagnosis. Grade A fistula refers to a biochemical leak, of minimal clinical consequence and is therefore no longer considered a true pancreatic fistula. Grade B fistula changes postoperative management in which continued observation with the drain in place for more than 3 weeks, or repositioning of the drain via endoscopic or percutaneous procedures is required. Grade C fistulas refer to those that lead to one or multiple organ system failure, and require reoperation.[45] Although reoperation is reserved for patients who have failed or are too unstable for other treatment options, a large review has shown a success rate of up to 92%, with a mortality of 6%–9%.[46]

NONOPERATIVE MANAGEMENT

Medical treatment is reserved for those unwilling, or unable to undergo surgery or for unresectable metastatic disease. Medical treatment requires small frequent meals, and control of hypoglycemia with medications such as diazoxide, somatostatin analogs, and glucocorticoids in refractory cases. Diazoxide is a nondiuretic benzothiodiazine that acts on pancreatic β-cells to decrease insulin secretion. Patients can be given 150–200 mg in two or three doses divided throughout the day with a maximum dose of 400 mg/day.[47] It is the most effective drug in controlling hypoglycemia and can be effective in approximately 50% of patients with insulinoma in controlling blood glucose.[48] Side effects of dioxide include edema, weight gain, renal impairment, and hirsutism. In refractory cases, glucocorticoids such as prednisolone can also be effective as well. In tumors that express somatostatin receptor subtype-2, somatostatin analogs such as octreotide may be used to help prevent hypoglycemia, but may exacerbate symptoms in those with tumors without receptor expression.[49] Octreotide also suppresses the release of glucagon and growth hormone, and therefore can intrinsically lower blood sugars.[50,51] Long-term side effects of octreotide treatment mimic patients observed with somatostatinomas include mild diabetes, cholelithiasis, malabsorption, and weight loss.[52] Select cases have also been medically managed with interferon-α.

Stereotactic radiosurgery (CyberKnife) is a minimally invasive procedure delivering large doses of ionizing radiation to a well-defined target. This technique has been reported to be used in a patient with pancreatic insulinoma. The authors report continued glycemic control at 3 years following treatment therefore adding this approach in select high-risk patients who are otherwise not eligible for surgery.[53]

EUS-guided alcohol ablation of insulinoma has also been performed safely with efficacy in patients who are poor surgical candidates, refuse surgery, or after incomplete surgical resection.[54] A case report of 95% ethanol solution injected endoscopically into a well-localized insulinoma results in resolution of hypoglycemia symptoms as well as no discrete tumor recurrence at 34 months.[55]

PATHOLOGY

Certain macroscopic, microscopic, and immunohistochemical findings support the diagnosis of insulinoma to allow for appropriate classification. Microscopically, evaluation of mitotic index and Ki67 is required.[49] Histologically, malignant insulinomas are difficult to distinguish and the diagnosis often occurs when there is evidence of metastatic disease.[56]

MALIGNANT INSULINOMA

Only 5%–10% of insulinomas are malignant; however, median disease-free survival after curative resection is 5 years with recurrent tumors in less than 2 years.[57] Metastatic disease occurs most commonly to the liver. Palliative resection may prolong survival, and adjunctive palliative debulking procedures such as radiofrequency ablation, cryotherapy, hepatic artery embolization, and chemoembolization have been used.[58] Systemic chemotherapy including combination doxorubicin and streptozocin can also result in significant tumor regression and remission of hypoglycemic symptoms, durable to 18 months.[59] For PNETs in general, including insulinoma, first-line capecitabine plus temozolomide has reported favorable results achieving a 70% objective tumor response with dacarbazine used as second-line therapy.[60] Mammalian target of rapamycin mTOR has been identified as abnormally active in PNETs. Therefore, Everolimus, an mTOR inhibitor, has also been shown to be an effective new treatment for metastatic insulinoma with the additional benefit of treating refractory hypoglycemia.[61,62] Peptide receptor radiotherapy (PRRT) requires the presence of somatostatin receptor subtypes on tumor cells to effectively bind the radioligand, but has been shown to have some efficacy in treating hyperinsulinism and maintaining euglycemia in insulinoma patients.[61]

OUTCOMES

The overall 5-year survival after insulinoma is excellent at 97%, with 100% disease-specific survival, and 90% disease-free survival. Most patients with benign disease can expect a normal lifespan after successful surgical resection.[1] A 25-year experience reported from the Massachusetts General Hospital revealed only lymphovascular invasion on multivariate analysis to be predictive of disease recurrence, with most recurrences occurring within the first 5 years.[63] The Mayo clinic series of 224 patients who underwent surgery for insulinoma found that 87% of patients were asymptomatic at 6 months postoperatively, with a recurrence of hypoglycemia of 6% at 10 years and 8% at 20 years. Patients who underwent insulinoma resection also showed no difference in overall survival compared to the general population. The reported incidence of developing diabetes mellitus postoperatively was 5%. In MEN-1 patients, the recurrence rates at 10 and 20 years were both 21%.[1]

REFERENCES

1. Service FJ, McMahon MM, O'Brien PC, Ballard DJ. Functioning insulinoma–incidence, recurrence, and long-term survival of patients: a 60-year study. *Mayo Clin Proc.* 1991;66(7):711–719.
2. Oberg K, Eriksson B. Endocrine tumours of the pancreas. *Best Pract Res Clin Gastroenterol.* 2005;19(5):753–781.
3. Sotoudehmanesh R, Hedayat A, Shirazian N, et al. Endoscopic ultrasonography (EUS) in the localization of insulinoma. *Endocrine.* 2007;31(3):238–241.
4. Whipple AO, Frantz VK. Adenoma of islet cells with hyperinsulinism: a review. *Ann Surg.* 1935;101(6):1299–1335.
5. Banting FG, Best CH. The internal secretion of the pancreas. 1922. *Indian J Med Res.* 2007;125(3):251–266.
6. Mansour JC, Chen H. Pancreatic endocrine tumors. *J Surg Res.* 2004;120(1):139–161.
7. Hough DM, Stephens DH, Johnson CD, Binkovitz LA. Pancreatic lesions in von Hippel-Lindau disease: prevalence, clinical significance, and CT findings. *AJR Am J Roentgenol.* 1994;162(5):1091–1094.
8. Larsson C, Skogseid B, Oberg K, Nakamura Y, Nordenskjöld M. Multiple endocrine neoplasia type 1 gene maps to chromosome 11 and is lost in insulinoma. *Nature.* 1988;332(6159):85–87.
9. Shen HC, He M, Powell A, et al. Recapitulation of pancreatic neuroendocrine tumors in human multiple endocrine neoplasia type I syndrome via Pdx1-directed inactivation of Men1. *Cancer Res.* 2009;69(5):1858–1866.
10. Wang H, Bender A, Wang P, et al. Insights into beta cell regeneration for diabetes via integration of molecular landscapes in human insulinomas. *Nat Commun.* 2017; 8(1):767.
11. Merimee TJ, Tyson JE. Hypoglycemia in man pathologic and physiologic variants. *Diabetes.* 1977;26(3):161–165.
12. Hirshberg B, Livi A, Bartlett DL, et al. Forty-eight-hour fast: the diagnostic test for insulinoma. *J Clin Endocrinol Metab.* 2000;85(9):3222–3226.
13. Marrack D, Rose FC, Marks V. Glucagon and tolbutamide tests in the recognition of insulinomas. *Proc Roy Soc Med.* 1961;54:749–752.
14. Trump D, Farren B, Wooding C, et al. Clinical studies of multiple endocrine neoplasia type 1 (MEN1). *QJM.* 1996;89(9):653–669.
15. Tucker ON, Crotty PL, Conlon KC. The management of insulinoma. *Br J Surg.* 2006;93(3):264–275.
16. Owen NJ, Sohaib SA, Peppercorn PD, et al. MRI of pancreatic neuroendocrine tumours. *Br J Radiol.* 2001;74(886): 968–973.
17. Ardengh JC, Rosenbaum P, Ganc AJ, et al. Role of EUS in the preoperative localization of insulinomas compared with spiral CT. *Gastrointest Endosc.* 2000;51(5):552–555.
18. Guettier JM, Kam A, Chang R, et al. Localization of insulinomas to regions of the pancreas by intraarterial calcium stimulation: the NIH experience. *J Clin Endocrinol Metab.* 2009;94(4):1074–1080.
19. Hiramoto JS, Feldstein VA, LaBerge JM, Norton JA. Intraoperative ultrasound and preoperative localization detects all occult insulinomas. *Arch Surg.* 2001;136(9): 1020–1025; discussion 1025-6.
20. Pasieka JL, McLeod MK, Thompson NW, Burney RE. Surgical approach to insulinomas. Assessing the need for preoperative localization. *Arch Surg.* 1992;127(4): 442–447.
21. Gaeke RF, Kaplan EL, Rubenstein A, Starr J, Burke G. Insulin and proinsulin release during calcium infusion in a patient with islet-cell tumor. *Metabolism.* 1975;24(9): 1029–1034.
22. Kaplan EL, Rubenstein AH, Evans R, Lee CH, Klementschitsch P. Calcium infusion: a new provocative test for insulinomas. *Ann Surg.* 1979;190(4):501–507.
23. Zimmer T, Stölzel U, Bäder M, et al. Endoscopic ultrasonography and somatostatin receptor scintigraphy in the preoperative localisation of insulinomas and gastrinomas. *Gut.* 1996;39(4):562–568.
24. Kayani I, Bomanji JB, Groves A, et al. Functional imaging of neuroendocrine tumors with combined PET/CT using 68Ga-DOTATATE (DOTA-DPhe1,Tyr3-octreotate) and 18F-FDG. *Cancer.* 2008;112(11):2447–2455.
25. Haug AR, Cindea-Drimus R, Auernhammer CJ, et al. The role of 68Ga-DOTATATE PET/CT in suspected neuroendocrine tumors. *J Nucl Med.* 2012;53(11):1686–1692.
26. Srirajaskanthan R, Kayani I, Quigley AM, Soh J, Caplin ME, Bomanji J. The role of 68Ga-DOTATATE PET in patients with neuroendocrine tumors and negative or equivocal findings on 111In-DTPA-octreotide scintigraphy. *J Nucl Med.* 2010;51(6):875–882.
27. Nockel P, Babic B, Millo C, et al. Localization of insulinoma using 68Ga-DOTATATE PET/CT scan. *J Clin Endocrinol Metab.* 2017;102(1):195–199.
28. Wilder RM. Hypoglycemia. *Diabetes.* 1952;1(3):183–187.
29. Shin JJ, Gorden P, Libutti SK. Insulinoma: pathophysiology, localization and management. *Future Oncol.* 2010; 6(2):229–237.
30. Thompson GB, Service FJ, van Heerden JA, et al. Reoperative insulinomas, 1927 to 1992: an institutional experience. *Surgery.* 1993;114(6):1196–1204; discussion 1205-1196.
31. Berends FJ, Cuesta MA, Kazemier G, et al. Laparoscopic detection and resection of insulinomas. *Surgery.* 2000; 128(3):386–391.
32. Briggs CD, Mann CD, Irving GR, et al. Systematic review of minimally invasive pancreatic resection. *J Gastrointest Surg.* 2009;13(6):1129–1137.
33. Fernandez Ranvier GG, Shouhed D, Inabnet WB. Minimally invasive techniques for resection of pancreatic neuroendocrine tumors. *Surg Oncol Clin.* 2016;25(1): 195–215.
34. Winer J, Can MF, Bartlett DL, Zeh HJ, Zureikat AH. The current state of robotic-assisted pancreatic surgery. *Nat Rev Gastroenterol Hepatol.* 2012;9(8):468–476.
35. Kang CM, Kim DH, Lee WJ, Chi HS. Conventional laparoscopic and robot-assisted spleen-preserving pancreatectomy: does da Vinci have clinical advantages? *Surg Endosc.* 2011;25(6):2004–2009.

36. Hirshberg B, Libutti SK, Alexander HR, et al. Blind distal pancreatectomy for occult insulinoma, an inadvisable procedure. *J Am Coll Surg.* 2002;194(6):761−764.

37. Zeiger MA, Shawker TH, Norton JA. Use of intraoperative ultrasonography to localize islet cell tumors. *World J Surg.* 1993;17(4):448−454.

38. Böttger TC, Junginger T. Is preoperative radiographic localization of islet cell tumors in patients with insulinoma necessary? *World J Surg.* 1993;17(4):427−432.

39. Proye C, Pattou F, Carnaille B, Lefebvre J, Decoulx M, d'Herbomez M. Intraoperative insulin measurement during surgical management of insulinomas. *World J Surg.* 1998;22(12):1218−1224.

40. Demeure MJ, Klonoff DC, Karam JH, Duh QY, Clark OH. Insulinomas associated with multiple endocrine neoplasia type I: the need for a different surgical approach. *Surgery.* 1991;110(6):998−1004; discussion 1004-1005.

41. O'Riordain DS, O'Brien T, van Heerden JA, Service FJ, Grant CS. Surgical management of insulinoma associated with multiple endocrine neoplasia type I. *World J Surg.* 1994;18(4):488−493; discussion 493-484.

42. Boukhman MP, Karam JH, Shaver J, Siperstein AE, Duh QY, Clark OH. Insulinoma−experience from 1950 to 1995. *West J Med.* 1998;169(2):98−104.

43. Brandi ML, Gagel RF, Angeli A, et al. Guidelines for diagnosis and therapy of MEN type 1 and type 2. *J Clin Endocrinol Metab.* 2001;86(12):5658−5671.

44. Bassi C, Butturini G, Molinari E, et al. Pancreatic fistula rate after pancreatic resection. The importance of definitions. *Dig Surg.* 2004;21(1):54−59.

45. Bassi C, Marchegiani G, Dervenis C, et al. The 2016 update of the International Study Group (ISGPS) definition and grading of postoperative pancreatic fistula: 11 Years after. *Surgery.* 2017;161(3):584−591.

46. Alexakis N, Sutton R, Neoptolemos JP. Surgical treatment of pancreatic fistula. *Dig Surg.* 2004;21(4):262−274.

47. Fajans SS, Vinik AI. Insulin-producing islet cell tumors. *Endocrinol Metab Clin N Am.* 1989;18(1):45−74.

48. Goode PN, Farndon JR, Anderson J, Johnston ID, Morte JA. Diazoxide in the management of patients with insulinoma. *World J Surg.* 1986;10(4):586−592.

49. de Herder WW, Niederle B, Scoazec JY, et al. Well-differentiated pancreatic tumor/carcinoma: insulinoma. *Neuroendocrinology.* 2006;84(3):183−188.

50. Maton PN. The use of the long-acting somatostatin analogue, octreotide acetate, in patients with islet cell tumors. *Gastroenterol Clin N Am.* 1989;18(4):897−922.

51. Maton PN, Gardner JD, Jensen RT. Use of long-acting somatostatin analog SMS 201-995 in patients with pancreatic islet cell tumors. *Dig Dis Sci.* 1989;34(suppl 3):28S−39S.

52. Krejs GJ, Orci L, Conlon JM, et al. Somatostatinoma syndrome. Biochemical, morphologic and clinical features. *N Engl J Med.* 1979;301(6):285−292.

53. Huscher CG, Mingoli A, Sgarzini G, Mereu A, Gasperi M. Image-guided robotic radiosurgery (CyberKnife) for pancreatic insulinoma: is laparoscopy becoming old? *Surg Innovat.* 2012;19(1):NP14−17.

54. Yang D, Inabnet WB, Sarpel U, DiMaio CJ. EUS-guided ethanol ablation of symptomatic pancreatic insulinomas. *Gastrointest Endosc.* 2015;82(6):1127.

55. Jürgensen C, Schuppan D, Neser F, Ernstberger J, Junghans U, Stölzel U. EUS-guided alcohol ablation of an insulinoma. *Gastrointest Endosc.* 2006;63(7):1059−1062.

56. Hirshberg B, Cochran C, Skarulis MC, et al. Malignant insulinoma: spectrum of unusual clinical features. *Cancer.* 2005;104(2):264−272.

57. Danforth DN, Gorden P, Brennan MF. Metastatic insulin-secreting carcinoma of the pancreas: clinical course and the role of surgery. *Surgery.* 1984;96(6):1027−1037.

58. O'Toole D, Maire F, Ruszniewski P. Ablative therapies for liver metastases of digestive endocrine tumours. *Endocr Relat Cancer.* 2003;10(4):463−468.

59. Rougier P, Mitry E. Chemotherapy in the treatment of neuroendocrine malignant tumors. *Digestion.* 2000;62(suppl 1):73−78.

60. de Herder WW, van Schaik E, Kwekkeboom D, Feelders RA. New therapeutic options for metastatic malignant insulinomas. *Clin Endocrinol.* 2011;75(3):277−284.

61. Yao JC, Shah MH, Ito T, et al. Everolimus for advanced pancreatic neuroendocrine tumors. *N Engl J Med.* 2011;364(6):514−523.

62. Bernard V, Lombard-Bohas C, Taquet MC, et al. Efficacy of everolimus in patients with metastatic insulinoma and refractory hypoglycemia. *Eur J Endocrinol.* 2013;168(5):665−674.

63. Nikfarjam M, Warshaw AL, Axelrod L, et al. Improved contemporary surgical management of insulinomas: a 25-year experience at the Massachusetts General Hospital. *Ann Surg.* 2008;247(1):165−172.

CHAPTER 19

Advances in the Diagnosis and Management of Gastrinoma

BRENDAN M. FINNERTY, MD • THOMAS J. FAHEY III, MD

INTRODUCTION

Gastrinoma is a functional neuroendocrine tumor (NET) that overproduces gastrin hormone resulting in gastric acid hypersecretion and its clinical sequelae known as Zollinger–Ellison syndrome (ZES). The initial report, published in 1955, described ZES based on three clinical manifestations: (1) peptic ulcer disease (PUD) in unusual locations, such as distal duodenum or proximal jejunum, (2) notable gastric acid hypersecretion refractory to intervention, and (3) presence of pancreatic islet cell tumor.[1] Astute recognition of this disease is essential for two main reasons. First, there exists a 60%–90% risk of malignancy, as defined by local invasion of the primary tumor and/or presence of metastatic disease. Second, unrecognized ZES can lead to complications associated with severe peptic ulcer disease (PUD) and gastroesophageal reflux disease (GERD), such as perforation, gastrointestinal hemorrhage, and stricture.[2]

Epidemiology

Gastrinoma is the second-most common functional NET after insulinoma with an incidence of 0.5–3 cases per million per year.[3] There is a slight male predominance and the median age at onset is in the 4th–5th decades of life. Unfortunately, there is an average delay in diagnosis of ZES from disease onset of approximately 5.5 years. As a result, upwards of 70% of patients present with a history of ulcerations, with a number of patients already having suffered a perforation (5%) or gastric outlet obstruction (12%).[4] Approximately 75% of gastrinomas arise sporadically, whereas 25% are associated with multiple endocrine neoplasia type I (MEN1).[5] Conversely, gastrinomas occur in approximately one-half of patients with MEN1 and are the most common functional NET in this condition.[6] Anatomically, 80% of tumors are located within the gastrinoma triangle, which is bounded by the junctions of the cystic duct and common bile duct superiorly, the second and third portion of the duodenum inferiorly, and the neck and body of the pancreas medially.[7] Historically, these tumors were thought to be most commonly located in the pancreas; however, reports from several decades ago began to challenge that dictum with an increasing detection of duodenal primary tumors.[8] In fact, a subsequent larger series reported that only 25%–40% of primary tumors are located in pancreas.[4] Compared to pancreatic tumors, duodenal tumors typically have a smaller diameter (<1 cm), similar risk of lymph node metastasis, and a lower risk of liver metastasis.[9,10] According to an international consensus, the distribution of duodenal tumors also varies between sporadic and MEN1 gastrinomas (50%–88% vs. 70%–100%, respectively).[11] Importantly, 10% of sporadic gastrinomas (but 0% of MEN1 gastrinomas) have been postulated to arise as a lymph node primary tumor—among these, 25% are multifocal but most are still found within the gastrinoma triangle.[12] Whether gastrinomas identified as "lymph node primary" are true primary tumors arising in lymph nodes or represent lymph node metastases from an occult duodenal or pancreatic primary remains uncertain.

Clinical Presentation

Symptoms of ZES are secondary to high gastric acid output resulting from gastrin's secretory effect on acid-producing parietal cells and histamine-producing enterochromaffin-like cells of the stomach. Thus, the most common symptoms include epigastric abdominal pain (75%), chronic diarrhea (73%), heartburn from gastroesophageal reflux (44%), nausea/emesis (30%), and weight loss (17%). Given the high intraluminal gastric acid content in ZES, most patients will present with multiple symptoms—in fact, nearly 30% will present with >4 symptoms. The distribution of

Advances in Treatment and Management in Surgical Endocrinology. https://doi.org/10.1016/B978-0-323-66195-9.00019-4

symptoms is roughly equivalent between sporadic and MEN1-associated gastrinoma; however, MEN1 patients present less frequently with abdominal pain (66%), and instead may display signs of concomitant hyperparathyroidism or pituitary adenoma. Of note, chronic diarrhea in this setting is multifactorial—high volumes of gastric acid cannot be fully reabsorbed by intestinal epithelium and may inhibit sodium and water absorption. In addition, the overall low intraluminal pH results in inactivation of pancreatic digestive enzymes leading to steatorrhea.[4,13]

A significant number of patients may present with complications secondary to chronic exposure to gastric acid hypersecretion. Over two-thirds of patients will present with confirmed evidence of peptic ulcer disease, typically recurrent and refractory to medical therapy; of note, ulcerations distal to the duodenal bulb should raise index of suspicion. Other impactful sequelae include gastrointestinal bleeding (25%), duodenal or pyloric scarring (10%), and digestive tract perforations (5%). As a result, most patients will present already having been started on a proton-pump inhibitor (PPI) or H2 blocker, and approximately 10% of patients will have even undergone a gastric acid-reducing operation.[13] Unfortunately, only 7% of gastrinoma patients are accurately diagnosed at initial presentation, therefore accounting for the average delay in diagnosis of 5.5 years. Instead, approximately 70% of patients are misdiagnosed with chronic idiopathic peptic ulcer disease. Other common misdiagnoses include chronic idiopathic GERD, chronic idiopathic diarrhea, inflammatory bowel disease, and irritable bowel syndrome.[4,13]

Tumor Classification

Histologically, gastrinomas appear similar to other pancreatic neuroendocrine tumors—they are typically well-differentiated tumors with a low ki-67 < 2% characterized by cells with uniform nuclei, salt-and-pepper chromatin, and fine granular cytoplasm. Although they tend to be slow growing, 60%–90% are malignant as defined by localized or distant metastasis. Nearly 25% of patients are classified has having "aggressive" pathology associated with poorer prognosis. As compared to the "nonaggressive" phenotype, these tumors are associated with female gender, markedly elevated fasting gastrin levels, larger diameters (>3 cm), pancreatic primary location, and liver metastases (20%)—as expected, 10-year survival rates are significantly lower in the "aggressive" phenotype (30% vs. 96%).[14] Regardless of classification, the most important predictor of patient survival is presence and extent of liver metastasis.[15] In the absence of liver metastasis, patients have a 20-year survival of 95%, whereas those with solitary or limited liver burden have a 15-year survival of 60%–70%, and those with diffuse liver burden have a 10-year survival of 15%. Although 30%–70% of gastrinomas will have lymph node metastasis, this does not appear to impact survival.[4,10,15]

Genetics

Approximately 25% of gastrinoma patients harbor the germline autosomal-dominant MEN1 mutation responsible for MEN1 syndrome, resulting in multigland primary hyperparathyroidism, pancreatic NETs, and pituitary adenomas. MEN1 encodes menin, a nuclear scaffold protein that serves as a transcriptional regulator via chromatin remodeling; it is also an essential component of a histone methyltransferase complex implicated in epigenetic modification.[16] The remainder of gastrinomas is sporadic, and unfortunately there is a severe paucity of data describing the genomics of these tumors. Loss of heterozygosity at the MEN1 locus (11q13) has been found in a wide range of sporadic tumors, and up to 40% of these tumors harbor nongermline MEN1 mutations.[17,18] However, the presence of an MEN1 gene mutation does not appear to correlate with any clinicopathologic characteristics or differences in outcomes of patients with gastrinoma.[19] Hypermethylation of p16^{INK4a} has also been observed in half of gastrinoma cases and has been implicated as a potential early event in tumorigenesis.[20] More comprehensive genomic analyses have begun to describe the genetic alterations driving pancreatic NET tumorigenesis, namely in nonfunctional tumors. Specifically, mutations of genes involved with chromatin remodeling and the mammalian target of rapamycin (mTOR) pathway account for most genetic alterations in a large nonfamilial pancreatic NET cohort.[21] In addition to MEN1, other prevalent mutations in chromatin remodeling genes included death-domain-associated protein (DAXX) and α-thalassemia/mental retardation syndrome X-linked (ATRX), which have been associated with worse prognosis in pancreatic NETs.[22] However, until more analyses regarding gastrinoma-specific genomic alterations become available, it is difficult to draw concrete conclusions translating these data.

DIAGNOSIS

The crux of early detection of ZES rests on a high index of suspicion based on the clinical features described earlier, particularly in the setting of multiple presenting symptoms. A thorough history and physical is prudent with careful attention to ZES symptomatology, medical comorbidities including possible misdiagnoses, prior abdominal operations and endoscopic procedures, family history of peptic ulcer disease or MEN1, and medication history of acid-reducing therapies. *Helicobacter pylori* testing should be documented, as well as inquiry into prior NSAID usage. A classic scenario is a patient presenting with chronic abdominal pain, diarrhea, and weight loss with a history of recurrent ulcerations refractory to PPI therapy, perhaps in the setting of negative *H. pylori* infection and absence of NSAID usage. A suggested algorithm for the diagnosis and treatment of ZES is depicted in Fig. 19.1.

Biochemical Evaluation

The first step in diagnosis is to obtain a fasting serum gastrin (FSG) level to evaluate for hypergastrinemia. Importantly, this should not preclude treatment of any ulceration, for fear of bleeding or perforation. Thus, *treat the ulcer first*, and then pursue a gastrinoma workup.

Nonetheless, it is imperative to have a comprehensive differential diagnosis regarding hypergastrinemia, which is typically defined as FSG >100 pg/mL in most assays.[4] Elevated gastrin levels should be evaluated with consideration to the level of gastric acid production. Hypergastrinemia associated with *decreased gastric acid production* (i.e., appropriate physiologic response) occurs with H2-blocker or PPI usage, *H. pylori* infection (pan-gastritis), atrophic gastritis, chronic renal failure, and prior vagotomy without antrectomy. Hypergastrinemia associated with *increased or normal gastric acid production* (i.e., inappropriate physiologic response) occurs with gastrinoma, retained gastric antrum syndrome, *H. pylori* infection (antral-predominant), antral G-cell hyperplasia, and gastric outlet obstruction.[23,24] Most of these clinical states produce only mild-to-moderate gastrin elevations that need to be differentiated from gastrinoma, especially as only approximately 35% of gastrinoma patients will present with the pathognomonic elevated gastrin level >1000 pg/mL, or 10 times the upper limit of normal. Conversely, a normal gastrin level is an effective test to rule out gastrinoma, as this occurs in only 0.3%–3% of gastrinoma patients.[4] Lastly, it is important to note that there is a wide variability in gastrin assays, and that only 5 of 12 kits appear to be truly accurate and reliable.[25,26] Thus, repeating an FSG may be prudent if the diagnosis is unclear and there is concern for a spurious value. Intraluminal gastric acid analysis has historically been a crucial adjunct to diagnosis of ZES. Basal acid output (BAO) is a direct measurement of gastric acid secretion obtained by aspiration of intraluminal gastric contents via nasogastric tube over the course of 1 h (units in mEq/h). Maximal acid output (MAO) is the same measurement after

stimulation with pentagastrin. However, these tests are uncommonly utilized due to limited accessibility across centers as well as unavailability of pentagastrin in the United States.[24] Alternative methods of measuring gastric pH include trans-nasal pH probe monitoring or intraluminal gastric fluid analysis using pH indicator paper. Table 19.1 outlines the biochemical interpretation of FSG and gastric acid levels, which largely reflects the results of two large NIH studies analyzing FSG, BAO, and MAO in ZES patients.[4,27] In general, ZES can be diagnosed by either an FSG >1000 pg/mL with gastric pH < 2, or, any FSG elevation with BAO >15 mEq/h.[4] Of note, in patients with FSG >1000 pg/mL and gastric pH < 2, retained gastric antrum syndrome should be ruled out before diagnosing a patient with ZES by taking a thorough history regarding prior gastrectomy—this includes critically reviewing operative reports and potentially obtaining a sodium pertechnetate scan if necessary.[28] Lastly, to ensure accurate biochemical diagnosis, PPI medications should be held 1–2 weeks before all testing—it is imperative that the physician and patient are mindful of the signs and symptoms of PUD exacerbation and complications during this hiatus. To help prevent this, patients should be bridged with high-dose ranitidine until 24 h before biochemical evaluation, which includes FSG, BAO, gastric pH, and even provocative testing if possible.

Approximately two-thirds of patients will present with equivocal biochemical results and thus require provocative testing with either secretin or calcium to confirm diagnosis of ZES. In the secretin stimulation test (SST), 2 units/kg of secretin are administered intravenously and FSG is measured serially before, during, and at 2, 5, 10, 15, and 30 min after injection. In normal gastric G-cells, secretin has an inhibitory effect on gastrin secretion, whereas the converse is true in gastrinoma cells (typically within 10 mins). A large series published by the NIH detected an optimal cutoff for diagnosis—an increase in gastrin levels >120 pg/mL has a sensitivity and specificity for ZES of 94% and 100%, respectively.[29] Clinicians should be aware that a false positive rate of 15% exists in the setting of hypo- and achlorhydria secondary to PPIs or atrophic gastritis.[30] The calcium infusion test has a similar protocol but is less robust when compared to SST—calcium is administered at a rate of 5 mg/kg/h and FSG levels are serially measured before, during, and at 1, 2, and 3 h after initiation. An increase in calcium >395 pg/mL has a sensitivity of only 62% (specificity 100%), thus, this test has largely been abandoned in favor of SST for provocative testing. However, as 38%–50% of patients with negative SST

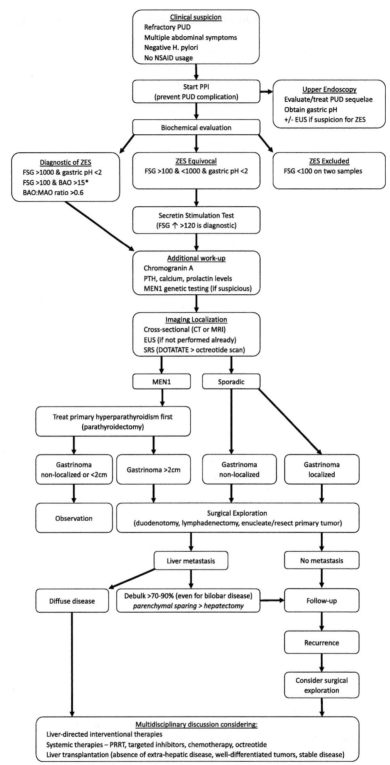

FIG. 19.1 A suggested algorithm for the diagnosis and treatment of ZES. * >5 if history of acid-reducing surgery. *BAO*, Basal acid output (mEq/h); *CT*, Computed tomography; *EUS*, Endoscopic ultrasound; *FSG*, fasting serum gastrin (pg/mL); *MAO*, maximal acid output (mEq/h); *MRI*, Magnetic resonance imaging; *PPI*, Proton pump inhibitor; *PRRT*, Peptide receptor radionuclide therapy; *PTH*, Parathyroid hormone; *PUD*, Peptic ulcer disease; *ZES*, Zollinger–Ellison syndrome.

TABLE 19.1
Biochemical Interpretation of Gastrinoma.

Gastrin Level (pg/mL)	Gastric Acid Level	Interpretation
>1000	pH < 2	Diagnostic of ZES
100–1000	pH < 2	Pursue additional testing[a] (e.g., secretin-stim or BAO)
>100	BAO > 15 mEq/h (no history of gastric surgery)	Diagnostic of ZES
>100	BAO > 5 mEq/h (history of gastric acid-reducing surgery)	Diagnostic of ZES
>100	BAO:MAO ratio > 0.6[b]	Diagnostic of ZES
Normal	–	Repeat → if normal, then ZES excluded

BAO: Basal acid output; ZES: Zollinger–Ellison syndrome.
[a] Off proton-pump inhibitor for 1–2 weeks.
[b] After subcutaneous pentagastrin stimulation.

will test positive on calcium infusion, this test should be used if clinical suspicion for ZES is high but SST is negative.[29]

Chromogranin A (CgA) is the only tumor marker relevant to gastrinomas. It is a protein located in secretory dense core granules of neuroendocrine tumors that have been used as a serum and immunohistochemical marker for NETs—rising levels have been correlated with NET progression and liver metastases.[31] However, in gastrinomas, CgA can be elevated in 90%–100% of cases even with localized and limited tumor burden.[32,33] A prospective study of gastrinoma patients from the NIH showed chromogranin A to be a highly sensitive (92%), but not specific (67%), marker for disease; moreover, it did not correlate with tumor growth or extent.[34] CgA decreases appropriately after gastrinoma resection, but it is neither sensitive nor specific for detecting increasing (62% and 53%, respectively) or stable (42% and 69%, respectively) tumor burden.[35] Importantly, elevations in both serum CgA and gastrin are associated with PPI therapy and *H. pylori* infection, but not H2-blocker therapy.[36–38]

Lastly, as 25% of gastrinomas are associated with MEN1, the diagnostic workup should include serum calcium, parathyroid hormone, and prolactin levels. Confirmation DNA-based *MEN1* genetic testing can be performed in cases suspicious for the syndrome.

Endoscopic Evaluation

Esophagogastroduodenoscopy (EGD) should be performed in all suspected ZES cases to first evaluate for evidence of PUD. Biopsy of ulcers and suspicious lesions should be performed, and treatment of bleeding ulcers should be addressed. Prominent rugal folds secondary to the trophic effects of gastrin are observed in over 90% of ZES cases and there may also be evidence of reflux esophagitis, while esophageal stricture and pyloric or duodenal scarring will be seen in only 10% of cases.[13] Signs indicating alternative etiologies for hypergastrinemia should be kept in mind during endoscopy, such as atrophic gastric mucosa indicative of pernicious anemia. Gastric fluid can be obtained during EGD for pH testing as described earlier. Tumor localization should be attempted by direct visualization and with endoscopic ultrasound (EUS) to identify duodenal, pancreatic, or peripancreatic lesions. EUS is 75%–100% sensitive and 95% specific for pancreatic lesions and is particularly useful for detecting small (<2 cm) intrapancreatic tumors; however, it has a poor sensitivity (38%–63%) for detecting duodenal tumors.[39–42] Fine-needle aspiration of masses can be performed to pursue cytologic diagnosis, but is not necessary.

Imaging for Tumor Localization

Upon biochemical diagnosis of ZES, the gastrinoma primary tumor must be localized and assessed for metastasis. In addition to endoscopy with EUS, this should include cross-sectional imaging with computed tomography (CT), magnetic resonance imaging (MRI), and/or somatostatin receptor scintigraphy (SRS).

CT of the abdomen with intravenous contrast is an excellent modality to detect pancreatic tumors >1 cm and liver metastases, but a poor modality for detecting subcentimeter extrapancreatic tumors—its sensitivity ranges from 59% to 78% with a specificity from 95% to 98%.[42,43] Gastrinomas will typically enhance on arterial phase due to their hypervascularity. MRI of the abdomen is also highly specific (88%–100%) for detecting gastrinomas and is better at detecting liver metastases than the primary tumor—its historic sensitivity in identifying primary lesions was only 20%–25% in early series.[44,45] However, more recent data demonstrate a much improved sensitivity of 85% for detecting primary tumors <2 cm, thus consideration for MRI as a first line imaging modality over CT is reasonable.[46] Gastrinomas typically have a high T2 signal and low T1 signal compared to surrounding organs on MRI.

SRS originally became a standard modality in the late 1990s after several prospective studies demonstrated an improved sensitivity in detecting gastrinomas using [111In-DTPA-D-Phe1]-octreotide (primary tumor 58%–78%, metastases 92%–100%) as compared to other imaging modalities, which altered management in nearly half of patients.[47–49] It was also shown to detect 64% of lesions <2 cm and 30% of lesions <1 cm, which was a diagnostic improvement at the time, but it still missed primarily small duodenal tumors.[47] More recently, several somatostatin analogues have been labeled with positron-emitting radionuclides (usually ^{68}Ga), most commonly known as tracers ^{68}Ga-DOTATOC, ^{68}Ga-DOTATATE, and ^{68}Ga-DOTANOC, which can be used for somatostatin receptor PET-CT imaging. A recent systematic review and meta-analysis calculated a pooled sensitivity and specificity of 93% and 96%, respectively, of the ability of somatostatin receptor PET-CT imaging to detect pulmonary or gastroenteropancreatic NETs.[50] This imaging modality has been reported to alter management in approximately half of patients with NETs.[51–53] In gastrinoma, only one small series evaluated the efficacy of ^{68}Ga-DOTANOC as compared to contrast-enhanced CT: ^{68}Ga-DOTANOC identified tumors in 36% and 93% of negative and equivocal CT scan results, respectively.[54] Thus, consideration for somatostatin receptor PET-CT should be included for tumor localization.

If cross-sectional imaging, EUS, and somatostatin receptor imaging fail to localize the tumor, then surgery should be pursued for intraoperative localization by ultrasound, transillumination, and manual palpation. Duodenal tumors are often missed by EUS and imaging modalities due to their small diameters and submucosal location. Surgery can detect gastrinoma in 98% of patients with negative localization studies, which is associated with a long-term cure rate of nearly 50% (mean follow-up 9.4 years).[55] In this series, compared to patients with positive preoperative localization, those with negative localization more often had a small duodenal tumor and thus a key component to operative exploration is wide duodenal mobilization and duodenotomy near the junction of the second and third portions.

THERAPY

Historically, total gastrectomy was the sole effective treatment to treat ZES by removing the end-organ target of gastrin. The advent of H2-blockers in the 1970s reduced the need for gastrectomy; however, patients required aggressive dose escalation to maintain BAO <10 mEq/h.[56] Failure rates approached 60% in some series, and many patients still required either gastrectomy or acid-reducing procedures (e.g., vagotomy) to control their disease. This management approach changed dramatically in the 1980s when PPIs became available due to their highly effective acid reduction and minimal need for aggressive dose escalation.[2] Long-term outcomes regarding improved symptomatology, reduced BAO, and the avoidance of complications secondary to gastric acid hypersecretion were reported in 90% of patients treated with PPIs, with annual relapse rates <5%.[57,58] The side-effect profile is safe, with the rare exceptions of vitamin B12 deficiency, bone fractures, dementia, micronutrient deficiencies (iron, calcium, magnesium), and intraabdominal infection (including *Clostridium difficile*).[59–61] PPI therapy remains the gold-standard therapy for pre- and postoperative gastric acid control, as 40% of patients who achieve curative resection will still require antisecretory therapy likely due to excess residual parietal cells from the longstanding trophic effects of gastrin.[62,63] Thus, the first step of treating patients with gastrinoma is to control gastric acid hypersecretion to improve symptoms and prevent negative sequelae of severe PUD. If acid output measurements are attainable, the dose of PPI should be titrated to reduce BAO below 15 mEq/h (or < 5mEq/h in those with a history of prior acid-reducing surgery).

In patients with MEN1, management of primary hyperparathyroidism should be addressed first. Hypercalcemia is known to increase serum gastrin levels and decrease response to acid-reducing therapy in patients with ZES.[64,65] Thus, normalizing calcium levels with parathyroidectomy lowers BAO and gastrin levels, thereby minimizing potential risks of severe PUD exacerbations.[66,67] Operative approach remains controversial—subtotal parathyroidectomy (removing 3.5 glands) is preferred by some groups with expected persistence and recurrence rates of 12% and 44%, respectively, during a mean follow up of 17 years.[67] However, other studies report higher long-term recurrence rates with subtotal parathyroidectomy, specifically 67% at 8 years.[68] Thus, total parathyroidectomy with autograft is advocated by some groups given its lower rates of persistence (0%) and recurrence (10%–50%), though, surgeons should be wary of its higher rate of permanent hypoparathyroidism as compared to subtotal parathyroidectomy (22% vs. 10%).[67,69,70]

All patients with sporadic ZES should be evaluated by a surgeon and offered surgical exploration for possible curative resection. Immediate postoperative disease-free rates approach 60%, with about one-half of these patients recurring by 5 years.[71,72] In patients with sporadic gastrinomas, approximately one-half and one-third of patients will be disease-free at 5 and 10 years, respectively, with overall a survival rate of 95% at 10 years in some series.[72,73] Compared to nonoperative management, surgery offers a major survival advantage from an oncologic perspective—surgical patients have a significantly less chance of developing liver metastases (5% vs. 29%), and thus have improved 20-year disease-specific survival (98% vs. 77%) and overall survival (81% vs. 55%) rates.[72]

There are several essential technical components during operative exploration. First, an extensive Kocher maneuver must be performed to expose the duodenum and pancreatic head, and the gastrocolic ligament must be divided to fully expose the pancreatic neck, body, and tail. In addition to palpation, intraoperative ultrasound is a useful adjunct to aid in identification of tumors in the duodenum, pancreas, and liver. Thorough duodenal examination should include endoscopic transillumination and a 3 cm longitudinal duodenotomy at the anterolateral surface of the second portion of the duodenum to facilitate visualization and palpation of subcentimeter tumors (closed transversely if possible). Duodenal tumors should be locally excised followed by durable primary closure. Surgical exploration with duodenotomy increases the success rate of finding the gastrinoma from 76% up to 98%, namely driven by the increased rate of duodenal tumor detection (62% vs. 18%) compared to no duodenotomy. It is associated with a better immediate postoperative cure rate (65% vs. 44%) as well as long-term cure rate (52% vs. 26%) after nearly 9 years of follow-up.[74] Enucleation of pancreatic (and peripancreatic) tumors is preferable over formal resection such as pancreaticoduodenectomy, unless there is pancreatic duct involvement or bulky disease not amenable to pancreas-preserving resection. Due to the 30%–70% risk of lymph node metastasis in gastrinoma, lymphadenectomy should also be performed during exploration with adequate sampling of lymph nodes from the peripancreatic, pancreaticoduodenal, hepatoduodenal ligament, and aortocaval basins. In a retrospective cohort, systematic lymphadenectomy with 10 or more lymph nodes excised was associated with a higher biochemical cure rate (100% vs. 64%), prolonged disease-specific survival, and reduced risk of mortality (0% vs. 29%).[75] Lastly, prophylactic cholecystectomy should be performed to avoid gallstone complications secondary to somatostatin analog therapy or gallbladder necrosis from potential future liver-ablative therapies for recurrent metastatic disease.[76]

Patients with MEN1 have tumor burden that is more difficult to control surgically compared to sporadic tumors, likely due to their multifocality, small size, and predilection for lymph node metastasis. MEN1 is associated with lower rates of immediate disease-free status (50% vs. 15%), 5-year disease-free survival (40% vs. 4%), and 10-year disease-free survival (34% vs. 0%); however, importantly, there are no differences in 10-year disease-specific or overall survival between sporadic and MEN1-associated gastrinoma.[73,77] Instead, the most important predictor of worse survival is liver metastasis, which is associated with tumors >2 cm.[10,15,77,78] Additionally, observing nonfunctional NETs <2 cm has been associated with safe oncologic outcomes in MEN1 patients.[79,80] As surgical cure is so rare in MEN1 tumors and ZES symptoms can be typically controlled by PPIs and parathyroidectomy, the main goal of treatment is to reduce the risk of liver metastasis—thus, resection of gastrinomas in these patients is indicated only when there is an identifiable tumor on imaging >2 cm. Using this approach, 15-year survival rates for patients with tumors <2.5 cm treated nonoperatively, tumors >2.5 cm treated operatively, and diffuse hepatic metastases treated nonoperatively are 100%, 89%–100%, and 52%, respectively.[81] Some groups recommend more aggressive anatomic resections in MEN1 with pancreaticoduodenectomy, but the utility of this approach is controversial given the good long-term survival associated with the algorithm and surgical approach described earlier.[82]

Given its complexity, recurrent and metastatic disease should be managed by a multidisciplinary team. Surgery should be considered for recurrent disease—operable recurrences occur in about one-quarter of ZES patients who undergo a curative-intent index resection with a mean time to reoperation of 6 years after initial surgery. Over one-third of patients will be immediately disease-free postoperatively, and one-quarter will remain disease-free after 8 years of follow-up.[77] During reoperation, the same principles of duodenotomy, adequate lymphadenectomy must be performed, and either enucleation or formal resection of all recurrent primary tumors must be pursued.

Liver metastases will be present in at least 25% of patients at presentation, with less than 25% of these patients having disease confined to one lobe.[4,15] Despite this, cytoreductive surgery with the goal of debulking 70%–90% of tumor burden has been associated with good long-term outcomes in mixed cohorts of functional and nonfunctional NETs with liver metastasis, particularly with disease-specific survival rates up to 90%.[83–85] Surgical approach in most series report a combination of formal hepatic resection and parenchymal-sparing nonanatomic resections with or without ablation, thus allowing for aggressive surgical management of bilobar liver disease while attempting to preserve adequate liver remnant. Interestingly, in one large series of surgically managed hepatic NETs, nearly all patients recurred by 5 years, but overall survival at 5 and 10 years was acceptable at 74% and 51%, respectively.[86] Additionally, R2 margin status occurred in 33% of the cohort and was not associated with worse survival on multivariate analysis. Other series report 5- and 10-year survival rates of 90% and 70% in patients undergoing hepatic resection of well-differentiated NET metastases, with surgical intervention being an independent predictor of survival (compared to nonoperative management options).[87] Thus, even if positive margins are encountered, patients with NET liver metastases have good long-term survival as cytoreductive surgery appears to "reset the clock."

The management of diffuse hepatic disease is controversial. Liver transplantation is one option for carefully selected patients in the management of metastatic NETs—a review of several series reports a wide variability in 5-year overall survival (33%–90%) and disease-free survival (9%–77%). Consideration for transplant should only include patients with extensive unresectable hepatic metastases of well-differentiated histology who have already undergone primary tumor resection—patients should have demonstrated stable disease for 6 months and have no evidence of extrahepatic metastases.[88] Other interventional liver-directed therapies include radiofrequency ablation, microwave ablation, transarterial chemoembolization, and selective internal radiation therapy, but none have emerged as a superior intervention for improving survival.[89] These therapies are best reserved to treat unresectable disease and hepatic recurrences after surgical management.

There are several systemic treatment options for metastatic NETs as well, although their treatment effects are less robust and studies evaluating response rates in gastrinomas alone are limited. Somatostatin analogues have been associated with improved progression-free survival in metastatic NETs, although they may not be effective as liver burden increases.[90,91] Chemotherapy regimens historically have been based on either streptozocin plus doxorubicin, but more recently temozolomide-based regimens (± capecitabine) have been used with objective response rates widely ranging from 15% to 70%.[92–94] The mTOR-inhibitor, everolimus, has been shown to increase progression-free

survival to 11 months from approximately 4 months in both metastatic pancreatic and extrapancreatic NETs, and has a positive hepatic treatment effect in the latter group.[95,96] The multitargeted tyrosine kinase inhibitor, sunitinib, has also demonstrated an improved progression-free survival from 5.5 to 11.4 months in metastatic pancreatic NETs, with improved objective response (9% vs. 0%) and mortality (10% vs. 25%) rates as compared to placebo.[97] Lastly, peptide receptor radionuclide therapy (PRRT) may be the most promising systemic therapy, as it has been shown to have an improved progression-free survival rate at 20 months (65% vs. 11%), objective response rate (18% vs. 3%), and overall survival (interim analysis) as compared to long-acting octreotide in inoperable somatostatin-receptor positive metastatic midgut NETs.[98] Interestingly, in a separate small retrospective cohort of 11 patients with progressive malignant gastrinomas, PRRT improved symptoms and decreased mean serum gastrin levels in all patients.[99] It also demonstrated complete response in 1 patient (9%) and partial response in 5 (45%), with an antitumor effect duration of 14 months in 7 patients (64%). Although the 36% of patients who died in this study originally presented with extensive liver disease, these data suggest that PRRT may play a role in inoperable metastatic gastrinoma and further study is warranted.

PROGNOSIS

Despite a majority of gastrinoma tumors being malignant, 20-year and 30-year overall survival rates are 84% and 68%, respectively. Even in patients who have operable recurrent tumors, disease-specific mortality is only 13%.[77] Prognosis of malignant gastrinoma is mainly dependent on presence and burden of liver metastasis (Fig. 19.1).[10,15] Patients with localized disease have an excellent 20-year survival of 95%. However, 10-year survival rates decrease dramatically from 90%–96% to 16%–30% if diffuse liver metastasis is present.[10,15] Additionally, patients who initially present with liver metastasis have a much worse 10-year survival rate (26%) than those who develop liver disease later on (85%).[15] Patients with risk factors for liver metastasis include pancreatic primary location and size of the primary tumor—increasing diameter from 1 to 3 cm increases the risk of metastasis from 4% to 62% in one series.[10] As mentioned earlier, approximately 25% of patients are classified with an "aggressive" pathology, which is associated with poorer prognosis. These factors include female gender, markedly elevated gastrin levels, tumor size >3 cm, pancreatic primary tumor, and liver metastases—10-year survival rates are significantly lower in the "aggressive" phenotype when compared to patients without these factors (30% vs. 96%).[14] Notably, survival does not appear to be affected independently by lymph node metastasis or MEN1 status.[10] The most common causes of ZES-related death include liver tumor-induced cachexia and hepatic failure from tumor burden.[15]

SUMMARY

Gastrinomas typically present as refractory PUD with multiple symptoms associated with high gastric acid output, such as abdominal pain, diarrhea, and weight loss. Astute recognition of this disease is critical to avoid the catastrophic complications of severe PUD (i.e., gastrointestinal perforation or bleeding) and to expeditiously treat this frequently malignant tumor. Immediate treatment of PUD with PPIs is of utmost importance, followed by a methodical workup including *H. pylori* testing, fasting serum gastrin levels, and upper endoscopy with either gastric pH testing or basal acid output measurements. Patients with equivocal results should undergo secretin stimulation testing for biochemical diagnosis, and MEN1 screening should be considered by evaluating calcium, PTH, and prolactin levels (with or without genetic testing). In MEN1 patients, treatment of hyperparathyroidism with parathyroidectomy should be addressed first to decrease gastric acid output. Imaging modalities that can assist in tumor localization include CT, MRI, EUS, and/or somatostatin receptor scintigraphy (preferably ^{68}Ga-DOTATATE PET-CT, if available). Nonlocalized patients with sporadic disease should undergo surgical exploration, with attention to the gastrinoma triangle; MEN1 patients should undergo exploration only if a tumor >2 cm is identified on imaging. Duodenotomy and locoregional lymphadenectomy should be performed routinely intraoperatively to minimize the risk of persistent disease. Primary tumors can be typically managed with enucleation, with formal pancreatic resection being reserved for bulky disease or duct involvement. Liver metastases portend the worst prognosis, but surgical management should be considered to achieve 70%–90% debulking. Recurrent disease may be amenable for surgical reexploration, but extensive metastases should be evaluated in a multidisciplinary setting for consideration of nonsurgical liver-directed treatments and/or system therapies such as PRRT.

REFERENCES

1. Zollinger R, Ellison E. Primary peptic ulcerations of the jejunum associated with islet cell tumors of the pancreas. *Ann Surg.* 1955;142(4):709–723.
2. Norton J, Foster D, Ito T, Jensen R. Gastrinomas: medical or surgical treatment. *Endocrinol Metab Clin North Am.* 2018; 47(3):577–601. https://doi.org/10.1016/j.ecl.2018.04.009.
3. Öberg K. Pancreatic endocrine tumors. *Semin Oncol.* 2010;37(6): 594–618. https://doi.org/10.1053/j.seminoncol.2010.10.014.
4. Berna MJ, Hoffmann KM, Serrano J, Gibril F, Jensen RT. Serum gastrin in Zollinger-Ellison syndrome: I. Prospective study of fasting serum gastrin in 309 patients from the National Institutes of Health and comparison with 2229 cases from the literature. *Medicine (Baltimore).* 2006;85(6):295–330. https://doi.org/10.1097/01.md.00 00236956.74128.76.
5. Jensen RT, Berna MJ, Bingham DB, Norton JA. Inherited pancreatic endocrine tumor syndromes: advances in molecular pathogenesis, diagnosis, management, and controversies. *Cancer.* 2008;113(suppl 7):1807–1843. https://doi.org/10.1002/cncr.23648.
6. Gibril F, Schumann M, Pace A, Jensen RT. Multiple endocrine neoplasia type 1 and Zollinger-Ellison syndrome: a prospective study of 107 cases and comparison with 1009 cases from the literature. *Medicine (Baltimore).* 2004;83(1):43–83. https://doi.org/10.1097/01.md.0000 112297.72510.32.
7. Stabile BE, Morrow DJ, Passaro E. The gastrinoma triangle: operative implications. *Am J Surg.* 1984;147(1):25–31. https://doi.org/10.1016/0002-9610(84)90029-1.
8. Pipeleers-Marichal M, Somers G, Willems G, et al. Gastrinomas in the duodenums of patients with multiple endocrine neoplasia type 1 and the Zollinger-Ellison syndrome. *N Engl J Med.* 1990;322(11):723–727.
9. Kisker O, Bastian D, Bartsch D, Nies C, Rothmund M. Localization, malignant potential, and surgical management of gastrinomas. *World J Surg.* 1998;22(7):651–657. https://doi.org/10.1007/s002689900448.
10. Weber HC, Venzon DJ, Lin JT, et al. Determinants of metastatic rate and survival in patients with Zollinger-Ellison syndrome: a prospective long-term study. *Gastroenterology.* 1995;108(6):1637–1649. https://doi.org/10.1016/0016-5085(95)90124-8.
11. Jensen RT, Cadiot G, Brandi ML, et al. ENETS consensus guidelines for the management of patients with digestive neuroendocrine neoplasms: functional pancreatic endocrine tumor syndromes. *Neuroendocrinology.* 2012;95(2): 98–119. https://doi.org/10.1159/000335591.
12. Norton JA, Alexander HR, Fraker DL, Venzon DJ, Gibril F, Jensen RT. Possible primary lymph node gastrinoma: occurrence, natural history, and predictive factors: a prospective study. *Ann Surg.* 2003;237(5):650–657. https://doi.org/10.1097/01.SLA.0000064375.51939.48.
13. Roy PK, Venzon DJ, Shojamanesh H, et al. Zollinger-Ellison syndrome. Clinical presentation in 261 patients. *Med.* 2000;79(6):379–411. https://doi.org/10.1097/ 00005792-200011000-00004.

14. Norton JA, Jensen RT. Resolved and unresolved controversies in the surgical management of patients with Zollinger-Ellison syndrome. *Ann Surg.* 2004;240(5):757−773. https://doi.org/10.1097/01.sla.0000143252.02142.3e.

15. Yu F, Venzon DJ, Serrano J, et al. Prospective study of the clinical course, prognostic factors, causes of death, and survival in patients with long-standing Zollinger-Ellison syndrome. *J Clin Oncol.* 1999;17(2):615−630. https://doi.org/10.1200/JCO.1999.17.2.615.

16. Hughes CM, Rozenblatt-Rosen O, Milne TA, et al. Menin associates with a trithorax family histone methyltransferase complex and with the hoxc8 locus. *Mol Cell.* 2004;13(4):587−597. https://doi.org/10.1016/S1097-2765(04)00081-4.

17. Lemos M, Thakker R. Multiple endocrine neoplasia type 1 (MEN1): analysis of 1336 mutations reported in the first decade following identification of the gene. *Hum Mutat.* 2008;29(1):22−32.

18. Debelenko LV, Zhuang Z, Emmert-Buck MR, et al. Allelic deletions on chromosome 11q13 in multiple endocrine neoplasia type 1-associated and sporadic gastrinomas and pancreatic endocrine tumors. *Cancer Res.* 1997;57(11):2238−2243.

19. Goebel S, Heppner C, Burns A, et al. Genotype/phenotype correlation of multiple endocrine neoplasia type 1 gene mutations in sporadic gastrinomas. *J Clin Endocrinol Metab.* 2000;85(1):116−123. https://doi.org/10.1210/jcem.85.1.6260.

20. Serrano J, Goebel S, Peghini P, Lubensky I, Gibril F, Jensen R. Alterations in the p16INK4a/CDKN2A tumor suppressor gene in gastrinomas. *J Clin Endocrinol Metab.* 2000;85(11):4146−4156. https://doi.org/10.1210/jcem.85.11.6970.

21. Jiao Y, Shi C, Edil BH, et al. DAXX/ATRX, MEN1, and mTOR pathway genes are frequently altered in pancreatic neuroendocrine tumors. *Science.* 2011;331(6021):1199−1203. https://doi.org/10.1126/science.1200609.

22. Marinoni I, Kurrer AS, Vassella E, et al. Loss of DAXX and ATRX are associated with chromosome instability and reduced survival of patients with pancreatic neuroendocrine tumors. *Gastroenterology.* 2014;146(2):453−460. https://doi.org/10.1053/j.gastro.2013.10.020.

23. Dacha S, Razvi M, Massaad J, Cai Q, Wehbi M. Hypergastrinemia. *Gastroenterol Rep (Oxf).* 2015;3(3):201−208. https://doi.org/10.1093/gastro/gov004.

24. Metz D, Cadiot G, Poitras P, Ito T, Jensen R. Diagnosis of Zollinger-Ellison syndrome in the era of PPIs, faulty gastrin assays, sensitive imaging and limited access to acid secretory testing. *Int J Endocr Oncol.* 2017;4(4):167−185. https://doi.org/10.2217/ije-2017-0018.

25. Rehfeld JF, Gingras MH, Bardram L, Hilsted L, Goetze JP, Poitras P. The Zollinger-Ellison syndrome and mismeasurement of gastrin. *Gastroenterology.* 2011;140(5):1444−1453. https://doi.org/10.1053/j.gastro.2011.01.051.

26. Rehfeld JF, Bardram L, Hilsted L, Poitras P, Goetze JP. Pitfalls in diagnostic gastrin measurements. *Clin Chem.* 2012;58(5):831−836. https://doi.org/10.1373/clinchem.2011.179929.

27. Roy PK, Venzon DJ, Feigenbaum KM, et al. Gastric secretion in Zollinger-Ellison syndrome. Correlation with clinical expression, tumor extent and role in diagnosis–a prospective NIH study of 235 patients and a review of 984 cases in the literature. *Medicine (Baltimore).* 2001;80(3):189−222. https://doi.org/10.1097/00005792-200105000-00005.

28. Lee CH, P'eng FK, Yeh PHH. Sodium pertechnetate Tc 99m antral scan in the diagnosis of retained gastric antrum. *Arch Surg.* 1984;119(3):309−311. https://doi.org/10.1001/archsurg.1984.01390150047012.

29. Berna MJ, Hoffmann KM, Long SH, Serrano J, Gibril F, Jensen RT. Serum gastrin in Zollinger-Ellison syndrome: II. prospective study of gastrin provocative testing in 293 patients from the National Institutes of Health and comparison with 537 cases from the literature. evaluation of diagnostic criteria, proposal of new criteria, and correlations with clinical and tumoral features. *Medicine (Baltimore).* 2006;85(6):331−364. https://doi.org/10.1097/MD.0b013e31802b518c.

30. Shah P, Singh MH, Yang YX, Metz DC. Hypochlorhydria and achlorhydria are associated with false-positive secretin stimulation testing for Zollinger-Ellison syndrome. *Pancreas.* 2013;42(6):932−936. https://doi.org/10.1097/MPA.0b013e3182847b2e.

31. Bajetta E, Ferrari L, Martinetti A, et al. Chromogranin A, neuron specific enolase, carcinoembryonic antigen, and hydroxyindole acetic acid evaluation in patients with neuroendocrine tumors. *Cancer.* 1999;86(5):858−865. https://doi.org/10.1002/(SICI)1097-0142(19990901)86:5<858::AID-CNCR23>3.0.CO;2-8.

32. Nobels FRE, Kwekkeboom DJ, Coopmans W, et al. Chromogranin A as serum marker for neuroendocrine neoplasia: comparison with neuron-specific enolase and the alpha-subunit of glycoprotein hormones. *J Clin Endocrinol Metab.* 1997;82(8):2622−2628. https://doi.org/10.1210/jc.82.8.2622.

33. Tomassetti P, Migliori M, Simoni P, et al. Diagnostic value of plasma chromogranin A in neuroendocrine tumours. *Eur J Gastroenterol Hepatol.* 2001;13(1):55−58.

34. Goebel SU, Serrano J, Yu F, Gibril F, Venzon DJ, Jensen RT. Prospective study of the value of serum chromogranin A or serum gastrin levels in the assessment of the presence, extent, or growth of gastrinomas. *Cancer.* 1999;85(7):1470−1483. https://doi.org/10.1002/(SICI)1097-0142(19990401)85:7<1470::AID-CNCR7>3.0.CO;2-S.

35. Abou-Saif A, Gibril F, Ojeaburu JV, et al. Prospective study of the ability of serial measurements of serum chromogranin A and gastrin to detect changes in tumor burden in patients with gastrinomas. *Cancer.* 2003;98(2):249−261. https://doi.org/10.1002/cncr.11473.

36. Pregun I, Herszényi L, Juhász M, et al. Effect of proton-pump inhibitor therapy on serum chromogranin A level. *Digestion.* 2011;84(1):22–28. https://doi.org/10.1159/000321535.

37. Raines D, Chester M, Diebold AE, et al. A prospective evaluation of the effect of chronic proton pump inhibitor use on plasma biomarker levels in humans. *Pancreas.* 2012;41(4):508–511. https://doi.org/10.1097/MPA.0b013e318243a0b6.

38. Sanduleanu S, Stridsberg M, Jonkers D, et al. Serum gastrin and chromogranin A during medium- and long-term acid suppressive therapy: a case-control study. *Aliment Pharmacol Ther.* 1999;13(2):145–153. https://doi.org/10.1046/j.1365-2036.1999.00466.x.

39. Proye C, Malvaux P, Pattou F, et al. Noninvasive imaging of insulinomas and gastrinomas with endoscopic ultrasonography and somatostatin receptor scintigraphy. *Surgery.* 1998;124(6):1134–1143. https://doi.org/10.1067/msy.1998.93109.

40. Rösch T, Lightdale CJ, Botet JF, et al. Localization of pancreatic endocrine tumors by endoscopic ultrasonography. *N Engl J Med.* 1992;326(26):1721–1726. https://doi.org/10.1056/NEJM199206253262601.

41. Anderson MA, Carpenter S, Thompson NW, Nostrant TT, Elta GH, Scheiman JM. Endoscopic ultrasound is highly accurate and directs management in patients with neuroendocrine tumors of the pancreas. *Am J Gastroenterol.* 2000;95(9):2271–2277. https://doi.org/10.1111/j.1572-0241.2000.02480.x.

42. Mendelson AH, Donowitz M. Catching the zebra: clinical pearls and pitfalls for the successful diagnosis of zollinger-ellison syndrome. *Dig Dis Sci.* 2017;62(9):2258–2265. https://doi.org/10.1007/s10620-017-4695-7.

43. Wank SA, Doppman JL, Miller DL, et al. Prospective study of the ability of computed axial tomography to localize gastrinomas in patients with Zollinger-Ellison syndrome. *Gastroenterology.* 1987;92(4):905–912. https://doi.org/10.1016/0016-5085(87)90963-2.

44. Frucht H, Doppman J, Norton J, et al. Gastrinomas: comparison of MR imaging with CT, angiography, and US. *Radiology.* 1989;171(3):713–717. https://doi.org/10.1148/radiology.171.3.2655004.

45. Pisegna JR, Doppman JL, Norton JA, Metz DC, Jensen RT. Prospective comparative study of ability of MR imaging and other imaging modalities to localize tumors in patients with Zollinger-Ellison syndrome. *Dig Dis Sci.* 1993;38(7):1318–1328. https://doi.org/10.1007/BF01296084.

46. Thoeni RF, Mueller-Lisse UG, Chan R, Do NK, Shyn PB. Detection of small, functional islet cell tumors in the pancreas: selection of MR imaging sequences for optimal sensitivity. *Radiology.* 2000;214(2):483–490. https://doi.org/10.1148/radiology.214.2.r00fe32483.

47. Alexander HR, Fraker DL, Norton JA, et al. Prospective study of somatostatin receptor scintigraphy and its effect on operative outcome in patients with Zollinger-Ellison syndrome. *Ann Surg.* 1998;228(2):228–238. https://doi.org/10.1097/00000658-199808000-00013.

48. Termanini B, Gibril F, Reynolds JC, et al. Value of somatostatin receptor scintigraphy: a prospective study in gastrinoma of its effect on clinical management. *Gastroenterology.* 1997;112(2):335–347. https://doi.org/10.1053/gast.1997.v112.pm9024287.

49. Gibril F, Reynolds JC, Doppman JL, et al. Somatostatin receptor scintigraphy: its sensitivity compared with that of other imaging methods in detecting primary and metastatic gastrinomas. A prospective study. *Ann Intern Med.* 1996;125(1):26–34. https://doi.org/10.7326/0003-4819-125-1-199607010-00005.

50. Geijer H, Breimer L. Somatostatin receptor PET/CT in neuroendocrine tumours: update on systematic review and meta-analysis. *Eur J Nucl Med Mol Imaging.* 2013;40(11):1770–1780. https://doi.org/10.1007/s00259-013-2482-z.

51. Hofman M, Kong G, Neels O, Eu P, Hong E, Hicks R. High management impact of Ga-68 DOTATATE (GaTate) PET/CT for imaging neuroendocrine and other somatostatin expressing tumours. *J Med Imaging Radiat Oncol.* 2012;56(1):40–47. https://doi.org/10.1111/j.1754-9485.2011.02327.x.

52. Frilling A, Sotiropoulos G, Radtke A, et al. The impact of 68Ga-DOTATOC positron emission tomography/computed tomography on the multimodal management of patients with neuroendocrine tumors. *Ann Surg.* 2010;252(5):850–856. https://doi.org/10.1097/SLA.0b013e3181fd37e8.

53. Froeling V, Elgeti F, Maurer M, et al. Impact of Ga-68 DOTATOC PET/CT on the diagnosis and treatment of patients with multiple endocrine neoplasia. *Ann Nucl Med.* 2012;26(9):738–743. https://doi.org/10.1007/s12149-012-0634-z.

54. Naswa N, Sharma P, Soundararajan R, et al. Diagnostic performance of somatostatin receptor PET/CT using 68Ga-DOTANOC in gastrinoma patients with negative or equivocal CT findings. *Abdom Imag.* 2013;38(3):552–560. https://doi.org/10.1007/s00261-012-9925-z.

55. Norton JA, Fraker DL, Alexander HR, Jensen RT. Value of surgery in patients with negative imaging and sporadic Zollinger-Ellison syndrome. *Ann Surg.* 2012;256(3):509–517. https://doi.org/10.1097/SLA.0b013e318265f08d.

56. Raufman JP, Collins SM, Pandol SJ, et al. Reliability of symptoms in assessing control of gastric acid secretion in patients with Zollinger-Ellison syndrome. *Gastroenterology.* 1983;84(1):108–113. https://doi.org/10.1016/S0016-5085(83)80173-5.

57. Hirschowitz BI, Simmons J, Mohnen J. Clinical outcome using lansoprazole in acid hypersecretors with and without Zollinger-Ellison syndrome: a 13-year prospective study. *Clin Gastroenterol Hepatol.* 2005;3(1):39–48. https://doi.org/10.1016/S1542-3565(04)00606-8.

58. Hirschowitz BI, Simmons J, Mohnen J. Long-term lansoprazole control of gastric acid and pepsin secretion in ZE and non-ZE hypersecretors: a prospective 10-year study. *Aliment Pharmacol Ther.* 2001;15(11):1795–1806. https://doi.org/10.1046/j.1365-2036.2001.01097.x.

59. Termanini B, Gibril F, Sutliff VE, Yu F, Venzon DJ, Jensen RT. Effect of long-term gastric acid suppressive therapy on serum vitamin B12 levels in patients with Zollinger-Ellison syndrome. *Am J Med.* 1998;104(5):422–430.

60. Ito T, Jensen RT. Association of long-term proton pump inhibitor therapy with bone fractures and effects on absorption of calcium, vitamin B12, iron, and magnesium. *Curr Gastroenterol Rep.* 2010;12(6):448–457. https://doi.org/10.1007/s11894-010-0141-0.

61. Freedberg DE, Kim LS, Yang Y-X. The risks and benefits of long-term use of proton pump inhibitors: expert review and best practice advice from the American gastroenterological association. *Gastroenterology.* 2017;152(4):706–715. https://doi.org/10.1053/j.gastro.2017.01.031.

62. Metz D, Benya R, Fishbeyn V, et al. Prospective study of the need for long-term antisecretory therapy in patients with Zollinger-Ellison syndrome following successful curative gastrinoma resection. *Aliment Pharmacol Ther.* 1993;7(3):247–257. https://doi.org/10.1111/j.1365-2036.1993.tb00095.x.

63. Fraker DL, Norton JA, Saeed ZA, Maton PN, Gardner JD, Jensen RT. A prospective study of perioperative and postoperative control of acid hypersecretion in patients with Zollinger-Ellison syndrome undergoing gastrinoma resection. *Surgery.* 1988;104(6):1054–1063. doi:0039-6060(88)90168-7 [pii].

64. Jansen J, Lamers C. Effect of changes in serum calcium on secretin-stimulated serum gastrin in patients with Zollinger-Ellison syndrome. *Gastroenterology.* 1982;83(1):173–178.

65. McCarthy DM, Peikin SR, Lopatin RN, et al. Hyperparathyroidism–a reversible cause of cimetidine-resistant gastric hypersecretion. *Br Med J.* 1979;1(6180):1765–1766. https://doi.org/10.1136/bmj.1.6180.1765.

66. Norton J, Cornelius M, Doppman J, Maton P, Gardner J, Jensen R. Effect of parathyroidectomy in patients with hyperparathyroidism, Zollinger-Ellison syndrome, and multiple endocrine neoplasia type I: a prospective study. *Surgery.* 1987;102(6):958–966.

67. Norton JA, Venzon DJ, Berna MJ, et al. Prospective study of surgery for primary hyperparathyroidism (HPT) in multiple endocrine neoplasia-type 1 and Zollinger-Ellison syndrome: long-term outcome of a more virulent form of HPT. *Ann Surg.* 2008;247(3):501–510. https://doi.org/10.1097/SLA.0b013e31815efda5.

68. Burgess JR, David R, Parameswaran V, Greenaway TM, Shepherd JJ. The outcome of subtotal parathyroidectomy for the treatment of hyperparathyroidism in multiple endocrine neoplasia type 1. *Arch Surg.* 1998;133(2):126–129. https://doi.org/10.1001/archsurg.133.2.126.

69. Tonelli F, Marcucci T, Fratini G, Tommasi MS, Falchetti A, Brandi ML. Is total parathyroidectomy the treatment of choice for hyperparathyroidism in multiple endocrine neoplasia type 1? *Ann Surg.* 2007;246(6):1075–1082. https://doi.org/10.1097/SLA.0b013e31811f4467.

70. Hubbard J, Sebag F, Maweja S, Henry J. Subtotal parathyroidectomy as an adequate treatment for primary hyperparathyroidism in multiple endocrine neoplasia type 1. *Arch Surg.* 2006;141(3):235–239. https://doi.org/10.1001/archsurg.141.3.235.

71. Norton JA, Doppman JL, Jensen RT. Curative resection in Zollinger-Ellison syndrome. Results of a 10-year prospective study. *Ann Surg.* 1992;215(1):8–18.

72. Norton JA, Fraker DL, Alexander HR, et al. Surgery increases survival in patients with gastrinoma. *Ann Surg.* 2006;244(3):410–419. https://doi.org/10.1097/01.sla.0000234802.44320.a5.

73. Norton JA, Fraker DL, Alexander HR, et al. Surgery to cure the Zollinger-Ellison syndrome. *N Engl J Med.* 1999;341(9):635–644. https://doi.org/10.1056/NEJM199908263410902.

74. Norton JA, Alexander HR, Fraker DL, Venzon DJ, Gibril F, Jensen RT. Does the use of routine duodenotomy (DUODX) affect rate of cure, development of liver metastases, or survival in patients with Zollinger-Ellison syndrome? *Ann Surg.* 2004;239(5):617–625. https://doi.org/10.1097/01.sla.0000124290.05524.5e.

75. Bartsch DK, Waldmann J, Fendrich V, et al. Impact of lymphadenectomy on survival after surgery for sporadic gastrinoma. *Br J Surg.* 2012;99(9):1234–1240. https://doi.org/10.1002/bjs.8843.

76. Norlén O, Hessman O, Stålberg P, Åkerström G, Hellman P. Prophylactic cholecystectomy in midgut carcinoid patients. *World J Surg.* 2010;34(6):1361–1367. https://doi.org/10.1007/s00268-010-0428-1.

77. Norton J, Krampitz G, Poultsides G, et al. Prospective evaluation of results of reoperation in Zollinger-Ellison syndrome. *Ann Surg.* 2018;267(4):782–788. https://doi.org/10.1097/SLA.0000000000002122.

78. Maire FR, Sauvanet A, Couvelard A, et al. Recurrence after surgical resection of gastrinoma: who, when, where and why? *Eur J Gastroenterol Hepatol.* 2012;24(4):368–374. https://doi.org/10.1097/MEG.0b013e328350f816.

79. Triponez F, Sadowski S, Pattou F, et al. Long-term follow-up of MEN1 patients who do not have initial surgery for Small ≤2 cm Nonfunctioning Pancreatic Neuroendocrine Tumors, an AFCE and GTE Study: association Francophone de Chirurgie Endocrinienne & Groupe d'Etude des Tumeurs Endocrines. *Ann Surg.* 2018;268(1):158–164. https://doi.org/10.1097/SLA.0000000000002191.

80. Triponez F, Goudet P, Dosseh D, et al. Is surgery beneficial for MEN1 patients with small (< or = 2 cm), nonfunctioning pancreaticoduodenal endocrine tumor? An analysis of 65 patients from the GTE. *World J Surg.* 2006;30(5):654–662. https://doi.org/10.1007/s00268-005-0354-9.

81. Norton JA, Alexander HR, Fraker DL, Venzon DJ, Gibril F, Jensen RT. Comparison of surgical results in patients with advanced and limited disease with multiple endocrine neoplasia type 1 and Zollinger-Ellison syndrome. *Ann Surg.* 2001;234(4):495–505. http://www.pubmedcentral.nih.gov/articlerender.fcgi?artid=1422073&tool=pmcentrez&rendertype=abstract.

82. Tonelli F, Fratini G, Nesi G, et al. Pancreatectomy in multiple endocrine neoplasia type 1-related gastrinomas and pancreatic endocrine neoplasias. *Ann Surg.* 2006;244(1):61–70. https://doi.org/10.1097/01.sla.0000218073.77254.62.

83. Sarmiento JM, Heywood G, Rubin J, Ilstrup DM, Nagorney DM, Que FG. Surgical treatment of neuroendocrine metastases to the liver: a plea for resection to increase survival. *J Am Coll Surg.* 2003;197(1):29–37. https://doi.org/10.1016/S1072-7515(03)00230-8.

84. Graff-Baker AN, Sauer DA, Pommier SJ, Pommier RF. Expanded criteria for carcinoid liver debulking: maintaining survival and increasing the number of eligible patients. *Surgery.* 2014;156(6):1369–1376. https://doi.org/10.1016/j.surg.2014.08.009.

85. Morgan RE, Pommier SEJ, Pommier RF. Expanded criteria for debulking of liver metastasis also apply to pancreatic neuroendocrine tumors. *Surgery.* 2018;163(1):218–225. https://doi.org/10.1016/j.surg.2017.05.030.

86. Mayo SC, De Jong MC, Pulitano C, et al. Surgical management of hepatic neuroendocrine tumor metastasis: results from an international multi-institutional analysis. *Ann Surg Oncol.* 2010;17(12):3129–3136. https://doi.org/10.1245/s10434-010-1154-5.

87. Fairweather M, Swanson R, Wang J, et al. Management of neuroendocrine tumor liver metastases: long-term outcomes and prognostic factors from a large prospective database. *Ann Surg Oncol.* 2017;24(8):2319–2325. https://doi.org/10.1245/s10434-017-5839-x.

88. Rossi R, Burroughs A, Caplin M. Liver transplantation for unresectable neuroendocrine tumor liver metastases. *Ann Surg Oncol.* 2014;21(7):2398–2405. https://doi.org/10.1245/s10434-014-3523-y.

89. Keutgen X, Schadde E, Pommier R, Halfdanarson T, Howe J, Kebebew E. Metastatic neuroendocrine tumors of the gastrointestinal tract and pancreas: a surgeon's plea to centering attention on the liver. *Semin Oncol.* 2018. https://doi.org/10.1053/j.seminoncol.2018.07.002 [Epub ahead of print].

90. Rinke A, Müller H, Schade-Brittinger C, et al. Placebo-controlled, double-blind, prospective, randomized study on the effect of octreotide LAR in the control of tumor growth in patients with metastatic neuroendocrine midgut tumors: a report from the PROMID Study Group. *J Clin Oncol.* 2009;27(28):4656–4663. https://doi.org/10.1200/JCO.2009.22.8510.

91. Caplin ME, Pavel M, Ćwikła JB, et al. Lanreotide in metastatic enteropancreatic neuroendocrine tumors. *N Engl J Med.* 2014;371(3):224–233. https://doi.org/10.1056/NEJMoa1316158.

92. Chan JA, Stuart K, Earle CC, et al. Prospective study of bevacizumab plus temozolomide in patients with advanced neuroendocrine tumors. *J Clin Oncol.* 2012;30(24):2963–2968. https://doi.org/10.1200/JCO.2011.40.3147.

93. Kulke MH, Stuart K, Enzinger PC, et al. Phase II study of temozolomide and thalidomide in patients with metastatic neuroendocrine tumors. *J Clin Oncol.* 2006;24(3):401–406. https://doi.org/10.1200/JCO.2005.03.6046.

94. Strosberg JR, Fine RL, Choi J, et al. First-line chemotherapy with capecitabine and temozolomide in patients with metastatic pancreatic endocrine carcinomas. *Cancer.* 2011;117(2):268–275. https://doi.org/10.1002/cncr.25425.

95. Yao JC, Shah MH, Ito T, et al. Everolimus for advanced pancreatic neuroendocrine tumors. *N Engl J Med.* 2011;364(6):514–523. https://doi.org/10.1056/NEJMoa1009290.

96. Yao J, Fazio N, Singh S, et al. Everolimus for the treatment of advanced, non-functional neuroendocrine tumours of the lung or gastrointestinal tract (RADIANT-4): a randomised, placebo-controlled, phase 3 study. *Lancet.* 2016;387(10022):968–977. https://doi.org/10.1016/S0140-6736(15)00817-X.

97. Raymond E, Dahan L, Raoul J-L, et al. Sunitinib malate for the treatment of pancreatic neuroendocrine tumors. *N Engl J Med.* 2011;364(6):501–513. https://doi.org/10.1056/NEJMoa1003825.

98. Strosberg J, El-Haddad G, Wolin E, et al. Phase 3 trial of 177Lu-dotatate for midgut neuroendocrine tumors. *N Engl J Med.* 2017;376(2):125–135. https://doi.org/10.1056/NEJMoa1607427.

99. Grozinsky-Glasberg S, Barak D, Fraenkel M, et al. Peptide receptor radioligand therapy is an effective treatment for the long-term stabilization of malignant gastrinomas. *Cancer.* 2011;117(7):1377–1385. https://doi.org/10.1002/cncr.25646.

CHAPTER 20

Advances in the Diagnosis and Management of Nonfunctional Pancreatic Neuroendocrine Tumors

AMANDA M. LAIRD, MD, FACS • STEVEN K. LIBUTTI, MD, FACS

INTRODUCTION

Pancreatic neuroendocrine tumors (PNETs) are tumors of the endocrine pancreas arising either from the islet cells of Langerhans or neuroendocrine cells that originate from pancreatic ductal epithelium. PNETs are relatively rare tumors with approximately 1000 new cases in the United States annually comprising 3%−5% of all pancreatic cancers.[1] Thought of previously as rare, the incidence has nearly doubled in the last 40 years.[2] Outcomes are determined from tumor grade, ranging from low to intermediate to high grade, as well as stage. Among gastroenteropancreatic neuroendocrine neoplasms as a whole, PNETs comprise 7.0% and tend to have a lower 5-year survival (<40%) than those of the remainder of the GI tract.[3]

PNETs may be functional or nonfunctional, meaning that they may or may not produce a hormone in excess including insulin, gastrin, glucagon, vasoactive intestinal peptide, and somatostatin. Hormone excess leads to symptoms that aid in diagnosis, but nonfunctional PNETs are more often discovered incidentally. Additionally, they may occur within a genetic syndrome including multiple endocrine neoplasia and von Hippel Lindau.[2,4] Presence or absence of any of these factors may influence medical and surgical decision making.

Traditionally, PNETs were managed surgically with pancreatic resection with or without metastatectomy. However, with widespread use of cross-sectional imaging, PNETs are discovered incidentally potentially at an early stage. Recent guidelines suggest that a more conservative approach may be used with similar outcomes.[5−7] This chapter focuses on diagnosis of sporadic nonfunctional PNETs and tumor-specific factors that influence treatment.

DIAGNOSIS

Clinical Features of PNETs

PNETs are traditionally called islet cell tumors thought to arise from the islet cells of Langerhans in the pancreas. More recent evidence suggests that they arise from precursor cells that originate from pancreatic ductal epithelium.[3] Nonfunctional PNETs do not secrete endocrine hormones such as insulin, gastrin, or somatostatin, but most produce other peptides, which may aid in follow-up. These include chromogranin A, neuron-specific enolase, and synaptophysin.[8,9] Most PNETs express somatostatin receptors (SSTR). SSTR are also present in other neuroendocrine tumor types, other endocrine glands, and throughout the gastrointestinal tract.[10] Five types of SSTR have been characterized and are present in greater number in well-differentiated PNETs rather than in those that are of high grade.[11] This tumor feature plays a role not only in diagnosis, but in management as well.

Because nonfunctional PNETs do not secrete excess hormones that would lead to symptoms, most patients present with larger tumors at a later stage.[12,13] Some patients are truly asymptomatic, and their tumors are discovered incidentally.[14] Others may present with one or more symptom including abdominal pain in the majority (35%−78%), weight loss (20%−35%), anorexia, and nausea (45%). Less frequent symptoms include intraabdominal hemorrhage (4%−20%), jaundice (17%−50%), or a mass palpable on physical exam (7%−40%).[15] In most patients the diagnosis is delayed because either they may be asymptomatic for many years or symptoms may be attributed to other conditions. In a survey of 758 patients with NETs of all types, the average length of time to diagnosis from the onset of

Advances in Treatment and Management in Surgical Endocrinology. https://doi.org/10.1016/B978-0-323-66195-9.00020-0

symptoms was 59 months. Patients saw an average of 5.7 physicians before arriving at a diagnosis.[16]

Tumor grade as well as stage at presentation correlates with outcomes. In a population-based study, the presence of metastases predicted worse survival more so than tumor size, and patients who underwent resection of any type had improved survival even in the setting of metastases.[17] A recent evaluation of data from the surveillance, epidemiology, and end results (SEER) program revealed that although the incidence and prevalence of NETs overall is increasing, there have been significant improvements in survival in patients with local disease as well as metastatic disease. The presence of lymph node metastases and distant metastases still predict reduced survival, however.[18]

Classification and Staging of PNETs

PNETs may be either functional or nonfunctional with nonfunctional PNETs comprising 90%.[19] They are further characterized by the presence or absence of a genetic mutation, which may influence treatment.

Similar to other malignancies, PNETs may be staged by a traditional staging system using tumor size, nodal status, and presence of metastases (TNM) to understand the clinical course and predict development of metastases. There is evidence that suggests, perhaps, the most important determinant of outcomes is tumor grade, which ultimately influences treatment.[20] The 2010 World Health Organization incorporates grade into staging of PNETs.[21] This classification system has been included in the most recent management guidelines published by the European Neuroendocrine Tumor Society (ENETS).[22] Determinants of grade include mitotic rate and Ki-67 index, a marker of proliferation. Ki-67 index, expressed as a percentage, provides critical prognostic information. In a series of patients with NETs, Ki-67 index used to categorize tumor grade predicts both progression-free survival as well as overall survival.[23] Low-grade tumors have a mitotic rate of <2 per high power field (HPF) and Ki-67 index of 0%–2%; intermediate-grade tumors have a mitotic rate of 2–20 per HPF and a Ki-67 index of 3%–20%; high-grade tumors, which may also be poorly differentiated, have a mitotic rate >20 per HPF and a Ki-67 index >20%. The higher of the two of mitotic rate and Ki-67 index determines grade.[7]

Pathologic stage is determined by the American Joint Committee on Cancer (AJCC) staging system, which employs TNM (tumor node metastasis) staging.[24] Although grade may ultimately determine prognosis and influence treatment decision making, the AJCC system is useful to define clinical stage, which aids in determining surgical candidacy as well as for planning type and extent of operation.

IMAGING OF PNETS

Many improvements have been made in imaging for PNETs over the last several years, not only as quality of computed tomography (CT) and magnetic resonance imaging (MRI) have improved, but with use of alternative imaging methods such as somatostatin receptor scintigraphy (SRS) and introduction of gallium-68 somatostatin analog positron emission tomography (^{68}GaSA-PET). Initial evaluation often begins with cross-sectional imaging, including CT or MRI, although either may have been obtained for another reason, as most PNETs are discovered incidentally.[25] Beyond making an initial diagnosis, imaging also is critical to surgical planning to determine resectability and appropriateness of surgery in the setting of metastases to lymph nodes and distant organs. In addition to traditional imaging, endoscopic ultrasound (EUS) is necessary for obtaining a tissue diagnosis but may also play a role in follow-up. There is variability of sensitivity and specificity of each, but all may play an important role in evaluation and treatment.

Somatostatin Receptor Scintigraphy

SRS is nuclear scintigraphy that was once the gold standard for imaging of NETs. The somatostatin analog octreotide is administered as indium-labeled octreotide, which binds to somatostatin receptors.[26] Planar images are acquired 24 h after injection, and the addition of single photon emission computed tomography with computed tomography (SPECT/CT) can localize abnormalities better than planar imaging or SPECT alone.[27,28] Sensitivity ranges from 70% to 90% with a specificity approaching 100%.[29,30] Different from strictly anatomic imaging, SRS has the advantage of being whole-body imaging and it is also widely available. It is limited, however, by its resolution and is limited by its ability to detect lesions smaller than 1 cm.[30] Furthermore, SRS does not provide enough anatomic detail to determine resectability in planning for potential surgery.[9]

Computed Tomography

CT is probably the most widely used imaging modality not only because of its accessibility, but because 90% of PNETs are discovered incidentally, it may be the initial test that leads to further evaluation.[25] CT has a similar sensitivity to SRS in the detection of both primary lesions as well as metastases but may be slightly better

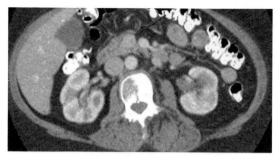

FIG. 20.1 Computed tomography of the abdomen in portal venous phase, pancreas mass indicated by arrow.

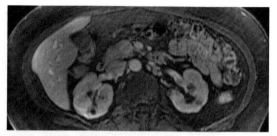

FIG. 20.2 Magnetic resonance imaging of the abdomen with contrast, pancreas mass indicated by arrow with contrast enhancement.

than SRS at detecting extrahepatic metastases.[31] Ideally, CT should be done as an early arterial-phase CT to demonstrate those imaging characteristics, which are typical of PNETs. Typically, lesions are isodense on precontrast images, then enhance in the arterial phase, with contrast washout on portal venous phase[32] as in Fig. 20.1. Large tumors may be centrally necrotic, heterogeneous, and contain calcifications and may not possess typical imaging characteristics.[32,33] Compared to other modalities, however, CT has the most advantage in understanding tumor relationship to surrounding structures and aids in surgical planning.

Magnetic Resonance Imaging

Similar to CT, MRI may be used to determine the anatomic relationship of the primary tumor to surrounding structures, thereby aiding in surgical planning. MRI also has the advantage of not exposing the patient to ionizing radiation, which may be of concern over a long period of follow-up.[34] MRI done with gadolinium with precontrast, arterial phase, and portal venous phase imaging is similar in sensitivity to CT.[35,36] On MRI, PNETs are hypo- or isodense on precontrast T1 images and are hyperdense on T2 images with enhancement postcontrast administration as in Fig. 20.2.[37,38]

Gallium-68 Somatostatin Analogs

Although positron emission tomography (PET) has been available, scanning with administration of a gallium-68 labeled somatostatin analog ([68]GaSA) is the latest addition for imaging of neuroendocrine tumors. Somatostatin analogs used include DOTATATE (tetraazacyclododecane tetraacetic acid-octreotate) and DOTATOC (DOTA[0]-D-Phe[1]-Tyr[3]-octreotide).[39] Much like octreotide in SRS, [68]GaSA has an affinity for somatostatin receptors types 2 and 5 but to a greater degree than octreotide. [68]GaSA-PET images are also fused with CT to improve sensitivity. Sensitivity is approximately 80% with a specificity of 90%,[40,41] and

when used to evaluate for disease beyond the pancreas, specificity approaches 100% for metastases.[42] Compared to SRS, [68]GaSA-PET/CT detects a greater number of primary and metastatic lesions.[43,44] Findings on [68]GaSA-PET may lead to changes in management. In a single-institution study where [68]GaSA-PET was compared to traditional imaging, findings led to a change in management in 19%—33% of patients influencing the decision to either proceed with or defer surgery.[42,45] In addition to providing useful anatomic information, [68]GaSA may be used to guide therapy because in patients with PNETs that take up [68]GaSA, somatostatin analogs may be effective.[46] Sensitivity may be limited by accumulation of [68]GaSA in the uncinate process of the pancreas or inflammation, which can lead to false-positive studies, Fig. 20.3.[47]

Fluorodeoxyglucose Positron Emission Tomography

Traditionally, PNETs that are low or intermediate grade do not take up fluorodeoxyglucose (FDG) readily; therefore, FDG positron emission tomography (FDG-PET) has less utility than other types of imaging. Standard uptake values (SUVs) are generally lower in low- or intermediate-grade PNETs.[48] FDG-PET may, however, be better for high-grade PNETs as they tend to take up glucose more readily and have higher SUVs.[49]

Endoscopic ultrasound

EUS is critical to the evaluation of PNETs as it is a way to not only characterize the tumor by ultrasound, but also enables a tissue diagnosis after identification of a lesion on cross-sectional imaging. A fine-needle aspiration (FNA) may be done at the time of EUS and provides critical information to confirm tumor type and to establish grade by obtaining tissue that can be stained and a Ki-67 index can thus be determined.[50] Although EUS cannot provide information regarding distant metastatic disease, it may provide additional detail not seen

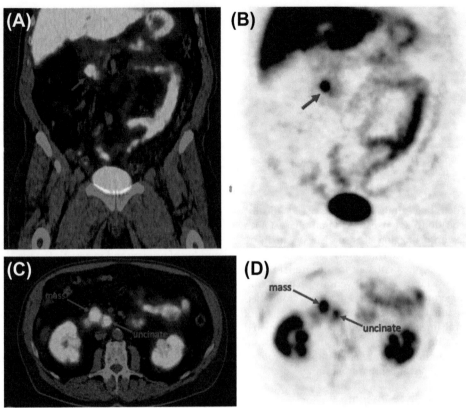

FIG. 20.3 ^{68}Ga-DOTATATE PET of a nonfunctional PNET; **(A)** fused CT and PET coronal image, tumor indicated by arrow; **(B)** planar image, tumor indicated by arrow; **(C)** fused CT and PET axial image demonstrating both tumor and physiologic uptake in uncinate process of the pancreas, indicated by arrow; **(D)** planar image, tumor, and uncinate process indicated by arrow.

on either CT or MRI to help determine resectability. It allows for improved visualization of margins with the superior mesenteric artery and other adjacent structures.[51] It is generally not used for surveillance for sporadic nonfunctional PNETs.[52]

CLINICAL GUIDELINES

Guidelines for management of PNETs are published by the North American Neuroendocrine Tumor Society (NANETS),[6] the ENETS,[7] the American Association of Clinical Endocrinologists and American College of Endocrinology (AACE/ACE),[5] and the National Comprehensive Cancer Network (NCCN).[53] Each of these outline management from initial diagnosis through decision making for either surgical or medical management. Although many recommendations are similar, there are some differences, specifically with respect to surgical management.

All published guidelines are relatively similar regarding imaging recommendations and testing of serum biomarkers. All recommend initial imaging, and CT is the preferred method with MRI depending on the individual clinical situation. It is recommended that all pancreas masses presumed to be PNETs on imaging be biopsied via endoscopic ultrasound-guided fine-needle aspiration (EUS-FNA). This allows for confirmation of the diagnosis by obtaining tissue, and staining for and obtaining a Ki-67 index is recommended by all. Obtaining serum biomarkers, specifically chromogranin A (CGA), is recommended; testing for additional levels including pancreatic polypeptide (PP) and 5-hydroxyindoleacetic acid (5-HIAA) is recommended based on clinical features. These are listed in Table 20.1.

There is variability regarding recommendations for surgery. Both AACE/ACE and ENETS recommendations for surgical resection vary based on the T-stage of the

TABLE 20.1
Comparison of Guidelines Recommendations.

	NANETS	ENETS	AACE/ACE	NCCN
Imaging	CT MRI, consider SRS recommended	CT MRI, consider ^{68}Ga versus SRS	CT MRI, consider [68]Ga ± EUS	CT MRI [68]Ga (preferred) versus SRS EUS, consider
Biopsy	FNA via EUS Obtain Ki-67 index	FNA via EUS Obtain Ki-67 index	FNA via EUS Obtain Ki-67 index	FNA via EUS Obtain Ki-67 index
Laboratory testing	CGA, 5-HIAA	CGA	CGA, ±PP	CGA, ±PP
Surgical recommendations	Surgery, no role for observation	Observation: <2 cm, G1 or low G2, asymptomatic Surgery: >2 cm, G2, symptomatic	Observation: <2 cm, G1, asymptomatic, no evidence of LN metastases Surgery: >2 cm, G2, symptomatic	Surgery for all Observation if <2 cm and patient high risk for surgery

[68]Ga, [68]GaSA PET/CT; CGA, Chromogranin A; CT, Computed tomography; EUS, Endoscopic ultrasound; FNA, Fine-needle aspiration; MRI, Magnetic resonance imaging; PP, Pancreatic polypeptide; SRS, Somatostatin receptor scintigraphy.

tumor as well as tumor grade. T1 tumors (<2 cm) that are low grade (G1) and are asymptomatic may be observed with close follow-up. ENETS further includes low-G2 tumors, with a Ki-67 index at the lower end of the G2 range, as potential candidates for observation. This is based on evidence that small nonfunctional, sporadic PNETs tend not to grow or metastasize. Two separate series of data compared patients managed with surgery versus observation. All had proven PNETs either by FNA biopsy or by imaging with characteristics typical of a PNET. In one, patients managed nonoperatively had a mean tumor size of 1 cm, and after a mean of 45 months of follow-up, there was no tumor progression and no evidence of metastatic disease.[54] In another single-institution series, those patients with T1, low-grade tumors observed for a median of 27.8 months demonstrated no tumor progression and no evidence of metastases.[55] Surgery is thus reserved to limit the potential for metastatic spread, more likely to occur in larger, intermediate-grade tumors.

NANETS and NCCN guidelines recommend resection regardless of size unless patient comorbidities are severe enough that the risk of operation would outweigh the benefit in the setting of a T1, low-grade PNET. A single-institution series of 139 patients, all managed surgically for sporadic nonfunctional PNETs, revealed that even in tumors <2 cm, 8% either had eventual development of metastasis or recurrence. Surgical morbidity rate was 44% and it is unknown if resection of PNETs in this series impacted survival given

the lack of a nonoperative control group for comparison.[56]

High-grade PNETs (G3) are generally managed similarly to those that are intermediate grade. Separate guidelines from ENETS and NANETS recommend the same imaging including CT and/or MRI including the chest, abdomen, and pelvis to evaluate for metastatic disease. Furthermore, FDG-PET should be performed if surgery is considered to evaluate for disease outside of the pancreas. Surgery is not recommended for G3 PNETs in the setting of metastases. Surgery is recommended for PNETs that are resectable without evidence of metastases, followed by adjuvant cytotoxic chemotherapy.[6,57,58] There is some evidence that suggests all G3 PNETs may not be the same and that Ki-67 index may help to determine which are high G3 but well differentiated and which are poorly differentiated neuroendocrine carcinoma (NEC).[59,60] Regardless of Ki-67 index, management is surgical if the tumor is resectable, though survival is worse in the setting of a G3 NEC ranging from 5 to 38 months depending on stage at presentation.[61]

SURGICAL MANAGEMENT
Operative Versus Nonoperative Management
In patients who have PNETs that are not invading adjacent structures, which would render them unresectable, surgery is preferred for patients who meet criteria. As outlined in the previous section, guidelines for

management vary, though it is the opinion of these authors that observation is appropriate for small (<2 cm) nonfunctional sporadic (not related to a genetic mutation) PNETs. Patients with T1 tumors may undergo surgery if they are G2 or G3, symptomatic, or have features that suggest potential for more aggressive behavior, such as lymph node metastases by imaging or biopsy. Our recommendation for those patients managed with observation is serial imaging with early arterial-phase CT of the abdomen every 6 months for a period of at least 2 years and then every 12 months thereafter if no growth, similar to the AACE/ACE guidelines.[5] CGA levels are obtained at the same intervals, and observation is continued provided that the PNET is stable in size. Surgery is recommended if there is tumor growth[5,7] as defined by response evaluation criteria in solid tumors (RECIST).[62]

Extent of Surgical Resection—Anatomic Resection Versus Enucleation

Alternatives for surgical resection include enucleation or central pancreatectomy (CP) as parenchyma-preserving procedures versus anatomic resection including pancreaticoduodenectomy (PD), distal pancreatectomy (DP) with or without splenectomy, and total pancreatectomy (TP).[63,64] Enucleation preserves pancreatic tissue while anatomic resection has the advantage of including adjacent fatty tissue containing lymph nodes, which allows for complete staging. There are no randomized data comparing outcomes of tumors managed with enucleation or CP to anatomic resection of any type. However, the goal of surgical resection for nonfunctional sporadic PNETs is to limit tumor spread based on their malignant potential.[65] Furthermore, single-institution data suggest that immediate postoperative outcomes and complication rates between enucleation and anatomic resection are similar despite enucleation being a more limited procedure.[65,66] Understanding presence or absence of lymph node metastases is useful as presence of lymph node metastases predict survival, and this information impacts postoperative treatment.[67] It is our opinion that no less than an anatomic resection should be performed for sporadic nonfunctional PNETs >2 cm in size.

Approaches to resection of any type include traditional open surgical (OS) approaches versus minimally invasive surgery (MIS). The most common operations for resection are PD and DP, reserving TP for recurrent disease. There are no randomized data comparing OS to MIS, and most data also include pancreatic adenocarcinoma, which may confound results regarding outcome. Regardless, MIS techniques have been introduced in pancreas surgery with the goals of reducing length of stay (LOS) and reducing postoperative pain while still achieving comparable surgical outcomes.[68] Most PDs are done open; those done as MIS tend to be done in academic medical centers with a higher 30-day mortality, no difference in LOS, and a conversion rate of approximately 30%.[69] Average LOS for MIS PD ranges from 12 to 18 days in other series.[70,71] For tumors in the tail or for some tumors in the body of the pancreas, DP (or extended DP) is the most appropriate procedure. Patients undergoing MIS DP compared to OS for PNETs specifically have a shorter LOS and fewer perioperative complications without impact on survival.[72] Few data compare robotic approaches to traditional MIS but in some series LOS and operative time are comparable.[73,74] Given the lack of randomized data, the use of MIS techniques over OS should be based on surgeon experience with those techniques and the specific clinical situation.

Surgery in Stage IV Disease

The decision to operate on a patient with a solitary PNET provided the tumor is resectable is much more straightforward than in the setting of stage IV disease. Different from other solid tumors, debulking to achieve cytoreduction may influence survival in patients with PNETs. Surgery is not recommended if there are metastases to other locations such as to lungs or bone. As normal hepatic parenchyma is replaced by tumor, the risk of liver failure increases and is a primary source of mortality in these situations.[75] The goal of surgery is to remove enough tumor from the liver to achieve at least a 70% cytoreduction as recommended by guidelines.[76] Options for resection include formal hepatic lobectomy and segmentectomy or parenchyma-sparing techniques including wedge resection and enucleation or local ablative techniques such as radiofrequency ablation (RFA). Survival following parenchyma-sparing techniques is similar to that following lobectomy and segmentectomy while preserving hepatic function.[77,78] A pooled population of patients with both PNETs and small bowel neuroendocrine tumors undergoing cytoreductive surgery achieving at least 70% cytoreduction have improved overall survival and progression-free survival (PFS).[79] A small series of patients with PNETs and liver metastases demonstrated a PFS of 11 months with at least 70% cytoreduction.[78] Data regarding liver resection for metastatic PNETs are limited and most series include functional PNETs, which may confound outcomes. If an operation is performed for an advanced PNET, that is, in the setting of metastases, cholecystectomy should be considered at the time of operation if the patient may receive a somatostatin analog (SSA) as part of therapy as they are at risk for developing cholelithiasis and cholecystitis.[53]

Other locoregional therapies for liver metastases include hepatic artery embolization (HAE), RFA, and radioembolization (RE) with yttrium-90. Data are limited given the rare nature of PNETs in general and lack of randomization of therapies. HAE may be useful for patients who are poor surgical candidates and is generally safe.[80] RFA may be performed either percutaneously or laparoscopically on even larger lesions with low morbidity though there is no data regarding survival advantage.[81,82] RE involves intraarterial hepatic injection of yttrium-90 microspheres, but utility is limited to smaller tumors of approximately 1 cm and data are limited.[83] Guidelines do not make any specific recommendations for or against any of these treatments.[84]

MEDICAL MANAGEMENT

Patients with R0-resected PNETs that are G1 or G2 should have follow-up imaging every 3—6 months and every 2—3 months if G3.[6,85] Postoperative therapy for G3 well-differentiated PNETs and for NEC of the pancreas includes cytotoxic chemotherapy consisting of cisplatin or carboplatin and etoposide.[86,87] There is no second-line chemotherapy though other regimens have been used in gastrointestinal neuroendocrine carcinomas with either partial response or tumor nonprogression.[88] Treatment with somatostatin analogs is not recommended for G3 PNETs.[85]

Recommendations for additional treatment following R0 resection of PNETs that are low or intermediate grade are less clear. Patients with complete resections have improved survival compared to those who present with liver metastases even without additional therapy following surgery.[89] SSA may be useful in controlling symptoms in the case of hormone-producing PNETs or in patients with symptoms of carcinoid syndrome in the case of advanced disease,[90] but their benefit as adjuvant treatment after initial complete resection is not established.[85] As many PNETs follow a more indolent course, observation after initial resection may be most appropriate.[91]

Somatostatin Analogs

SSAs as monotherapy for PNETs have not been evaluated prospectively against placebo separately from other gastrointestinal NETs. Their use may be used to control symptoms of carcinoid syndrome, but more recent data reveal promising results. There is one trial

that compared the SSA octreotide to octreotide plus interferon-α that included both PNETs and other types of gastrointestinal NETs. However, addition of interferon-α was not superior to treatment with octreotide alone.[92] The largest trial of SSA therapy for NETs is the Controlled Study of Lanreotide Antiproliferative Response in Neuroendocrine Tumors (CLARINET) trial inclusive of both PNETs and gastrointestinal NETs. The study was placebo-controlled, double-blind, and multinational. Patients with G1 PNETs and some G2 were included if they had not previously received an SSA, radioembolization, or chemotherapy. Outcomes were not reported based on primary tumor source. PFS was not reached in the lanreotide group and was 18 months in the placebo group. Estimated survival at 24 months was nearly 2 times greater in the lanreotide group, 65.1% versus 33% in the placebo group. Safety was equivalent between groups. Given its efficacy and safety, lanreotide is approved for treatment of metastatic neuroendocrine tumors that are SSTR-positive.

Molecular Targeted Therapies

In some patients, however, even those with well-differentiated G1 tumors, metastases either develop over time or are known at the time of initial diagnosis. When advanced disease is present at the time of diagnosis and surgical resection is not feasible, the recommendation is then treatment and multiple options are available for G1 and G2 tumors including observation in the absence of symptoms and with low-volume disease, everolimus, sunitinib, capecitabine/temozolamide, and others. Cytotoxic chemotherapy is reserved for progressive disease after failing other therapy and for G3 PNETs.[6,85] The treating physicians should consider discussion of care as part of a multidisciplinary approach to offer best available therapy as part of a tailored treatment plan. These types of therapeutic options for PNETs have been evaluated in clinical trials, each with some advantages over others. There are no trials comparing treatment options; therefore, each option must be evaluated individually and there is not a specific order to follow for selection of the appropriate option. The selection is continued if there is either response to therapy or disease nonprogression, and treatment is reevaluated if there is disease progression on follow-up imaging.[6]

The RADIANT-3 trial (RAD001 in Advanced Neuroendocrine Tumors) evaluated the oral mTOR inhibitor everolimus as a single agent therapy versus placebo for G1 and G2 PNETs in the setting of metastases. Approximately 400 patients were included over a 2-year period. After a median follow up of 17 months,

PFS was 11 months in the everolimus group compared to 4.6 months in the placebo group. Furthermore, tumor size was decreased in the treatment group. This represented a significant development in the management of advanced PNETs as before this only streptozocin either alone or along with doxorubicin was approved for use in these cases.[93] The tyrosine kinase inhibitor sunitinib has also been evaluated as a single agent. In a placebo-controlled randomized trial, 171 patients were evaluated. The trial was discontinued early due to serious adverse events in the placebo group combined with favorable outcomes with the use of sunitinib. PFS was 11.4 versus 5.5 months comparing sunitinib to placebo.[94] A more recent analysis of these data was performed confirming the initial results with PFS of 12.6 months in the treated group and 5.8 months in the placebo group. After 5 years, overall survival was 38.6 versus 29.1 months in those patients treated; however, there was significant crossover to the sunitinib arm.[95]

Cytotoxic Chemotherapy

Finally, there are chemotherapeutic regimens used for G1 and G2 PNETs in patients with progressive disease or for selected clinical situations. Capecitabine and temozolomide (CAPTEM) given in combination have a response rate of 54%−61% with a PFS of 14 months.[96,97] Another option in the setting of progressive disease is streptozocin in combination with 5-FU or doxorubicin.[85] In a single-institution retrospective evaluation, patients with advanced PNETs treated with this regimen had a median PFS of 16 months and overall survival of 28 months. Ki-67 index was a predictor of response with an inverse relationship of index to response rate.[98]

Peptide Receptor Radiotherapy

A recent advance in the treatment of metastatic NETs of the gastrointestinal tract and pancreas is the targeted radiopharmaceutical, [177]Lutecium-DOTATATE (^{177}Lu-DOTATATE). [177]Lu works by emitting beta radiation after binding to the SSTR of the tumor. Recently FDA approved, it is indicated in advanced G1 and G2 GI and PNETs that express somatostatin receptors. The phase 3 Neuroendocrine Tumors Therapy (NETTER-1) trial evaluated response of therapy in patients treated with ^{177}Lu-DOTATATE plus octreotide versus octreotide alone. Inclusion criteria for the trial were patients with G1 or G2 GI NETs that were SSTR-positive, which progressed on therapy with any SSA. Patients received ^{177}Lu-DOTATATE every 8 weeks for a total of four treatments and long-acting octreotide monthly. Over a

4-year period, 229 patients were recruited and randomized. Group characteristics were similar. PFS was not reached during follow-up for the ^{177}Lu group compared to 8.4 months in the control group. At 20 months, PFS was 65.2% for the ^{177}Lu-DOTATATE group compared to 10.2% in the control group.[99] After FDA approval, indications are similar and now include G1 and G2 PNETs. It is not indicated for G3 PNETs as these typically do not express SSTR.

CONCLUSION

Pancreatic neuroendocrine tumors are rare neoplasms. Behavior may be predicted by grade and stage, although even apparent well-differentiated tumors that appear benign at initial presentation may ultimately behave more aggressively. Surgery remains the most effective therapy for patients who are candidates even in the setting of advanced disease. Multiple treatment options exist for those patients who are not candidates for surgery with emerging therapies available. Multidisciplinary evaluation and management allow for developing a thoughtful treatment plan for both intervention and follow-up.

REFERENCES

1. Ries LAG, Young JL, Keel GE, et al. *SEER Survival Monograph: Cancer Survival Among Adults: US SEER Program, 1988–2001, Patient and Tumor Characteristics*. Bethesda, MD: National Cancer Institute; 2007.
2. Lawrence B, Gustafsson BI, Chan A, et al. The epidemiology of gastroenteropancreatic neuroendocrine tumors. *Endocrinol Metab Clin N Am.* 2011;40(1):1–18. vii.
3. Reid MD, Balci S, Saka B, et al. Neuroendocrine tumors of the pancreas: current concepts and controversies. *Endocr Pathol.* 2014;25(1):65–79.
4. Norton JA, Krampitz G, Jensen RT. Multiple endocrine neoplasia: genetics and clinical management. *Surg Oncol Clin.* 2015;24(4):795–832.
5. Herrera MF, Akerstrom G, Angelos P, et al. AACE/ACE disease state clinical review: pancreatic neuroendocrine incidentalomas. *Endocr Pract.* 2015;21(5):546–553.
6. Kunz PL, Reidy-Lagunes D, Anthony LB, et al. Consensus guidelines for the management and treatment of neuroendocrine tumors. *Pancreas.* 2013;42(4):557–577.
7. Falconi M, Eriksson B, Kaltsas G, et al. ENETS consensus guidelines update for the management of patients with functional pancreatic neuroendocrine tumors and nonfunctional pancreatic neuroendocrine tumors. *Neuroendocrinology.* 2016;103(2):153–171.
8. Dickson PV, Behrman SW. Management of pancreatic neuroendocrine tumors. *Surg Clin.* 2013;93(3):675–691.
9. Kuo JH, Lee JA, Chabot JA. Nonfunctional pancreatic neuroendocrine tumors. *Surg Clin.* 2014;94(3):689–708.

10. Chan JA, Kulke MH. Neuroendocrine tumors–current and future clinical advances. *Hematol Oncol Clin N Am.* 2016; 30(1). xiii–xiv.

11. Cives M, Strosberg J. The expanding role of somatostatin analogs in gastroenteropancreatic and lung neuroendocrine tumors. *Drugs.* 2015;75(8):847–858.

12. Halfdanarson TR, Rabe KG, Rubin J, et al. Pancreatic neuroendocrine tumors (PNETs): incidence, prognosis and recent trend toward improved survival. *Ann Oncol.* 2008;19(10):1727–1733.

13. Franko J, Feng W, Yip L, et al. Non-functional neuroendocrine carcinoma of the pancreas: incidence, tumor biology, and outcomes in 2,158 patients. *J Gastrointest Surg.* 2010; 14(3):541–548.

14. Cheema A, Weber J, Strosberg JR. Incidental detection of pancreatic neuroendocrine tumors: an analysis of incidence and outcomes. *Ann Surg Oncol.* 2012;19(9): 2932–2936.

15. Falconi M, Plockinger U, Kwekkeboom DJ, et al. Well-differentiated pancreatic nonfunctioning tumors/carcinoma. *Neuroendocrinology.* 2006;84(3):196–211.

16. Wolin EM, Leyden J, Goldstein G, et al. Patient-reported experience of diagnosis, management, and burden of neuroendocrine tumors: results from a large patient survey in the United States. *Pancreas.* 2017;46(5):639–647.

17. Genc CG, Klumpen HJ, van Oijen MGH, et al. A nationwide population-based study on the survival of patients with pancreatic neuroendocrine tumors in The Netherlands. *World J Surg.* 2018;42(2):490–497.

18. Dasari A, Shen C, Halperin D, et al. Trends in the incidence, prevalence, and survival outcomes in patients with neuroendocrine tumors in the United States. *JAMA Oncol.* 2017;3(10):1335–1342.

19. Liu JB, Baker MS. Surgical management of pancreatic neuroendocrine tumors. *Surg Clin.* 2016;96(6): 1447–1468.

20. Kim JY, Hong SM. Recent updates on neuroendocrine tumors from the gastrointestinal and pancreatobiliary tracts. *Arch Pathol Lab Med.* 2016;140(5):437–448.

21. Kim BS, Park YS, Yook JH, et al. Comparison of the prognostic values of the 2010 WHO classification, AJCC 7th edition, and ENETS classification of gastric neuroendocrine tumors. *Medicine (Baltimore).* 2016;95(30):e3977.

22. Kloppel G, Rindi G, Perren A, et al. The ENETS and AJCC/UICC TNM classifications of the neuroendocrine tumors of the gastrointestinal tract and the pancreas: a statement. *Virchows Arch.* 2010;456(6):595–597.

23. Dhall D, Mertens R, Bresee C, et al. Ki-67 proliferative index predicts progression-free survival of patients with well-differentiated ileal neuroendocrine tumors. *Hum Pathol.* 2012;43(4):489–495.

24. AJCC Cancer Staging Manual, 8th ed. Vol 1. Chicago, IL: Springer; 2017.

25. Vagefi PA, Razo O, Deshpande V, et al. Evolving patterns in the detection and outcomes of pancreatic neuroendocrine neoplasms: the Massachusetts General Hospital experience from 1977 to 2005. *Arch Surg.* 2007;142(4):347–354.

26. Lamberts SW, Reubi JC, Krenning EP. Somatostatin receptor imaging in the diagnosis and treatment of neuroendocrine tumors. *J Steroid Biochem Mol Biol.* 1992;43(1–3): 185–188.

27. Balon HR, Brown TL, Goldsmith SJ, et al. The SNM practice guideline for somatostatin receptor scintigraphy 2.0. *J Nucl Med Technol.* 2011;39(4):317–324.

28. Corleto VD, Scopinaro F, Angeletti S, et al. Somatostatin receptor localization of pancreatic endocrine tumors. *World J Surg.* 1996;20(2):241–244.

29. Gibril F, Jensen RT. Diagnostic uses of radiolabelled somatostatin receptor analogues in gastroenteropancreatic endocrine tumours. *Dig Liver Dis.* 2004;36(suppl 1): S106–S120.

30. Kwekkeboom DJ, Krenning EP. Somatostatin receptor imaging. *Semin Nucl Med.* 2002;32(2):84–91.

31. Kumbasar B, Kamel IR, Tekes A, et al. Imaging of neuroendocrine tumors: accuracy of helical CT versus SRS. *Abdom Imag.* 2004;29(6):696–702.

32. Reznek RH. CT/MRI of neuroendocrine tumours. *Cancer Image.* 2006;6:S163–S177.

33. Pelage JP, Soyer P, Boudiaf M, et al. Carcinoid tumors of the abdomen: CT features. *Abdom Imag.* 1999;24(3): 240–245.

34. Fletcher JG, Kofler JM, Coburn JA, et al. Perspective on radiation risk in CT imaging. *Abdom Imag.* 2013;38(1): 22–31.

35. Ichikawa T, Peterson MS, Federle MP, et al. Islet cell tumor of the pancreas: biphasic CT versus MR imaging in tumor detection. *Radiology.* 2000;216(1):163–171.

36. Thoeni RF, Mueller-Lisse UG, Chan R, et al. Detection of small, functional islet cell tumors in the pancreas: selection of MR imaging sequences for optimal sensitivity. *Radiology.* 2000;214(2):483–490.

37. Semelka RC, Custodio CM, Cem Balci N, et al. Neuroendocrine tumors of the pancreas: spectrum of appearances on MRI. *J Magn Reson Imaging.* 2000;11(2):141–148.

38. Tamm EP, Kim EE, Ng CS. Imaging of neuroendocrine tumors. *Hematol Oncol Clin N Am.* 2007;21(3):409–432. vii.

39. Yu R, Wachsman A. Imaging of neuroendocrine tumors: indications, interpretations, limits, and pitfalls. *Endocrinol Metab Clin N Am.* 2017;46(3):795–814.

40. Haug AR, Cindea-Drimus R, Auernhammer CJ, et al. The role of 68Ga-DOTATATE PET/CT in suspected neuroendocrine tumors. *J Nucl Med.* 2012;53(11):1686–1692.

41. Haug AR, Cindea-Drimus R, Auernhammer CJ, et al. Neuroendocrine tumor recurrence: diagnosis with 68Ga-DOTATATE PET/CT. *Radiology.* 2014;270(2):517–525.

42. Naswa N, Sharma P, Kumar A, et al. Gallium-68-DOTA-NOC PET/CT of patients with gastroenteropancreatic neuroendocrine tumors: a prospective single-center study. *AJR Am J Roentgenol.* 2011;197(5):1221–1228.

43. Gabriel M, Decristoforo C, Kendler D, et al. 68Ga-DOTA-Tyr3-octreotide PET in neuroendocrine tumors: comparison with somatostatin receptor scintigraphy and CT. *J Nucl Med.* 2007;48(4):508–518.

44. Srirajaskanthan R, Kayani I, Quigley AM, et al. The role of 68Ga-DOTATATE PET in patients with neuroendocrine tumors and negative or equivocal findings on 111In-DTPA-octreotide scintigraphy. *J Nucl Med.* 2010;51(6):875–882.

45. Ilhan H, Fendler WP, Cyran CC, et al. Impact of (68)Ga-DOTATATE PET/CT on the surgical management of primary neuroendocrine tumors of the pancreas or ileum. *Ann Surg Oncol.* 2015;22(1):164–171.

46. Koch W, Auernhammer CJ, Geisler J, et al. Treatment with octreotide in patients with well-differentiated neuroendocrine tumors of the ileum: prognostic stratification with Ga-68-DOTA-TATE positron emission tomography. *Mol Imag.* 2014;13:1–10.

47. Moradi F, Jamali M, Barkhodari A, et al. Spectrum of 68Ga-dota TATE uptake in patients with neuroendocrine tumors. *Clin Nucl Med.* 2016;41(6):e281–287.

48. Panagiotidis E, Alshammari A, Michopoulou S, et al. Comparison of the impact of 68Ga-DOTATATE and 18F-FDG PET/CT on clinical management in patients with neuroendocrine tumors. *J Nucl Med.* 2017;58(1):91–96.

49. Squires 3rd MH, Volkan Adsay N, Schuster DM, et al. Octreoscan versus FDG-PET for neuroendocrine tumor staging: a biological approach. *Ann Surg Oncol.* 2015;22(7):2295–2301.

50. Zilli A, Arcidiacono PG, Conte D, et al. Clinical impact of endoscopic ultrasonography on the management of neuroendocrine tumors: lights and shadows. *Dig Liver Dis.* 2018;50(1):6–14.

51. Fujimori N, Osoegawa T, Lee L, et al. Efficacy of endoscopic ultrasonography and endoscopic ultrasonography-guided fine-needle aspiration for the diagnosis and grading of pancreatic neuroendocrine tumors. *Scand J Gastroenterol.* 2016;51(2):245–252.

52. van Asselt SJ, Brouwers AH, van Dullemen HM, et al. EUS is superior for detection of pancreatic lesions compared with standard imaging in patients with multiple endocrine neoplasia type 1. *Gastrointest Endosc.* 2015;81(1), 159-167.e152.

53. Shah MH, Goldner WS, Halfdanarson TR, et al. NCCN guidelines insights: neuroendocrine and adrenal tumors, version 2.2018. *J Natl Compr Cancer Netw.* 2018;16(6):693–702.

54. Lee LC, Grant CS, Salomao DR, et al. Small, nonfunctioning, asymptomatic pancreatic neuroendocrine tumors (PNETs): role for nonoperative management. *Surgery.* 2012;152(6):965–974.

55. Rosenberg AM, Friedmann P, Del Rivero J, et al. Resection versus expectant management of small incidentally discovered nonfunctional pancreatic neuroendocrine tumors. *Surgery.* 2016;159(1):302–309.

56. Haynes AB, Deshpande V, Ingkakul T, et al. Implications of incidentally discovered, nonfunctioning pancreatic endocrine tumors: short-term and long-term patient outcomes. *Arch Surg.* 2011;146(5):534–538.

57. Garcia-Carbonero R, Sorbye H, Baudin E, et al. ENETS consensus guidelines for high-grade gastroenteropancreatic neuroendocrine tumors and neuroendocrine carcinomas. *Neuroendocrinology.* 2016;103(2):186–194.

58. Haugvik SP, Janson ET, Osterlund P, et al. Surgical treatment as a principle for patients with high-grade pancreatic neuroendocrine carcinoma: a nordic multicenter comparative study. *Ann Surg Oncol.* 2016;23(5):1721–1728.

59. Basturk O, Yang Z, Tang LH, et al. The high-grade (WHO G3) pancreatic neuroendocrine tumor category is morphologically and biologically heterogenous and includes both well differentiated and poorly differentiated neoplasms. *Am J Surg Pathol.* 2015;39(5):683–690.

60. Heetfeld M, Chougnet CN, Olsen IH, et al. Characteristics and treatment of patients with G3 gastroenteropancreatic neuroendocrine neoplasms. *Endocr Relat Cancer.* 2015;22(4):657–664.

61. Sorbye H, Strosberg J, Baudin E, et al. Gastroenteropancreatic high-grade neuroendocrine carcinoma. *Cancer.* 2014;120(18):2814–2823.

62. Eisenhauer EA, Therasse P, Bogaerts J, et al. New response evaluation criteria in solid tumours: revised RECIST guideline (version 1.1). *Eur J Cancer.* 2009;45(2):228–247.

63. Haugvik SP, Labori KJ, Edwin B, et al. Surgical treatment of sporadic pancreatic neuroendocrine tumors: a state of the art review. *ScientificWorldJournal.* 2012;2012:357475.

64. D'Haese JG, Tosolini C, Ceyhan GO, et al. Update on surgical treatment of pancreatic neuroendocrine neoplasms. *World J Gastroenterol.* 2014;20(38):13893–13898.

65. Jilesen AP, van Eijck CH, Busch OR, et al. Postoperative outcomes of enucleation and standard resections in patients with a pancreatic neuroendocrine tumor. *World J Surg.* 2016;40(3):715–728.

66. Jilesen AP, van Eijck CH, in't Hof KH, et al. Postoperative complications, in-hospital mortality and 5-year survival after surgical resection for patients with a pancreatic neuroendocrine tumor: a systematic review. *World J Surg.* 2016;40(3):729–748.

67. Krampitz GW, Norton JA, Poultsides GA, et al. Lymph nodes and survival in pancreatic neuroendocrine tumors. *Arch Surg.* 2012;147(9):820–827.

68. Zeh 3rd HJ, Bartlett DL, Moser AJ. Robotic-assisted major pancreatic resection. *Adv Surg.* 2011;45:323–340.

69. Adam MA, Choudhury K, Dinan MA, et al. Minimally invasive versus open pancreaticoduodenectomy for cancer: practice patterns and short-term outcomes among 7061 patients. *Ann Surg.* 2015;262(2):372–377.

70. Staudacher C, Orsenigo E, Baccari P, et al. Laparoscopic assisted duodenopancreatectomy. *Surg Endosc.* 2005;19(3):352–356.

71. Gagner M, Palermo M. Laparoscopic Whipple procedure: review of the literature. *J Hepatobiliary Pancreat Surg.* 2009;16(6):726–730.

72. Xourafas D, Tavakkoli A, Clancy TE, et al. Distal pancreatic resection for neuroendocrine tumors: is laparoscopic really better than open? *J Gastrointest Surg.* 2015;19(5):831–840.

73. Wayne M, Steele J, Iskandar M, et al. Robotic pancreatic surgery is no substitute for experience and clinical judgment: an initial experience and literature review. *World J Surg Oncol.* 2013;11:160.

74. Giovanardi RO, Giovanardi HJ, Ali MR, et al. Laparoscopic pancreatic resection without advanced laparoscopic devices. *Hepato-Gastroenterology.* 2013;60(125):1206–1210.

75. Givi B, Pommier SJ, Thompson AK, et al. Operative resection of primary carcinoid neoplasms in patients with liver metastases yields significantly better survival. *Surgery.* 2006;140(6):891–897; discussion 897-898.

76. Howe JR, Cardona K, Fraker DL, et al. The surgical management of small bowel neuroendocrine tumors: consensus guidelines of the North American neuroendocrine tumor society. *Pancreas.* 2017;46(6):715–731.

77. Mayo SC, de Jong MC, Pulitano C, et al. Surgical management of hepatic neuroendocrine tumor metastasis: results from an international multi-institutional analysis. *Ann Surg Oncol.* 2010;17(12):3129–3136.

78. Morgan RE, Pommier SJ, Pommier RF. Expanded criteria for debulking of liver metastasis also apply to pancreatic neuroendocrine tumors. *Surgery.* 2018;163(1):218–225.

79. Scott AT, Breheny PJ, Keck KJ, et al. Effective cytoreduction can be achieved in patients with numerous neuroendocrine tumor liver metastases (NETLMs). *Surgery.* 2018.

80. Gupta S, Johnson MM, Murthy R, et al. Hepatic arterial embolization and chemoembolization for the treatment of patients with metastatic neuroendocrine tumors: variables affecting response rates and survival. *Cancer.* 2005; 104(8):1590–1602.

81. Hellman P, Ladjevardi S, Skogseid B, et al. Radiofrequency tissue ablation using cooled tip for liver metastases of endocrine tumors. *World J Surg.* 2002;26(8):1052–1056.

82. Siperstein A, Garland A, Engle K, et al. Local recurrence after laparoscopic radiofrequency thermal ablation of hepatic tumors. *Ann Surg Oncol.* 2000;7(2):106–113.

83. Rhee TK, Lewandowski RJ, Liu DM, et al. 90Y Radioembolization for metastatic neuroendocrine liver tumors: preliminary results from a multi-institutional experience. *Ann Surg.* 2008;247(6):1029–1035.

84. Falconi M, Bartsch DK, Eriksson B, et al. ENETS Consensus Guidelines for the management of patients with digestive neuroendocrine neoplasms of the digestive system: well-differentiated pancreatic non-functioning tumors. *Neuroendocrinology.* 2012;95(2):120–134.

85. Pavel M, Baudin E, Couvelard A, et al. ENETS Consensus Guidelines for the management of patients with liver and other distant metastases from neuroendocrine neoplasms of foregut, midgut, hindgut, and unknown primary. *Neuroendocrinology.* 2012;95(2):157–176.

86. Moertel CG, Kvols LK, O'Connell MJ, et al. Treatment of neuroendocrine carcinomas with combined etoposide and cisplatin. Evidence of major therapeutic activity in the anaplastic variants of these neoplasms. *Cancer.* 1991; 68(2):227–232.

87. Fjallskog ML, Granberg DP, Welin SL, et al. Treatment with cisplatin and etoposide in patients with neuroendocrine tumors. *Cancer.* 2001;92(5):1101–1107.

88. Welin S, Sorbye H, Sebjornsen S, et al. Clinical effect of temozolomide-based chemotherapy in poorly differentiated endocrine carcinoma after progression on first-line chemotherapy. *Cancer.* 2011;117(20):4617–4622.

89. Thompson GB, van Heerden JA, Grant CS, et al. Islet cell carcinomas of the pancreas: a twenty-year experience. *Surgery.* 1988;104(6):1011–1017.

90. Wynick D, Bloom SR. Clinical review 23: the use of the long-acting somatostatin analog octreotide in the treatment of gut neuroendocrine tumors. *J Clin Endocrinol Metab.* 1991;73(1):1–3.

91. Jensen RT. Carcinoid and pancreatic endocrine tumors: recent advances in molecular pathogenesis, localization, and treatment. *Curr Opin Oncol.* 2000;12(4):368–377.

92. Arnold R, Rinke A, Klose KJ, et al. Octreotide versus octreotide plus interferon-alpha in endocrine gastroenteropancreatic tumors: a randomized trial. *Clin Gastroenterol Hepatol.* 2005;3(8):761–771.

93. Yao JC, Shah MH, Ito T, et al. Everolimus for advanced pancreatic neuroendocrine tumors. *N Engl J Med.* 2011; 364(6):514–523.

94. Raymond E, Dahan L, Raoul JL, et al. Sunitinib malate for the treatment of pancreatic neuroendocrine tumors. *N Engl J Med.* 2011;364(6):501–513.

95. Faivre S, Niccoli P, Castellano D, et al. Sunitinib in pancreatic neuroendocrine tumors: updated progression-free survival and final overall survival from a phase III randomized study. *Ann Oncol.* 2017;28(2):339–343.

96. Cives M, Ghayouri M, Morse B, et al. Analysis of potential response predictors to capecitabine/temozolomide in metastatic pancreatic neuroendocrine tumors. *Endocr Relat Cancer.* 2016;23(9):759–767.

97. Fine RL, Gulati AP, Krantz BA, et al. Capecitabine and temozolomide (CAPTEM) for metastatic, well-differentiated neuroendocrine cancers: the Pancreas Center at Columbia University experience. *Cancer Chemother Pharmacol.* 2013; 71(3):663–670.

98. Krug S, Boch M, Daniel H, et al. Streptozocin-based chemotherapy in patients with advanced neuroendocrine neoplasms–predictive and prognostic markers for treatment stratification. *PLoS One.* 2015;10(12):e0143822.

99. Strosberg J, El-Haddad G, Wolin E, et al. Phase 3 trial of (177)Lu-dotatate for midgut neuroendocrine tumors. *N Engl J Med.* 2017;376(2):125–135.

FURTHER READING

1. Dierdorf SF. Carcinoid tumor and carcinoid syndrome. *Curr Opin Anaesthesiol.* 2003;16(3):343–347.

2. Mancuso K, Kaye AD, Boudreaux JP, et al. Carcinoid syndrome and perioperative anesthetic considerations. *J Clin Anesth.* 2011;23(4):329–341.

3. Modlin IM, Oberg K, Chung DC, et al. Gastroenteropancreatic neuroendocrine tumours. *Lancet Oncol.* 2008;9(1): 61–72.

4. Kinney MA, Warner ME, Nagorney DM, et al. Perianaesthetic risks and outcomes of abdominal surgery for metastatic carcinoid tumours. *Br J Anaesth.* 2001;87(3):447−452.

5. Parris WC, Oates JA, Kambam J, et al. Pre-treatment with somatostatin in the anaesthetic management of a patient with carcinoid syndrome. *Can J Anaesth.* 1988;35(4):413−416.

6. Seymour N, Sawh SC. Mega-dose intravenous octreotide for the treatment of carcinoid crisis: a systematic review. *Can J Anaesth.* 2013;60(5):492−499.

7. Condron ME, Pommier SJ, Pommier RF. Continuous infusion of octreotide combined with perioperative octreotide bolus does not prevent intraoperative carcinoid crisis. *Surgery.* 2016;159(1):358−365.

8. Massimino K, Harrskog O, Pommier S, et al. Octreotide LAR and bolus octreotide are insufficient for preventing intraoperative complications in carcinoid patients. *J Surg Oncol.* 2013;107(8):842−846.

CHAPTER 21

Pituitary Adenomas: Evaluation and Management From a Surgical Perspective

WILLIAM W. MAGGIO, MD, FACS, FAANS •
JOSEF SHARGORODSKY, MD, MPH, FAAOA

Pituitary adenomas are a very common group of benign tumors. Based on autopsy or imaging series, 10.4%−16.7% of the general population may harbor a pituitary adenoma.[1,2] Although most of these are small and incidental, some of these tumors may cause nonspecific, subtle symptoms. It is rare for a small incidental tumor to grow to a clinically significant tumor. The prevalence of large or macroadenomas is about 1 in 600 persons.[2] Clinically significant pituitary tumors account for 17.5% of all brain tumors diagnosed between 2011 and 2015, making pituitary tumors one of the most common brain tumors.[3] The average age adjusted annual incidence of clinically significant pituitary tumors is 4.19 per 100,000, and the incidence appears to be increasing.[3,4] Moreover, 2.7% of pituitary adenoma patients will have multiple endocrine neoplasia type 1 (MEN1), and 40% of MEN1 patients have a pituitary adenoma.[5,6]

Based on immunohistochemistry (IHC), the World Health Organization classifies pituitary adenomas as somatotroph, lactotroph, thyrotroph, corticotroph, gonadotroph, null cell, pleurihormonal, and double adenomas.[7] A tumor with a particular IHC profile may be functioning or nonfunctioning. Functioning, or secretory, adenomas are associated with hormone hypersecretion and often a characteristic endocrine syndrome. A nonfunctioning pituitary adenoma (NFPA), although usually IHC positive for one or more of the pituitary hormones, is not associated with the hypersecretion of any hormone. Lactotroph adenomas, defined as IHC positive for prolactin, secrete prolactin and are commonly called prolactinomas. Prolactinomas are the most common functional adenoma, accounting for 30%−50% of all adenomas. Moreover, 10%−20% of pituitary adenomas are functioning somatotroph

adenomas that secrete growth hormone (GH) and are associated with acromegaly. Cushing's disease is caused by elevated adrenocorticotrophic hormone (ACTH) secreted by corticotroph adenomas, accounting for about 15% of tumors. Gonadotroph adenomas, defined by IHC staining, are common but usually nonfunctional. Thyrotroph adenomas are rare. Furthermore, 14%−53% of adenomas are nonfunctioning, making NFPA one of the most common pituitary adenomas.[8]

Pituitary adenomas are also classified according to size and invasiveness. Microadenomas are less than 10 mm in diameter; macroadenomas are greater than 10 mm. Tumors over 4 cm are usually considered giant tumors. Microadenomas are generally confined to the sella; Macroadenomas can, and often do, extend beyond the sella to the suprasellar area, cavernous sinus, or into the sphenoid sinus. Invasive tumors are defined by the degree of growth into the cavernous sinus.[8,9]

Symptomatic pituitary adenomas present with neurologic complaints and or endocrinopathy. Vision complaints result from tumor compression of the optic nerves, chiasm, or the cranial nerves in the cavernous sinus. Bitemporal hemianopia is the classic finding with compression of the optic chasm by a pituitary macroadenoma; however, other vision problems may occur. Oculomotor palsies causing diplopia or pupil abnormalities may be seen with adenomas invading or compressing the cavernous sinus. The patient may not be aware of the visual impairment, so formal ophthalmological evaluation is recommended in all macroadenoma patients. Headache is a common mass effect symptom.

The pituitary hormonal axis should be completely evaluated in every patient suspected of having a pituitary

Advances in Treatment and Management in Surgical Endocrinology. https://doi.org/10.1016/B978-0-323-66195-9.00021-2

adenoma. Blood work should consist of prolactin, GH, insulin-like growth factor 1 (IGF-1), am cortisol, and ACTH, free L-thyroxine (T4), thyroid-stimulating hormone (TSH), follicle-stimulating hormone (FSH), and luteinizing hormone (LH). In addition to an overt clinical syndrome, such as acromegaly or Cushing's disease, this initial profile will indicate hormonal hypersecretion and hypopituitarism. Hypopituitarism, the deficiency of one or more pituitary hormone, is found in up to 87% of pituitary adenomas.[10] Panhypopituitarism is rare. Hypopituitarism of one hormone axis can coexist with hypersecretion in another. GH hyposecretion is the most common, and it is usually asymptomatic. Deficiencies of the gonadotropin, thyrotropin, and ACTH axes may be present and symptomatic.[11] Provocative or dynamic response tests may be needed to further characterize these endocrinopathies.

The standard imaging modality for pituitary adenomas is the dedicated pituitary MRI with dynamic coronal T1 postcontrast imaging. Both the normal pituitary and adenomas enhance with contrast, but there is a difference in timing of the enhancement that is exploited by dynamic imaging. The normal pituitary and infundibulum enhance within less than 60 s of contrast injection, and adenomas enhance after 60 s.[12,13] On coronal imaging, stalk deviation away from the adenoma or asymmetrical elevation of the sellar diaphragm can be supportive of the diagnosis of microadenoma, but the finding can be misleading if no obvious tumor is demonstrated.[14] The differential in timing of contrast enhancement is important for identifying microadenomas but is less useful for visualizing macroadenomas, which are more readily apparent due to their size.

Treatment is determined by neurologic issues, endocrinopathy, and imaging findings. Although usually benign, some adenomas may be aggressive with early recurrence and failure with multiple therapeutic modalities. Malignant pituitary tumors marked by systemic or craniospinal distant metastasis are very rare. Pituitary apoplexy is a rare but graphic complication of pituitary adenoma caused by infarction or hemorrhage into the tumor with acute mass effect and often hypopituitarism.

PRINCIPLES OF ENDOSCOPIC PITUITARY SURGERY

The indications for surgical intervention vary depending on the type of adenoma. Visual impairment or the threat of impairment is an indication for surgical intervention regardless of the tumor type. Apoplexy is also an indication to intervene surgically. Surgery is the treatment of choice to control hypersecretion except for prolactinomas. Hypopituitarism correction is a less certain indication for surgery.

Surgery for pituitary tumors involves either a craniotomy or a transsphenoidal approach. The transsphenoidal approach provides access to the sella, suprasellar, and medial cavernous sinus without the risk of brain manipulation. The transsphenoidal approach is preferred for almost all pituitary adenomas. Giant adenomas with significant intracranial extension may require staging both craniotomy and transsphenoidal approaches for removal.

Transsphenoidal pituitary surgery is done either microscopically or endoscopically. The microscopic technique requires a nasal speculum to retract the nasal structures and maintain a straight, narrow surgical corridor for instruments, line of sight, and light. Transnasal transsphenoidal endoscopy, the newer approach, has become more popular since it was first described in 1992.[15] Studies comparing microscopic with endoscopic approaches find similar overall outcomes in terms of extent of resection, recurrence, and complications.[16-20] Although there is some evidence that the endoscopic technique results in more cerebrospinal fluid (CSF) leaks and more postoperative diabetes insipidus (DI),[21] these complications probably reflect the tendency to be more aggressive with dissection and tumor removal with the endoscope. The endoscopic approach has the advantage of wider exposure of the sphenoid sinus and sella with less trauma to the nasal structures. It also seems to be better for large and potentially invasive adenomas.[22,23] In one study, the endoscope was used at the end of a microsurgical operation. The endoscope found more tumor 40% of the time and removed more tumor 36% of the time.[24] The surgical team usually consists of a neurosurgeon and otorhinolaryngologist working through both nostrils with the scope in one and instruments through the other.

Preoperatively, it is imperative to correct any thyroid or cortisol deficiencies and control any cardiovascular or metabolic issues that are related to hypersecretion syndromes to minimize the surgical risks. Visualization of a microadenoma on imaging may be difficult, but is important for successful surgery. For macroadenomas, the degree of suprasellar extension or cavernous sinus invasion is important both for predicting the likelihood of complete removal and the risk of CSF leak. Appreciation of the highly variable sphenoid sinus anatomy is critical for a safe and successful approach. The relationship of the tumor and the carotid arteries to any septations of the sinus is important.

The surgeon should also assess the risk of CSF leak. The size of the tumor and the degree of suprasellar extension on the preop MRI is related to the risk of CSF leak. Tumors larger than 2.5 cm or having greater than 1 cm of suprasellar extension are at a higher risk for postoperative CSF leak and will generally require nasal septal flap reconstruction and lumbar drainage.[25] Elevated body mass index (BMI) is one of the most significant risk factors for the development of a CSF leak after transsphenoidal surgery. Patients with a BMI greater than 25 kg/m² are at a higher risk for this complication.[26]

Lumbar drainage is usually not necessary. When a problematic CSF leak is anticipated, the drain can be placed at the beginning of operation, allowing for intrathecal injection of fluorescein dye that facilitates detecting CSF leaks during surgery.[27] The abdomen is routinely prepped and draped in the event fat, and fascia is required for the repair. The procedure is done with intraoperative stereotactic image guidance.

With the endoscope tracking along the septum from anterior to posterior, the middle turbinate is encountered followed by the superior turbinate just posterior. The superior turbinate is followed posteriorly to the sphenoethmoidal recess until the sphenoid ostium is visualized. A wide sphenoidotomy is then performed. If anticipated, a pedicled septal mucosal flap, based on the posterior septal branch of the sphenopalatine artery, is harvested and tucked away for later reconstruction. The posterior septectomy is performed next, identifying the contralateral sphenoid. The sphenoidotomy is completed to provide a wide opening into the sinus. The sphenoid septa are removed as needed to widely visualize the bone over the entire sella turcica, bilateral opticocarotid recess, and the sphenoid roof and floor. If necessary, an ipsilateral or even bilateral ethmoidectomy with possible middle turbinectomy can provide additional visualization and space for instrumentation. The sphenoid mucosa is then stripped and the bone over the sella is removed either with a drill or with a curette. At this point, the otolaryngologist holds the scope in one nostril while the neurosurgeon works bimanually via the other nostril.

Within the sphenoid sinus, there are very important landmarks that the surgeon must appreciate before opening the sella. The location of the carotid arteries within the cavernous sinuses, optic nerves, and floor of the sella must be identified. The lateral and medial opticocarotid recesses must also be identified bilaterally. Image guidance and preoperative study of the sphenoid sinus septations can be helpful if these structures are not immediately apparent. To widely expose

the sella contents, the bone removal should routinely extend to the medial cavernous sinuses bilaterally, to the tuberculum sella superiorly, and include the floor of the sella inferiorly. Next, the dura is opened widely. The surgeon needs to appreciate the location of the tumor and normal pituitary. With microadenomas, the tumor may not be immediately apparent and incision into the normal appearing gland may be necessary. This incision is guided by the location of the microadenoma on imaging. Removal of the tumor is guided by remaining oriented to the capsule. Macroadenomas are more obvious on opening the dura. Large adenomas usually require some internal decompression before removing the peripheral portions. We prefer to dissect the inferior tumor off the floor and dorsum first, followed by the two sides and leaving the superior portion to last. Dissection of the superior portion can sometimes be hampered by collapse of the arachnoid and normal pituitary into the field. The superior dissection is often when CSF leaking occurs. Once the tumor is completely removed, the sella can be inspected with the angled endoscope. Bleeding within the sella and cavernous sinus is frequent but readily controlled with routine hemostatic techniques.

At the completion of the pituitary tumor resection, the surgeon has to make a decision about the reconstruction of the sella defect. The biggest deciding factor is the level of suspicion for a cerebrospinal fluid leak. The defect can be left open if there is no visible leak and the risk is low given the extent of dissection. Several reconstructive options exist if a leak is seen or suspected. Underlay graft options to place within the sella defect include abdominal fat, a free fascia graft, harvested from rectus abdominus fascia, fascia lata, or temporalis fascia. Commercially available allografts are effective alternatives. Overlay graft options include the nasal septal pedicled flap, either a middle turbinate or septal mucosal free grafts, a fascial free graft, or a collagen-derived allograft. Depending on the method of reconstruction, temporary nasal packing may be needed until graft integration occurs over the defect.

Postoperatively, patients should be carefully monitored for the development of DI, hypocortisolism, hyponatremia, and CSF leak. Lumbar drainage, if necessary, is usually continued for a few days after surgery. Following surgery, extensive mucus and exudate crusting forms in the posterior nasal cavity along the mucosal edges and the exposed bone. Gentle saline irrigation becomes important to soften the crusts. After approximately 1 month, careful debridement of the posterior nasal cavity under endoscopic visualization helps to clear the crusting and restore sinonasal mucosal function. Failure to clear the crusting predisposes the patient to bacterial overgrowth, scarring along the sinus openings and nasal inflammation. Regular surveillance and further debridement is indicated until healthy mucosalization of the surgical site is complete. We will do the first postoperative surveillance MRI at 3–4 months after surgery.

The most common complications are endocrine. The incidence of transient DI is 8.4%–17%, permanent DI is 2.3%–4.3%, symptomatic hyponatremia is 4.2%, and new hypopituitarism is 3.6%. Cerebrospinal fluid leak occurs in 1.7%–11% or cases. Vision deterioration is seen in less than 2% of patients. Epistaxis, hematoma, meningitis, new cranial nerve deficit, carotid artery injury, stroke, and hydrocephalus occur less than 1% of the time. Medical complications were also very low with less than 1% incidence of pneumonia, myocardial infarction, thromboembolic disease, or sepsis.[16,17,19,20,28–31]

PRINCIPLES OF STEREOTACTIC RADIOSURGERY FOR PITUITARY ADENOMAS

Stereotactic radiosurgery (SRS) and other precisely targeted radiation techniques have supplanted conventional fractionated radiation therapy in the management of pituitary adenomas. SRS is administered as a single treatment (12–30 Gy to the margin). In hypofractionated SRS (HSRS), a higher total marginal dose of 20–25 Gy is given over 2–5 fractions. Fractionated SRS (FSRS) gives total marginal doses of 45–60 Gy in 20–30 fractions. All three approaches have been shown to have similar tumor control rates and complications. The choice between these three methods depends on patient convenience as well as balancing tumor control with complications.[32] These techniques are usually considered second-line treatments, but have been used with some success as initial treatment.[33,34] The complications of SRS techniques are radiation-induced hypopituitarism, visual impairment, and cavernous sinus cranial nerve impairments. Outcomes are related to adenoma type, and secreting tumors require a larger dose of radiation for control.[34]

Hypopituitarism is the most common complication after SRS; it is documented to occur 31.3% of the time over the 10 years after radiosurgery with most cases occurring within 5 years.[35] Most patients developing hypopituitarism have impairment of only one hormone axis; hypothyroidism is the most common. The incidence of hypopituitarism after FSRS or HSRS is

about 15%–22%. Panhypopituitarism is rare after SRS, HSRS, or FSRS.[32,36,37]

The risk of injury to the optic nerve and chiasm with SRS is a concern with tumors compressing or abutting these structures. The risk of radiation-induced optic neuropathy (RION) from a single SRS treatment is about 1% if the nerve is exposed to 10 Gy or less. The risk of RION escalates with SRS doses above the 8–10 Gy range.[38–41] Patient age and prior irradiation increase the risk of RION; prior irradiation increases the risk of RION 10-fold.[38] The latency period from SRS to the development of RION is 6–50 months with 90% of the cases manifesting before 3 years.[42] Most practitioners recommend trying to keep the exposure of the optic nerve and chasm to less than 8 Gy.[34] To minimize the exposure of optic nerve and chasm, it is recommended that tumors should be more than 3 mm from the optic nerve or chiasm to be safely treated with single fraction SRS. Tumors that are closer to the optic system should be considered for surgical debulking, HFRS, or FSRS.[40] With HFRS, the risk of RION is <1% for 20 Gy in three fractions or 25 Gy in five fractions.[38] The cranial nerves III, IV, V, and VI within the cavernous sinus appear to be less sensitive to radiation damage. With SRS doses to the cavernous sinus less than 30 Gy, cranial neuropathy is rare. However, with doses of 40 Gy, there is about an 8% risk of new cranial neuropathy. There is a 3–41 month latency between SRS and the development of cavernous sinus cranial nerve deficits.[41,42]

PROLACTINOMAS

Lactotroph adenomas, commonly referred to as prolactinomas, are defined by the IHC expression of prolactin. Almost all prolactinomas are associated with hyperprolactinemia. Hyperprolactinemia causes amenorrhea and galactorrhea in females and loss of libido in males. The symptoms may be overlooked in males.

Microprolactinomas will generally have prolactin elevations of 100–250 ng/mL. Macroadenomas usually have a prolactin level greater than 250 ng/mL, and very large tumors can have prolactin levels over 1000 ng/mL.[43] The diagnosis of prolactinoma is made with an elevated serum prolactin and a corresponding pituitary tumor on imaging.

There are some pitfalls to keep in mind in the interpretation of an elevated prolactin. There is a normal elevation related to pregnancy, breast feeding, exercise, and stress. Physiologic prolactinemia rarely exceeds 40 ng/mL. Medications, such as neuroleptics, antipsychotics, antidepressants, antihypertensives, metoclopramide, and H-2 blockers, can cause mild hyperprolactinemia (<100 ng/mL).[43,44] Macroprolactin, a complex of prolactin and immunoglobulins, can be responsible for an elevated prolactin but is usually not associated with hyperprolactinemia symptoms.[45] Primary hypothyroidism can also cause hyperprolactinemia.

Large tumors other than prolactinomas in the sella and suprasellar area can cause an elevated prolactin level by the "stalk effect," which is the result of compromise of the infundibulum connecting the hypothalamus to the pituitary that interrupts the normal dopaminergic inhibition of prolactin secretion by the pituitary. Hyperprolactinemia from the stalk effect is usually less than 150 ng/mL. The "Hook effect" is an artifactual low prolactin level associated with macroprolactinomas. This happens because the prolactin radioimmunoassay is overwhelmed by an extremely high concentration of prolactin. The Hook effect can be corrected for by performing a dilution on the serum sample used to measure the prolactin. The clinician should suspect either the stalk or Hook effect when a large pituitary adenoma is associated with a prolactin that is normal or less than 150 ng/mL.[43,44]

Regardless of the choice of treatment, the important prognostic indicators are pretreatment prolactin level, size, and cavernous sinus invasion on imaging. The higher the pretreatment prolactin level the more difficult it is to normalize the prolactin with medication, surgery, or irradiation.[44,46–48] It is more difficult to achieve successful treatment of macroadenomas than microadenomas regardless of treatment. Invasion into the cavernous sinus is an independent predictor of treatment failure.

The decision to treat a prolactinoma is dependent on the presence of symptoms of hyperprolactinemia and size of the tumor. An asymptomatic or minimally symptomatic microadenoma may be managed by observation. Microadenomas rarely grow to become macroadenomas.[44,49] The decision to observe a patient with hyperprolactinemia must be balanced against the increased risk of osteoporosis in patients with long-term hyperprolactinemia.[43] Microadenomas may be monitored by regular check of serum prolactin. Imaging is repeated if the prolactin level increases or new symptoms develop. The goals of treatment of prolactinoma are normalization of serum prolactin, normal menstruation, fertility, normalization of libido, shrinkage of a macroadenoma, preventing osteoporosis, and minimizing side effects of treatment.

Medical management with the dopamine agonist, cabergoline, is the treatment of choice for prolactinomas.[43,44,46,49,50] Cabergoline will normalize prolactin levels in 92% of patients with microadenomas and 77% of those with macroadenomas.[46,49] Moreover, 89% of women will have resumption of normal menstrual cycles. About 67% of patients with macroadenomas will experience greater than 50% reduction of tumor size within a year.[44,51,52]

Cabergoline intolerance, usually refractory nausea and vomiting, occurs in only 3% of patients.[44,49] The standard cabergoline dose of less than 2 mg per week is highly effective and safe. At much higher doses, there may be a risk of cardiac valve disease, so patients requiring higher doses of cabergoline may need echocardiogram monitoring.[44,49,53,54]

Bromocriptine is an effective second-line drug for prolactinoma, normalizing serum prolactin levels in 77.8% microadenomas and 72.5% in macroadenomas. Ovulation will resume in about 80%–90% of patients.[44,50,55] The drawbacks of bromocriptine are frequent, severe and refractory nausea, and vomiting and inconvenience because the drug must often be taken more than twice a day.

Pregnancy is often the goal of treatment for women with prolactinomas. Both bromocriptine and cabergoline are considered safe during pregnancy.[56] It is still recommended to stop dopamine agonist therapy as soon as the patient is aware of being pregnant.[44] The risk of growth during pregnancy is minimal for microadenomas; however, macroadenomas may enlarge and cause neurologic symptoms. It is currently recommended to monitor patients for clinical symptoms during pregnancy and image them if they develop neurologic complaints. If there is evidence of symptomatic tumor enlargement, dopamine agonist therapy can be reinstituted.[57] Medical treatment is considered safer for the mother and unborn child than surgery during pregnancy.

Because the dopamine agonists are so effective, transsphenoidal surgery for prolactinoma is a second-line treatment. Surgery may be indicated for medication intolerance, dopamine agonist resistance, or in the setting of precipitous vision decline associated with apoplexy. Surgery may also to be considered in patients who require a high dose of cabergoline to normalize their prolactin levels, because of the risk of serious cardiac valve disease. Prophylactic surgery may have a role in the patient that suffered symptomatic growth of her prolactinoma during a prior pregnancy and she is considering a subsequent pregnancy.

Surgery can achieve a postop normalization of prolactin levels in 78%–90% of patients with microprolactinomas and 50%–75% of macroprolactinomas. Only

27% of patients with cavernous sinus invasion achieved a normal postoperative prolactin.[58,59] There is a 16%−50% late recurrence rate in hyperprolactinemia over the 4−5 years after surgery.[59] The long-term control for a microprolactinoma is 90%−94%, and for macroprolactinoma the rate is 50%−75%.[58,60] A postoperative day 1 prolactin level of less than 10 ng/mL is predictive of long-term cure.[58] The likelihood of achieving remission is inversely related to pretreatment prolactin level, size, and cavernous sinus invasion.[58,59]

Prolactinomas resistant to dopamine agonists are also difficult to control with surgery. The surgical control rate for hyperprolactinemia is only 27%−63% in this situation. Dopamine agonist response may improve after surgery.[61−63] Prolactinomas in men tend to be large, invasive, and resistant to dopamine agonist therapy, and therefore, are more difficult to control with surgery.[64]

SRS is used primarily as an adjunct to surgery or medication. Control of the growth of prolactinomas with SRS, HSRS, or FSRS can be achieved 89%−100% of the time with actual tumor shrinkage 46%−84.6% of the time.[36,37,48,65−70] The median time to reduction of tumor size is about 3 years.[33] The response can include complete disappearance of the tumor. These are similar to the responses for other types of pituitary adenomas. Normalization of prolactin levels is less certain. Prolactin levels are normalized off dopamine agonist therapy in 17.4%−46.6% of patients, and the mean latency to normalization is 24−96 months.[34,68] One long-term study did not find any recurrences of hypersecretion once normalization was achieved.[68]

NONFUNCTIONING PITUITARY ADENOMAS

Based on IHC, NFPAs represent a heterogeneous group of pituitary adenomas defined by the lack of hypersecretion of any pituitary hormone. About 80% of NFPAs stain for gonadotropins, 15% stain for corticotropin, 2%−3% stain for somatotropin, and the rest may be silent thyrotroph, lactotroph, mixed lactotroph and somatotroph, and null cell tumors. Recognition of the IHC findings is important as silent corticotroph, silent sparsely granulated somatotroph, and mixed tumors are more aggressive.[71] 15%−37% of pituitary adenomas are NFPA, and about 80% of macroadenomas are NFPA.[6,11,16,18,33−36]

The presentation of NFPA is almost always due to mass effect or an incidental finding on imaging. The most common symptoms are headache and vision complaints. Vision impairment, usually field defects, acuity impairment and motility problems, are found in 13%−60.8% of patients. A complete ophthalmologic exam including formal visual fields is indicated in all macroadenomas as part of their pretreatment evaluation because asymptomatic visual deficits are common.[29,72] Symptomatic NFPAs are usually macroadenomas; most microadenomas are asymptomatic incidentalomas. The diagnosis is made with MRI. They often have suprasellar extension and invasion into the cavernous sinus. NFPA is the most common pituitary adenoma associated with apoplexy.[73]

The most common endocrinopathies associated with NFPA are hypopituitarism and hyperprolactinemia. These abnormalities may be the presenting complaint. Hypopituitarism is found in 37%−85% of NFPA patients. Growth hormone deficiency is most common, occurring in 61%−100% of patients. Hypogonadism is found in 36%−95% of patients. Adrenal insufficiency and hypothyroidism are also common and can be life threatening.[10] Hyperprolactinemia is found in 25%−65% of patients; the mean prolactin level is 39 ng/mL.[10] A mildly elevated prolactin level associated with a macroadenoma is due to stalk effect or Hook effect. The Hook effect, if not appreciated, may cause a macroprolactinoma to be misdiagnosed as an NFPA.

The treatment of NFPAs is primarily surgical; alternatives are observation, SRS, HSRS, and FSRS. Medical management has not been proven to be effective. A complete endocrine and ophthalmological evaluation should be performed before deciding on treatment. The indication for surgery of NFPA is to relieve mass effect. Mass effect may cause visual loss, oculomotor palsies, headache, and hypopituitarism. Anatomic signs on imaging of impending vision loss, such as significant suprasellar extension, and abutting or displacing the optic nerves or chiasm, are considered indications for surgical intervention even with a normal vision exam.[29,30] Hypopituitarism is a relative indication for surgical intervention because the recovery of pituitary function with surgery is uncertain.[74]

Although observation of incidental microadenomas is usually the best course of action, it needs to be more carefully considered for macroadenomas. The risks of growth, apoplexy, and the development of new hormonal deficits must be considered in the decision to observe NFPA. There is a 10% risk of growth with a microadenoma, a 23%−40% risk of growth with a macroadenoma over 1−8 years, and a 1.2%−9.5% risk of apoplexy over this time period.[74,75] Moreover, 21% of macroadenomas required surgical intervention within 3 years of the start of observation[75]; 7% of micro and 12% of macro NFPAs may actually get smaller while under observation.[74]

With endoscopic transnasal pituitary surgery, a gross total resection of an NFPA macroadenoma can be achieved in 64%—90% of patients.[29,30,59,76] The predictors of total resection are of size less than 2 cm and lack of cavernous sinus invasion by imaging or surgical findings. After total resection, there is a 12%—19% recurrence rate over a median follow-up of 53 months.[29,59,76] With subtotal resection, the risk of radiographic progression is 61% and symptomatic progression is 17%.[29]

Surgery is effective in relieving the symptoms of mass effect regardless of the extent of resection. There is improvement in preoperative headache in 89.7% of patients. 75%—91% pf patients with impaired vision report improvement after surgery.[30] In patients with some form of hypopituitarism preop, 19.6% became normal and 30%—50% had some form of improvement.[29,30,59] There is an overall complication rate of about 9.1% and mortality of 0.6%.[18]

SRS treatment of NFPAs is considered an adjunct to surgery, although it is useful in patients who do not wish to have surgery or are poor candidates for surgery because of comorbidities.[77—79] The choice of SRS, HSRS, or FSRS generally depends on size the tumor and proximity of the optic nerve and chiasm.[37,77,80—82]

SRS achieves a median tumor control rate of 90%—95% at 5 years and shrinkage of tumor in 20%—60%. Vision can improve in 25%. New or worsening hormonal deficits are seen in 10%—40%, and vision deficits are seen in 1%—4% when the optic nerve exposure is less than 10 Gy.[78,81] Similar result and safety profiles are seen with FSRS with total doses of 45—50 Gy in 1.8—2 Gy fractions in tumors that are within 2 mm of the optic nerve and, therefore, considered unsafe to treat with single dose SRS.[81] In known subtotal resections, prophylactic postop SRS seems to provide a better long-term tumor control than when SRS is withheld until growth of residual tumor is observed.[83]

SOMATOTROPH PITUITARY ADENOMAS: ACROMEGALY

Chronic excess of GH results in gigantism in children and acromegaly in adults. The incidence of acromegaly is estimated to be 10 cases per million with a prevalence of 125—137 cases per million.[84,85] The characteristic physical stigmata of acromegaly are marked by soft tissue and bone overgrowth, with enlargement and coarsening of hands, feet, and facial features. Patients with acromegaly usually have associated diabetes, hypertension, cardiomyopathy, arrhythmia and coronary artery

disease related to the effects of excess GH and IGF-1. Patients with acromegaly have 2—3 times the age-matched mortality of the general population.[84,86] Over 95% of patients with acromegaly have a GH-secreting pituitary adenoma. GH-secreting adenomas may be IHC positive for and even secrete other pituitary hormones, with prolactin being the most common.[85,87]

The presentation of acromegaly is often insidious. Patients are rarely aware of the physical stigmata, although they are almost invariably present.[88,89] The patients usually seek medical attention for associated medical, dental, or orthopedic issues. They may also present with pituitary tumor mass effect symptoms.

Elevated GH and IGF-1 levels combined with MRI demonstration of a pituitary tumor are diagnostic. Normal GH levels spike several times a day to as high as 30 ng/mL from a baseline of less than 1 ng/mL, so a random GH level can be misleading. The IGF-1 level is more consistent, and so an elevated random IGF-1 level is often more helpful in establishing the diagnosis of acromegaly. Because glucose suppresses GH secretion, the oral glucose tolerance test (OGTT) is important in the diagnosis of acromegaly. Within 2 h of an oral glucose load, GH level of less than 1 ng/mL excludes the diagnosis. A random GH level of less than 0.4 ng/mL also excludes the diagnosis.[84] Elevated prolactin can also be seen in about a third of patients with acromegaly. The cause may either be stalk effect or cosecretion of prolactin by a mammosomatotroph adenoma or mixed somatotroph and lactotroph adenoma. The complete pituitary axis needs evaluation because hypopituitarism and hypersecretion of other pituitary hormones may occur.

The goal of successful treatment of acromegaly is relieving any mass effect caused by the somatotroph adenoma and normalizing GH and IGF-1. Surgery is the most effective and expeditious way to achieve that goal. Somatostatin receptor ligands (SRLs) and GH antagonists may ameliorate the symptoms of acromegaly, but are not considered primary therapy. SRS modalities are useful adjunct or salvage therapy. Effective treatment can often involve employing more than one modality in a given patient.

Regardless of the modalities employed, if the GH levels cannot be brought under 2.5 ng/mL, the mortality from acromegaly remains high.[84,86] Remission is defined as random GH level of less than 1 ng/mL, a GH level of less than 0.4 ng/mL during OGTT, in addition to a normal IGF-1.[90] With surgery, a GH level of less than 2.5 ng/mL on the first postop day predicts remission.[91—94] A greater than 50% decrease in the IGF-1 level at 1 month postop is also predictive of eventual remission. It may take 6 months after surgery to achieve remission.[91–94]

Because many patients with acromegaly have associated cardiovascular and endocrine problems, a careful assessment and timely correction of medical comorbidities is important to minimize medical complications of surgery. The pretreatment GH and IGF-1 levels, as well as size and cavernous sinus invasion as assessed by imaging are factors in predicting surgical success. Preoperative IGF-1 levels less than 625 ng/mL were associated with 100% rate of remission and when the levels were above 825 ng/mL the rate of remission was only 31.6%. Similarly, if the GH level was less than 4.5 ng/mL, the remission rate was 100%. Moreover, when the GH level was over 30 ng/mL, the rate was only 18.2%.[91]

The surgical remission rate for somatotroph microadenomas is 74%–100%.[22,86,91] In macroadenomas without evidence of cavernous sinus invasion, the remission rate is 60%–67%.[22,86,91–93] Cavernous sinus invasion is associated with remission rates of 5%–54%.[22,91,93] In patients achieving remission, there is a 3%–7% recurrence rate over 10 years.[84,93] There is a 2%–5% risk of persistent DI, 2%–5.4% risk of adrenal insufficiency, and a 1%–29% risk of new hypogonadism in men and 1%–17% chance of new hypogonadism in women after surgery.[91,92]

There are two types of medications used to control the effects of excess GH secretion, SRLs, and GH antagonists. SRL work by mimicking the negative effect of somatostatin on tumor somatotroph cells. GH antagonists block the effect of GH to decrease IGF-1 production. SRLs include octreotide, lanreotide, and pasireotide. Long-acting formulations of these SRLs can be administered once a month. SRLs, as first line or after surgery, achieve control of GH about 55% and normalize IGF-1 about 56% of the time regardless of the particular SRL.[95,96] Octreotide can shrink somatotroph adenomas to a noticeable degree about 66% of the time. In studies where there was quantification of the shrinkage, octreotide achieved a mean reduction of 50%; however, tumor shrinkage did not coincide with biochemical control.[90,97] SRL can improve many of the symptoms of acromegaly such as headache; however, the mortality of the disease cannot be improved unless the GH can be lowered to less than 2.5 ng/mL.[84,86]

Pegvisomant, the only GH receptor antagonist available to date, requires a daily subcutaneous injection. It has no direct effect on the tumor or GH levels, but is effective in normalizing IGF-1 about 65% of the time. It is effective in relieving many of the symptoms of acromegaly as well.[95,98] There have been no reports of tumor growth or shrinkage on pegvisomant, but regular surveillance imaging is recommended.[84,95,98] There has been no documentation of the effect of pegvisomant on the mortality of acromegaly. The dopamine agonist, cabergoline, has been used in acromegaly. Cabergoline can control of GH levels in one-third of patients, but it requires high doses.[84]

SRS techniques are usually employed as adjuncts to surgery. The published results using SRS as primary therapy in acromegaly are inferior to those published for surgery.[99] There is also a higher risk of complications because higher SRS marginal doses are required for control of secreting tumors compared to NFPAs.[34,35] Current criteria for remission after SRS are normal IGF-1 and GH suppression to <1.0 ng/mL on OGTT.[100] It is recommended to stop any pituitary suppression medications 1 month before SRS.[100,101]

The overall remission rate in terms of GH secretion and normalization of IGF-1 after SRS is 50%–65.4% over a median follow-up of 36–61.5 months with tumor marginal doses of 18–30 Gy.[100,101] Remission may be delayed years after SRS.[100] Tumor control in terms of size on imaging can be attained 98.5%–100% over the same median follow-up of 3–5 years; however, 1.5% may start growing years after SRS. Higher pretreatment IGF-1 levels and treatment with SRL at time of SRS are associated with lower remission rates.[100,101] The higher the dose of radiation, the more likely remission.[100]

With the higher doses of radiation required for SRS control, there is a 31.6% incidence of new pituitary hormone deficiencies over 5 years. Although most involve only one axis, there are a few cases of panhypopituitarism. Similar to remission, deficiencies may take 8 or more years to manifest. Higher radiation doses and larger tumors (>2.5 mL) are associated with higher risk of new hormone deficits. There is about a 3% risk of vision deterioration over 5 years after SRS for acromegaly.[100]

CORTICOTROPH PITUITARY ADENOMAS: CUSHING'S DISEASE

Cushing's syndrome (CS) is caused by sustained elevated cortisol levels associated with characteristic changes in appearance, hypertension, diabetes, obesity, osteoporosis, vascular disease, and early death. The causes of Cushing's syndrome are exogenous steroid administration, an ACTH-secreting pituitary adenoma, ectopic ACTH-secreting tumor, and adrenal tumor; ACTH-secreting pituitary tumor is the most common cause of endogenous CS, accounting for 70%–80% of cases. Cushing's disease (CD) is CS caused by ACTH-secreting pituitary adenoma. The prevalence of CD is about 39.1/million population, and the incidence is 1.2−2.4 cases/million per year. Untreated CD has a standard mortality of 1.9−4.8. The primary treatment of CD is surgery. Successful surgery results in immediate biochemical remission.[102]

Because there is no one single highly reliable test to diagnose CS or CD the diagnosis is a several step process relying on the convergence of the clinical data in an individual case. The diagnosis of CS requires verification of elevated cortisol by at least two different screening tests. The screening tests employed for CS are the 24-h urinary free cortisol (UFC), late-night salivary cortisol test, and the low-dose dexamethasone suppression test. Once CS is established, then further tests are required to establish CD as the cause.

The diagnosis of CD as the cause of CS requires establishing associated elevated ACTH secretion from the pituitary. Provocative tests rely on the underlying ACTH pituitary adenoma not being completely autonomous, and still somewhat responsive to stimulation by corticotropin-releasing hormone (CRH) and suppression by high doses of dexamethasone. Ectopic ACTH-secreting tumors are not responsive to these stimulations. Normal individuals will have the same response profile to CRH and high-dose dexamethasone, so it is critical to firmly establish CS before proceeding with these provocative tests for CD.

Blood ACTH levels in the setting of CS should be unmeasurable if the hypercortisolism is not driven by oversecretion of ACTH, so normal or elevated ACTH levels strongly support the diagnosis of ACTH-dependent CS. If the ACTH is greater than 10−20 pg/mL then the cause is either an ACTH-secreting pituitary adenoma or an ectopic ACTH-secreting tumor.[103] Ectopic ACTH tumors tend to produce higher ACTH levels than pituitary tumors; however ACTH pituitary adenomas are the most common cause of CS. Equivocal situations require CRH stimulation testing or high-dose dexamethasone suppression testing. Ectopic ACTH tumors usually do not respond to these tests, but there are some false negatives and positives.

All patients suspected of CD should have a dedicated pituitary MRI. High-resolution spoiled gradient-recalled imaging can enhance the detection of small ACTH-secreting adenomas.[104,105] ACTH adenomas can be either microadenomas or macroadenomas. The adenoma can be too small to be seen on imaging; 12%−40% of patients with CD may have a normal pituitary MRI. Most of the pituitaries that appear normal on imaging will harbor small adenomas.[106,107] There is

also a possibility that the lesion on the MRI may be an incidentaloma, unrelated to the CD.[105]

If it cannot be decided if the patient has CD or an ectopic ACTH with the above testing sequences and imaging, then selective, bilateral inferior petrosal sinus sampling (IPSS) should be done. IPSS is usually indicated when the pituitary MRI is normal or equivocal.[107] Simultaneous blood samples of both inferior petrosal sinuses and peripheral blood are analyzed for ACTH. Significant elevation of the petrosal sinus ACTH level relative to the peripheral level indicates CD. The test is able to correctly predict the side in only about 70% of cases.[102] CRH stimulation during IPSS may also enhance the sensitivity of the test.

Once the diagnosis of Cushing's disease has been made, surgery is indicated even if the imaging is normal. The patient with CD has a demonstrable microadenoma, a macroadenoma, or normal imaging with confirmatory IPSS. Invasion into the cavernous sinus may be evident on imaging, but the surgeon should be aware that invasion may occur even with microadenomas[31] and that MRI has a high false-negative rate for predicting invasion.[107] Therefore, the surgical approach for patients with ACTH adenomas in the lateral gland should include inspection of the medial wall of the cavernous sinus and resection of the dura if invasion is suspected.[108]

Transsphenoidal pituitary surgery for CD can expect to produce remission up to 90% of the time. The remission rate for microadenomas is 65%−90% with a recurrence rate of 10%−20% at 10 years. Macroadenomas have a lower remission rate of less than 65% and a higher recurrence rate of 12%−45%.[109] Recent series give initial remission rates of 89%−97% for microadenomas and 63%−87% for macroadenomas.[31,102,106,110]

In patients with normal preop imaging, a microadenoma is often found on exploration and the reported subsequent remission rates are 84%−100%.[31,106] With a normal MRI, the exploration is directed by the IPSS results. Because 85% of microadenomas are in the lateral anterior pituitary, exploration starts with examining the lateral surfaces of the gland, followed by dissection and exploration within the gland itself. If no adenoma is found, then some degree of hypophysectomy should be considered.

After successful surgery, the cortisol levels fall immediately. Remission after surgery requires postoperative cortisol levels of 2−5 mcgm/dL or UFC less than 20 mcgm/24 h. A cortisol level less than 2 mcgm/dL on the first postop morning is highly predictive of lasting remission and low recurrence rate.[109] Postop hypocortisolism is to be expected and is also predictive of remission. Most patients will need to have cortisol replacement for 6–12 months. The incidence of postop CSF leak and pituitary dysfunction are similar to other transsphenoidal surgeries for pituitary adenomas. However, the overall surgical complication rate of 13% is higher for CD patients because of medical complications, such as thromboembolic disease.[111]

Second-line treatments employed after failure of surgery for CD are SRS, medications and bilateral adrenalectomy. SRS requires higher doses of radiation than for NFPA to achieve remission in CD. After failed surgery, SRS can achieve remission in 70% of patients after 5 years.[112] There is a 15.6% recurrence rate and 36% incidence of new endocrine deficits. There is also a 5.2% incidence of new or worsening cranial nerve deficits, but these are usually in patients receiving more than one radiation treatment.[112] A small, multicenter study of patients treated upfront with SRS found a remission rate of 81% over a median time of 12.7 months and a 9.7% recurrence rate. New pituitary dysfunction occurred in 20%, and there was a 4.7% incidence of cranial nerve dysfunction.[99]

Medical management is usually not a satisfactory permanent solution for patients with CD. Side effects and toxicity are common. Medications are generally used to control hypercortisolism until surgery or SRS can induce remission. The medications are useful for improving clinical parameters associated with CD, but less effective in normalizing serum cortisol levels. There are three categories of drugs used to control CD: steroidogenesis inhibitors that block steroid synthesis in the adrenal, glucocorticoid receptor antagonists that block the systemic responses to excess cortisol, and pituitary directed drugs that work to decrease the tumor and ACTH levels. Ketoconazole is the most commonly used inhibitor of steroidogenesis. Ketoconazole alone will normalize UFC in 49% of patients. Mifepristone, a glucocorticoid receptor blocker, improves the clinical signs and symptoms of CD, but it causes the ACTH and cortisol levels to rise and it may cause adenoma progression.[113]

Pasireotide and cabergoline are the two medications having a direct action on the tumor that have received the most study. Pasireotide is a somatostatin analog that, different from the other somatostatin analogs, selectively binds to a subtype of somatostatin receptor expressed on corticotroph adenomas of CD. When used alone, pasireotide will normalize UFC in about 25%–29% of patients at 6–12 months. Pasireotide may also shrink the tumor.[114] Hyperglycemic events are a problem with pasireotide. Cabergoline has been shown to normalize UFC in 25%–40% of patients, but a significant number of patients escape control over time.[113] With the poor control rates and side effects of monotherapy, there has been interest in combination therapies. The most promising combination so far involves the sequential addition of pasireotide, cabergoline, and ketoconazole in which 88% of patients ultimately achieved normalization of UFC.[115]

As a last resort bilateral, adrenalectomy may be used to control the hypercortisol effects of CD. The procedure achieves remission 95% of the time, but carries a significant surgical mortality and morbidity mainly due to stroke and cardiac complications. There is an 8%–29% risk of Nelson's syndrome after adrenalectomy for CD. The pituitary tumor of Nelson's syndrome can be very difficult to control.[102,109]

CONCLUSION

Pituitary tumors are common and present with a combination of neurologic and endocrine problems. The most common tumors are prolactinomas, NFPA, somatotroph adenomas, and corticotroph adenomas. Each tumor type has a unique presentation, natural history, and response to treatment. Although these are benign tumors, they carry morbid and life-shortening consequences unless properly managed. Complications of pituitary adenomas may sometimes be immediately life threatening. The proper management requires careful endocrine, neurologic, and anatomic evaluation. These tumors usually require a multidisciplinary management team.

REFERENCES

1. Buurman H, Saeger W. Subclinical adenomas in postmortem pituitaries: classification an correlation to clinical data. *Eur J Endocrinol.* 2006;154:753–758.
2. Ezzat S, Asa SL, Couldwell WT, et al. The prevalence of pituitary adenomas: a systematic review. *Cancer.* 2004;101(3):613–619.
3. Ostrom QT, Gittleman H, Liao P, et al. Central Brain Tumor Registry of the United States (CBTRUS) Statistical report: primary brain and other central nervous system tumors diagnosed in the United States in 2011–2015. *Neuro Oncol.* 2018;19(suppl 5):iv1–86.
4. Gittleman H, Ostrom QT, Farah PD, et al. Descriptive epidemiology of pituitary tumors in the United States, 2004–2009. *J Neurosurg.* 2014;121:527–535.
5. Scheithauer BW, Laws ER, Kovacs K, Horvath E, Randall RV, Carney JA. Pituitary adenomas of the multiple endocrine neoplasia type I syndrome. *Semin Diagn Pathol.* 1987;4(3):205–211.
6. Daly AF, Tichomirowa MA, Beckers A A. The epidemiology and genetics of pituitary adenomas. *Best Pract Res Clin Endocrinol Metabol.* 2009;23:543–554.

7. Osamura RY, Grossman A, Korbonits M, et al. Pituitary adenoma. In: Lloyd RV, Osamura RY, Kloppel G, Rosai J, eds. *WHO Classification of Tumors of Endocrine Organs*. 4th ed. Lyon: International Agency for Research on Cancer; 2017:14–18.

8. Micko ASG, Wohrer A, Wolfsberger S, Knosp E. Invasion of the cavernous sinus space in pituitary adenomas: endoscopic verification and and its correlation with an MRI-based classification. *J Neurosurg*. 2015;122:803–811.

9. Connor SEJ, Wilson F, Hogarth K. Magnetic resonance imaging criteria to predict complete excision of parasellar pituitary macroadenoma on postoperative imaging. *J Neurol Surg B*. 2014;75:41–46.

10. Fleseriu M, Bodach ME, Tumialan LM, et al. Congress of Neurological Surgeons systematic review and evidence based guideline for pretreatment endocrine evaluation of patients with nonfunctioning pituitary adenomas. *Neurosurgery*. 2016;79(4):E527–E529.

11. Chen L, White WL, Spetzler RF, Xu B. A prospective study of nonfunctioning pituitary adenomas: presentation, management, and clinical outcomes. *J Neuro Oncol*. 2011;102:129–138.

12. Sakamoto Y, Takahashi M, Korogi Y, Bussaka H, Ushio Y. Normal and abnormal pituitary glands: gadopentetate dimeglumine-enhanced MR imaging. *Radiology*. 1991; 178:441–445.

13. Chaudhary V, Bano S. Imaging of the pituitary: recent advances. *Indian J Endocrinol Metab*. 2011;15(suppl 3): s216–s223.

14. Ahmadi H, Larsson EM, Jenkins JR. Normal pituitary gland: coronal MR imaging of infundibular tilt. *Radiology*. 1990;177:389–392.

15. Jankowski R, Auque J, Simon C, Marchal JC, Hepner H, Wayoff M. Endoscopic pituitary tumor surgery. *Laryngoscope*. 1992;102:198–203.

16. Agam MS, Wedemeyer MA, Wrobel B, Weiss MH, Carmichael JD, Zada G. Complications associated with microscopic and endoscopic transsphenoidal pituitary surgery: experience of 1153 consecutive cases treated at a single tertiary care pituitary center. *J. Neurosurg*. 2018. https://thejns.org/doi/abs/10.3171/2017.12JNS172318.

17. Ammirati M, Wei L, Ciric I. Short-term outcome of endoscopic versus microscopic pituitary adenoma surgery: a systematic review and meta-analysis. *J Neurol Neurosurg Psychiatry*. 2013;84:843–849.

18. Halvorsen H, Ramm-Pettersen J, Josefsen R, et al. Surgical complications after transsphenoidal microscopic and endoscopic surgery for pituitary adenoma: a consecutive series of 506 procedures. *Acta Neurochir*. 2014;156: 441–449.

19. Dallapiazza R, Bond AE, Grober Y, et al. Retrospective analysis of a concurrent series of microscopic versus endoscopic transsphenoidal surgeries for Knosp grades 0-2 nonfunctioning pituitary macroadenomas at a single institution. *J Neurosurg*. 2014;121:511–517.

20. Messerer M, De battista JC, Raverot G, et al. Evidence of improved surgical outcome following endoscopy for nonfunctioning pituitary adenoma removal: personal experience and review of the literature. *Neurosurg Focus*. 2011;30(4):E11.

21. Asemota AO, Ishii M, Brem H, Gallia GL. Comparison of complications, trends and costs in endoscopic vs microscopic pituitary surgery: analysis from a US health claims database. *Neurosurgery*. 2017;81:458–472.

22. Dorward NL. Endocrine outcomes in endoscopic pituitary surgery: a literature review. *Acta Neurochir*. 2010; 152:1275–1279.

23. Komotar RJ, Starke RM, Raper DMS, Anand VK, Schwartz TH. Endoscopic endonasal compared with microscopic transsphenoidal and open transcranial resection of giant pituitary adenomas. *Pituitary*. 2012;15:150–159.

24. McLaughlin N, Eisenberg AA, Cohan P, Chaloner CB, Kelly DF. Value of endoscopy for maximizing tumor removal in endonasal transsphenoidal pituitary adenoma surgery. *J Neurosurg*. 2013;118:613–620.

25. Patel KS, Komotar RJ, Szentirmai O, et al. Case-specific protocol to reduce cerebrospinal fluid leakage after endonasal endoscopic surgery. *J Neurosurg*. 2013;119: 661–668.

26. Dlouhy BJ, Madhavan K, Clinger JD, et al. Elevated body mass index and risk of postoperative CSF leak following transsphenoidal surgery. *J Neurosurg*. 2012;116: 1311–1317.

27. Placantonakis DG, Tabaee A, Anand VK, Hiltzik D, Schwartz TH. Safety of low-dose intrathecal fluorescein in endoscopic cranial base surgery. *Neurosurgery*. 2007; 61. ONS 161- ONS 166.

28. Iglesias P, Arcano K, Trivino V, et al. Non-functioning pituitary adenoma underwent surgery: a multicenter retrospective study over the last four decades (1977–2015). *Eur J Intern Med*. 2017;41:62–67.

29. Penn DL, Burke WT, Laws ER. Management of nonfunctioning pituitary adenomas: surgery. *Pituitary*. 2018; 21:145–153.

30. Lucas JW, Bodach ME, Tumialan LM, et al. Congress of Neurological Surgeons systematic review and evidence based guideline on primary management of patients with nonfunctioning pituitary adenomas. *Neurosurgery*. 2016;79:E533–E535.

31. Starke RM, Reames DL, Chen C-J, Laws ER, Jane JA. Endoscopic transsphenoidal surgery for Cushing's disease: techniques, outcomes, and predictors of remission. *Neurosurgery*. 2013;72:240–247.

32. Minniti G, Clarke E, Scaringi C, Enrici RM. Stereotactic radiotherapy and radiosurgery for non-functioning and secreting pituitary adenomas. *Rep Practical Oncol Radiother*. 2016;21:370–378.

33. Pamir MN, Kilic T, Belirgen M, Abacioglu U, Karabekiroglu N. Pituitary adenomas treated with gamma knife radiosurgery: volumetric analysis of 100 cases with minimum 3 year follow-up. *Neurosurgery*. 2007;61:270–280.

34. Sheehan JP, Pouratian N, Steiner L, Laws ER, Vance ML. Gamma knife surgery for pituitary adenomas: factors related to radiological and endocrine outcomes. *J Neurosurg*. 2011;114:303–309.

35. D. Cordeiro, Z. Xu, G. U. Mehta, D. Ding, M. L. Vance, H. Kano, N. Sisterson, H. Yang, D. Kondziolka, L. D. Lunsford, D. Mathieu, G. H. Barnett, V. Chiang, J. Lee, P. Sneed, Y. Su, C. Lee, M. Krsek, R. Liscak, A. M. Nabeel, A. El-Shehaby, K. A. Karim, W. A. Reda, N. Martinez-Moreno, R. Martinez-Alvarez, K. Blas, I. Grills, K. C. Lee, M. Kosak, C. P. Cifarelli, G. A. Katsevman, J. P. Sheehan, Hypopituitarism after gamma knife radiosurgery for pituitary adenomas: a multicenter, international study. *J Neurosurg.* (published online November 9, 2018); 1–9, https://doi.org/10.3171/2018.5.JNS18509.

36. Minniti G, Traish D, Ashley S, Gonsalves A, Brada M. Fractionated stereotactic conformal radiotherapy for secreting and nonsecreting pituitary adenomas. *Clin Endocrinol.* 2006;64:542–548.

37. Barber SM, Teh BS, Baskin DS. Fractionated stereotactic radiotherapy for pituitary adenomas: single-center experience in 75 consecutive patients. *Neurosurgery.* 2015;0: 1–12. https://doi.org/10.1227/NEU0000000000001155.

38. Milano MT, Grimm J, Soltys SG, et al. Single- and multi-fraction stereotactic radiosurgery dose tolerances of the optic pathways. *Int J Radiat Oncol Biol Phys.* 2018: 1–13. https://doi.org/10.1016/j.ijrobp.2018.01.053.

39. Mayo C, Martel MK, Marks LB, Flickinger J, Nam J, Kirkpatrick J. Radiation dose-volume effects of optic nerves and chiasm. *International Journal of Radiation Oncology Biology Physics.* 2010;76(3):S28–S35.

40. Sheehan JP, Niranjan A, Sheehan JM, et al. Stereotactic radiosurgery for pituitary adenomas: an intermediate review of its safety, efficacy and role in the neurosurgical treatment armamentarium. *J Neurosurg.* 2005;102:678–691.

41. Tishler RB, Loeffler JS, Lunsford LD, et al. Tolerance of cranial nerves of the cavernous sinus to radiosurgery. *International Journal of Radiation Oncology Biology Physics.* 1993;27:215–221.

42. Leber KA, Bergloff J, Pendl G. Dose-response tolerance of the visual pathways and cranial nerves of the cavernous sinus to stereotactic radiosurgery. *J Neurosurg.* 1998; 88(1):43–50.

43. Coppens JR, Couldwell WT. Prolactinomas and apoplexy. In: Schwartz TH, Anand VK, eds. *Endoscopic Pituitary Surgery: Endocrine, Neuro-Ophthalmologic, and Surgical Management.* New York: Theime; 2012:87–96 (Chapter 9).

44. Gillam MP, Moltich ME. Prolactinoma. In: Melmed S, ed. *The Pituitary.* 3rd ed. London: Elsevier, Academic Press; 2011:475–531 (Chapter 15).

45. Kasum M, Pavicic-Baldani D, Stanic P, et al. The importance of macroprolactinemia in hyperprolactinemia. *Eur J Obstet Gynecol Reprod Biol.* 2014;183:28–32.

46. Verhelst J, Abs R, Maiter D, Van den Bruel A, Vandewegh M, et al. Cabergoline in the treatment of hyperprolactinemia: a study in 455 patients. *J Endocrinol Metab.* 1999;84:2518–2522.

47. Gillam MP, Molitch ME, Lombardy G, Colao A. Advances in the treatment of prolactinomas. *Endocr Rev.* 2006;27: 485–534.

48. Castinetti F, Nagai M, Morange I, et al. Long-term results of stereotactic radiosurgery in secretory pituitary adenomas. *J Clin Endocrinol Metab.* 2009;94(9): 3400–3407.

49. Maiter D, Primeau V. 2012 update in the treatment of prolactinomas. *Ann Endocrinol.* 2012;73:90–98.

50. Webster J, Piscitelli G, Polli A, Ferrari C, Ismail I, Scanlon M. A comparison of cabergoline and bromocriptine in the treatment of hyperprolactinemic amenorrhea. *N Engl J Med.* 1994;331:904–909.

51. Colao A, Di Sarno A, L Landi M, et al. Macroprolactinoma shrinkage during cabergoline treatment is greater in naive patients than in patients pretreated with other dopamine agonists: a prospective study in 110 patients. *J Clin Endocrinol Metab.* 2000;85:2247–2252.

52. Delgrange E, Daems T, Verhelst J, Albs R, Maiter D. Characterization of resistance to the prolactin-lowering effects of cabergoline in macroprolactinomas: a study in 122 patients. *Eur J Endocrinol.* 2009;160:747–752.

53. Melmed S, Cassanueva FF, Hoffman AR, et al. Diagnosis and treatment of hyperprolactinemia: an Endocrine Society clinical practice guideline. *J Clin Endocrinol Metab.* 2011;96:273–288.

54. Schade R, Andersohn F, Suissa S, Haverkamp W, Garb E. Dopamine agonists and the risk of cardiac-valve regurgitation. *N Engl J Med.* 2007;356:29–38.

55. Bergh T, Nillius SJ, Wide L. Bromocriptine treatment of 42 hyperprolactinemic women with secondary amenorrhea. *Acta Endocrinol.* 1978;88:435–451.

56. Maiter D. Prolactinoma and pregnancy: from the wish of conception to lactation. *Ann Endocrinol.* 2016;77: 128–134.

57. Mancini T, Casanueva F, Giustina A. Hyperprolactinemia and prolactinomas. *Endocrinol Metab Clin N Am.* 2008;37: 67–99.

58. Amar AP, Couldwell WT, Chen JCT, Weis MH. Predictive value of serum prolactin levels measured immediately after transsphenoidal surgery. *J Neurosurg.* 2002;97: 307–314.

59. Losa M, Mortini P, Barzaghi R, et al. Early results of surgery in patients with nonfunctioning pituitary adenoma and analysis of the risk of tumor recurrence. *J Neurosurg.* 2008;108:525–532.

60. Babey M, Sahli R, Vajtai I, Andres RH, Seiler RW. Pituitary surgery for small prolactinomas as an alternative to treatment with dopamine agonists. *Pituitary.* 2011;14: 222–230.

61. Kristof RA, Schramm J, Redel L, Neuloh G, Wichers M, Klingmuller D. Endocrinological outcome following first time transsphenoidal surgery for GH-, ACTH-, and PRL-secreting pituitary adenomas. *Acta Neurochir.* 2002;144: 555–561.

62. Hamilton DK, Vance ML, Boulos PT, Laws ER. Surgical outcomes in hyporesponsive prolactinomas: analysis of patients with resistance or intolerant to dopamine agonists. *Pituitary.* 2005;8:53–60.

63. Primeau V, Raftopoulos C, Maiter D. Outcomes of transsphenoidal surgery in prolactinomas: improvement of hormonal control in dopamine agonist-agonist-resistant patients. *Eur. J Endocrinol.* 2012;166: 779–786.

64. Liu W, Shraiky Zahr R, McCartney S, Cetas JS, Dogan A, Fleseriu M. Clinical outcomes in male patients with lactotroph adenomas who require pituitary surgery: a retrospective single center study. *Pituitary*. 2018;21:454−462.

65. Pouratian N, Sheehan J, Jagannathan J, Laws ER, Steiner L, Vance ML. Gamma knife radiosurgery for medically and surgically refractory prolactinomas. *Neurosurgery*. 2006;59:255−266.

66. Pollock B, Brown P, Nippoldt T, Young W. Pituitary tumor type affects the chance of biochemical remission after radiosurgery of hormone-secreting pituitary adenomas. *Neurosurgery*. 2008;62(6):1271−1278.

67. Kajiwara K, Saito K, Yoshikawa K, et al. Stereotactic radiosurgery/radiotherapy for pituitary adenomas: a review of recent literature. *Neurol Med Chir*. 2010;50:749−755.

68. Jezkova J, Hana V, Krsek M, et al. Use of the Leksell gamma knife in the treatment of prolactinoma patients. *Clin Endocrinol*. 2009;70:732−741.

69. Puataweepong P, Dhanachai M, Hansasuta A, et al. The clinical outcome of hypo fractionated stereotactic radiotherapy with CyberKnife robotic radiosurgery for perioptic pituitary adenoma. *Technol Canc Res Treat*. 2016; 15(6):NP10−NP15.

70. Yoon S, Suh T, Jang H, et al. Clinical results of 24 pituitary macro adenomas with linac-based stereotactic radiosurgery. *Int J Radiat Oncol Biol Phys*. 1998;41(4): 849−853.

71. Manojlovic-Gacic E, Engstrom BE, Casar-Borota O. Histopathological classification of non-functioning pituitary neuroendocrine tumors. *Pituitary*. 2018;21:119−129.

72. Newman SA, Turbin RE, Bodach ME, et al. Congress of Neurological Surgeons systematic review and evidence based guideline on pretreatment ophthalmology evaluation in patients with suspected nonfunctioning pituitary adenomas. *Neurosurgery*. 2016;79(4):E530−E532.

73. Wildemberg LE, Glezer A, Bronstein MD, Gadelha MR. Apoplexy in nonfunctioning pituitary adenomas. *Pituitary*. 2018;21:138−144.

74. Huang W, Moltich ME. Management of nonfunctioning pituitary adenomas (NFAs): observation. *Pituitary*. 2018;21:162−167.

75. Arita K, Tominaga A, Sugiyama K, et al. Natural course of incidentally found nonfunctioning pituitary adenoma, with special reference to pituitary apoplexy during follow-up examination. *J Neurosurg*. 2006;104:884−891.

76. Dallapiazza RF, Grober Y, Starke RM, Laws ER, Jane JA. Long-term results of endonasal endoscopic transsphenoidal resection of nonfunctioning pituitary macroadenomas. *Neurosurgery*. 2015;76:42−53.

77. Sheehan JP, Starke RM, Mathieu D, et al. Gamma knife radiosurgery for the management of nonfunctioning pituitary adenomas: a multicenter study. *J Neurosurg*. 2013;119:446−456.

78. Starke RM, Williams BJ, Jane JA, Sheehan JP. Gamma knife surgery for patients with nonfunctioning pituitary macroadenomas: predictors of tumor control, neurological deficits, and hypopituitarism. *J Neurosurg*. 2012; 117:129−135.

79. Losa M, Valle M, Mortini P, et al. Gamma knife surgery for treatment of residual nonfunctioning pituitary adenomas after surgical debulking. *J Neurosurg*. 2004;100:438−444.

80. Sheehan J, Lee C-C, Bodach ME, et al. Congress of Neurological Surgeons systematic review and evidence based guideline for the management of patients with residual or recurrent nonfunctioning pituitary adenomas. *Neurosurgery*. 2016;79:E539−E540.

81. Minniti G, Flickinger J, Tolu B, Paolini S. Management of nonfunctioning pituitary tumors: radiotherapy. *Pituitary*. 2018;21:154−161.

82. Iwata H, Sato K, Tatewaki K, et al. Hypofractionated stereotactic radiotherapy with CyberKnife for nonfunctioning pituitary adenoma: high local control with low toxicity. *Neuro Oncol*. 2011;13(8):916−922.

83. Pomeraniec IJ, Kano H, Xu Z, et al. Early versus late Gamma Knife radiosurgery following transsphenoidal surgery for nonfunctioning pituitary macroadenomas: a multicenter matched-cohort study. *J Neurosurg*. 2018; 129:648−657.

84. Melmed S. Acromegaly. In: Melmed S, ed. *The Pituitary*. 3rd ed. London: Elsevier, Academic Press; 2011: 433−474 (Chapter 14).

85. Mete O, Korbonits M, Osamura RY, Trouilas J, Yamada S. Somatotroph adenoma. In: Lloyd RV, Osamura RY, Kloppel G, Rosai J, eds. *WHO Classification of Tumors of Endocrine Organs*. 4th ed. Lyon: International Agency for Research on Cancer; 2017:19−23.

86. Snyder BJ, Post KD. Acromegaly. In: Schwartz TH, Anand VK, eds. *Endoscopic Pituitary Surgery: Endocrine, Neuro-Ophthalmologic, and Surgical Management*. New York: Thieme; 2012:97−108 (Chapter 10).

87. Ben-Shlomo A, Melmed S. Acromegaly. *Endocrinol Metab Clin N Am*. 2008;37:101−122.

88. Nabarro JDN. Acromegaly. *Clin Endocrinol*. 1987;26: 481−512.

89. Molitch ME. Clinical manifestations of acromegaly. *Endocrinol Metab Clin N Am*. 1992;21(3):597−614.

90. Giustina A, Chanson P, Bronstein MD, et al. A consensus criteria for cure of acromegaly. *J Clin Endocrinol Metab*. 2010;95:3141−3148.

91. Jane JA, Starke RM, Elzoghby MA, et al. Endoscopic transsphenoidal surgery for acromegaly: remission using modern criteria, complications, and predictors of outcome. *J Clin Endocrinol Metab*. 2011;96:2732−2740.

92. Hazer DB, Isik S, Berker D, et al. Treatment of acromegaly by endoscopic transsphenoidal surgery: surgical experience in 214 cases and cure rates according to current consensus criteria. *J Neurosurg*. 2013;119:1467−1477.

93. Babu H, Ortega A, Nuno M, et al. Long-term endocrine outcomes following endoscopic endonasal transsphenoidal surgery for acromegaly and associated prognositc factors. *Neurosurgery*. 2017;81:357−366.

94. Nishioka H, Fukuhara N, Horiguchi K, Yamada S. Aggressive transsphenoidal resection of tumors invading the cavernous sinus in patients with acromegaly: predictive factors, strategies, and outcomes. *J Neurosurg*. 2014;121: 505−510.

95. Melmed S. New therapeutic agents for acromegaly. *Nat Rev Endocrinol*. 2016;12:90–98.

96. Carmichael JD, Bonert VS, Nuno M, Ly D, Melmed S. Acromegaly clinical trial methodology impact on reported biochemical efficacy rates of somatostatin receptor ligand treatments: a meta-analysis. *J Clin Endocrinol Metab*. 2014;99:1825–1833.

97. Giustina A, Mazziotti G, Torri V, Spinello M, Floriani I, Melmed S. Meta-analysis on the effects of octreotide on tumor mass in acromegaly. *PLoS One*. 2012;7(5):e36411.

98. Tritos NA, Biller BMK. Pegvisomant: a growth hormone receptor antagonist used in the treatment of acromegaly. *Pituitary*. 2017;20:129–135.

99. Gupta A, Xu Z, Kano H, et al. Upfront Gamma Knife radiosurgery for Cushing's disease and acromegaly: a multi center, international study. *J Neurosurg*. 2018. https://doi.org/10.3171/2018.3.JNS18110.

100. Lee C-C, Vance ML, Xu Z, et al. Stereotactic radiosurgery for acromegaly. *J Clin Endocrinol Metab*. 2014;99: 1273–1281.

101. Pollock BE, Jacob JT, Brown PD, Nippoldt TB. Radiosurgery of growth hormone-producing adenomas: factors associated with biochemical remission. *J Neurosurg*. 2007;106:833–838.

102. Lonser RR, Nieman L, Oldfield EH. Cushing's disease: pathobiology, diagnosis, and management. *J Neurosurg*. 2017;126:404–417.

103. Pivonello R, De Martino MC, De Leo M, Lombardi G, Colao A. Cushing's syndrome. *Endocrinol Metab Clin N Am*. 2008;37:135–149.

104. Kasaliwal R, Sankhet SS, Lila AR, et al. Volume interpolated 3D-spoiled gradient echo sequence is better than dynamic contrast spin echo sequence for MRI detection of corticotropin secreting pituitary microadenomas. *Clin Endocrinol*. 2013;78:825–830.

105. Grober Y, Grober H, Wintermark M, Jane JA, Oldfield EH. Comparison of MRI techniques for detecting micro adenomas in Cushing's disease. *J Neurosurg*. 2018;128: 1051–1057.

106. Johnston PC, Kennedy L, Hamrahian AH, et al. Surgical outcomes in patients with Cushing's disease: the cleveland clinic experience. *Pituitary*. 2017. https://doi.org/10.1007/s11102-017-0802-1.

107. Lonser RR, Ksendzovsky A, Wind JJ, Vortmeyer AO, Oldfield EH. Prospective evaluation of the characteristics and incidence of adenoma-associated dural invasion in Cushing's disease. *J Neurosurg*. 2012;116:272–279.

108. Oldfield EH. Editorial: management of invasion by pituitary adenomas. *J Neurosurg*. 2014;121:501–504.

109. Biller BMK, Grossman AB, Stewart PM, et al. Treatment of adrenocorticotropin-dependent Cushing's syndrome: a consensus statement. *J Clin Endocrinol Metab*. 2008; 93(7):2454–2462.

110. Ciric I, Zhao J-C, Du H, et al. Transsphenoidal surgery for Cushing's disease: experience with 136 patients. *Neurosurgery*. 2012;70:70–81.

111. Bertagna X, Guignat L, Raux-Demay MC, Guilhaume B, Girard F. Cushing's disease. In: Melmed S, ed. *The Pituitary*. 3rd ed. London: Elsevier, Academic Press; 2011: 533–617 Chapter 16.

112. Sheehan JP, Xu Z, Salvetti DJ, Schmitt PJ, Vance ML. Results of gamma knife surgery for Cushing's disease. *J Neurosurg*. 2013;119:1486–1492.

113. Creemers SG, Hofland LJ, Lamberts SWJ, Feelders RA. Cushing's syndrome: an update on current pharmacotherapy and future directions. *Expert Opin Pharmacother*. 2015;16(12):1829–1844.

114. Colao A, Petersenn S, Newell-Price J, et al. A 12-month phase 3 study of pasireotide in Cushing's disease. *N Engl J Med*. 2012;366:914–924.

115. Feelders RA, de Bruin C, Pereira AM, et al. Pasireotide alone or with cabergoline and ketoconazole in Cushing's disease. *N Engl J Med*. 2010;362(19): 1846–1848.

CHAPTER 22

Advances in the Orbital Decompressive Surgery for the Treatment of Graves' Ophthalmopathy

TUSHAR R. PATEL, MD, FACS • JORDAN N. HALSEY, MD

Graves' disease is an autoimmune disorder that affects production of thyroid hormone, leading to decreased thyroid-stimulating hormone (TSH) and/or an increase in serum levels of triiodothyronine (T3) and thyroxine (T4) leading to symptoms of hyperthyroidism. In the United States, Graves' disease affects 13.9/100,000 patients, most commonly women under the age of 40. It can be spontaneous or familial and is often associated with other autoimmune diseases. Environmental factors, notably tobacco use, have been associated with the development of Graves' disease. Specific genes such as human leukocyte antigen and CTLA-4 have also been implicated in susceptibility of Graves' disease development.[1]

Patients with Graves' disease can present with a variety of systemic manifestations. Many patients develop enlargement of their thyroid gland, which is called diffuse thyrotoxic goiter. This can affect breathing and swallowing and can become grossly visible on physical examination. Other manifestations of Graves' disease include weight loss, insomnia, palpitations, shortness of breath, skin changes, hair loss, and muscle weakness. Notably, the most common extrathyroidal manifestation of Graves' disease is Graves' ophthalmopathy, which usually appears within 18 months of initial diagnosis. Ocular changes in Graves' disease are clinically relevant in 50% of patients.[2]

In patients with Graves' ophthalmopathy, there is no correlation between thyroid levels and the degree of progression, although euthyroid patients who are adequately treated have been shown to have better outcomes than patients with uncontrolled hormone levels. It is therefore essential for Graves' ophthalmology patients to be closely followed by their endocrinologist and to remain compliant with their medical treatment. The first-line treatments of choice for Graves' disease are methimazole, carbimazole, and propylthiouracil. These medications act to diminish the overproduction of thyroid hormone. Other treatment options that are less-often utilized include radioiodine therapy and thyroidectomy.[3]

Graves' ophthalmopathy has a bimodal peak in the 5th and 7th decades of life. A recent study performed in Iran showed that increasing age was associated with increased severity of ophthalmopathy symptoms.[4] Graves' ophthalmopathy affects four times as many females as males, although men with Graves' ophthalmopathy are more likely to present with severe symptoms.[5] Racial differences in disease prevalence have also been observed; Caucasians have been shown to be more likely to develop Graves' ophthalmopathy than patients of Asian descent.[6] As previously mentioned, smoking has been shown to be associated with development and progression of ophthalmopathy. Patients who smoke tobacco also tend to present with more severe symptoms than nonsmokers and are more refractory to medical treatment.[7]

Patients with Graves' ophthalmopathy demonstrate varying degrees of eyelid retraction along with the appearance of "bulging" eyes, called exophthalmos. In addition to symptoms related to increased globe exposure such as dry eyes and keratitis, patients are often bothered by the change in their facial appearance. Their aesthetic change in appearance often leads to the patient's desire for correction. The significant physical manifestations associated with Graves' ophthalmopathy can be devastating for patients. For this reason, Graves' ophthalmopathy does not only impact the patient clinically, but can also lead to impaired quality of life and decreased socioeconomic status.[8] More than other autoimmune diseases that directly affect visual acuity and cause blindness, Graves' ophthalmopathy

Advances in Treatment and Management in Surgical Endocrinology. https://doi.org/10.1016/B978-0-323-66195-9.00022-4

has been shown to have a significant effect on patient functionality because of the combined effect of the clinical symptoms and the psychologic implications related to their disfigurement.

Patients with Graves' ophthalmopathy typically undergo periods of disease progression and latency over a period of one to 3 years, which usually initiates soon after initial diagnosis. Following an early period of active, worsening disease, patients will typically enter a stable phase where disease progression ceases. Graves' ophthalmopathy can infrequently become reactivated during this stable period where patients reenter the active disease stage; these infrequent occurrences are usually associated with radioactive iodine treatment or cigarette smoking.[9] In 3%–5% of patients, Graves' ophthalmopathy will progress rapidly to its most severe form, termed malignant exophthalmos. These patients typically require emergent surgical decompression due to rapid compression of the optic nerve.

Graves' ophthalmopathy patients often initially present to their endocrinologist or primary care physician with visual complaints of diplopia and prominent exophthalmos. These symptoms occur as a direct result of increased periorbital fat and the hypertrophy and eventual fibrosis of the extraocular muscles that develop as a part of the Graves' disease process. The orbital vault volume decreases due to the expansion of the periorbital fat and edematous extraocular muscles, leading to extrusion of the globe. A variety of other ocular symptoms are often also present during initial presentation, including conjunctivitis, photophobia, lagophthalmos, chemosis, excess tearing, keratitis, and corneal ulcerations. In some cases, an acute increase in the intraocular pressure can occur, leading to acute glaucoma and optic neuropathy. The German Society of Endocrinology developed a classification system of orbital clinical findings in Graves' ophthalmopathy, which can be seen in Table 22.1.

As previously mentioned, the pathogenesis of Graves' ophthalmopathy is related to the mechanical compression of orbital contents by expanding fat and muscle hypertrophy. It has been shown that patients under the age of 40 tend to have more fat expansion, while older patients have more swelling of their extraocular muscles.[10] Orbital connective tissue contains autoantigens called thyroid-stimulating hormone receptor-like proteins (TSH-R) and insulin growth factor-1 (IGF-1), which show immunologic cross-reactivity with antigens expressed in the thyroid. These are targeted as a part of the Graves' disease autoimmune response leading to excess cytokine and glycosaminoglycan production. The cytokines attract T and B lymphocytes, which attack the orbital tissues in an autoimmune fashion. Additionally, it is thought that

TABLE 22.1 Modified Werner Classification of Endocrine Ophthalmopathy.[1]	
Grade I	Noninfiltrative lid symptomatology Upper lid retraction (Dalrymple sign) Upper lid stare, when looking down (Graefe Rare lid close (Stellwag)
Grade II	Infiltrative lid symptomatology Swelling of lid, epiphora Chemosis, keratitis, conjunctivitis Photophobia
Grade III	Protrusion of the bulb: With or without lid swelling Pathologic Hertel index
Grade IV	Extraocular muscle involvement Diplopia Convergence weakness (Möbius) Strabismus
Grade V	Corneal involvement (because of lagophthalmos) Corneal stippling (extremely painful) Corneal ulcer (not painful)
Grade VI	Sight loss up to blindness Caused by compression of optic nerve/thrombosinusitis

the thyroid receptor antibodies activate fibroblasts directly, leading to swelling and fibrosis.[11]

The compressive effect of the expanding periocular tissues leads to orbital congestion and venous obstruction. Ultimately, the eye becomes grossly proptotic and the upper and lower eyelids retract, leading to increased scleral show, fat herniation, and increased tension on the optic nerve. Over time, the extraocular muscles become fibrotic and even atrophic, limiting extraocular muscular function and leading to worsening diplopia. The pathogenesis of Graves' ophthalmopathy can be visualized in Fig. 22.1.

The diagnosis of Graves' ophthalmopathy is usually clinical, based on the patient's clinical appearance and symptoms in the context of a diagnosis of Graves' disease. The severity of Graves's ophthalmopathy can be characterized by the degree of functional deficit the patient experiences. The European Group of Graves' Orbitopathy (EUGOGO) developed a rating system to classify patient severity according to both subjective and objective findings[7]:

1. **Mild:** Graves' ophthalmopathy has only a minor impact on daily life, insufficient to justify immunosuppression or surgery. Patients may have <2 mm lid

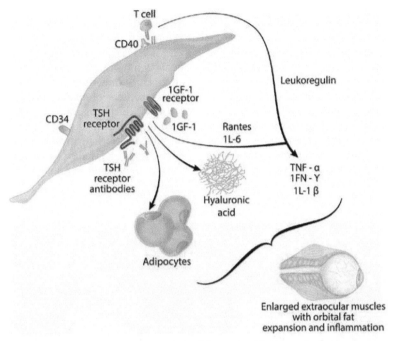

FIG. 22.1 Pathogenesis of Graves' ophthalmopathy.[5]

retraction, exophthalmos <3 mm above normal, transient diplopia, and corneal exposure that responds to lubricants.

2. **Moderate—Severe:** Graves' ophthalmopathy symptoms are nonemergent, but symptoms do affect daily life. Immunosuppression is recommended in the active/acute stage, which can be combined with radiation therapy. Elective surgery is suggested in patient's refractory to immunosuppression. Patients typically present with significant lid retraction, exophthalmos ≥3 mm above normal, and diplopia.

3. **Vision threatening:** Emergent surgery is required for acute vision changes that occur in Graves' ophthalmopathy. Indications for acute surgical intervention include significant corneal breakdown, orbital subluxation, and optic neuropathy.

A full eye examination should be performed on all patients who present with Graves' ophthalmopathy symptoms. Patients should be evaluated by an ophthalmologist as soon as possible to undergo a thorough ocular examination. The retina should be assessed for microvascular changes, extraocular muscles and visual fields tested, visual acuity should be assessed, active and passive diplopia should be noted, and fluorescein should be used to evaluate for corneal injury in suspected cases. It is important to make a precise

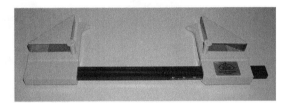

FIG. 22.2 Hertel exophthalmometer.

evaluation of exophthalmos in Graves' ophthalmopathy patients, for both the initial diagnosis and to monitor for clinical improvement. A Hertel exophthalmometer (Fig. 22.2) can be used to measure the degree of forward eye displacement in exophthalmos. The instrument measures the distance of the lateral orbital wall to the front of the cornea, normal is < 18 mm. Many studies have shown the Hertel exophthalmometer is a very reliable tool, even when used by different examiners. A study from the Netherlands showed that 96% of the Hertel values measured by two separate examiners were within 2 mm of agreement.[12]

Although ophthalmologists can perform an excellent examination of the patient's visual acuity and the changes that occur in the structures pertaining to the globe itself, it is essential that either the ophthalmologist or plastic surgeon involved also performs a thorough examination of the eyelids and periorbital structures. Clinically, the degree of palpebral fissure widening, the margin-reflex distance (MRD-1/MRD-2), and the amount of lagophthalmos present should be assessed. Additionally, the tone of the eyelids should be examined using the snap-back test and the medial and lateral canthi laxity tests should be performed.

Multiple imaging techniques can be used to assess ocular changes and disease progression in patients with Graves' ophthalmopathy. Ultrasound can reveal the presence of inflamed or fibrotic extraocular muscles.[13] Computed tomography (CT) scans and magnetic resonance imaging (MRI) of the orbits are useful in visualizing the extraocular muscle enlargement along with the increase in periorbital fat (Fig. 22.3). MRI is especially useful in the assessment of the optic nerve, which can be affected in Graves' ophthalmopathy. Three-dimensional CT imaging analysis allows for a precise, volumetric analysis of orbital fat and muscles, which can evaluate active disease and also be used for surgical planning. Quantifying the amount of fat and muscle hypertrophy using imaging can accurately reveal episodes of active inflammation and show therapeutic response following medical

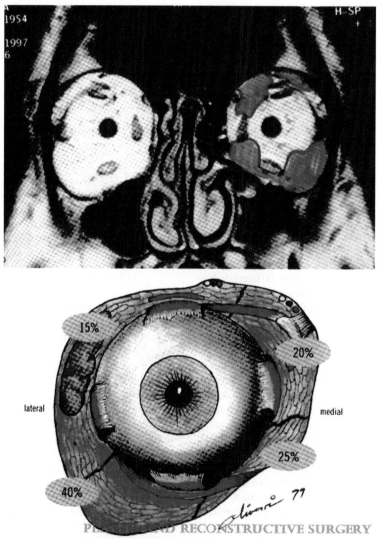

FIG. 22.3 Volumetric analysis of periorbital fat.[2]

treatment.[14] Interestingly, imaging of bilateral orbits in patients who only have unilateral clinically significant disease often shows subclinical fat hypertrophy and extraocular muscle enlargement.[15]

Color Doppler flow imaging can also be used as a noninvasive method to assess orbital vessel blood flow. Interestingly, ophthalmic and central retinal artery peak systolic and end diastolic velocities have been shown to correlate with increased intraocular pressure and extraocular muscle hypertrophy in Graves' disease.[16] Patients with active Graves' ophthalmopathy have been shown to have increased retinal microvascular density, which could also contribute to decreased visual acuity in these patients.[17]

Treatment of Graves' ophthalmopathy differs for active versus inactive stages of disease except when surgical emergencies such as acute optic nerve compression, globe subluxation, or significant corneal injury are present. During active stage of disease, medical treatment of Graves' disease along with immunosuppressive medications and radiation are the indicated treatments. During inactive stages of disease, defined as when clinical improvement by nonsurgical means reaches a plateau, rehabilitative surgical decompression of the orbit becomes the treatment of choice to correct the physical manifestations of Graves' ophthalmopathy.

The first step in the treatment of active Graves' ophthalmopathy involves optimizing medical treatment of Graves' disease. Patients with uncontrolled thyroid function have been shown to have worse symptoms than patients who are euthyroid,[18] although once ophthalmopathy symptoms are present, thyroidectomy and antithyroid drug therapies have not been shown to improve Graves' ophthalmopathy outcomes.[19] Radioactive iodine therapy, which is often employed to combat the significant hyperthyroid symptoms of Graves's disease, has been associated with the development or worsening of ophthalmopathy symptoms in approximately 15% of patients.[20] This can be combatted with the use of corticosteroids for 3 months following radioactive iodine treatment.

Mild cases of Graves' ophthalmopathy often resolve with medical treatment and do not require additional immunosuppression or surgical therapy. If corneal exposure is present, lubrication and ointments are recommended to prevent abrasion. Head elevation can also decrease eyelid swelling and Botox has been shown to be a useful adjunctive treatment for patients with lid retraction, through direct relaxation of the orbicularis oculi and levator muscles.[21] Selenium supplementation for 6 months has also been advocated by EUGOGO. Selenium was shown in a multicenter, randomized, double blind, placebo-controlled trial to lead to a significant improvement in quality of life and ophthalmopathy symptoms, along with a lower rate of disease progression.[22]

Moderate-to-severe active Graves' ophthalmopathy is typically treated with intravenous and/or oral corticosteroids. There has been great debate in the literature whether pulsed high-dose intravenous steroids are more efficacious than oral steroid use. The choice to use steroids should be a judicious one, as prolonged steroid use is not without potential complications, including weight gain, Cushingoid symptoms, hyperglycemia, and osteoporosis. Patients using steroids beyond 3 months should be prescribed antiosteoporosis medications. Cyclosporine, azathioprine, methotrexate, and many newer immunosuppressive agents are also often used and can be given in combination with steroids to combat the inflammatory effects of Graves' ophthalmopathy.

The pathogenesis of Graves' ophthalmopathy is related to the expression of TSH-R and IGF-1 by orbital tissues, leading to inflammatory cytokine production and the recruitment of lymphocytes. The advantage of immunotherapy for Graves' ophthalmopathy is that the medications directly attack specific receptors, cytokines, and/or lymphocytes, leading to a potent and targeted physiologic response. Many of these agents are still in the research and development stage, although there are some agents that have begun to be used clinically and have shown promising results.

Drugs targeting the TSH-R and IGF-1 are currently under various stages of development. Notably, teprotumumab, a monoclonal antibody that targets IGF-1 receptors has been used in a placebo-controlled, multicenter clinical trial for patients with active, severe Graves' ophthalmopathy.[23] The results of this trial, which was completed in 2017, were very promising and showed improvement of proptosis >2 mm and clinical appearance of exophthalmos after only 6 weeks of therapy. Although more safety and efficacy studies are currently being performed, based on the results of the trial, the US Food and Drug Administration designated teprotumumab with "breakthrough" status. This drug will likely play a role in the treatment of Graves' ophthalmopathy in the future.[23]

Cytokine-based monoclonal antibody therapies have been shown to be useful in other autoimmune diseases such as rheumatoid arthritis and Crohn's disease, especially in patients that were refractory to other treatments. Interleukin-6 receptor antagonists, tocilizumab and atlizumab, have shown promise in the treatment of juvenile rheumatoid arthritis and have been proposed to be used in Graves' ophthalmopathy due to the potent IL-6 cytokine production during active stages of disease. TNF-α inhibitors such as etanercept have also been shown to be effective for Graves' ophthalmopathy in preliminary studies.[24,25]

Monoclonal/polyclonal antibodies have been shown to be effective in combating the lymphocytic response seen in Graves' ophthalmopathy. The best-studied drug in this class is rituximab, a monoclonal antibody that attacks CD-20 on B-lymphocytes.[26] A clinical trial performed in Europe showed rituximab to be equivalent to methylprednisolone in its disease-modifying effects, with 100% response rate. However, a similar trial conducted in the United States showed rituximab was equivalent to placebo in the treatment of Graves' ophthalmopathy. It is thought that small sample sizes in these randomized controlled trials are the reason for the conflicting results, thus larger studies are needed to better understand the role of rituximab in the treatment of Graves' ophthalmopathy. Importantly, both studies did demonstrate greater immunosuppression when earlier treatment was initiated.[26]

The use of orbital irradiation in conjunction with immunosuppressive therapy has shown promising results in patients with Graves' ophthalmopathy. Low-dose radiation allows for a targeted antiinflammatory and immunosuppressive effect without the systemic toxicity associated with chronic steroid use. Radiation decreases the adhesion of leukocyte-endothelial cells, induces apoptosis in proinflammatory cells, decreases the nitric oxide and reactive oxygen species, and increases expression of antiinflammatory cytokines (IL-10, TGF-α).[27] Typical dose used in Graves' ophthalmopathy is 10−20 Gy, which is administered in 10 daily doses for 2 weeks.

Radiation has been shown to improve diplopia and eye motility, especially when used within the first year of symptom development. It is likely that the ineffectiveness of radiation beyond the first year is related to fibrosis that occurs in the extraocular muscles over time.[28] Studies have demonstrated radiation to be an effective therapy when compared with oral steroids as treatment for moderate−severe Graves' ophthalmopathy. However, most studies indicate that radiation is especially useful in combination with steroid use.[29]

The low doses used in radiation therapy for Graves' ophthalmopathy have a much better side-effect profile than what is typically observed in high-dose therapy for cancer treatment. The most commonly observed side effect is dry eyes,[29] although radiation-induced cancers, retinopathy, and cataract formation have been described in rare cases. It is recommended to not use radiation in patients less than 35 years old and in patients with uncontrolled hypertension or diabetes, as the radiation could worsen any retinopathy that is already present.[28] Another complication associated with the use of radiation is scarring and fibrosis that could make dissection during subsequent surgical procedures more difficult.

Nonsurgical treatment options have been shown to have a 65% response rate with modest improvement of clinical symptoms when used during the active stage of disease progression.[1] When medical treatment plateaus, surgical treatment options should be discussed with the patient. Orbital decompression surgery can address exophthalmos, proptosis, and lid retraction that is unrelieved by conservative measures. Importantly, in some cases, surgical treatment for Graves' ophthalmopathy must be performed emergently. Acute surgical treatment is indicated when patients show signs of optic nerve compression, as emergent surgical decompression has been shown to allow for improvement of visual symptoms in 70%−90% of patients.[30] Optic neuropathy in most patients manifests as total sudden vision loss, though some patients have partial or intermittent vision loss that can make diagnosis of optic nerve injury difficult. Other conditions such globe subluxation or significant corneal ulceration also mandate emergent evaluation and surgical treatment.

In most cases, high-dose intravenous corticosteroids are given as initial therapy for acute optic nerve compression and are also administered perioperatively before emergent surgery. Studies have shown that improvement of optic nerve function is typically observed within 1−2 weeks when high-dose steroids are used either alone or in combination with surgical procedures.[31] A small randomized controlled trial performed by Wakelkamp et al. in the Netherlands showed that pulse steroids were equivalent to surgical treatment in patients with optic neuropathy and often both therapies were required in combination. In their study, 82% of surgically treated patients did not have full resolution of their symptoms with surgery alone, but nearly 100% resolved when surgery was combined with high-dose steroids. Conversely, 45% of patients treated with steroids alone did not fully improve until they were treated with surgical decompression.[32] Any patient with Graves' disease who experiences acute loss of vision or acute onset of severe visual disturbance should be evaluated in an emergent manner to prevent long-term sequelae, including permanent vision loss.

In most cases, surgical treatment of Graves' ophthalmopathy is performed on an elective basis. As mentioned previously, patients typically seek surgery when their symptoms and clinical appearance become refractory to the use of other therapies. However, primary surgical decompression can also be completed for first-line treatment for Graves' ophthalmopathy. A majority of patients will significantly benefit from orbital decompression as a primary treatment method without subjecting the patient to refractory medical management and the associated side effects. The goals of surgical decompression procedures are to address the orbital congestion, pain, disfiguring proptosis, and lid malposition exhibited in Graves' ophthalmopathy. Patients who are candidates for orbital decompression surgery should be euthyroid for 3 months preoperatively and should plan at least a 2-week interval between addressing the first and second eye. An artist's rendition of the preoperative appearance of a patient with Graves' ophthalmopathy, an intraoperative diagram showing periorbital fat and medial/inferior orbital walls that are targeted for removal, and postoperative outcome can be observed in Figs. 22.4–22.6, respectively.

Orbital decompression procedures, whether emergent or elective, involves excision of periorbital fat and osseous expansion of the orbit by bony excision of the medial, lateral, and/or inferior orbital walls. These procedures can be performed before or in combination with other surgical procedures to address eyelid retraction, decreased eyelid tone, and strabismus. Orbital decompression procedures can be performed through a variety of incisions and approaches.[33] In the 1950s, transbuccal incisions were commonly used to access the inferior orbital rim because they were

less visible. In the late 1960s, Tessier proposed that orbital decompression surgeries should be performed through a coronal incision, which allow for full visibility of the orbital walls. This incision, although much larger than the transbuccal incision, can be hidden in the hairline. This technique popularized in the 1980s has now been largely replaced by periorbital approaches. Inferior fornix incisions are often used to approach the inferior and medial orbital walls and the inferior periorbital fat. Lateral orbital wall osteotomies can be performed through well-hidden upper lid skin crease or a blepharoplasty incision. The "swinging eyelid technique" is a transconjunctival approach that offers full access to the bony orbit along with the fat compartments.[1] Most surgeons tailor their incision patterns to their patient's specific pathology, often with a combination of periorbital incisions.

The Olivari technique is a well-described method of surgical treatment for Graves' ophthalmopathy. This technique involves removal of extraconal and intraconal fat in the periorbital region to decompress the globe. Because the volume of periorbital tissue is roughly 14cc, resecting only a small amount of fat can lead to a significant clinical effect.[1] It is essential to resect intraconal fat directly surrounding the globe because even a small fat resection in the region of the extraocular muscles can improve eye mobility and reduce diplopia symptoms. Intraconal fat must be excised in a symmetric manner around the globe to prevent globe malposition.

Other described surgical techniques include osseous expansion of the orbit via one to modified three wall

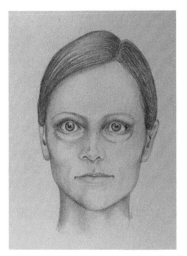 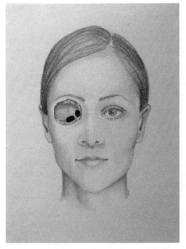 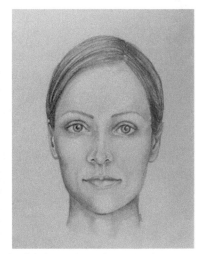

FIGS. 22.4–22.6 (LtoR): (4) Preoperative photo of a patient with Graves' ophthalmopathy pathognomonic features. (5) Excessive periorbital fat with inferior/medial orbital walls marked for planned removal. (6) Postoperative result with improvement of exophthalmos and lid retraction.

removal combination. Orbital decompression by orbital wall removal was initially described by Tessier for the treatment of patients with significant exophthalmos that even significant fat reduction would not fully correct.[13] Bony expansion allows the globe to return to a more physiologic position, addressing both the aesthetic and often functional concerns associated with exophthalmos (Fig. 22.3). An example of a pre- and postoperative result following orbital decompression by both fat removal and osseous expansion can be seen in Fig. 22.7.

A recent article published in Plastic and Reconstructive Surgery by Doumit et al. suggests a three-tier approach to surgical treatment in Graves' ophthalmopathy.[34] According to their algorithm, mild proptosis should be treated with intra/extraconal fat excision alone. Moderate-to-severe proptosis, where the Hertel values exceed 28 mm,[1] should be treated with fat excision combined with orbital wall removal. In cases of severe proptosis in patients with a negative vector, that is, when the malar eminence is posterior to the anterior aspect of the cornea, the malar eminence should undergo malar augmentation with or without a midface lift to establish a neutral or positive vector.

For all Graves' ophthalmopathy patients who undergo surgical decompression, it is essential to excise intraconal and extraconal orbital fat. To perform this using the Olivari technique, blepharoplasty incisions are made through skin and orbicularis oculi muscles on both the upper and lower eyelid to allow for exposure of the orbital septum encasing the eyelid fat compartments. Using this excision method, excess extraconal fat can be removed from the central and medial compartments of the upper lid and the lateral, medial, and middle compartments of the lower lid. The upper lid is typically approached first. After the initial eyelid crease incision, the orbital septum is encountered and incised on the medial aspect to allow for fat excision from both the medial and central compartments. Caution must be taken during fat excision in the central compartment of the upper lid, as lateral to this is the lacrimal gland. If there is significant hypertrophy of the lacrimal gland, Olivari et al. recommends attaching the gland to the Whitnall ligament and carefully

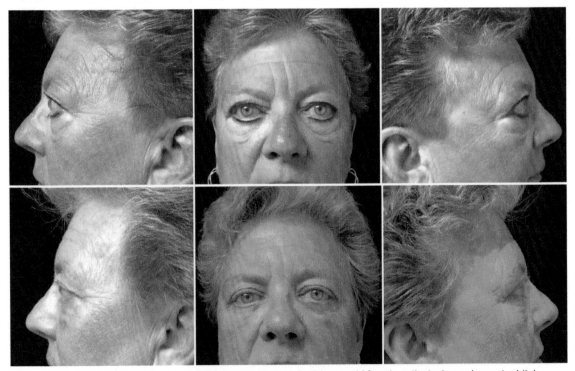

FIGS. 22.7 AND 22.8 (7, Top) Preoperative photos of a 54-year-old female patient who underwent orbital decompression surgery. (8, Bottom) Postoperative result, showing improvement of exophthalmos and improved eyelid position.

reducing its volume using bipolar cautery. It is essential to use the bipolar carefully during all aspects of the surgery to prevent hyperthermic damage to the periorbital structures. Of note, the central compartment of the upper lid typically has more yellow-appearing fat than the medial compartment, allowing for fat from these compartments to be easily distinguished from each other. The fat should be carefully teased out of each compartment, carefully coagulating the small vessels within the compartment as fat is retracted to maintain hemostasis throughout the procedure.

During fat excision from the compartments of the upper eyelid, the medial rectus will become eventually exposed deep to the superficial fat within the compartment; this should be left undamaged. Other deeper structures such as the superior oblique muscle and the supratrochlear artery and nerve will likely also be visualized and should be protected. At the base of the upper lid fat compartments lies the tenon fascia that surrounds the globe. Incising the deep fibrous-appearing tenon allows for exposure of the softer intraconal fat that is clinically different than the extraconal fat initially encountered. The globe must be carefully protected during this part of the surgery and care must be taken to not damage the extraocular muscles during intraconal fat excision. The anesthesiologist should be made aware when the globe is retracted or manipulated at any point, as bradycardia resulting from the oculocardiac reflex may occur. To prevent hollowing, intraconal fat can also be manipulated at this stage to appropriately fill any empty-appearing areas after fat resection. All periorbital fat resection should be symmetric to prevent postoperative globe malposition.

The approach of the lower lid is nearly analogous to the upper lid. Once the initial subciliary incision is made through the skin and orbicularis muscle, the orbital septum is dissected and exposed down to the arcus marginalis. Incisions can be made in this septum as needed to excise fat from the lateral, middle, and medial fat compartments. The first incision is typically made between the central and medial compartments allowing removal of fat from either compartment through a single incision. Just as in the upper lid, the fat excised from the medial compartment of the lower lid appears paler than the yellow-appearing fat of the middle compartment. The inferior oblique muscle will be visualized in the base of the medial fat compartment. To expose the deeper intraconal fat, an incision must again be made in the deep tenon fascia and should be approached between the inferior and medial recti. Periorbital fat can be carefully excised all the way

to the orbital apex. Hemostasis should be maintained with bipolar cautery during fat excision and the globe should be carefully retracted to prevent injury.

The middle fat compartment of the lower lid typically has the greatest amount of fat when compared to all compartments of both the upper and lower eyelid. After fat from the lateral compartment is excised, an additional incision can be made in the thick tenon fascia between the lateral and inferior recti exposing the lateral aspect of the lower orbit, allowing for the excision of more intraconal fat. The tenon fascia incisions and incisions made in the orbital septum do not require suture closure. The orbicularis oculi muscle is also not typically closed as a distinct layer. Skin closure of the upper and lower eyelids can then be performed.

Before skin closure, some authors advocate performing adjunctive eyelid procedures concurrent with orbital decompression. In patients with significant upper eyelid retraction, Olivari et al. advocates elongating the levator muscle by sectioning the lateral three quarters of the muscle along the Müller's muscle. Strabismus correction can also be performed, as the extraocular muscles are easily exposed during the surgery. Alternatively, these procedures can be performed under local anesthesia on a later date. Performing the surgery during a second-stage allows for any edema that may present to settle and for exophthalmos and proptosis to resolve before addressing the eyelids. Moreover, using local anesthesia and keeping the patient awake during fine-tuning procedures of eyelid positioning can allow for precise lid adjustment with patient cooperation.

With regard to lower eyelid malposition and retraction, Olivari et al. does not advocate performing any corrective surgeries at the time of the initial decompression procedure; rather, the lower lid is addressed 3–6 months following the orbital decompression. Other surgeons advocate performing the lower eyelid correction at the time of decompressive surgery to potentially decrease the need of an additional procedure and to allow for a quicker recovery for patients.[35] A canthopexy/tarsal strip procedure can easily be performed following lower eyelid fat excision during the orbital decompression surgery in cases where the patient demonstrates excessive lower lid laxity. The suggested treatment of lower eyelid retraction involves placing a solid graft in a retroseptal pocket extending from tarsus to the arcus marginalis to keep the lower eyelid in a stable nonretracted position. Materials that have been described for use in the lower eyelid include ear cartilage, hard palate mucosa, acellular dermal matrix, and polydioxanone foil.[36,37] The graft can be sutured to the inferior aspect of the tarsal plate with permanent suture, while the inferior margin of the graft is left free to maintain appropriate eyelid mobility.

In severe cases of Graves' ophthalmopathy, orbital floor and lateral/medial wall ostectomies are performed, during fat resection for a more exaggerated orbital decompression. A variety of lower eyelid approaches can be utilized to expose the orbital bones, and they are often combined with a lateral canthal incision to allow for wider visualization. The swinging eyelid technique can be especially useful when bony decompression is necessary. Dissection should proceed in a retroseptal plane down to the arcus marginalis. The arcus marginalis is then excised and blunt subperiosteal dissection from the medial to the lateral orbital walls is performed extending posteriorly toward the orbital apex.[36] The posterior aspect of the lateral orbital wall is then removed using a drill. The posterior aspect of the medial orbital wall can be excised either using a drill or by infracturing the ethmoid air cells with an osteotome. The orbital floor is then excised if needed, though the anterior aspect of the floor and the inferior orbital rim should remain intact. Pre- and postoperative photos from the author's experience can be visualized in Figs. 22.7–22.8.

Orbital decompression surgeries take approximately 2 h and require general anesthesia. Patients may develop significant chemosis and periorbital edema by the end of the case. Patients should be counseled that their swollen appearance will take several days to improve. The use of perioperative corticosteroids and persistent head elevation can be useful in improving postoperative edema. Additionally, a temporary Frost suture can be placed at the end of the case into the lower lid margin and secured to superior orbital rim to prevent ectropion and lagophthalmos that may initially occur postoperatively. An upper and lower eyelid tarsorrhaphy may be performed to improve ectropion prevention.

Recently, several centers have begun to perform minimally invasive endoscopic orbital decompression procedures. Yang and Ye, at the Zhongshan Ophthalmic Centre in China, perform bony decompression of the medial orbital wall endoscopically through a transnasal approach. The medial orbital wall can be easily approached using this method and fractured through the ethmoid air cells. The primary advantage of this minimally invasive approach is to avoid an external incision scar; however, additional incisions may be needed if lateral/inferior wall decompression is necessary. This newer technique requires a higher cost for equipment and has been shown to have a high incidence of esotropia due to inadvertent extraocular muscle damage because of poor visualization.[38] This technique also does not allow for fat excision to be performed unless additional incisions are made.

In general, orbital decompression surgeries carry a similar risk profile as other periorbital procedures. The most common complications of orbital decompression surgeries include conjunctivitis/chemosis, hematoma, diplopia, supraorbital nerve paresis, and infection. Dry eyes and temporary diplopia often resolve over time without need for further treatment. Bleeding can occur perioperatively and in severe cases, such as retrobulbar hematoma, may require emergent reexploration. Hypertrophic scarring and keloid formation can occur with any type of incisional approach. Transconjunctival incisions can lead to lower eyelid entropion, while subciliary incisions can lead to ectropion. Coronal approaches predispose patients to temporal hollowing. Newer endoscopic approaches can lead to postobstructive sinusitis, mucoceles, and cerebrospinal fluid leak.[39] Hypoesthesia and neuroma formation along branches of the trigeminal nerve in the periorbital region can also occur.[11,12]

Following recovery from orbital decompression procedures, some patients may require subsequent surgeries to address strabismus, eyelid retraction that was not fully corrected by decompression, and any excess skin that may now be evident in the periorbital region. Postoperative assessment of eyelid laxity should be performed using the lid snap-back test and also by the assessment of canthal patency. Revision surgeries should not be performed until at least 6 months to 1 year following the initial procedure to wait for full resolution of periorbital edema and for the initial stages of wound healing to subside. Complete improvement in proptosis generally can be appreciated 6–18 months postoperatively. All patients should be counseled appropriately in the time necessary to allow orbit relocation and ultimately meet expectations.

In conclusion, Graves' ophthalmopathy is the most common extrathyroidal manifestation of Graves' disease and can be a significant source of morbidity in this population. The significant ocular prominence from the increase in orbital fat and muscular hypertrophy can lead to vision changes, decreased ocular motility, and disfiguring proptosis that is debilitating. Patients with Graves' disease that begin to show signs of ophthalmopathy development should be evaluated and begin medical treatment to stunt the active stage of the disease process. In patients that fail medical management or experience significant or progressive visual symptoms, surgical decompression can be a useful treatment modality. The author's preferred technique for operative orbital decompression for moderate-to-severe Graves' ophthalmopathy is as follows:

1. Upper eyelid extraconal and intraconal fat excision from the central and medial compartments via a blepharoplasty incision;
2. Lower eyelid extraconal and intraconal fat excision from the medial, middle, and lateral compartments via a subciliary incision;
3. Inferior orbital floor and medial orbital wall excision if indicated;
4. Lower eyelid canthopexy, upper and lower eyelid tarsorrhaphy, and lower eyelid Frost stitch.

Orbital decompression surgery can provide functional and aesthetic improvement of symptoms for patients with Graves' ophthalmopathy.

REFERENCES

1. Richter DF, Stoff A, Olivari N. Transpalpebral decompression of endocrine ophthalmopathy by intraorbital fat removal (Olivari Technique): experience and progression after more than 3000 operations over 20 years. *Plast Reconstr Surg.* 2007;120:109.
2. Wiersinga WM, Smit T, van der Gaag R, Koornneef L. Temporal relationship between onset of Graves' ophthalmopathy and onset of thyroidal Graves' disease. *J Endocrinol Investig.* 1988;11:615−619.
3. Ruchała M, Sawicka-Gutaj N. Advances in the pharmacological treatment of Graves' orbitopathy. *Expert Rev Clin Pharmacol.* 2016;9(7):981−989.
4. Gharib S, Moazezi Z, Bayani MA. Prevalence and severity of ocular involvement in Graves' disease according to sex and age: a clinical study from Babol, Iran. *Caspian J Int Med.* 2018;9(2):178−183.
5. Bahn RS. Current insights into the pathogenesis of Graves' ophthalmopathy. *Horm Metab Res.* 2015;47(10): 773−778.
6. Tellez M, Cooper J, Edmonds C. Graves' ophthalmopathy in relation to cigarette smoking and ethnic origin. *Clin Endocrinol.* 1992;36:291−294.
7. Baltalena L, Baldeschi L, Dickinson A, et al. Consensus statement of the European Group on Graves' orbitopathy (EUGOGO) on management of GO. *Eur J Endocrinol.* 2008;158:273−285.
8. Bruscolini A, Sacchetti M, La Cava M, et al. Quality of life and neuropsychiatric disorders in patients with Graves' Orbitopathy: current concepts. *Autoimmun Rev.* 2018; 17(7):639−643.
9. Smith TJ. Challenges in orphan drug development: identification of effective therapy for thyroid-associated ophthalmopathy. *Annu Rev Phannacol Toxicol.* 2019;59: 129−148.
10. Koumas L, Smith TJ, Feldon S, et al. Thy-1 expression in human fibroblast subsets defines myofibroblastic or lipofibroblastic phenotypes. *Am J Pathol.* 2003;163: 1291−1300.
11. Bahn RS. Thyrotropin receptor expression in orbital adipose/connective tissues from patients with thyroid-associated ophthalmopathy. *Thyroid.* 2002;12:193−195.
12. Mourits MP, Lombardo SH, van der Sluijs FA, et al. Reliability of exophthalmos measurement and the exophthalmometry value distribution in a healthy Dutch population and in Graves' patients. An exploratory study. *Orbit.* 2004; 23(3):161−168.
13. Clauser L, Galie M, Sarti E, et al. Rationale of treatment in Graves' ophthalmopathy. *Plast Reconstr Surg.* 2001;108: 1880.
14. Byun JS, Moon NJ, Lee JK. Quantitative analysis of orbital soft tissues on computed tomography to assess the activity of thyroid-associated orbitopathy. *Graefes Arch Clin Exp Ophthalmol.* 2017;255(2):413−420.
15. Wiersinga WM, Smit T, van der Gaag R, et al. Clinical presentation of Graves' ophthalmopathy. *Ophthalmic Res.* 1989;21(2):73−82.
16. Perri P, Campa C, Costagliola C, et al. Increased retinal blood flow in patients with active Graves' ophthalmopathy. *Curr Eye Res.* 2007;32:985−990.
17. Ye L, Zhou S-S, Yang W-L, et al. Retinal microvascular alteration in active thyroid-associated ophthalmopathy. *Endocr Pract.* July 2018;24(7):658−667.
18. Prummel MF, Wiersinga WM, Mourits MP, Koornneef L, Berghout A, van der Gaag R. Effect of abnormal thyroid function on the severity of Graves' ophthalmopathy. *Arch Intern Med.* 1990;150:1098−1101.
19. Bartalena L, Marcocci C, Bogazzi F, Manetti L, Tanda ML, Dell'Unto E, Bruno-Bossio G, Nardi M, Bartolomei MP, Lepri A, Rossi G, Martino E & Pinchera A. Relation between therapy for hyperthyroidism and the course of Graves' ophthalmopathy. *N Engl J Med,* 1998;338:73−78.
20. Bartalena L, Marcocci C, Bogazzi F, Panicucci M, Lepri A, Pinchera A. Use of corticosteroids to prevent progression of Graves' ophthalmopathy after radioiodine therapy for hyperthyroidism. *N Engl J Med.* 1989;321: 1349−1352.
21. Uddin JM, Davies PD. Treatment of upper eyelid retraction associated with thyroid eye disease with subconjunctival botulinum toxin injection. *Ophthalmology.* 2002;109: 1183−1187.
22. Marcocci C, Marinò M. Treatment of mild, moderate-to-severe and very severe Graves' orbitopathy. *Best Pract Res Clin Endocrinol Metabol.* 2012;26:325−337.
23. Smith TJ, Kahaly GJ, Ezra DG, et al. Teprotumumab for thyroid-associated ophthalmopathy. *N Engl J Med.* 2017; 376:1748−1761.
24. Rajaii F, McCoy AN, Smith TJ. Cytokines are both villains and potential therapeutic targets in thyroid-associated ophthalmopathy: from bench to bedside. *Expert Rev Ophthalmol.* 2014;9(3):227−234.
25. Salvi M, Vannucchi G, Currò N, et al. Efficacy of B-cell targeted therapy with rituximab in patients with active moderate to severe Graves' orbitopathy: a randomized controlled study. *J Clin Endocrinol Metab.* 2015;100: 422−431.

26. Strianese D. Efficacy and safety of immunosuppressive agents for thyroid eye disease. *Ophthalmic Plast Reconstr Surg.* 2018;34(4S suppl 1):S56–S59.

27. San Miguel I, Arenas M, Carmona R, et al. Review of the treatment of Graves' ophthalmopathy: the role of the new radiation techniques. *Saudi J Ophthalmol.* 2018; 32(2):139–145.

28. Schaefer U, Hesselmann S, Micke O, Schueller P, Bruns F, Palma C. A long-term follow-up study after retro-orbital irradiation for Graves' ophthalmopathy. *Int J Radiat Oncol Biol Phys.* 2002;52(1):192–197.

29. Perros P, Krassas GE. Orbital irradiation for thyroid-associated orbitopathy: conventional dose, low dose or no dose? *Clin Endocrinol.* 2002;56(6):689–691.

30. Prummel MF, Bakker A, Wiersinga WM, et al. Multi–center study on the characteristics and treatment strategies of patients with Graves' orbitopathy: the first European Group on Graves' Orbitopathy experience. *Eur J Endocrinol.* 2003;148:491–495.

31. Hart Frantzco RH, Kendall-Taylor P, Crombie A, Perros P. Early response to intravenous glucocorticoids for severe thyroid-associated ophthalmopathy predicts treatment outcome. *J Ocul Pharmacol Ther.* 2005;21:328–336.

32. Wakelkamp IM, Baldeschi L, Saeed P, et al. Surgical or medical decompression as a first–line treatment of optic neuropathy in Graves' ophthalmopathy? A randomized controlled trial. *Clin Endocrinol.* 2005;63(3):323–328.

33. Baldeschi L. Small versus coronal incision orbital decompression in Graves' orbitopathy. *Orbit.* 2010;29(4): 177–182.

34. Doumit G, Abouhassan W, Yaremchuk M. Aesthetic refinements in the treatment of Graves' ophthalmopathy. *Plast Reconstr Surg.* 2014;134:519.

35. Taban MR. Combined orbital decompression and lower eyelid retraction surgery. *J Curr Ophthalm.* 2018;30(2): 169–173.

36. Olivari N, Richter DF, Eder EF. *Endocrine Orbitopathy, Surgical Therapy.* Germany: Kaden Verlag; 2001.

37. Kim KY, Woo YJ, Jang SY, et al. Correction of lower eyelid retraction using acellular human dermis during orbital decompression. *Ophthalmic Plast Reconstr Surg.* 2017; 33(3):168–172.

38. Yang HS, Ye HJ. Orbital decompression for thyroid associated ophthalmopathy: transnasal endoscopic approach or external orbital approach? *Zhonghua Yan Ke Za Zhi.* 2018; 54(7):484–487.

39. Antisdel JL, Gumber D, Holmes J, et al. Management of sinonasal complications after endoscopic orbital decompression for Graves' orbitopathy. *Laryngoscope.* 2013; 123(9):2094–2098.

FURTHER READING

1. Sellari-Franceschini S, Dallan I, Bajrakatari A. Surgical complications in orbital decompression for Graves' orbitopathy. *Acta Otorhinolaryngol Ital.* 2016;36(4):265–274.

2. Baldeschi L, Saeed P, Regensburg NI. Traumatic neuroma of the infraorbital nerve subsequent to inferomedial orbital decompression for Graves' orbitopathy. *Eur J Ophthalmol.* 2010;20(2):481–484.

CHAPTER 23

Advances in the Minimally Invasive Surgical Approaches to Thyroid, Parathyroid, and Adrenal Disorders

MARCO RAFFAELLI • DE CREA CARMELA • PENNESTRÌ FRANCESCO • LOMBARDI CELESTINO PIO • BELLANTONE ROCCO

In recent years, since the first reported cases of endoscopic adrenalectomy[1] and parathyroidectomy,[2] several minimally invasive approaches in endocrine surgery have been developed[3–12].

The conventional surgery for neck endocrine diseases is generally performed using traditional Kocher incision characterized by a long skin incision that results in a visible scar in the neck. For the minimally invasive neck endocrine surgery, some techniques that require the use of endoscope[3–7] and others that do not need its use[13] have been proposed. The different minimally invasive techniques implying the use of the endoscope can be classified in purely endoscopic[2,4,5,12] and video-assisted[7–9] procedures. In the pure endoscopic techniques, surgical dissection is completely carried out under endoscopic vision.[14] This requires a continuous CO_2 insufflation[3,4,12] or the use of external devices (retractors) to maintain the operative space for dissection and trocar positioning.[14] The totally endoscopic approaches have as a major limit the more difficult dissection, mainly in the case of extracervical accesses. They are difficult to be reproduced in different settings, especially by not skilled endoscopic surgeons, and they are technically demanding.[14] Indeed, the totally endoscopic procedures encountered only limited diffusion.[15] On the other hand, minimally invasive video-assisted parathyroidectomy (MIVAP) and minimally invasive video-assisted thyroidectomy (MIVAT), short after their introduction during the late 1990s,[6,7] gained a quite large worldwide diffusion, maybe because these techniques combine the advantages related to the endoscopic magnification with those due to the close similarity with the conventional surgery that makes these surgical approaches safe and reproducible in different surgical settings. MIVAP and MIVAT are completely gasless procedures that reproduce all the steps of the conventional operation. The endoscope represents only a tool that allows to perform the same operation through a very minimal skin incision.[7,8,16,17]

Early after its introduction, endoscopic adrenalectomy showed several advantages over the open counterpart specifically consistent in less postoperative pain, improved patients' satisfaction, shorter hospital stay and recovery time..[18–20] These advantages have led to an evolution of indications for adrenalectomy and produced the broadening of the indications..[21–23] To date, laparoscopic adrenalectomy is the standard treatment for small to medium sized benign adrenal tumors.[24] Contemporary series of laparoscopic adrenalectomies show very rare peri- and postoperative mortality, an overall intraoperative complication rate of 7%, a minor postoperative complication rate (Clavien-Dindo I–II) of 1.2%–3.6%, and a major postoperative complication rate (III–IV) of 0%–1.4%. The Main indications for endoscopic adrenalectomy include benign appearing nonfunctioning tumors (36.8%–39.6%), pheochromocytomas (18.9%–27.4%), aldosterone-producing tumors (11.8%–17.9%), glucocorticosteroid-secreting tumors (15.4%–25.2%), and metastases to adrenal gland (4.6%). The conversion rate to an open approach is less than 2%, and the average length of hospital stay is 1.8–3.5 days.[24,25] Different minimally invasive approaches to adrenalectomy have been described, such as anterior/lateral laparoscopic and lateral/posterior retroperitoneoscopic approaches.[26] All procedures can be performed conventionally with multiple ports or with a multichannel single-site port. Additionally, all procedures can be performed with the assistance of a robot.[27]

Advances in Treatment and Management in Surgical Endocrinology. https://doi.org/10.1016/B978-0-323-66195-9.00023-6

MINIMALLY INVASIVE VIDEO-ASSISTED THYROIDECTOMY

The minimal access guarantees for an optimal cosmetic result (Fig. 23.1). Moreover, the absence of neck hyperextension and extensive dissections results in less postoperative pain. Several comparative studies have demonstrated the advantages of MIVAT in terms of reduced postoperative pain, better cosmetic result, and higher patients' satisfaction over the conventional thyroidectomy.[28–31] Furthermore, data from multicenter studies on large series of patients showed that MIVAT is a safe, effective, and reproducible technique.[29,32,33] Its low invasiveness and the similarity with the conventional procedure render this approach feasible also under locoregional anesthesia (cervical block),[34] showing the best results in patients with relative contraindications for general anesthesia such as pregnant patients with papillary thyroid carcinoma, because the strong patient's motivation plays a relevant role in the feasibility of the procedure. By the time, some concern about MIVAT was clarified. Indeed, in a published retrospective study,[35] we demonstrated that thyroid gland manipulation was similar between MIVAT and conventional thyroidectomy without additional risk of thyroid capsule rupture and thyroid cells seeding in patients who undergo MIVAT. Moreover, we as well as other authors[36–38] demonstrated the possibility and the feasibility to treat thyroid malignancy by a video-assisted approach. After an adequate period of validation and standardization of the technique, MIVAT has been successfully proposed for the surgical treatment of selected cases of papillary thyroid carcinoma. Some studies comparing the results of MIVAT and conventional thyroidectomy in terms of adequacy of surgical resection, showed that MIVAT is safe and effective for the treatment of small papillary thyroid carcinoma and has a similar oncological effectiveness of traditional thyroidectomy, at least at medium-term follow-up.[38]

An accurate patient's selection plays a key role to ensure the success of MIVAT. In the early experience with MIVAT, the indications were quite limited. Indeed, initial contraindications included thyroiditis and prior neck surgery.[14] With increasing experience, selection criteria for MIVAT have been widened, and patients with previous contralateral video-assisted neck surgery or thyroiditis no longer represented a contraindication to MIVAT. In our experience, patients who underwent video-assisted thyroid lobectomy needing a completion of thyroidectomy or patients with Basedow's disease were treated by a video-assisted approach. Some authors demonstrated that in selected patients with Graves' disease, MIVAT is feasible and can be performed safely and the results are comparable with open surgery.[39] In our experience, it has been possible to perform MIVAT also in the case of nodule >35 mm in diameter.[14]. Regarding the preoperative diagnosis, ideal candidates for MIVAT are patients with small nodules with indeterminate or suspicious cytology. In addition, small size hot nodules represent the best indication for this type of surgery. The results of MIVAT in the case of small "low-risk" papillary carcinoma are encouraging. Therefore, selected patients with papillary thyroid carcinoma could be eligible for MIVAT. On the contrary, we still believe that a preoperatively diagnosed lymph-node involvement represents a contraindication for MIVAT.[14] Patients carrying RET protooncogene (rearranged during transfection) mutation for familial forms of medullary thyroid carcinoma but not expressing the disease (absence of detectable nodules and basal/stimulated calcitonin in the normal range) are also excellent candidates for MIVAT.[40] Most part of surgical instruments required for MIVAT is usually available in almost all operating rooms, and it is not a source of additional costs. The only instruments not commonly used for a conventional thyroidectomy are small dedicated tools (2–3 mm in diameter) necessary for dissection (ad hoc designed spatulas and spatulas-shaped aspiration) that, however, are reusable. Ultrasound knife system is shown to be very useful in this type of operation in reducing the operative time.[41] The operative technique has

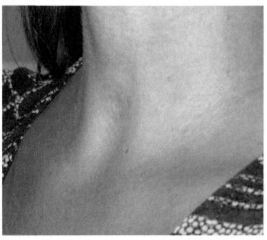

FIG. 23.1 Aesthetics results of MIVAT.

been previously described in detail[17] (Fig. 23.2A—D). The monitor is positioned at the head of the patients in front of the surgeons, who is positioned on the right side of the patient. A second monitor is usually positioned in front of the assistants who are on the left side of the patient. The endoscope is held by one of the two assistants. The absence of any external support allows modulating and changing the position of the endoscope in relation to the different steps of dissection. This represents an important advantage of the video-assisted procedure over purely endoscopic techniques. The tip of the endoscope is usually oriented toward the head of the patients, but it can be changed to expose and explore the upper mediastinum when, for example, a concomitant central compartment lymphadenectomy is required.

We published in 2009 a review of our experience[42] to evaluate the results obtained in a series of patients selected for MIVAT over a 10-year period. A total of 1363 video-assisted thyroidectomies were attempted in the time period considered. Conversion to the conventional procedure was necessary in seven cases. In 126 patients, the central neck nodes were removed through the same access. Pathological results showed benign disease in 986 cases, papillary thyroid carcinoma in 368 cases, C-cell hyperplasia in 1 case, and medullary microcarcinoma in 1 patient with RET germline mutation. Postoperative complications included 27 transient and 1 definitive recurrent laryngeal nerve palsies, 230 transient hypocalcemia, 10 definitive hypoparathyroidism, 4 postoperative hematoma, and 5 wound infections.

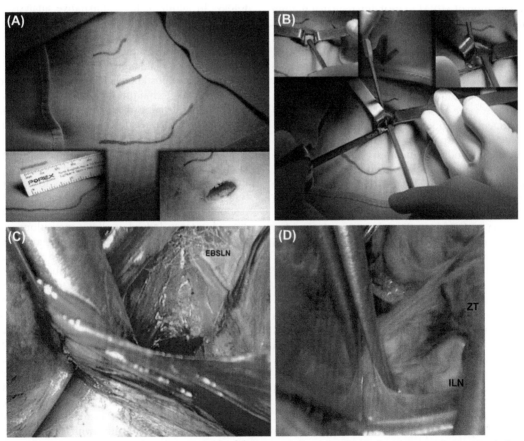

FIG. 23.2 **(A, B, C, D):** Skin incision: the thyroid lobe is medially retracted while the strap muscle are retracted laterally, using two little Farabeuf retractors; endoscope (5 mm—30 degrees) and the dedicated small surgical instruments are introduced through the single skin incision without any trocar utilization; the dissection is carried out by a blunt technique using two dedicated instruments called spatulas.

MINIMALLY INVASIVE VIDEO-ASSISTED NECK DISSECTION

Central compartment lymph-node metastases, often microscopic, are frequent in patients with papillary thyroid carcinoma[36–38] and in RET gene mutation carriers.[43] Nonetheless, according to the current guidelines, prophylactic central compartment dissection in the case of differentiated thyroid carcinoma is not mandatory.[44,45] A macroscopic preoperatively identified lymph-node involvement in the case of papillary thyroid carcinoma has been always considered an absolute contraindication for a video-assisted approach. However, it is difficult to assess, with accuracy, the status of central compartment in a preoperative setting, and the unexpected intraoperative finding of VI level lymph-node enlargement during thyroidectomy for cancer is rather frequent. In the cases, enlarged lymph node should be removed to clarify the node status and sometimes to obtain a node clearance. Since the first application of MIVAT to treat differentiated thyroid carcinomas with no preoperative evidence of lymph-node involvement, several times we have faced enlarged lymph nodes that required to be removed. After acquiring and adequate experience with the technique and supported by the evidence of safety and completeness of oncological resection of the video-assisted approach,[36,37] we described a video-assisted central compartment dissection (VA-CCD) in patients who underwent MIVAT for papillary thyroid carcinoma or suspicious thyroid nodules with unexpected intraoperative finding of lymph-node enlargement.

In 2002, we reported the result of our preliminary experience[46] on 5 patients who underwent removal of enlarged central neck lymph nodes incidentally discovered during MIVAT for papillary thyroid carcinoma. For what concerns operative time, lymph-node dissection added about 15 min to the time required for thyroidectomy in all the cases. We registered two cases of transient postoperative hypocalcemia. No other complications occurred. Through this first experience, VA-CCD demonstrated to be feasible and safe with no additional risk of complication and with additional advantages in terms of better cosmetic result and less postoperative discomfort. After this preliminary report, many other papers concerning the results of VA-CCD in case of patients with papillary thyroid carcinoma[36,37,47–51] and in RET gene mutation carriers[43] have been published. By the way, all of them represented the report of experiences of different centers on relatively small series of patients. Despite these encouraging results, some experts remained hesitant in accepting MIVAT as valid option to treat thyroid cancer.[15] The

lacking, in the literature, of comparative studies specifically addressing the oncological results of VA-CCD in comparison with the conventional procedure led us to compare two groups of patients with papillary thyroid carcinoma and similar epidemiologic and pathologic features who underwent, respectively, video-assisted and conventional central-node dissection.[52] The mean follow-up time was comparable. In all the included cases, the decision to perform the central neck-node dissection relied on the surgeon's intraoperative assessment of the nodal status. Indeed, all the patients were considered N0 (node negative) according to the preoperative evaluation. The incidence of node metastases was 50% and 46%, respectively, in video-assisted and conventional groups. No statistically significant differences were found between the two groups in terms of mean operative time, complication rate, lesion size, and number of removed lymph nodes as well as in terms of number of the metastatic lymph nodes at histology. In addition, the comparative analysis of the follow-up data showed no significant differences between the two groups in terms of mean sTg levels off LT4 suppressive treatment and mean postoperative quantitative ^{131}I ablation. The result of this study confirmed previous knowledge about the safety of the video-assisted technique and clearly demonstrated that the completeness of surgical resection of the two groups was similar, regardless of the surgical approach. The two techniques also showed the same results in terms of patient outcome at short-medium follow-up. Despite the results of this approach are encouraging, further controlled studies are necessary to evaluate the long-term results. From a pure technical point of view, it should be considered that the endoscope shows specific advantages. Indeed, it allows meticulous exploration of the central compartment, and enables identification of even slightly enlarged lymph nodes that might be overlooked at open surgery. The most widespread imaging technique used to assess the node status in patients with papillary thyroid carcinoma is ultrasonography, but it is operator dependent and it can identify only a small portion of lymph nodes found at surgical exploration because of the small size of lymph nodes, the interference of the thyroid gland for the certain unfavorable anatomic situations (e.g., obese patients, short neck, etc.).[53] The endoscope, with its optical magnification, guarantees a good exposure of the neck structures allowing for a careful dissection that is very important when dealing with structures at high risk of injury such as inferior laryngeal nerves and parathyroid glands that are extensively exposed and dissected when the central neck lymphadenectomy is carried on. The advantages that might be expected from VA-CCD are the same that have been already demonstrated for other video-assisted operations such as MIVAT.

Supported by the results of video-assisted approach for selected cases of differentiated thyroid carcinoma and encouraged by the results of VA-CCD, we also evaluated the feasibility of a minimally invasive video-assisted approach to the functional lateral neck dissection (VALNED) in patients with papillary thyroid carcinoma. We considered eligible two patients with low-risk papillary thyroid carcinoma and lateral neck nodal metastases <2 cm, without evidence of great vessels involvement. One patient underwent bilateral and one patient underwent unilateral VALNED. The mean number of removed nodes was 25 per side. Both patients experienced transient hypocalcemia. No other complications were registered. No evidence of residual tissue or recurrent disease was found at follow-up.[54] These results are encouraging but it should be considered a preliminary experience that shows only the feasibility of the technique.

An accurate patients' selection plays a relevant role to ensure the success of any video-assisted procedure, especially at the beginning of the experience. Now, ideal candidates for video-assisted approach are patients with small low-intermediate risk differentiated thyroid carcinoma and RET gene mutation carriers who have no preoperative evidence of lymph-node metastases. Among these, the results of the studies mentioned earlier demonstrated that VA-CCD can be carried out with equivalent outcomes of conventional operation if unexpected suspicious or simply enlarged lymph nodes are found out during MIVAT. Obviously to obtain the best results, with similar or even less complication rate than conventional intervention, a good patient selection is not sufficient. Surgeons, indeed, should be well trained in both endocrine and endoscopic surgery.[32,33,55]

VA-CCD represents the completion of MIVAT. Therefore, the endoscopic instruments are the same. The dissection is carried out by a blunt technique using the same two dedicated instruments called spatulas, previously mentioned for MIVAT. VA-CCD is carried out under endoscopic vision, selectively clipping and cutting, or directly cutting with energy devices the lymphatic vessels (Figs. 23.3 and 23.4). It is very important to accurately control the tip of the instruments to avoid any injury of the recurrent nerves and trachea.

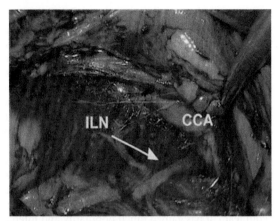

FIG. 23.3 The magnification (2–3-fold) of the endoscope permits a quite easy identification of the nerves and parathyroid glands. *CCA*, common carotid artery; *ILN*, inferior laryngeal nerve.

ROBOTIC TRANSAXILLARY THYROID SURGERY

The noncervical, remote access approaches originally developed primarily due to cosmetic considerations—poor wound healing of certain ethnic groups and the aversion in the Asian culture to neck scars.[56] Ikeda et al. in 2000 were the first to develop the transaxillary endoscopic approach to the thyroid.[57] With the introduction of the da Vinci robot (Intuitive Surgical, Sunnyvale, CA, USA), some surgeons have recognized its potential advantages. The South Korean team from

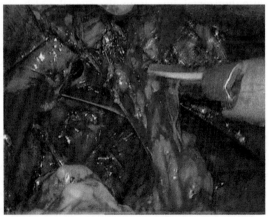

FIG. 23.4 The endoscope enables the identification of enlarged lymph nodes allowing a more accurate dissection.

Seoul, led by Chung, pioneered the transaxillary approach to the thyroid gland in late 2007.[58,59] The robotic-assisted transaxillary thyroid surgery (RATS) approach was first described in North America by Kupersmith and Holsinger in 2011.[60] As it was first introduced, more than 3000 RATS procedures were performed in South Korea, and more than 6000 worldwide.[61] Among the other robotic-assisted thyroidectomy approaches (facelift approach, bilateral-axillary breast approach), the transaxillary became the most popular. The initial RATS was performed via two incisions (axillary and anterior chest wall), but later the modification using a single axillary incision was described.[57,58] Since the first report of RATS by the Seoul team, it has gained much popularity and interest in other parts of the world. Several groups have published their initial successful experience.[62] However, as the conventional approach is safe, effective, and time honored, some surgeons doubt the value of using robotic thyroid surgery and its clinical use.[63] Robotic thyroidectomy, including RATS, remains controversial.[62]

Although several eligibility criteria to RATS were described, no standard selection criteria have been established.[64] Absolute contraindications are previous neck surgery or irradiation, retrosternal thyroid extension, and advanced thyroid disease (invasion of trachea, esophagus, and distant metastases). Relative contraindications are patients' comorbidities, age, obesity, very large goiters, well-differentiated carcinomas with a diameter larger than 2 cm, lateral neck metastases, and previous ipsilateral shoulder dysfunction.[57,65,66]

The axillary incision is defined in its inferior border by a horizontal line, from the sternal notch. The superior border, by an oblique line, is at a 60-degree angle from the thyroid notch. Following anesthesia, the patient's arm is placed in an extended position over the head, with 90-degree flexion of the elbow. The arm should be carefully rotated and padded. Following the axillary incision (5–6 cm), a dissection is performed in the subcutaneous plane, superficial to the pectoralis major muscle, to the clavicle (Figs. 23.5 and 23.6). At the sternoclavicular joint, the sternal and clavicular heads of the sternocleidomastoid muscle are identified. The dissection continues between these two heads to expose the strap muscles and deeper, the thyroid gland. Care should be taken during this step to avoid injury to the internal and external jugular veins. At this point, the retractor is inserted.[67] The da Vinci cart is placed in the contralateral side. All three arms are inserted through the axillary incision (Prograsp forceps, harmonic shears, and Maryland dissector), as

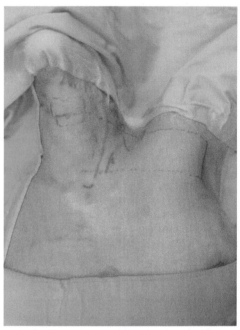

FIG. 23.5 Skin incision during robotic transaxillary thyroidectomy.

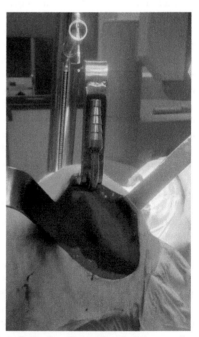

FIG. 23.6 Following the axillary incision, a dissection is performed in the subcutaneous plane, superficial to the pectoralis major muscle, to the clavicle.

well as the 30 degrees camera. The proper alignment of the robotic arms is crucial to avoid collision of the robotic arms inside the working space and the general success of the procedure. The thyroidectomy is performed in the classic fashion: first, dissecting and safely transecting the superior thyroid vessels; second, the lobe is retracted medially to help identify the parathyroid glands and the recurrent laryngeal nerve. After ligating the inferior thyroid vessels and identifying the trachea, the lobe is carefully dissected for Berry's ligament and extracted through the axillary incision. A drain is placed in the thyroid bed.[66,68]

The most obvious advantage of RATS over conventional cervical thyroidectomy is that it eliminates the need for any cervical incision. The cosmetic aspect makes RATS appealing especially to young female patients and those with a tendency toward keloid formation. The RATS has several technical advantages over the endoscopic approaches. First, the robotic system provides three-dimensional magnified visualization, which enables easier identification of the recurrent laryngeal nerve and parathyroid glands compared to the cervical approach. Second, it eliminates the natural surgeon tremor; and third, it enables, a wider range of motion through the robot's EndoWrist and the articulations of the arms. All of these result in minimal complication rates and excellent cancer control and functional results. In addition, the improved visualization and surgical ergonomics provide for reduced musculoskeletal discomfort to the surgeon compared with open or endoscopic surgery. RATS was found to yield better patient outcomes, including reduced pain and increased cosmetic satisfaction, as well as lower rates of paresthesia, postoperative voice change, and swallowing discomfort.[59,69] On the other hand, due to the new approach to the surrounding anatomy and the loss of tactile sensation, RATS introduces potential new complications such as tracheal and esophageal injury. Very few studies accounted for such complications and then only a minor way with no need to convert to open thyroidectomy.[58] In addition, due to ipsilateral arm position, there is a risk of brachial plexus neuropathy. This risk can be reduced by placing the arm in a flexed overhead 90 degrees position, thereby reducing the chance of stretching the nerves. Intraoperative monitoring of the ulnar, radial, and median nerves may further reduce the possibility of brachial plexus injury, by identifying any impending damage to these nerves and enabling the patient to be repositioned.[58] Another disadvantage of RATS is the longer operative time due to the creation of the working space and the robot docking. However,

several studies have examined the learning curve of the robotic thyroidectomy and show that increased experience led to decreased total operative time.[58] RATS involves a steep learning curve, compared to the conventional approach. However, it has been demonstrated that compared to the endoscopic approach that requires 55–60 procedures, the robotic thyroidectomy required only 35–40 procedures.[59] Another disadvantage of RAT is the limitation in the body habitus and BMI. Although obese patients (BMI > 30 kg/m^2) make the operation (particularly the working space preparation) challenging, it has been demonstrated that, in skilled hands, this obstacle can safely be overcome.[58,70,71] In terms of cost, the robotic thyroidectomy is a more expensive procedure compared to the open and the endoscopic thyroidectomy, due to the cost of the equipment and the longer operative time. However, some studies have pointed out that robotic thyroidectomy eliminated the need for an additional surgical assistant, and, combined with the potentially shorter hospital stay and the expected decrease in the maintenance cost of the robot, this may eventually result in an equally cost-effective procedure.[67]

In 2011, Lee et al. published their experience with robotic thyroidectomy on 1043 patients with low-risk well-differentiated thyroid carcinoma. They showed that the RATS was feasible and offered outcomes similar to conventional and endoscopic thyroidectomies.[72] Another study published recently explored the efficacy of RATS in North American population with thyroid cancer, compared to the conventional approach—they found similar operative times and blood loss, with negative margins for malignancy and similar thyroglobulin levels.[73] Ban et al. have described the surgical complications in their experience of 3000 patients who underwent robotic thyroidectomy for thyroid cancer. Hypocalcemia was the most common complication—1% permanent; recurrent laryngeal nerve injury—0.27% permanent; tracheal injury—0.2%; carotid artery injury—0.03%; skin flap injury—0.1%, and brachial plexopathy—0.13%. The mortality rate was 0%.[74] Male gender, overweight BMI, a large thyroid gland, and coexistent thyroiditis are factors that were found to adversely affect the surgical outcome of robotic thyroidectomy in differentiated thyroid carcinoma cases, namely longer operative times.[61] The resection of contralateral thyroid lobe in total or subtotal thyroidectomy is challenging via a single axillary incision. Therefore, some surgeons doubted the surgical completeness of RATS. A recently published meta-analysis compared the surgical completeness and oncological outcome between robotic thyroidectomy and conventional open thyroidectomy in low-risk differentiated thyroid carcinoma. Ten studies were analyzed, including 752 patients who had robotic thyroidectomy and 1453 who had open thyroidectomy. Robotic thyroidectomy was associated with fewer central lymph-node retrieval and less-complete resection (based on Tg levels), compared to open thyroidectomy, probably due to residual tissue in the contralateral side. Nevertheless, no locoregional recurrence was found in the robotic thyroidectomy group; therefore, the authors concluded that using robotic thyroidectomy was unlikely to compromise the outcome of low-risk differentiated thyroid carcinoma.[62] Several other studies investigated the completeness of the thyroidectomy, comparing it to conventional thyroidectomy using stimulated thyroglobulin levels, RAI uptake, and postoperative sonography. These studies ultimately demonstrated that the surgical completeness of robotic thyroidectomy is comparable to conventional thyroidectomy, if performed by experienced surgeons.[75-78]

ROBOTIC FACELIFT THYROIDECTOMY

The ability to perform thyroid surgery without any visible cervical incision became more feasible with the introduction of the da Vinci robot (Intuitive Surgical, Sunnyvale, CA, USA), which allowed the development of a gasless transaxillary approach.[79] As surgeons in the United States began to implement this approach, concerns emerged over the safety of the technique in patients with a larger Western body habitus.[60,71,80-83] The approach also required placement of drains and necessitated hospital admission, which represented a step backward from advances made in minimally invasive thyroid surgery during the period decade. An alternative robotic remote access approach, the robotic facelift thyroidectomy (RFT), was developed to help overcome the concern and limitations of robotic axillary thyroidectomy in the Western patient population.[84,85] Development of the RFT approach with cadaver dissection to assess the feasibility of the procedure.[86] Terris et al. reported the first use of the RFT approach in patients in 2011, with a series of 14 patients undergoing 18 RFT procedures.[87] One patient had a total thyroidectomy through bilateral incisions, and three patients had a second contralateral RFT procedure to address malignancies identified at the initial surgery. The mean operative time was 155 min, and there were no conversions to an anterior cervical approach. The first patient treated with this technique received a drain and was admitted, but all subsequent procedures were

performed without drains in the outpatients' setting. There were two seromas and one patient with transient vocal fold weakness in this series, and all of these resolved spontaneously without intervention. All patients reported temporary hypesthesia of the great auricular nerve distribution that severs weeks. Permanent vocal fold weakness and hypoparathyroidism did not occur. Remote-access thyroidectomy approaches offer the distinct advantage over anterior cervical approaches of eliminating a visible neck scar. The anatomy and vector of dissection are familiar to head and neck surgeons and the brachial plexus is not a risk for injury as it is with the robotic axillary approach.[60,80,85] The decreased area of dissection in the RFT approach compared to the axillary approach permits outpatient without drains.[84,86] Once the procedure was developed for a unilateral thyroid lobectomy, surgeons have developed robotic techniques to perform total thyroidectomy, bilateral central neck dissection, and an ipsilateral modified neck dissection through a unilateral retroauricular incision.[88] Although this approach is feasible, it has only been evaluated in a small series of 4 patients. Even in the most experienced hands, this approach took a considerable amount of time and planning and is still considered experimental. Despite these advantages, the technique is not without limitations. Transient hypesthesia in the distribution of the great auricular nerve is universal, and through it is temporary, patients need to be counseled appropriately because this does not occur through the conventional anterior approach. One main disadvantage of the RFT approach is the increased operative time over a conventional lobectomy.[84] Another significant disadvantage is the additional cost of the procedure.[89]

Stringent patient selection criteria for RFT have been created to maximize the likelihood of surgical success while minimizing the risk of complications.[87] Patients should not be morbidly obese to avoid difficulty retracting an excessively thick skin flap, yet patients who are extremely thin are also challenging because elevating a thin flap requires very delicate dissection. There should be no prior history of neck surgery, as previous scarring can compromise flap integrity. In addition to favorable patients' characteristics, the thyroid condition being addressed must also be appropriate for the approach.[87] The thyroid disease should be one that is normally treated with unilateral surgery such as an enlarging or symptomatic benign nodule, a follicular lesion, or follicular lesion of undetermined significance that is being removed for diagnostic purposes. The nodule size should not exceed 4 cm in greatest dimension, and there should be no thyroiditis or history of thyroid compartment surgery in the past. The thyroid lobe should have no substernal extension, and there should be no evidence of a high grade of malignancy such as extrathyroidal extension or pathological lymphadenopathy.[89]

The occipital hairline is shaved 1 cm posteriorly, and the facelift incision is marked behind the hairline so that it will be concealed once the hair regrows. The incision begins near the inferior extent of the lobule in the postauricular crease and is carried superiorly and posteriorly into the shaved region of the occipital hairline in a gentle curve. The incision is carried posteriorly and inferiorly as far as necessary to allow adequate exposure. The skin is incised with a scalped and the diathermy is used to develop a subplatysmal flap. The sternocleidomastoid muscle (SCM) is identified, and dissection continues anteriorly and inferiorly along the SCM. The first important structure identified is the great auricular nerve. Dissection superficial to the great auricular nerve reveals the external jugular vein and subsequently the anterior border of the SCM. The muscular triangle border by the SCM, the omohyoid, and the sternohyoid is defined. The omohyoid, sternohyoid, and sternothyroid muscles are then retracted ventrally, and the superior pole of the thyroid gland is exposed. The modified Chung retractor (Marina Medical, Sunrise, USA) is secured on the contralateral side of the operating table and then positioned so that the strap muscles are retracted ventrally. A Singer hook (Medtronic, Jacksonville, FL) attached to a Greenberg retractor (Codman & Shurtleff, Inc., Raynham, USA) secured to the ipsilateral side of the operating table retracts the SCM laterally and dorsally and provides a stable operative field. The robotic console is positioned on the contralateral side of the patients, with the pedestal angled 30 degrees away from the operating table. The robotic portion of the procedure begins with the division of the superior pedicle with the harmonic device. The superior thyroid pole is retracted inferiorly and ventrally to expose the inferior constrictor muscle. The muscle is dissected inferiorly to its lower border, and the superior laryngeal nerve is avoided. The superior parathyroid gland is identified on the posterior aspect of the thyroid and dissected so that the blood supply is preserved. The recurrent laryngeal nerve is then identified. The ligament of Berry is exposed and then transected with the harmonic device. The isthmus is divided, and the middle thyroid vein is ligated. The inferior parathyroid gland is identified and then dissected away from the thyroid gland with its blood supply intact. Lastly, the inferior thyroid vasculature is transected with the harmonic device, any remaining attachments between the thyroid lobe and the surrounding tissue are lysed, and the specimen is removed from the field.

TRANSORAL THYROIDECTOMY

Endoscopic thyroidectomy has been carefully investigated since 2008 with a natural orifice transluminal endoscopic surgery (NOTES) throughout a sublingual, or via a transtracheal approach to perfect cosmesis, which is an entire scarless benefit in the skin.[90–93] In 2013, a new NOTES procedure with an inferior three-incision vestibular approach has been popularized for thyroid gland surgery in Thailand.[94] The main benefit and indication for transoral thyroidectomy (TOT) is the cosmetic result. TOT in comparison to both conventional and other endoscopic thyroidectomy has the advantage of no visible incision in the skin, in the neck, and/or in other areas of the patient body.[94–96] The three surgical incisions are weaved in the vestibular, lower lip. Therefore, no physical or physiological complication related to scar such as keloid, hypertrophic scar, contracture formation, and dehiscence.[97–99]

TOT convoy a strict, precise yet wide inclusion criteria, that is, a preoperative ultrasonographically estimated gland size <10 cm; thyroid volume <45 mL; dominant nodule size ≤50 mm; a benign lesion such as thyroid cyst, single-nodule goiter, or multinodular goiter; Bethesda 3 or 4 lesion; papillary microcarcinoma without any evidence of metastasis.[94–103] The inclusion criteria are certainly broader than the other endoscopic or robotic procedures.[94] Exclusion criteria comprise patients who are unfit for surgery; cannot tolerate general anesthesia; had antecedent radiation in the area of the head, neck, and/or upper mediastinum; had previous neck surgery; recurrent or huge goiter; thyroid gland volume >45 mL; dominant nodule size >50 mm; evidence of lymph-node or distant metastases; tracheal/esophageal invasion; preoperative recurrent laryngeal nerve palsy; biochemical or ultrasonographically sign of hyperthyroidism and oral abscess.[94–103]

TOT is a minimally invasive procedure as its vestibular access is near to the thyroid gland, the length of dissection guarantees less operation.[94] The route to reach neck is close, shorter than that from the axilla, or breast, or retroauricular.[101–104] The transoral approach respects surgical anatomical subplatysmal planes.[94] The flap dissection is similar to that of conventional surgery.[104] TOT is through a central-median approach, thus it provides the required secure bilateral view and exposure of thyroid gland, and the two-sided procedure can be performed in safety without additional incisions.[104] Otherwise other endoscopic and robotic-assisted approaches that have a lateral remote access (as in the axilla, or retroauricular), TOT approach provides a midline access (Figs. 23.7 and 23.8A,B) and main laid line exposure to the isthmus, both the right and the left thyroid lobes in their completeness (superior and inferior pole, posterior gland), pyramidal lobe, the two inferior laryngeal nerves and superior laryngeal nerves, parathyroid glands and the lymph nodes in the central compartments (level VI), trachea and esophagus.[96–98] Central compartment inspection, dissection, with complete lymphadenectomy was described and is feasible and safe.[94–103] TOT represents an appreciable opportunity over the other remote techniques (bilateral-axillary breast approach), in which approaching the contralateral thyroid lobe, central compartment lymph node, and pyramidal lobe is actually demanding even for the experienced surgeons.[82] Robot is not executed widely in neck thyroid surgery because of obstacles in the economy.[82] The rating use of routine conventional laparoscopic endoscopic instrumentation for TOT seems to be a more feasible option for wide adaption of this new technique. TOT can be carried with or without the aid of the robot, and safely with only the use of conventional endoscopic instruments. De facto, TOT is done fully endoscopic using conventional endoscopic instruments with less overall operative time.[102]

MINIMALLY INVASIVE VIDEO-ASSISTED PARATHYROIDECTOMY

Bilateral neck exploration with identification of four parathyroid glands and removal of all hyperfunctioning

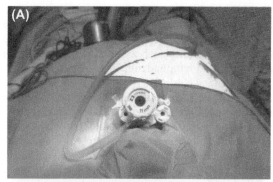

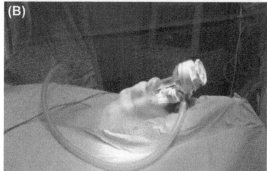

FIG. 23.8 **(A,B):** Transoral thyroidectomy—trocars position.

tissue has been considered the "gold standard" for the treatment of primary hyperparathyroidism (pHPT), achieving a cure in more than 95% of cases with a complication rate generally less than 3%.[14] During the last 3 decades, the improved preoperative localization studies[105] and the introduction of the clinical practice of intraoperative PTH (IO-PTH) assay[14] led to the development of the targeted approaches to parathyroidectomy.[106] MIVAP was first described by Miccoli et al.[6] Early after its description, MIVAP gained a large worldwide acceptance in different surgical settings, due to its reproducibility and its similarity with the conventional technique for the parathyroidectomy.[107,108] Several comparative studies have demonstrated the advantages of MIVAP to reduce the postoperative pain and improve the cosmetic result and the patient satisfaction over both the conventional and open nonendoscopic minimally invasive parathyroidectomy.[109,110]

Patients with sporadic pHPT in whom a single adenoma is suspected based on preoperative imaging studies (MIBI-scan and ultrasonography) are ideal candidates for MIVAP. Parathyroid adenoma larger than 3 cm are usually excluded because of the theoretical risk of capsular effraction and consequent parathyromatosis due to difficult dissection and extraction.[111] At the beginning of the experience,

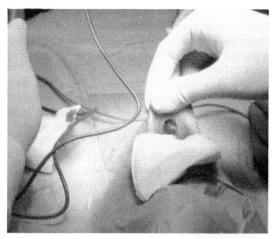

FIG. 23.7 Incision during transoral thyroidectomy.

exclusion criteria included the previous neck surgery, persistent or recurrent hyperparathyroidism, mediastinal adenomas, and concomitant large goiter that can undergo MIVAP if the usual inclusion criteria for the video-assisted thyroidectomy are met.[112] Moreover, in selected cases, patients with the previous neck surgery and intrathymic/retrosternal adenomas can be selected for MIVAP. Because bilateral neck exploration is possible through the same access, MIVAP can be performed both in patients with suspected multiglandular disease and in patients with uncertain preoperative localization.[111] The rates of patients with sporadic pHPT who are candidates for MIVAP varies (37%−71%)[29,42] due to different incidences of coexisting thyroid disease that may require a conventional approach.[113] MIVAP has also been proposed for patients with four glands hyperplasia (i.e., familial pHPT[114] and secondary and tertiary hyperparathyroidism.[43,107,108,111,112,114,115] However, these indications still need to be confirmed and validated by larger series and comparative studies.[14]

As for MIVAT also for MIVAP in selected cases, it is feasible under locoregional anesthesia (cervical block)[113] (Fig. 23.9). Instruments for MIVAP are the same that are used for MIVAT previously described. Thanks to the central access, MIVAP allows exploration of contralateral parathyroid glands through the same skin when necessary (suspicious of multiglandular disease because of inadequate IO-PTH decrease, two enlarged glands found at unilateral exploration, inadequate preoperative localization studies, etc.) (Fig. 23.10).

Several large retrospective series have reported on the short- and medium-term outcome of MIVAP. In 350 cases of MIVAP, in 6 years, Miccoli et al.[115]

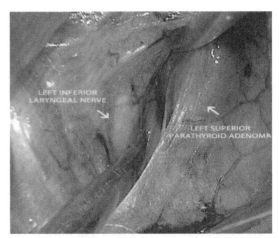

FIG. 23.10 MIVAP: Left inferior laryngeal nerve and left superior parathyroid adenoma.

reported a cure rate of 98.3%. At medium follow-up of 35.1 months, four patients had persistent disease due to a false-positive IO-PTH. Complications occurred in 14 patients: 2.7% transient hypocalcemia, 0.8% permanent nerve palsy, and 0.3% postoperative bleeding.[115] Others have reported similar results in smaller series.[107] In our previous published series of 107 cases of MIVAP, we reported a success rate of 98.1% with persistent disease in two patients (1.9%).[113] We reported 11.1% rate of temporary hypocalcemia with no permanent hypoparathyroidism and no other complications.[113] MIVAP could be considered, in selected cases and in experienced center, the standard treatment of sporadic pHPT.[113]

ENDOSCOPIC PARATHYROIDECTOMY WITHOUT ROBOTIC SYSTEM

Procedures that imply the utilization of the endoscope (totally endoscopic and video-assisted techniques) take advantages not only of the targeted approach, but also of the endoscopic magnification that allows performing the same intervention through a very minimal incision.[116,117] Although not supported by evidence-based data, it has been argued that the use of an endoscope was theoretically associated with a lower risk of complications due to optimal visualization of neck structures.[117] Parathyroid techniques using an endoscope can be classified into totally endoscopic and video-assisted procedures. Total endoscopic parathyroidectomy was described by Ganger et al. in 1996.[2] Initial technique was carried out entirely under a steady gas flow, using a 5 mm

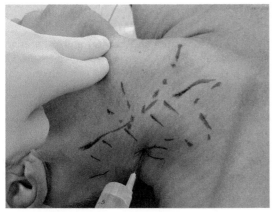

FIG. 23.9 Locoregional anesthesia (cervical block).

endoscope introduced through a central trocar, and two or three additional trocars for needlescopic instruments. The dissection was first performed beneath the platysma to obtain a good working space. The midline was then opened and the strap muscles were retracted to expose the thyroid lobe and explore the parathyroid gland after dissection of the thyroid from the fascia.[118] This initial approach using a central cervical access and gas insufflation has been subsequently modified over time but is currently rarely perfomed.[117,119] This evolution is mainly explained by the fact that this central approach with gas insufflation does not allow complete and easy exposure to parathyroid glands localized posteriorly.[117,119] Consequently, this surgical access has been considered to be well adapted for anteriorly locating parathyroid glands and when inferior parathyroid adenomas are located at the tip of the inferior pole of the thyroid, or along the thyrothymic ligament. However, this anterior access is not always suitable for the removal of parathyroid adenomas deeply and posteriorly located in the neck because thyroid volume may hamper the dissection. The lateral access (or back-door access) using the plane between the strap muscle medially and the carotid sheath laterally has been considered to be much more suitable for these posteriorly located parathyroid adenomas.[116,120] Totally endoscopic lateral approach was first described by Henry et al. in 1995.[121] A 10-mm incision is made at the anterior border of the SCM and deepened by sharp and blunt dissection to create a space lateral to the ipsilateral thyroid lobe and medial to the carotid artery and the internal jugular vein. Two 3-mm trocars are introduced cranially and caudally to the incision along the anterior SCM border and a 5-mm trocar with a 0-degree endoscope is placed in the initial incision, which is temporarily closed by a purse-string suture. Carbon dioxide is insufflated at a pressure of 8 mmHg to expand the artificial space, and dissection is performed with 3-mm instruments. During the procedure, identification of the recurrent laryngeal nerve and the ipsilateral parathyroid are often easily possible. For totally endoscopic lateral approach (Henry technique), evaluation has been made by five retrospective studies and one comparative study.[116,120,122−124] A prospective study including 200 patients showed that more than half of all patients (52%) with pHPT could undergo totally endoscopic lateral parathyroidectomy with a 98% cure rate. In this series, this approach was associated with a complication rate similar to conventional techniques.[118] There was no mortality. Transient recurrent laryngeal nerve palsy was observed in five patients

(2.5%) and remained permanent in one patient (0.5%). Eleven patients (5.5%) had a transient postoperative hypoparathyroidism.[122] However, conversion rate remained an important issue (28%) and patient selection, disease severity, and adenoma localization had no significant impact on conversion rate.[122] In another series evaluating medium-term result, Maweja et al. reported a cure rate of 98.5% with one case of recurrent disease in 394 totally endoscopic lateral procedures after a median follow-up of 20.5 months.[125] The main technical limitation of the techniques is considered to be the unilateral approach that prevents the possibility to accomplish bilateral exploration. Overall, totally endoscopic lateral approach is not widely performed, and studies evaluating this technique have remained unfrequented.[116,120,122,125] Besides those techniques with direct cervical access, other procedures with an extracervical endoscopic approach have also been proposed.[117,120] These approaches gained initial success mainly in the Asian surgical community, where avoiding any neck scar is culturally important. Hence, extracervical accesses from the chest wall, breast, oral cavity, retroauricular region (facelift incision), and axilla to perform parathyroidectomy have been reported.[124,126,127] All those endoscopic techniques are characterized by continuous CO_2 insufflation or mechanical external retraction to maintain the operative working space for retraction and trocar positioning.[117] All those extracervical endoscopic approaches provide optimal cosmetic results in the neck but are technically demanding, are associated with extracervical incisions with the need for extended dissection to reach the neck with potential related complications, and are difficult to be reproduced, especially by unskilled endoscopic surgeons.[117]

ENDOSCOPIC PARATHYROIDECTOMY WITH ROBOTIC SYSTEM

The inherent limitations of cervical and extracervical endoscopic approaches have led to the emergences of the robotic parathyroidectomy as an alternative option.[128] Reported experience with robotic parathyroidectomy is currently limited, and it corresponds mainly to extracervical approaches.[129] In 2011, Tolley et al. prospectively evaluated 11 selected patients with pHPT.[130] Patients with significant thyroiditis, large thyroid volume, and previous neck surgery were excluded. An ipsilateral infraclavicular incision and three small incisions in the ipsilateral anterior axillary line were performed. The parathyroid adenoma was successfully excised in all 11 patients and there were no complications. The recurrent laryngeal nerve was identified in all cases. Mean operative time was 61 min. One patient had persistent disease, and one patient required conversion to open surgery due to high body mass index.[130,131] The same year, Landry et al. reported two patients who underwent transaxillary robotic parathyroidectomy.[132] In this study, both patients had their adenoma localized preoperatively. Despite the long operative times (115 and 102 min, respectively), there were no complications with the parathyroid adenoma successfully excised in both cases. In 2012, Foley et al. compared four transaxillary robotic parathyroidectomy patients against 12 matched controls that underwent targeted open parathyroidectomy.[133] All robotic parathyroidectomy patients were cured, but the mean operative time in this study group of patients was significantly longer. This study concluded that improved cosmesis should be weighed against the length of robotic surgery parathyroidectomy. Noureldine et al. retrospectively evaluated nine patients who underwent transaxillary robotic parathyroidectomy by a single surgeon.[134] No complications were reported (with routine pre- and postoperative laryngoscopy). At 6-month follow-up, the overall cosmetic outcome was subjectively considered to be good with the incision scar located in the axilla area. Lastly, Karagkounis et al. retrospectively evaluated eight patients who underwent transaxillary robotic parathyroidectomy for a preoperatively localized cervical parathyroid adenoma.[135] All patients were cured of their disease with 6-month follow-up. The only complication was seroma formation in one patient (13%), and there was no need for conversion to open surgery. To date, no robotic procedure to perform parathyroidectomy for pHPT and using neck incision has been published. This is likely due to the fact that the robotic system is generally used to avoid neck scars as proposed by Asian groups for robotic thyroidectomy. However, Van Slycke et al. showed that the use of a robotic system to perform lateral endoscopic cervical parathyroidectomy as described by Henry et al. was feasible.[118] Robotic-assisted parathyroidectomy through a lateral cervical approach has shown to be a safe and feasible procedure especially in patients with posteriorly localized parathyroid adenomas.[118]

LAPAROSCOPIC TRANSABDOMINAL ADRENALECTOMY

During the last 2 decades, minimally invasive surgery has become the gold standard of treatment for the removal of benign functioning and nonfunctioning tumors of the adrenal glands.[136–138] Several factors explain the successful application of minimally invasive surgery to adrenals, for example, the endoscopic approach allows an adequate exposure of the glands, the magnification of the endoscope is particularly useful during the dissection of an anatomically complex and dangerous area, the gland's blood supply is well defined, surgery is most commonly performed for small lesions, there is a low incidence of malignant tumors, and the procedures are ablative and therefore do not require a reconstructive technique.[137,138] Transabdominal laparoscopic adrenalectomy (TLA) was first reported in 1992 by Gagner et al.,[1] who used a transperitoneal flank approach in the lateral decubitus position.[139] Multiple retrospective comparative studies have demonstrated the benefit of minimally invasive techniques in adrenalectomy, specifically the decreased requirement for analgesic, improvement in patients' satisfaction, and shorter hospital stay and recovery time when compared to open approach.[140–146] The lateral transperitoneal approach to the adrenal glands is currently the most wide practice route, as it provides a good overall view of the gland and surrounding structures and allows a wide operative field.[137,138] One of the main advantages of the lateral approach is to allow the gravity-facilitated exposure of the adrenals.[137,138] Moreover, this approach provides familiar landmarks that help the surgeon to localize the adrenal gland and a safe access and control of the vascular structures.[137,138] A further advantage of this route is to allow exploiting the abdominal cavity and to treat other abdominal pathologies simultaneously.[137,138] From a technical point of view, the primary prerequisite for a successful procedure are an adequate knowledge of anatomy, a delicate tissue handling, and a meticulous hemostasis technique to properly identify structures and prevent bleeding that could greatly complicate the surgical procedures.[137,138,147] In some cases, the left adrenalectomy can pose more challenges than the right, considering the reported difficulty to clearly identify the adrenal gland in the perineal fat, mainly in obese patients.[148] Despite body mass index correlated with TLA longer operative times,[149,150] obesity was not considered a contraindication to this approach.[146] Previous surgery, especially when performed on the kidney, pancreas, or spleen, can cause significant adhesion in the operative areas and may render the transperitoneal approach challenging especially for surgeons with limited laparoscopic experience. Nonetheless, in several series, up to 55% of patients have previous abdominal surgery, but conversions were very rarely attributed to adhesion.[18,146,151]

The patient is placed on the supine position first, until general anesthesia is induced. The patient is then turned to the lateral decubitus position (Fig. 23.11) with the side of the adrenal lesion up. The 10th rib is positioned at the level of the break point in the operating table. A soft axillary roll is placed underneath the chest wall to protect the axilla. A pillow is placed between the legs with the lower leg flexed and the upper leg straightened. The space between the lower costal margin and the iliac crest is then increased by flexing the bed. The patient is secured to the table with additional tape and padding placed over the lower extremities and pelvis. The monitors are placed at the patient's head and the surgeon and first assistant stand facing the abdominal wall of the patient. Access can be obtained by either the Veress needle, open Hasson techniques or optical access trocar. The initial trocar is placed at the anterior axillary line, 2 cm below the costal margin (Fig. 23.12). The next two ports are placed on either side of the first port with at least 8 cm of distance between them to allow freedom of movement of the instruments. At least one of these ports should be a 10/12-mm port to allow use of a clip applier or a stapling device to allow for control of the adrenal vein. The other ports can be 5 mm. For a right adrenalectomy, a fourth port is necessary for placement of a liver retractor. Occasionally, during a left adrenalectomy, a fourth port is required. This is usually placed after the splenic flexure is mobilized.

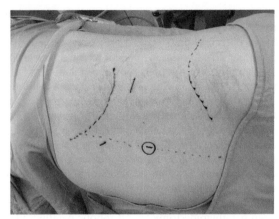

FIG. 23.12 TLA—trocars position.

Right adrenalectomy. The key factor for an adequate exposure is an effective dissection of the liver right triangular ligament and of the hepatoparietal ligament wide enough in order to achieve a complete mobilization of the liver, that can be retracted . After the effective liver mobilization, the adrenal gland and the vena cava are adequately exposed. Once the liver is mobilized, dissection of the medial border of the adrenal is begun. A plane is developed between the lateral aspect of the inferior vena cava and the medial border of the adrenal gland. The adrenal vein is identified and exposed with 10-mm right angle dissector. The vein can be divided by double clipping on either side or by using a stapler with a vascular load. Once the adrenal vein is divided, the dissection proceeds superiorly and inferiorly with the ultrasonic dissector. The specimen should then be mobilized posteriorly of the psoas muscle and the lateral attachments divided. Once the specimen has been mobilized, the specimen should be placed in an impermeable endocatch bag to avoid spillage in the event of an unsuspected malignancy and removed from the abdomen. Hemostasis is assured and the fascia is closed.

Left adrenalectomy. The dissection begins with the mobilization of the splenic flexure. The splenorenal ligament is then completely divided from the inferior pole of the spleen to the level of the diaphragm using the ultrasonic dissector. This allows complete mobilization of the spleen medially. The border of the adrenal gland should be mobilized from the left kidney until the adrenal vein is identified emptying into the left renal vein. The adrenal vein should be identified and exposed with the 10-mm right angel dissector. The vein can then be doubly clipped and divided. Once the adrenal vein is controlled, the gland

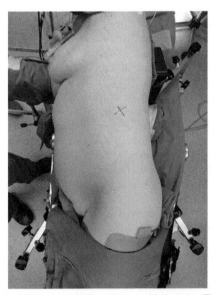

FIG. 23.11 Lateral decubitus position during TLA.

should be mobilized taking all the periadrenal tissue in block with the gland. Care should be taken to avoid the tail of the pancreas during this dissection.

Economopoulos et al.[152] attempted to determine if there were certain patient characteristics pertaining to a more difficult laparoscopic adrenalectomy. The author retrospectively analyzed 365 surgeries, 6 of which (1.6%) were converted to an open procedure. Unexpectedly, obesity and previous abdominal surgery did not result in higher conversion rates or postoperative complication rate. Obesity, previous abdominal surgery anatomically close to adrenal gland (i.e., nephrectomy, bowel/colon resection), bilateral adrenalectomy, male sex, and tumor size at least 4 cm led to a prolonged operative time; bilateral adrenalectomy, pheochromocytoma, and age prolonged lenght of hospital stay. The rate of postoperative complications and conversion was increased by tumor size greater than 8 cm only. The authors concluded that laparoscopic adrenalectomy can be safely performed by skilled endocrine surgeons despite obesity, previous abdominal surgery, or the need of bilateral adrenalectomy.[152]

POSTERIOR RETROPERITONEOSCOPIC ADRENALECTOMY

As with conventional operative procedures, different endoscopic approaches to the adrenals have been described. These include laparoscopic approaches with the patients in a supine (anterior approach) or lateral position (lateral approach) and a retroperitoneoscopic approach with the patient in a lateral (lateral approach) or prone position (posterior approach).[137,138] Although comparisons of the different endoscopic adrenalectomy approaches have been reported,[153–160] definitive conclusions about which procedures are optimal have yet to be drawn. Posterior retroperitoneoscopic adrenalectomy (PRA), first described by Mercan et al.[161] has been standardized by Walz et al.[162] and has recently increased in popularity and is currently adopted in about 20% of referral centers[80,138,163,164] (Fig. 23.13). It may provide more direct access to the adrenals, thus avoiding postoperative adhesions and the need for patient repositioning in bilateral adrenalectomy. Although it has been suggested to be feasible for large tumors,[165] large tumor size is indicated as the main limitation of PRA, mainly because of the small space available for dissection.

The patient is in prone position with the chest and the abdomen supported by the Wilson frame that allows the abdominal contents to full anteriorly (Fig. 23.14). The table is flexed in jack-knife position

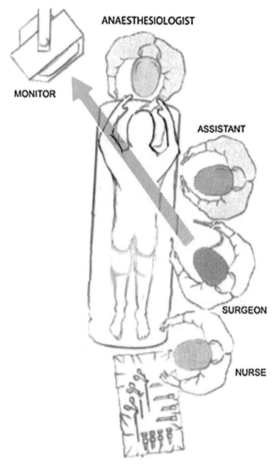

FIG. 23.13 Surgical team and equipment placement in a right posterior retroperitoneoscopic adrenalectomy.

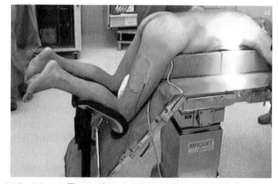

FIG. 23.14 The patient is in prone position with the chest and the abdomen supported by the Wilson frame. The table is flexed in jack-knife position with the back level.

allowing for opening the space between the posterior costal margin and the posterior iliac crest. A 1.5-cm transverse incision is performed just below the tip of the 12th rib. The retroperitoneal space is created by blunt and sharp dissection. A small cavity is prepared for the insertion of two standard trocars (5–10 mm), introduced with internal finger guidance 4–5 cm laterally (midaxillary line) and medially (sacrospinalis muscle) to the initial incision site, respecting the subcostal nerve. The finger guidance allows for a safe trocars placement. The retropneumoperitoneum is created by maintaining a CO_2 pressure of 20–25 mmHg. The endoscope (10 mm, 30 degrees) is introduced at the level of the central trocar. The Zuckerkandl's fascia is then opened under direct vision by blunt and sharp dissection: the dissection should be wide as far as possible, to allow an adequate access to the retroperitoneum. After opening the Zuckerkandl's fascia, the retroperitoneal fat must be dissected downward to expose para-vertebral muscles medially, diaphragm cranially, and peritoneum laterally (with the liver and the spleen, respectively, on the right and left side). This step is critical for the creation of an adequate working space. If the peritoneum is inadvertently opened at this time, the procedures could be continued. The kidney upper pole should be exposed and dissected. The kidney represents the most important landmark in the retroperitoneoscopic approach, crucial for the subsequent dissection of the adrenal gland. The dissection of the upper pole of the kidney should be as complete as possible, to allow an adequate exposure of the inferior aspect of the adrenal, crucial for an easy and safe identification of the main adrenal vein. The operative field is now delimited by the kidney upper pole caudally, diaphragm cranially, the spine and paraspinal muscles medially, the peritoneum laterally. The muscles of the posterior abdominal wall are the top of the space of dissection. The mobilization of the adrenal gland begins caudally. All adrenal gland manipulations must be performed carefully using blunt palpation probes to avoid any capsular rupture and/or adrenal tissue fragmentation. Dissection is continued medially between the diaphragmatic branch and adrenal gland. In this area on the right side, the adrenal gland arteries cross the vena cava posteriorly. These vessels are divided by clips or activated shears. After caudally and medially adrenal dissection, the gland can be lifted up to expose the vena cava in its retroperitoneal cranial aspect. The short right adrenal vein then becomes clearly visible running posteriorly and laterally. On the left side, the main adrenal vein must be prepared in the space between the adrenal gland and the diaphragmatic branch medial to the upper pole of the kidney. In this space, it is possible to identify the diaphragmatic vein joining the main adrenal vein. This represents an important landmark for identifying the left main adrenal vein. The adrenal gland is then laterally and cranially dissected. The resected adrenal gland is extracted by means of endoscopic specimen bags through the central trocar port.

Since its standardization in recent years,[162] PRA has emerged as a valid and attractive alternative to lateral transperitoneal laparoscopic adrenalectomy.[138,163,166] This approach allows direct access to the adrenals with minimal dissection of the surrounding structures, which has been suggested to shorten operative time.[162,163,168] Moreover, the retroperitoneal route allows endoscopic adrenalectomy to be performed easily and safely in cases where there are major abdominal adhesions related to previous procedures. The main disadvantage of this technique is the small working space, which limits the size of the lesions suitable for this approach. Many practitioners have advocated that retroperitoneoscopic posterior adrenalectomy should be the procedure of choice for adrenalectomy in cases of small-to medium-sized benign adrenal tumors owing to theoretical advantages over transperitoneal adrenalectomy, in terms of decreased operative time, low conversion rates, and minimal dissection of the surrounding tissues.[162,166] Although comparative analysis of the different endoscopic adrenalectomy approaches have been reported,[163,164] definitive conclusions about which procedures are optimal are yet to be drawn. The posterior approach appeared as a very attractive procedure for patients requiring bilateral adrenalectomy, as it eliminates the need to reposition the patient. The prone position exposes both the adrenal regions at the same time.[11,167] The technique for simultaneous posterior retroperitoneoscopic bilateral adrenalectomy has been described elsewhere[167]: two different surgical teams (surgeon, assistant, nurse) and sets of equipment (monitor, insufflator, camera, and surgical instrumentation) were assembled on each side of the patient.[167] In a multicenter comparative analysis of the three different approaches for bilateral adrenalectomy (transabdominal laparoscopic vs. simultaneous posterior retroperitoneoscopic vs. robot-assisted bilateral adrenalectomy), the posterior retroperitoneoscopic approach showed a significantly less operative time because it eliminates the need to reposition the patient.[11] In our experience, among a series of 563 adrenalectomies, 151 patients underwent unilateral posterior retroperitoneoscopic adrenalectomy (19 simultaneous bilateral posterior retroperitoneoscopic adrenalectomy). Overall, the mean operative time was 111.2 ± 51.1 min (range 30−285). Postoperative minor complications were registered in 12 cases. No mortality was registered in this series. Although retroperitoneoscopic adrenalectomy has also been proposed in the case of large adrenal lesions,[165] we believe that benign lesions ranging in size within 6 cm represent the ideal indication for this approach.[163] This group include most tumors of the adrenal gland, both functioning and nonfunctioning.[163,166,168]

ROBOTIC ADRENALECTOMY

In 1999, Piazza et al.[169] and Hubens et al.[170] described the first robotic-assisted adrenalectomy using the AESOP 2000, a commercially available robotic platform in Europe at that time. Subsequently, the da Vinci robotic system (Intuitive Surgical, Sunnyvale, CA, USA) has been introduced in the clinical practice. Surgical management of adrenal disorders has seen a paradigm change in its approach. Many centers have performed robotic-assisted adrenalectomy successfully, establishing it as a safe, feasible, and effective approach. With the use of the da Vinci robotic system, challenges and limitations associated with pure laparoscopic surgery are alleviated while preserving the benefits of minimally invasive surgery. The superior ergonomics, three-dimensional magnification of the operative field, tremor filtration, and the Endowrist technology of robotic instruments providing a greater range of motion as compared to the human hand has allowed for easier handling of the fragile adrenal gland surrounded by major vessels and viscera in a confined space. The lateral transperitoneal and the posterior retroperitoneal approaches are the commonest approaches adopted by most centers during robotic-assisted adrenalectomies.[171]

Robotic-assisted or conventional laparoscopic adrenalectomy can be performed via a transperitoneal or retroperitoneal approach. The transperitoneal approach provides greater working space, and facilitates orientation by providing readily identifiable anatomical landmarks and better visualization of surrounding anatomical structures. It also provides greater versatility in the angles of approach of laparoscopic trocars and instruments. In the lateral approach, peritoneal contents fall medially to give greater surgical exposure. For robotic-assisted transperitoneal adrenalectomy, most centers describe a lateral transperitoneal technique where patients are usually positioned in the lateral decubitus or modified lateral position with varying degrees of tilt of between 30 and 60 degrees.

Adrenalectomy can also be performed via the retroperitoneal approach. This approach mimics open surgery with its avoidance of the peritoneal cavity. This becomes the main advantage of this approach. There is also no entry into the peritoneal cavity, and complications associated with intraperitoneal access, such as intraperitoneal visceral injury, problems associated with pneumoperitoneum, and adhesion formation, are reduced. As such, it may be the preferred approach in patients requiring access to bilateral adrenal glands and in patients with multiple previous abdominal surgeries, where intraperitoneal surgery may be more challenging due to previous adhesion formation. The greatest limitation with retroperitoneal adrenalectomy, however, is the limitation in working space that increases the technical difficulties of the operation. Eight centers have described their techniques for robotic-assisted posterior retroperitoneal adrenalectomy.[128,172−179] In these centers, the patients are positioned in a prone position with the table flexed into a jack-knife position.

Port placement and the choice of port size is surgeon dependent. Most techniques describe a port placement configuration of 4 ports for left-sided adrenalectomy with one additional port required for right-sided adrenalectomy to aid in liver retraction. In recent years, laparoendoscopic single-site (LESS) adrenalectomy has been described based on the principle that with a smaller number of incisions and ports, enhancement of cosmesis and reduction of associated port-site complications can be attained. Both the retroperitoneal and transperitoneal approaches have been described for LESS adrenalectomy with variable strategies in terms of patient positioning, incision sites, and ports placement. Usually a 2−3-cm incision is required for the insertion of a multiport device, typically described to be placed at the umbilicus for cosmetic benefits. Careful preoperative assessment and patient selection are imperative in minimizing challenges during surgery, reducing complications and ensuring quality outcome. The disadvantages of LESS adrenalectomy include that of reduced distance between ports and loss of instrument triangulation resulting in cross over and paradoxical movement of instruments, as well as suboptimal approach to the adrenal gland and inadequate countertraction. Nozaki et al.[180] described their technique of intraumbilical access to solve the problem associated with crossover instrumentation during LESS adrenalectomy. This involves a longitudinal incision of the umbilicus and a wider area of subcutaneous tissue dissection to accommodate multiple ports. The incision length remains within the depression of the umbilicus therefore preserving normal umbilical appearance. Few centers have reported their experience with robotic-assisted single port adrenalectomy[178,179,181,182] performed via both the transperitoneal and the retroperitoneal approaches. Park et al.[178] reported their initial experience with robotic single-site posterior retroperitoneal approach, demonstrating its safety and feasibility. In their described technique, the operation is performed in the prone jack-knife position, with a 3-cm transverse skin incision made just below the lowest tip of the 12th rib. For the transperitoneal approach, the patient is placed in a flexed lateral decubitus position, with an ipsilateral middle quadrant incision made for the single-site port.

Some retrospective comparisons of laparoscopic retroperitoneal and transperitoneal approaches tend to favor the retroperitoneal approach. Several operative parameters have been found to favor adrenalectomy performed via the retroperitoneal approach. These include shorter hospital stay,[150,160,183,184] faster resumption of oral intake,[150,183] decreased analgesic requirement, and postoperative pain that in turn leads to earlier ambulation,[184,185] shorter operative time,[184,185] blood loss,[150,185] and morbidity[155] associated with the procedure. The major benefit of the retroperitoneal approach is that with the adrenal against the ribcage at the back, there was no need to move any other organs out of the way. By mimicking open surgery, the peritoneal cavity is avoided, eliminating bowel handling and potential for injury to the intraabdominal viscera. Walz et al.[186] reported that out of 142 patients who had posterior retroperitoneal adrenalectomy, half the patients did not require any postoperative analgesia and only five required pain medication for more than 24 h postoperatively. Faster resumption of oral intake, together with decreased analgesia requirement and postoperative pain, may all contribute toward a shorter convalescence and hospital stay. Although patients with smaller tumors, lower body mass index, and bilateral adrenal pathologies and having significant prior abdominal surgery tend to benefit from retroperitoneal approach, patients with a higher body mass index with larger tumors and no prior abdominal surgeries tend to benefit more from the lateral transperitoneal approach.[187] These two approaches were found to be complementing and not competitive to each other when certain patient selection criteria are followed. There have been descriptions of robotic-assisted posterior retroperitoneal adrenalectomy[175–177,188] including descriptions of robotic-assisted single port

retroperitoneal adrenalectomy.[178,179] In a comparison between robotic-assisted posterior retroperitoneal adrenalectomy and laparoscopic posterior retroperitoneal adrenalectomy, it was found that beyond the initial learning curve, robotic-assisted posterior retroperitoneal adrenalectomy shortens the skin-to-skin operative time by 28 min when compared with the laparoscopic approach. However, this may be nullified should there be additional intraoperative time used for transportation of the robotic unit to the operating room, starting up of the system, calibration of the robotic cameras, and draping of the robotic arms. There was also lower immediate postoperative pain level for patients who underwent robotic-assisted posterior retroperitoneal adrenalectomy.[188] Nevertheless, more randomized controlled trials need to be performed to study more meaningful outcomes and measures before this procedure can be justified.

Systematic reviews and meta-analyses of current evidence available have demonstrated the safety and efficacy of robotic-assisted adrenalectomy when compared to laparoscopic adrenalectomy.[171] In 2004, Morino et al.[189] in a prospective randomized controlled study comparing robotic and laparoscopic adrenalectomy concluded that laparoscopic adrenalectomy was superior to robotic-assisted adrenalectomy in terms of feasibility, morbidity and cost in view of longer operative time, higher 30-day complication rate, and a similar length of hospital stay. However, since then, many subsequent retrospective studies and meta-analyses have been performed comparing the outcomes of robotic versus laparoscopic adrenalectomy that demonstrates equivalence if not superior outcomes for robotic-assisted adrenalectomy. There is a wide range of operative times reported by different centers with a mean reported time of between 98 and 234.4 min. Brunaud et al.[190] identified several criteria that had an impact on operative time such as surgeon experience, first assistant training level, as well as tumor size, with tumors less than 4.5 cm having a shorter operative time. Longer operative times were typically demonstrated in the initial part of the learning curve. This can be partly attributed to time spent docking the robot. Once the ports are placed in traditional laparoscopic surgery, the operation commences. However, in robotic surgery, after the ports are placed, the robot tower must then be docked with instruments inserted, and this has been found to increase the operative time by between 15 and 40 min[191] with initial docking time reported to be as long as 1 h.[190] Although these can be streamlined with increasing experience, this is still an extra step when compared to laparoscopic surgery. However, beyond the initial learning curve, Agcaoglu et al.[172] reported a significant improvement in operative time after the 10th procedure, and the difference in operative time can be eliminated from as early as the 20th operative case.[190] They reported that the mean operative time decreased 134 min in the last 45 cases compared with the first 50 cases and by multiple regression analysis, surgeons experience, first assistant level, and tumor size were independent predictors of operative time. Brandao et al.[192] in a meta-analysis comparing robotic and laparoscopic adrenalectomy found no statistical difference between the operative times between the two procedures. Karabulut et al.[193] also found that the time spent for individual steps of procedure was similar between the laparoscopic and the robotic group and even though the tumor size was larger in the robotic groups. The duration of hospital stay in the robotic-assisted studies reported a mean range of 1.1–6.4 days. Perioperative outcome studies have reported a shorter hospital stay when robotic-assisted adrenalectomy is performed when compared to laparoscopic adrenalectomy.[174,192,193] Karabulut et al.[193] found that in their cohort of patients, the main reasons for hospital stay in the robotic group was for nausea, atelectasis, and the need for pain control, and all patients were discharged within 2 days. This is in comparison to their patients who underwent laparoscopic adrenalectomy who stayed between 1 and 4 days. This shorter hospital stay is possibly the result of a combination of various improved outcomes such as a shorter operative time and lesser blood loss, though hospital stay can be an unreliable outcome parameter for comparison as it can be confounded by many factors. One other significant outcome in favor of robotic surgery was the lower estimated blood loss. Reported mean blood loss ranged from less than 50 to 576 mL, with most centers reporting mean blood loss of less than 100 mL. Bilateral adrenalectomies tend to result in greater blood losses. Lee et al.[181] reported a mean of 1698 mL (150–6140 mL) in their five cases of bilateral robotic-assisted single-site adrenalectomy that were performed. Pineda-Solís et al.[194] in their retrospective study found that the blood loss tended to be lower in the robotic group versus the laparoscopic group (30 ± 5 mL vs. 55 ± 74 mL, $P = .07$) though this was not statistically significant. Other studies also reported equivalence in terms of intraoperative blood loss.[195,196] Brandao et al.[192] in their meta-analysis comparing outcomes between robotic-assisted adrenalectomy and laparoscopic adrenalectomy found that seven out of nine studies reported less bleeding for the robotic group with a statistically significant difference between the two groups. However, this difference may not be clinically significant and that both techniques can be performed with minimal associated blood loss. In the current literature, low conversion rates have been reported for both robotic and laparoscopic adrenalectomy.[192] Conversion rate for robotic-assisted adrenalectomy were reported to range between 0% and 40% for laparoscopic conversion and 0% and 10% for open conversion while open conversion rates in the laparoscopic studies ranged between 0% and 10.5%. Of note, in both groups, many studies reported a 0% conversion rate. Common reasons for conversion in robotic cases cited included adherence of the tumor to surrounding structures or adhesions (five cases) or bleeding (four cases). Other reasons included poor visualization of structures (two cases), technical difficulties resulting in incomplete isolation, camera malfunction, and failure to progress (one case each). Conversion rate for robotic cases was found to decrease with increasing surgical experience.[189] Studies comparing robotic and laparoscopic adrenalectomy reported same or superior results for the robotic group in postoperative complications rate (7% vs. 11%).[197] Meta-analysis[192] performed comparing these outcomes also showed a no statistically significant difference in a higher complication rate in the laparoscopic group (6.8% vs. 3.6%, $P = .05$). There were more reported severe complications in the laparoscopic groups including grade 4 and 5 complications according to the Clavien-Dindo classification system, which has gained popularity as the preferred grading system. Reported complications in the robotic group were generally of a lesser degree of severity.[192] Postoperative morbidity and mortality have been demonstrated to be comparable to conventional laparoscopy.[189] One of the major points of criticism with robotic surgery has always been the higher cost factor. Brunaud et al.[198] found that when cost evaluation was performed using baseline cost in their hospital, robotic adrenalectomy was 2.3 times more costly than laparoscopic adrenalectomy. (4102 euro vs. 1799 euro). Total cost was found to be most affected by the total number of robotic cases per year and depreciation of the robotic system. Operative time, in contrast, was found to only play a minor role in the overall cost. This finding was also echoed by Morino et al.[189] who found a difference of $729 excluding the capital investment of the da Vinci robot. This increased expense was mainly due to the use of semidisposable robotic instruments and longer operative time. However, it is to be noted that these studies were performed in the earlier era of robotic-assisted adrenalectomy. With increasing volumes and improved outcomes associated with robotic-assisted adrenalectomy, more up to date cost analysis studies should be performed to evaluate this parameter. Arghami et al.[182] analyzed the cost associated with single-port robotic adrenalectomy and found that in their health system, as there are no specific billing codes for robotic-assisted adrenalectomy with similar reimbursement compared to the laparoscopic technique, a robotic procedure adds about $950 to the cost compared to laparoscopic adrenalectomy. However, they found that the total bill cost for single port robotic adrenalectomy was 16% lesser than laparoscopic adrenalectomy, which may be related to shorter hospital stay and an approximately 50% reduction in narcotic use. Probst et al.[199] in a recent paper, comparing costs of robotic adrenalectomy and open adrenalectomy demonstrated that the additional costs of robotic surgery were equalized if at least 150 cases of robotic procedures were performed per year based on certain healthcare cost assumptions within the healthcare system. In terms of quality-of-life assessment, no significant difference was observed for all Short Form 36 health survey scores between patients after laparoscopic or robotic adrenalectomy except for role limitations due to emotional problems. These were increased after 6 weeks in patients who underwent robotic adrenalectomy. There was also no significant difference regarding state and trait anxiety, postoperative pain, quality of sleep, and sleep duration.[190]

REFERENCES

1. Gagner M, Lacroix A, Bolté E. Laparoscopic adrenalectomy in Cushing's syndrome and pheochromocytoma. *N Engl J Med.* 1992;327(14):1033. https://doi.org/10.1056/NEJM199210013271417.
2. Gagner M. Endoscopic subtotal parathyroidectomy in patients with primary hyperparathyroidism. *Br J Surg.* 1996;83(6):875. http://www.ncbi.nlm.nih.gov/pubmed/8696772.
3. Gagner M, Inabnet WB. Endoscopic thyroidectomy for solitary thyroid nodules. *Thyroid.* 2001;11(2):161–163. https://doi.org/10.1089/105072501300042848.
4. Yeung GH. Endoscopic surgery of the neck: a new frontier. *Surg Laparosc Endosc.* 1998;8(3):227–232. http://www.ncbi.nlm.nih.gov/pubmed/9649050.
5. Ikeda Y, Takami H, Tajima G, et al. Total endoscopic thyroidectomy: axillary or anterior chest approach. *Biomed Pharmacother.* 2002;56(suppl 1):72s–78s. http://www.ncbi.nlm.nih.gov/pubmed/12487257.
6. Miccoli P, Pinchera A, Cecchini G, et al. Minimally invasive, video-assisted parathyroid surgery for primary hyperparathyroidism. *J Endocrinol Investig.* 1997;20(7):429–430. https://doi.org/10.1007/BF03347996.
7. Bellantone R, Lombardi CP, Raffaelli M, Rubino F, Boscherini M, Perilli W. Minimally invasive, totally gasless video-assisted thyroid lobectomy. *Am J Surg.* 1999;177(4):342–343. http://www.ncbi.nlm.nih.gov/pubmed/10326857.
8. Miccoli P, Berti P, Bendinelli C, Conte M, Fasolini F, Martino E. Minimally invasive video-assisted surgery of the thyroid: a preliminary report. *Langenbeck's Arch Surg.* 2000;385(4):261–264. http://www.ncbi.nlm.nih.gov/pubmed/10958509.
9. Mourad M, Saab N, Malaise J, et al. Minimally invasive video-assisted approach for partial and total thyroidectomy. *Surg Endosc.* 2001;15(10):1108–1111. https://doi.org/10.1007/s004640090018.
10. Walz MK, Peitgen K, Hoermann R, Giebler RM, Mann K, Eigler FW. Posterior retroperitoneoscopy as a new minimally invasive approach for adrenalectomy: results of 30 adrenalectomies in 27 patients. *World J Surg.* 1996;20(7):769–774. http://www.ncbi.nlm.nih.gov/pubmed/8678949.
11. Raffaelli M, Brunaud L, De Crea C, et al. Synchronous bilateral adrenalectomy for Cushing's syndrome: laparoscopic versus posterior retroperitoneoscopic versus robotic approach. *World J Surg.* 2014;38(3):709–715. https://doi.org/10.1007/s00268-013-2326-9.
12. Inabnet III WB, Jacob BP, Gagner M. Minimally invasive endoscopic thyroidectomy by a cervical approach. *Surg Endosc.* 2003;17(11):1808–1811. https://doi.org/10.1007/s00464-002-8760-7.
13. Ferzli GS, Sayad P, Abdo Z, Cacchione RN. Minimally invasive, nonendoscopic thyroid surgery. *J Am Coll Surg.* 2001;192(5):665–668. http://www.ncbi.nlm.nih.gov/pubmed/11333106.
14. Sessa L, Lombardi CP, De Crea C, Raffaelli M, Bellantone R. Video-assisted endocrine neck surgery: state of the art. *Updates Surg.* 2017;69(2):199–204. https://doi.org/10.1007/s13304-017-0467-3.
15. Duh Q-Y. Presidential Address: minimally invasive endocrine surgery–standard of treatment or hype? *Surgery.* 2003;134(6):849–857. https://doi.org/10.1016/S0039.
16. Bellantone R, Lombardi CP, Raffaelli M, Boscherini M, De Crea C, Traini E. Video-assisted thyroidectomy. *J Am Coll Surg.* 2002;194(5):610–614. http://www.ncbi.nlm.nih.gov/pubmed/12022601.
17. Miccoli P, Berti P, Raffaelli M, Conte M, Materazzi G, Galleri D. Minimally invasive video-assisted thyroidectomy. *Am J Surg.* 2001;181(6):567–570. http://www.ncbi.nlm.nih.gov/pubmed/11513788.
18. Brunt LM, Moley JF, Doherty GM, Lairmore TC, DeBenedetti MK, Quasebarth MA. Outcomes analysis in patients undergoing laparoscopic adrenalectomy for hormonally active adrenal tumors. *Surgery.* 2001;130(4):629–635. https://doi.org/10.1067/msy.2001.116920.

19. Guazzoni G, Montorsi F, Bocciardi A, et al. Transperitoneal laparoscopic versus open adrenalectomy for benign hyperfunctioning adrenal tumors: a comparative study. *J Urol.* 1995;153(5):1597–1600. http://www.ncbi.nlm.nih.gov/pubmed/7714980.

20. Kebebew E, Siperstein AE, Duh Q-Y. Laparoscopic adrenalectomy: the optimal surgical approach. *J Laparoendosc Adv Surg Tech.* 2001;11(6):409–413. https://doi.org/10.1089/10926420152761941.

21. Chavez-Rodriguez J, Pasieka JL. Adrenal lesions assessed in the era of laparoscopic adrenalectomy: a modern day series. *Am J Surg.* 2005;189(5):581–585; discussion 585-6. https://doi.org/10.1016/j.amjsurg.2005.02.003.

22. Miccoli P, Raffaelli M, Berti P, Materazzi G, Massi M, Bernini G. Adrenal surgery before and after the introduction of laparoscopic adrenalectomy. *Br J Surg.* 2002; 89(6):779–782.   https://doi.org/10.1046/j.1365-2168.2002.02110.x.

23. Saunders BD, Wainess RM, Dimick JB, Upchurch GR, Doherty GM, Gauger PG. Trends in utilization of adrenalectomy in the United States: have indications changed? *World J Surg.* 2004;28(11):1169–1175. https://doi.org/10.1007/s00268-004-7619-6.

24. Pedziwiatr M, Wierdak M, Ostachowski M, et al. Single center outcomes of laparoscopic transperitoneal lateral adrenalectomy – lessons learned after 500 cases: a retrospective cohort study. *Int J Surg.* 2015;20:88–94. https://doi.org/10.1016/j.ijsu.2015.06.020.

25. Kang T, Gridley A, Richardson WS. Long-term outcomes of laparoscopic adrenalectomy for adrenal masses. *J Laparoendosc Adv Surg Tech.* 2015;25(3):182–186. https://doi.org/10.1089/lap.2014.0430.

26. Hupe MC, Imkamp F, Merseburger AS. Minimally invasive approaches to adrenal tumors: an up-to-date summary including patient position and port placement of laparoscopic, retroperitoneoscopic, robot-assisted, and single-site adrenalectomy. *Curr Opin Urol.* 2017;27(1):56–61. https://doi.org/10.1097/MOU.0000000000000339.

27. Nomine-Criqui C, Germain A, Ayav A, Bresler L, Brunaud L. Robot-assisted adrenalectomy: indications and drawbacks. *Updates Surg.* 2017;69(2):127–133. https://doi.org/10.1007/s13304-017-0448-6.

28. Miccoli P, Berti P, Raffaelli M, Materazzi G, Baldacci S, Rossi G. Comparison between minimally invasive video-assisted thyroidectomy and conventional thyroidectomy: a prospective randomized study. *Surgery.* 2001;130(6): 1039–1043. https://doi.org/10.1067/msy2001.118264.

29. Bellantone R, Lombardi CP, Bossola M, et al. Video-assisted vs conventional thyroid lobectomy: a randomized trial. *Arch Surg.* 2002;137(3):301–304; discussion 305. http://www.ncbi.nlm.nih.gov/pubmed/11888453

30. Gal I, Solymosi T, Szabo Z, Balint A, Bolgar G. Minimally invasive video-assisted thyroidectomy and conventional thyroidectomy: a prospective randomized study. *Surg Endosc.* 2008;22(11):2445–2449.   https://doi.org/10.1007/s00464-008-9806-2.

31. El-Labban GM. Minimally invasive video-assisted thyroidectomy versus conventional thyroidectomy: a

single-blinded, randomized controlled clinical trial. *J Minimal Access Surg.* 2009;5(4):97–102. https://doi.org/10.4103/0972-9941.59307.

32. Miccoli P, Bellantone R, Mourad M, Walz M, Raffaelli M, Berti P. Minimally invasive video-assisted thyroidectomy: multiinstitutional experience. *World J Surg.* 2002;26(8):972–975. https://doi.org/10.1007/s00268-002-6627-7.

33. Del Rio P, Sommaruga L, Cataldo S, Robuschi G, Arcuri MF, Sianesi M. Minimally invasive video-assisted thyroidectomy: the learning curve. *Eur Surg Res.* 2008; 41(1):33–36. https://doi.org/10.1159/000127404.

34. Lombardi CP, Raffaelli M, Modesti C, Boscherini M, Bellantone R. Video-assisted thyroidectomy under local anesthesia. *Am J Surg.* 2004;187(4):515–518. https://doi.org/10.1016/j.amjsurg.2003.12.030.

35. Lombardi CP, Raffaelli M, Princi P, et al. Safety of video-assisted thyroidectomy versus conventional surgery. *Head Neck.*   2005;27(1):58–64.   https://doi.org/10.1002/hed.20118.

36. Bellantone R, Lombardi CP, Raffaelli M, et al. Video-assisted thyroidectomy for papillary thyroid carcinoma. *Surg Endosc.* 2003;17(10):1604–1608. https://doi.org/10.1007/s00464-002-9220-0.

37. Lombardi CP, Raffaelli M, de Crea C, et al. Report on 8 years of experience with video-assisted thyroidectomy for papillary thyroid carcinoma. *Surgery.* 2007;142(6): 944–951. https://doi.org/10.1016/j.surg.2007.09.022.

38. Miccoli P, Elisei R, Materazzi G, et al. Minimally invasive video-assisted thyroidectomy for papillary carcinoma: a prospective study of its completeness. *Surgery.* 2002; 132(6):1070–1074. https://doi.org/10.1067/msy.2002.128694.

39. Berti P, Materazzi G, Galleri D, Donatini G, Minuto M, Miccoli P. Video-assisted thyroidectomy for Graves? disease: report of a preliminary experience. *Surg Endosc.* 2004;18(8):1208–1210.   https://doi.org/10.1007/s00464-003-9225-3.

40. Dralle H, Gimm O, Simon D, et al. Prophylactic thyroidectomy in 75 children and adolescents with hereditary medullary thyroid carcinoma: German and Austrian experience. *World J Surg.* 1998;22(7):744–750; discussion 750-1. http://www.ncbi.nlm.nih.gov/pubmed/9606292.

41. Miccoli P, Berti P, Raffaelli M, Materazzi G, Conte M, Galleri D. Impact of Harmonic Scalpel on operative time during video-assisted thyroidectomy. *Surg Endosc.* 2002;16(4):663–666. https://doi.org/10.1007/s00464-001-9117-3.

42. Lombardi CP, Raffaelli M, De Crea C, D'Amore A, Bellantone R. Video-assisted thyroidectomy: lessons learned after more than one decade. *Acta Otorhinolaryngol Ital.*   2009;29(6):317–320.   http://www.ncbi.nlm.nih.gov/pubmed/20463836.

43. Miccoli P, Elisei R, Donatini G, Materazzi G, Berti P. Video-assisted central compartment lymphadenectomy in a patient with a positive RET oncogene: initial experience. *Surg Endosc.* 2007;21(1):120–123. https://doi.org/10.1007/s00464-005-0642-3.

44. Kebebew E, Clark OH. Differentiated thyroid cancer: "complete" rational approach. *World J Surg*. 2000; 24(8):942–951. http://www.ncbi.nlm.nih.gov/pubmed/10865038.

45. Haugen BR, Alexander EK, Bible KC, Doherty GM, Mandel SJ, Nikiforov YE, Pacini F, Randolph GW, Sawka AM, Schlumberger M, Schuff KG, Sherman SI, Sosa JA, Steward DL, Tuttle RM. Wartofsky. 2015 American Thyroid Association Management Guidelines for Adult Patients with Thyroid Nodules and Differentiated Thyroid Cancer: The American Thyroid Association Guidelines Task Force on Thyroid Nodules and Differentiated Thyroid Cancer. *Thyroid*. 2016;26(1):1–133. https://doi.org/10.1089/thy.2015.0020.

46. Bellantone R, Lombardi CP, Raffaelli M, Boscherini M, Alesina PF, Princi P. Central neck lymph node removal during minimally invasive video-assisted thyroidectomy for thyroid carcinoma: a feasible and safe procedure. *J Laparoendosc Adv Surg Tech*. 2002;12(3):181–185. https://doi.org/10.1089/10926420260188074.

47. Lombardi CP, Raffaelli M, De Crea C, et al. Video-assisted thyroidectomy for papillary thyroid carcinoma. *J Oncol*. 2010;2010:1–5. https://doi.org/10.1155/2010/148542.

48. Miccoli P, Pinchera A, Materazzi G, et al. Surgical treatment of low- and intermediate-risk papillary thyroid cancer with minimally invasive video-assisted thyroidectomy. *J Clin Endocrinol Metab*. 2009;94(5): 1618–1622. https://doi.org/10.1210/jc.2008-1418.

49. Wu C-T, Yang L-H, Kuo S-J. Comparison of video-assisted thyroidectomy and traditional thyroidectomy for the treatment of papillary thyroid carcinoma. *Surg Endosc*. 2010;24(7):1658–1662. https://doi.org/10.1007/s00464-009-0826-3.

50. Seybt MW, Terris DJ. Minimally invasive thyroid cancer surgery. *Minerva Chir*. 2010;65(1):39–43. http://www.ncbi.nlm.nih.gov/pubmed/20212416.

51. Neidich MJ, Steward DL. Safety and feasibility of elective minimally invasive video-assisted central neck dissection for thyroid carcinoma. *Head Neck*. 2012;34(3):354–358. https://doi.org/10.1002/hed.21733.

52. Lombardi CP, Raffaelli M, De Crea C, Sessa L, Rampulla V, Bellantone R. Video-assisted versus conventional total thyroidectomy and central compartment neck dissection for papillary thyroid carcinoma. *World J Surg*. 2012;36(6):1225–1230. https://doi.org/10.1007/s00268-012-1439-x.

53. Mulla M, Schulte K-M. Central cervical lymph node metastases in papillary thyroid cancer: a systematic review of imaging-guided and prophylactic removal of the central compartment. *Clin Endocrinol*. 2012;76(1): 131–136. https://doi.org/10.1111/j.1365-2265.2011.04162.x.

54. Lombardi CP, Raffaelli M, Princi P, De Crea C, Bellantone R. Minimally invasive video-assisted functional lateral neck dissection for metastatic papillary thyroid carcinoma. *Am J Surg*. 2007;193(1):114–118. https://doi.org/10.1016/j.amjsurg.2006.02.024.

55. Papavramidis TS, Michalopoulos N, Pliakos J, et al. Minimally invasive video-assisted total thyroidectomy: an easy to learn technique for skillful surgeons. *Head Neck*. 2010;32(10):1370–1376. https://doi.org/10.1002/hed.21336.

56. Terris DJ. Surgical approaches to the thyroid gland. *JAMA Otolaryngol Neck Surg*. 2013;139(5):515. https://doi.org/10.1001/jamaoto.2013.289.

57. Ikeda Y, Takami H, Sasaki Y, Takayama J, Niimi M, Kan S. Clinical benefits in endoscopic thyroidectomy by the axillary approach. *J Am Coll Surg*. 2003;196(2):189–195. https://doi.org/10.1016/S1072-7515(02)01665-4.

58. Jackson NR, Yao L, Tufano RP, Kandil EH. Safety of robotic thyroidectomy approaches: meta-analysis and systematic review. *Head Neck*. 2014;36(1):137–143. https://doi.org/10.1002/hed.23223.

59. Lee J, Kang SW, Jung JJ, et al. Multicenter study of robotic thyroidectomy: short-term postoperative outcomes and surgeon ergonomic considerations. *Ann Surg Oncol*. 2011;18(9):2538–2547. https://doi.org/10.1245/s10434-011-1628-0.

60. Kuppersmith RB, Holsinger FC. Robotic thyroid surgery: an initial experience with North American patients. *Laryngoscope*. 2011;121(3):521–526. https://doi.org/10.1002/lary.21347.

61. Son H, Park S, Lee CR, et al. Factors contributing to surgical outcomes of transaxillary robotic thyroidectomy for papillary thyroid carcinoma. *Surg Endosc*. 2014; 28(11):3134–3142. https://doi.org/10.1007/s00464-014-3567-x.

62. Lang BH-H, Wong CKH, Tsang JS, Wong KP, Wan KY. A systematic review and meta-analysis evaluating completeness and outcomes of robotic thyroidectomy. *Laryngoscope*. 2015;125(2):509–518. https://doi.org/10.1002/lary.24946.

63. Chung WY. Pros of robotic transaxillary thyroid surgery: its impact on cancer control and surgical quality. *Thyroid*. 2012;22(10):986–987. https://doi.org/10.1089/thy.2012.2210.com1.

64. Lin H-S, Folbe AJ, Carron MA, et al. Single-incision transaxillary robotic thyroidectomy: challenges and limitations in a North American population. *Otolaryngol Head Neck Surg*. 2012;147(6):1041–1046. https://doi.org/10.1177/0194599812461610.

65. Perrier ND, Randolph GW, Inabnet WB, Marple BF, vanHeerden J, Kuppersmith RB. Robotic thyroidectomy: a framework for new technology assessment and safe implementation. *Thyroid*. 2010;20(12):1327–1332. https://doi.org/10.1089/thy.2010.1666.

66. Lee Y-M, Yi O, Sung T-Y, Chung K-W, Yoon JH, Hong SJ. Surgical outcomes of robotic thyroid surgery using a double incision gasless transaxillary approach: analysis of 400 cases treated by the same surgeon. *Head Neck*. 2013; 36(10). https://doi.org/10.1002/hed.23472. n/a-n/a.

67. Rabinovics N, Aidan P. Robotic transaxillary thyroid surgery. *Gland Surg*. 2015;4(5):397–402. https://doi.org/10.3978/j.issn.2227-684X.2015.04.08.

68. Holsinger FC, Chung WY. Robotic thyroidectomy. *Otolaryngol Clin.* 2014;47(3):373–378. https://doi.org/10.1016/j.otc.2014.03.001.

69. Sun GH, Peress L, Pynnonen MA. Systematic review and meta-analysis of robotic vs conventional thyroidectomy approaches for thyroid disease. *Otolaryngol Neck Surg.* 2014;150(4):520–532. https://doi.org/10.1177/0194599814521779.

70. Kandil E. Transaxillary gasless robotic Thyroidectomy A single surgeon's experience in North America. *Arch Otolaryngol Neck Surg.* 2012;138(2):113. https://doi.org/10.1001/archoto.2011.1082.

71. Kandil EH, Noureldine SI, Yao L, Slakey DP. Robotic transaxillary thyroidectomy: an examination of the first one hundred cases. *J Am Coll Surg.* 2012;214(4):558–564. https://doi.org/10.1016/j.jamcollsurg.2012.01.002.

72. Lee J, Yun JH, Nam KH, Choi UJ, Chung WY, Soh E-Y. Perioperative clinical outcomes after robotic thyroidectomy for thyroid carcinoma: a multicenter study. *Surg Endosc.* 2011;25(3):906–912. https://doi.org/10.1007/s00464-010-1296-3.

73. Noureldine SI, Jackson NR, Tufano RP, Kandil E. A comparative North American experience of robotic thyroidectomy in a thyroid cancer population. *Langenbeck's Arch Surg.* 2013;398(8):1069–1074. https://doi.org/10.1007/s00423-013-1123-0.

74. Ban EJ, Yoo JY, Kim WW, et al. Surgical complications after robotic thyroidectomy for thyroid carcinoma: a single center experience with 3,000 patients. *Surg Endosc.* 2014;28(9):2555–2563. https://doi.org/10.1007/s00464-014-3502-1.

75. Tae K, Song CM, Ji YB, Kim KR, Kim JY, Choi YY. Comparison of surgical completeness between robotic total thyroidectomy versus open thyroidectomy. *Laryngoscope.* 2014;124(4):1042–1047. https://doi.org/10.1002/lary.24511.

76. Yi O, Yoon JH, Lee Y-M, et al. Technical and oncologic safety of robotic thyroid surgery. *Ann Surg Oncol.* 2013;20(6):1927–1933. https://doi.org/10.1245/s10434-012-2850-0.

77. Lee S, Lee CR, Lee SC, et al. Surgical completeness of robotic thyroidectomy: a prospective comparison with conventional open thyroidectomy in papillary thyroid carcinoma patients. *Surg Endosc.* 2014;28(4):1068–1075. https://doi.org/10.1007/s00464-013-3303-y.

78. Lee J, Kwon IS, Bae EH, Chung WY. Comparative analysis of oncological outcomes and quality of life after robotic versus conventional open thyroidectomy with modified radical neck dissection in patients with papillary thyroid carcinoma and lateral neck node metastases. *J Clin Endocrinol Metab.* 2013;98(7):2701–2708. https://doi.org/10.1210/jc.2013-1583.

79. Kang S-W, Lee SC, Lee SH, et al. Robotic thyroid surgery using a gasless, transaxillary approach and the da Vinci S system: the operative outcomes of 338 consecutive patients. *Surgery.* 2009;146(6):1048–1055. https://doi.org/10.1016/j.surg.2009.09.007.

80. Landry CS, Grubbs EG, Warneke CL, et al. Robot-assisted transaxillary thyroid surgery in the United States: is it comparable to open thyroid lobectomy? *Ann Surg Oncol.* 2012;19(4):1269–1274. https://doi.org/10.1245/s10434-011-2075-7.

81. Perrier ND. Why I have abandoned robot-assisted transaxillary thyroid surgery. *Surgery.* 2012;152(6):1025–1026. https://doi.org/10.1016/j.surg.2012.08.060.

82. Dionigi G, Lavazza M, Wu C-W, et al. Transoral thyroidectomy: why is it needed? *Gland Surg.* 2017;6(3):272–276. https://doi.org/10.21037/gs.2017.03.21.

83. Dionigi G. Robotic thyroidectomy. *Otolaryngol Neck Surg.* 2013;148(1). https://doi.org/10.1177/0194599812469790, 178-178.

84. Terris DJ, Singer MC, Seybt MW. Robotic facelift thyroidectomy: II. Clinical feasibility and safety. *Laryngoscope.* 2011;121(8):1636–1641. https://doi.org/10.1002/lary.21832.

85. Terris DJ, Singer MC. Qualitative and quantitative differences between 2 robotic thyroidectomy techniques. *Otolaryngol Neck Surg.* 2012;147(1):20–25. https://doi.org/10.1177/0194599812439283.

86. Singer MC, Seybt MW, Terris DJ. Robotic facelift thyroidectomy: I. Preclinical simulation and morphometric assessment. *Laryngoscope.* 2011;121(8):1631–1635. https://doi.org/10.1002/lary.21831.

87. Terris DJ, Singer MC, Seybt MW. Robotic facelift thyroidectomy. *Surg Laparosc Endosc Percutaneous Tech.* 2011;21(4):237–242. https://doi.org/10.1097/SLE.0b013e3182266dd6.

88. Byeon HK, Holsinger FC, Tufano RP, et al. Robotic total thyroidectomy with modified radical neck dissection via unilateral retroauricular approach. *Ann Surg Oncol.* 2014;21(12):3872–3875. https://doi.org/10.1245/s10434-014-3896-y.

89. Bomeli SR, Duke WS, Terris DJ. Robotic facelift thyroid surgery. *Gland Surg.* 2015;4(5):403–409. https://doi.org/10.3978/j.issn.2227-684X.2015.02.07.

90. Witzel K, von Rahden BHA, Kaminski C, Stein HJ. Transoral access for endoscopic thyroid resection. *Surg Endosc.* 2008;22(8):1871–1875. https://doi.org/10.1007/s00464-007-9734-6.

91. Benhidjeb T, Wilhelm T, Harlaar J, Kleinrensink G-J, Schneider TAJ, Stark M. Natural orifice surgery on thyroid gland: totally transoral video-assisted thyroidectomy (TOVAT): report of first experimental results of a new surgical method. *Surg Endosc.* 2009;23(5):1119–1120. https://doi.org/10.1007/s00464-009-0347-0.

92. Wilhelm T, Metzig A. Endoscopic minimally invasive thyroidectomy: first clinical experience. *Surg Endosc.* 2010;24(7):1757–1758. https://doi.org/10.1007/s00464-009-0820-9.

93. Wilhelm T, Metzig A. Endoscopic minimally invasive thyroidectomy (eMIT): a prospective proof-of-concept study in humans. *World J Surg.* 2011;35(3):543–551. https://doi.org/10.1007/s00268-010-0846-0.

94. Anuwong A. Transoral endoscopic thyroidectomy vestibular approach: a series of the first 60 human cases. *World J Surg.* 2016;40(3):491–497. https://doi.org/10.1007/s00268-015-3320-1.

95. Liu E, Qadir Khan A, Niu J, Xu Z, Peng C. Natural orifice total transtracheal endoscopic thyroidectomy surgery: first reported experiment. *J Laparoendosc Adv Surg Tech*. 2015; 25(7):586–591. https://doi.org/10.1089/lap.2014.0452.

96. Woo SH. Endoscope-assisted transoral thyroidectomy using a frenotomy incision. *J Laparoendosc Adv Surg Tech*. 2014;24(5):345–349. https://doi.org/10.1089/lap.2014.0110.

97. Benhidjeb T, Stark M. Endoscopic minimally invasive thyroidectomy (eMIT): safety first!. *World J Surg*. 2011; 35(8):1936–1937. https://doi.org/10.1007/s00268-011-1077-8.

98. Clark JH, Kim HY, Richmon JD. Transoral robotic thyroid surgery. *Gland Surg*. 2015;4(5):429–434. https://doi.org/10.3978/j.issn.2227-684X.2015.02.02.

99. Lee HY, Richmon JD, Walvekar RR, Holsinger C, Kim HY. Robotic transoral periosteal thyroidectomy (TOPOT): experience in two cadavers. *J Laparoendosc Adv Surg Tech*. 2015;25(2):139–142. https://doi.org/10.1089/lap.2014.0543.

100. Lee HY, You JY, Woo SU, et al. Transoral periosteal thyroidectomy: cadaver to human. *Surg Endosc*. 2015; 29(4):898–904. https://doi.org/10.1007/s00464-014-3749-6.

101. Inabnet WB, Suh H, Fernandez-Ranvier G. Transoral endoscopic thyroidectomy vestibular approach with intraoperative nerve monitoring. *Surg Endosc*. 2017; 31(7). https://doi.org/10.1007/s00464-016-5322-y, 3030-3030.

102. Park J-O, Kim M-R, Kim DH, Lee DK. Transoral endoscopic thyroidectomy via the trivestibular route. *Ann Surg Treat Res*. 2016;91(5):269–272. https://doi.org/10.4174/astr.2016.91.5.269.

103. Witzel K, Hellinger A, Kaminski C, Benhidjeb T. Endoscopic thyroidectomy: the transoral approach. *Gland Surg*. 2016;5(3):336–341. https://doi.org/10.21037/gs.2015.08.04.

104. Udelsman R, Anuwong A, Oprea AD, et al. Trans-oral vestibular endocrine surgery: a new technique in the United States. *Ann Surg*. 2016;264(6):e13–e16. https://doi.org/10.1097/SLA.0000000000002001.

105. Mazzeo S, Caramella D, Lencioni R, et al. Comparison among sonography, double-tracer subtraction scintigraphy, and double-phase scintigraphy in the detection of parathyroid lesions. *AJR Am J Roentgenol*. 1996; 166(6):1465–1470. https://doi.org/10.2214/ajr.166.6.8633466.

106. Palazzo FF, Delbridge LW. Minimal-access/minimally invasive parathyroidectomy for primary hyperparathyroidism. *Surg Clin*. 2004;84(3):717–734. https://doi.org/10.1016/j.suc.2004.01.002.

107. Mourad M, Ngongang C, Saab N, et al. Video-assisted neck exploration for primary and secondary hyperparathyroidism. *Surg Endosc*. 2001; 15(10):1112–1115. https://doi.org/10.1007/s004640090017.

108. Hallfeldt KKJ, Trupka A, Gallwas J, Horn K. Minimally invasive video-assisted parathyroidectomy. *Surg Endosc*. 2001;15(4):409–412. https://doi.org/10.1007/s004640090042.

109. Barczyński M, Cichoń S, Konturek A, Cichoń W. Minimally invasive video-assisted parathyroidectomy versus open minimally invasive parathyroidectomy for a solitary parathyroid adenoma: a prospective, randomized, blinded trial. *World J Surg*. 2006;30(5):721–731. https://doi.org/10.1007/s00268-005-0312-6.

110. Miccoli P, Bendinelli C, Berti P, Vignali E, Pinchera A, Marcocci C. Video-assisted versus conventional parathyroidectomy in primary hyperparathyroidism: a prospective randomized study. *Surgery*. 1999;126(6): 1117–1121; discussion 1121-2. http://www.ncbi.nlm.nih.gov/pubmed/10598196.

111. Lombardi CP, Raffaelli M, Traini E, De Crea C, Corsello SM, Bellantone R. Video-assisted minimally invasive parathyroidectomy: benefits and long-term results. *World J Surg*. 2009;33(11):2266–2281. https://doi.org/10.1007/s00268-009-9931-7.

112. De Crea C, Raffaelli M, Traini E, et al. Is there a role for video-assisted parathyroidectomy in regions with high prevalence of goitre? *Acta Otorhinolaryngol Ital*. 2013; 33(6):388–392. http://www.ncbi.nlm.nih.gov/pubmed/24376294.

113. Lombardi CP, Raffaelli M, Traini E, et al. Advantages of a video-assisted approach to parathyroidectomy. *ORL J Otorhinolaryngol Relat Spec*. 2008;70(5):313–318. https://doi.org/10.1159/000149833.

114. Miccoli P, Minuto MN, Cetani F, Ambrosini CE, Berti P. Familial parathyroid hyperplasia: is there a place for minimally invasive surgery? description of the first treated case. *J Endocrinol Investig*. 2005;28(10):942–943. http://www.ncbi.nlm.nih.gov/pubmed/16419499.

115. Miccoli P, Berti P, Materazzi G, Massi M, Picone A, Minuto MN. Results of video-assisted parathyroidectomy: single Institution?s six-year experience. *World J Surg*. 2004;28(12):1216–1218. https://doi.org/10.1007/s00268-004-7638-3.

116. Henry J-F, Sebag F, Cherenko M, Ippolito G, Taieb D, Vaillant J. Endoscopic parathyroidectomy: why and when? *World J Surg*. 2008;32(11):2509–2515. https://doi.org/10.1007/s00268-008-9709-3.

117. Bellantone R, Raffaelli M, DE Crea C, Traini E, Lombardi CP. Minimally-invasive parathyroid surgery. *Acta Otorhinolaryngol Ital*. 2011;31(4):207–215. http://www.ncbi.nlm.nih.gov/pubmed/22065831.

118. Brunaud L, Li Z, Van Den Heede K, Cuny T, Van Slycke S. Endoscopic and robotic parathyroidectomy in patients with primary hyperparathyroidism. *Gland Surg*. 2016; 5(3):352–360. https://doi.org/10.21037/gs.2016.01.06.

119. Cougard P, Goudet P, Bilosi M, Peschaud F. Videoendoscopic approach for parathyroid adenomas: results of a prospective study of 100 patients. *Ann Chir*. 2001; 126(4):314–319. http://www.ncbi.nlm.nih.gov/pubmed/11413810.

120. Henry J-F, Thakur A. Minimal access surgery — thyroid and parathyroid. *Indian J Surg Oncol*. 2010;1(2): 200–206. https://doi.org/10.1007/s13193-010-0033-7.

121. Henry JF, Defechereux T, Gramatica L, De Boissezon C. Endoscopic parathyroidectomy via a lateral neck incision. *Ann Chir.* 1999;53(4):302−306. http://www.ncbi.nlm.nih.gov/pubmed/10327694.

122. Fouquet T, Germain A, Zarnegar R, et al. Totally endoscopic lateral parathyroidectomy: prospective evaluation of 200 patients. *Langenbeck's Arch Surg.* 2010;395(7):935−940. https://doi.org/10.1007/s00423-010-0687-1.

123. Gaborit B, Aron-Wisnewsky J, Salem J-E, Bege T, Frere C. Pharmacologic venous thromboprophylaxis After bariatric surgery. *Ann Surg.* 2017;XX(Xx):1. https://doi.org/10.1097/SLA.0000000000002536.

124. Ikeda Y, Takami H, Niimi M, Kan S, Sasaki Y, Takayama J. Endoscopic total parathyroidectomy by the anterior chest approach for renal hyperparathyroidism. *Surg Endosc Other Interv Tech.* 2002;16(2):320−322. https://doi.org/10.1007/s00464-001-8131-9.

125. Maweja S, Sebag F, Hubbard J, Giorgi R, Henry JF. Immediate and medium-term results of intraoperative parathyroid hormone monitoring during video-assisted parathyroidectomy. *Arch Surg.* 2004;139(12):1301−1303. https://doi.org/10.1001/archsurg.139.12.1301.

126. Ohgami M, Ishii S, Arisawa Y, et al. Scarless endoscopic thyroidectomy: breast approach for better cosmesis. *Surg Laparosc Endosc Percutaneous Tech.* 2000;10(1):1−4. http://www.ncbi.nlm.nih.gov/pubmed/10872517.

127. Myers EN, Kitano H, Fujimura M, et al. Endoscopic surgery for a parathyroid functioning adenoma resection with the neck region-lifting method. *Otolaryngol Neck Surg.* 2000;123(4):465−466. https://doi.org/10.1067/mhn.2000.105183.

128. Okoh AK, Berber E. Laparoscopic and robotic adrenal surgery: transperitoneal approach. *Gland Surg.* 2015;4(5):435−441. https://doi.org/10.3978/j.issn.2227-684X.2015.05.03.

129. Garas G, Holsinger FC, Grant DG, Athanasiou T, Arora A, Tolley N. Is robotic parathyroidectomy a feasible and safe alternative to targeted open parathyroidectomy for the treatment of primary hyperparathyroidism? *Int J Surg.* 2015;15:55−60. https://doi.org/10.1016/j.ijsu.2015.01.019.

130. Tolley N, Arora A, Palazzo F, et al. Robotic-assisted parathyroidectomy. *Otolaryngol Neck Surg.* 2011;144(6):859−866. https://doi.org/10.1177/0194599811402152.

131. Tolley N, Garas G, Palazzo F, et al. Long-term prospective evaluation comparing robotic parathyroidectomy with minimally invasive open parathyroidectomy for primary hyperparathyroidism. *Head Neck.* 2016;38(S1):E300−E306. https://doi.org/10.1002/hed.23990.

132. Landry CS, Grubbs EG, Stephen Morris G, et al. Robot assisted transaxillary surgery (RATS) for the removal of thyroid and parathyroid glands. *Surgery.* 2011;149(4):549−555. https://doi.org/10.1016/j.surg.2010.08.014.

133. Foley CS, Agcaoglu O, Siperstein AE, Berber E. Robotic transaxillary endocrine surgery: a comparison with conventional open technique. *Surg Endosc.* 2012;26(8):2259−2266. https://doi.org/10.1007/s00464-012-2169-8.

134. Noureldine SI, Lewing N, Tufano RP, Kandil E. The role of the robotic-assisted transaxillary gasless approach for the removal of parathyroid adenomas. *ORL J Otorhinolaryngol Relat Spec.* 2014;76(1):19−24. https://doi.org/10.1159/000353629.

135. Karagkounis G, Uzun DD, Mason DP, Murthy SC, Berber E. Robotic surgery for primary hyperparathyroidism. *Surg Endosc.* 2014;28(9):2702−2707. https://doi.org/10.1007/s00464-014-3531-9.

136. Smith CD, Weber CJ, Amerson JR. Laparoscopic adrenalectomy: new gold standard. *World J Surg.* 1999;23(4):389−396. http://www.ncbi.nlm.nih.gov/pubmed/10030863.

137. Henry JF. Minimally invasive adrenal surgery. *Best Pract Res Clin Endocrinol Metabol.* 2001;15(2):149−160. https://doi.org/10.1053/beem.2001.0132.

138. Gumbs AA, Gagner M. Laparoscopic adrenalectomy. *Best Pract Res Clin Endocrinol Metabol.* 2006;20(3):483−499. https://doi.org/10.1016/j.beem.2006.07.010.

139. Gagner M, Lacroix A, Bolte E, Pomp A. Laparoscopic adrenalectomy. The importance of a flank approach in the lateral decubitus position. *Surg Endosc.* 1994;8(2):135−138. http://www.ncbi.nlm.nih.gov/pubmed/8165486.

140. Prinz RA. A comparison of laparoscopic and open adrenalectomies. *Arch Surg.* 1995;130(5):489−492; discussion 492-4. http://www.ncbi.nlm.nih.gov/pubmed/7748086.

141. Brunt LM, Doherty GM, Norton JA, Soper NJ, Quasebarth MA, Moley JF. Laparoscopic adrenalectomy compared to open adrenalectomy for benign adrenal neoplasms. *J Am Coll Surg.* 1996;183(1):1−10. http://www.ncbi.nlm.nih.gov/pubmed/8673301.

142. Thompson GB, Grant CS, van Heerden JA, et al. Laparoscopic versus open posterior adrenalectomy: a case-control study of 100 patients. *Surgery.* 1997;122(6):1132−1136. http://www.ncbi.nlm.nih.gov/pubmed/9426429.

143. Dudley NE, Harrison BJ. Comparison of open posterior versus transperitoneal laparoscopic adrenalectomy. *Br J Surg.* 1999;86(5):656−660. https://doi.org/10.1046/j.1365-2168.1999.01110.x.

144. Imai T, Kikumori T, Ohiwa M, Mase T, Funahashi H. A case-controlled study of laparoscopic compared with open lateral adrenalectomy. *Am J Surg.* 1999;178(1):50−53; discussion 54. http://www.ncbi.nlm.nih.gov/pubmed/10456703.

145. Hallfeldt KKJ, Mussack T, Trupka A, Hohenbleicher F, Schmidbauer S. Laparoscopic lateral adrenalectomy versus open posterior adrenalectomy for the treatment of benign adrenal tumors. *Surg Endosc.* 2003;17(2):264−267. https://doi.org/10.1007/s00464-002-8810-1.

146. Assalia A, Gagner M. Laparoscopic adrenalectomy. *Br J Surg.* 2004;91(10):1259−1274. https://doi.org/10.1002/bjs.4738.

147. Prinz RA. Mobilization of the right lobe of the liver for right adrenalectomy. *Am J Surg.* 1990;159(3):336—338. http://www.ncbi.nlm.nih.gov/pubmed/2305943.

148. Marescaux J, Mutter D, Wheeler MH. Laparoscopic right and left adrenalectomies. Surgical procedures. *Surg Endosc.* 1996;10(9):912—915. http://www.ncbi.nlm.nih.gov/pubmed/8703150.

149. Naya Y, Nagata M, Ichikawa T, et al. Laparoscopic adrenalectomy: comparison of transperitoneal and retroperitoneal approaches. *BJU Int.* 2002;90(3):199—204. http://www.ncbi.nlm.nih.gov/pubmed/12133053.

150. Suzuki K, Kageyama S, Hirano Y, Ushiyama T, Rajamahanty S, Fujita K. Comparison of 3 surgical approaches to laparoscopic adrenalectomy: a nonrandomized, background matched analysis. *J Urol.* 2001;166(2):437—443. http://www.ncbi.nlm.nih.gov/pubmed/11458043.

151. MacGillivray DC, Whalen GF, Malchoff CD, Oppenheim DS, Shichman SJ. Laparoscopic resection of large adrenal tumors. *Ann Surg Oncol.* 2002;9(5):480—485. http://www.ncbi.nlm.nih.gov/pubmed/12052760.

152. Economopoulos KP, Mylonas KS, Stamou AA, et al. Laparoscopic versus robotic adrenalectomy: a comprehensive meta-analysis. *Int J Surg.* 2017;38:95—104. https://doi.org/10.1016/j.ijsu.2016.12.118.

153. Fernández-Cruz L, Saenz A, Benarroch G, Astudillo E, Taura P, Sabater L. Laparoscopic unilateral and bilateral adrenalectomy for Cushing's syndrome. Transperitoneal and retroperitoneal approaches. *Ann Surg.* 1996;224(6): 727—734; discussion 734-6. http://www.ncbi.nlm.nih.gov/pubmed/8968227.

154. Duh QY, Siperstein AE, Clark OH, et al. Laparoscopic adrenalectomy. Comparison of the lateral and posterior approaches. *Arch Surg.* 1996;131(8):870—875; discussion 875-6. http://www.ncbi.nlm.nih.gov/pubmed/8712912.

155. Terachi T, Yoshida O, Matsuda T, et al. Complications of laparoscopic and retroperitoneoscopic adrenalectomies in 370 cases in Japan: a multi-institutional study. *Biomed Pharmacother.* 2000;54(suppl 1):211s—214s. http://www.ncbi.nlm.nih.gov/pubmed/10915027.

156. Lezoche E, Guerrieri M, Feliciotti F, et al. Anterior, lateral, and posterior retroperitoneal approaches in endoscopic adrenalectomy. *Surg Endosc.* 2002;16(1):96—99. https://doi.org/10.1007/s004640090043.

157. Yagisawa T, Ito F, Ishikawa N, et al. Retroperitoneoscopic adrenalectomy: lateral versus posterior approach. *J Endourol.* 2004;18(7):661—664. https://doi.org/10.1089/end.2004.18.661.

158. Farres H, Felsher J, Brodsky J, Siperstein A, Gill I, Brody F. Laparoscopic adrenalectomy: a cost analysis of three approaches. *J Laparoendosc Adv Surg Tech.* 2004;14(1): 23—26. https://doi.org/10.1089/109264204322862315.

159. Gockel I, Kneist W, Heintz A, Beyer J, Junginger T. Endoscopic adrenalectomy: an analysis of the transperitoneal and retroperitoneal approaches and results of a prospective follow-up study. *Surg Endosc.* 2005;19(4):569—573. https://doi.org/10.1007/s00464-004-9085-5.

160. Rubinstein M, Gill IS, Aron M, et al. Prospective, randomized comparison of transperitoneal versus retroperitoneal laparoscopic adrenalectomy. *J Urol.* 2005;174(2):442—445. https://doi.org/10.1097/01.ju.0000165336.44836.2d; discussion 445.

161. Mercan S, Seven R, Ozarmagan S, Tezelman S. Endoscopic retroperitoneal adrenalectomy. *Surgery.* 1995; 118(6):1071—1075; discussion 1075-6. http://www.ncbi.nlm.nih.gov/pubmed/7491525.

162. Walz MK, Alesina PF, Wenger FA, et al. Posterior retroperitoneoscopic adrenalectomy—results of 560 procedures in 520 patients. *Surgery.* 2006;140(6):943—950. https://doi.org/10.1016/j.surg.2006.07.039.

163. Lombardi CP, Raffaelli M, De Crea C, et al. Endoscopic adrenalectomy: is there an optimal operative approach? Results of a single-center case-control study. *Surgery.* 2008;144(6):1008—1015. https://doi.org/10.1016/j.surg.2008.08.025.

164. De Crea C, Raffaelli M, D'Amato G, et al. Retroperitoneoscopic adrenalectomy: tips and tricks. *Updates Surg.* 2017; 69(2):267—270. https://doi.org/10.1007/s13304-017-0469-1.

165. Walz MK, Petersenn S, Koch JA, Mann K, Neumann HPH, Schmid KW. Endoscopic treatment of large primary adrenal tumours. *Br J Surg.* 2005;92(6):719—723. https://doi.org/10.1002/bjs.4964.

166. Perrier ND, Kennamer DL, Bao R, et al. Posterior retroperitoneoscopic adrenalectomy. *Trans Meet Am Surg Assoc.* 2008;126(4):309—317. https://doi.org/10.1097/SLA.0b013e31818a1d2a.

167. Lombardi CP, Raffaelli M, de Crea C, et al. ACTH-dependent Cushing syndrome: the potential benefits of simultaneous bilateral posterior retroperitoneoscopic adrenalectomy. *Surgery.* 2011;149(2):299—300. https://doi.org/10.1016/j.surg.2010.06.005.

168. Barczyński M, Konturek A, Gołkowski F, et al. Posterior retroperitoneoscopic adrenalectomy: a comparison between the initial experience in the invention phase and introductory phase of the new surgical technique. *World J Surg.* 2007;31(1):65—71. https://doi.org/10.1007/s00268-006-0083-8.

169. Piazza L, Caragliano P, Scardilli M, Sgroi AV, Marino G, Giannone G. Laparoscopic robot-assisted right adrenalectomy and left ovariectomy (case reports). *Chir Ital.* 1999; 51(6):465—466. http://www.ncbi.nlm.nih.gov/pubmed/10742897.

170. Hubens G, Ysebaert D, Vaneerdeweg W, Chapelle T, Eyskens E. Laparoscopic adrenalectomy with the aid of the AESOP 2000 robot. *Acta Chir Belg.* 1999;99(3): 125—127; discussion 127-9. http://www.ncbi.nlm.nih.gov/pubmed/10427347.

171. Teo XL, Lim SK. *Robotic Assisted Adrenalectomy: Is it Ready for Prime Time?.* 2016 https://doi.org/10.4111/icu.2016.57.S2.S130.

172. Agcaoglu O, Aliyev S, Karabulut K, Siperstein A, Berber E. Robotic vs laparoscopic posterior retroperitoneal adrenalectomy. *Arch Surg.* 2012;147(3):272. https://doi.org/10.1001/archsurg.2011.2040.

173. Giulianotti PC, Buchs NC, Addeo P, et al. Robot-assisted adrenalectomy: a technical option for the surgeon? *Int J Med Robot.* 2011;7(1):27—32. https://doi.org/10.1002/rcs.364.

174. Aksoy E, Taskin HE, Aliyev S, Mitchell J, Siperstein A, Berber E. Robotic versus laparoscopic adrenalectomy in obese patients. *Surg Endosc*. 2013;27(4):1233–1236. https://doi.org/10.1007/s00464-012-2580-1.

175. Ludwig AT, Wagner KR, Lowry PS, Papaconstantinou HT, Lairmore TC. Robot-assisted posterior retroperitoneoscopic adrenalectomy. *J Endourol*. 2010;24(8): 1307–1314. https://doi.org/10.1089/end.2010.0152.

176. Karabulut K, Agcaoglu O, Aliyev S, Siperstein A, Berber E. Comparison of intraoperative time use and perioperative outcomes for robotic versus laparoscopic adrenalectomy. *Surgery*. 2012;151(4):537–542. https://doi.org/10.1016/j.surg.2011.09.047.

177. Berber E, Mitchell J, Milas M, Siperstein A. Robotic posterior retroperitoneal adrenalectomy. *Arch Surg*. 2010; 145(8):781. https://doi.org/10.1001/archsurg.2010.148.

178. Park JH, Walz MK, Kang S-W, et al. Robot-assisted posterior retroperitoneoscopic adrenalectomy: single port access. *J Korean Surg Soc*. 2011;81(suppl 1):S21. https://doi.org/10.4174/jkss.2011.81.Suppl1.S21.

179. Park JH, Kim SY, Lee C-R, et al. Robot-assisted posterior retroperitoneoscopic adrenalectomy using single-port access: technical feasibility and preliminary results. *Ann Surg Oncol*. 2013;20(8):2741–2745. https://doi.org/10.1245/s10434-013-2891-z.

180. Nozaki T, Ichimatsu K, Watanabe A, Komiya A, Fuse H. Longitudinal incision of the umbilicus for laparoendoscopic single site adrenalectomy: a particular intraumbilical technique. *Surg Laparosc Endosc Percutaneous Tech*. 2010;20(6):e185–e188. https://doi.org/10.1097/SLE.0b013e3181f70a2a.

181. Lee GS, Arghami A, Dy BM, McKenzie TJ, Thompson GB, Richards ML. Robotic single-site adrenalectomy. *Surg Endosc*. 2016;30(8):3351–3356. https://doi.org/10.1007/s00464-015-4611-1.

182. Arghami A, Dy BM, Bingener J, Osborn J, Richards ML. Single-port robotic-assisted adrenalectomy: feasibility, safety, and cost-effectiveness. *JSLS J Soc Laparoendosc Surg*. 2015;19(1):e2014. https://doi.org/10.4293/JSLS.2014.00218, 00218.

183. Mohammadi-Fallah MR, Mehdizadeh A, Badalzadeh A, et al. Comparison of transperitoneal versus retroperitoneal laparoscopic adrenalectomy in a prospective randomized study. *J Laparoendosc Adv Surg Tech*. 2013; 23(4):362–366. https://doi.org/10.1089/lap.2012.0301.

184. Bonjer HJ, Hazebroek EJ, Kazemier G, Giuffrida MC, Meijer WS, Lange JF. Open versus closed establishment of pneumoperitoneum in laparoscopic surgery. *Br J Surg*. 1997;84(5):599–602. http://www.ncbi.nlm.nih.gov/pubmed/9171741.

185. Chen W, Li F, Chen D, et al. Retroperitoneal versus transperitoneal laparoscopic adrenalectomy in adrenal tumor. *Surg Laparosc Endosc Percutaneous Tech*. 2013;23(2):121–127. https://doi.org/10.1097/SLE.0b013e3182827b57.

186. Walz MK, Peitgen K, Walz MV, et al. Posterior retroperitoneoscopic adrenalectomy: lessons learned within five years. *World J Surg*. 2001;25(6):728–734. http://www.ncbi.nlm.nih.gov/pubmed/11376407.

187. Berber E, Tellioglu G, Harvey A, Mitchell J, Milas M, Siperstein A. Comparison of laparoscopic transabdominal lateral versus posterior retroperitoneal adrenalectomy. *Surgery*. 2009;146(4):621–626. https://doi.org/10.1016/j.surg.2009.06.057.

188. Agcaoglu O. Robotic vs laparoscopic posterior retroperitoneal adrenalectomy. *Arch Surg*. 2012;147(3):272. https://doi.org/10.1001/archsurg.2011.2040.

189. Morino M, Benincà G, Giraudo G, Del Genio GM, Rebecchi F, Garrone C. Robot-assisted vs laparoscopic adrenalectomy: a prospective randomized controlled trial. *Surg Endosc*. 2004;18(12):1742–1746. https://doi.org/10.1007/s00464-004-9046-z.

190. Brunaud L, Ayav A, Zarnegar R, et al. Prospective evaluation of 100 robotic-assisted unilateral adrenalectomies. *Surgery*. 2008;144(6):995–1001. https://doi.org/10.1016/j.surg.2008.08.032.

191. Akarsu C, Dural AC, Kankaya B, et al. The early results of our initial experience with robotic adrenalectomy. *Ulus cerrahi Derg*. 2014;30(1):28–33. https://doi.org/10.5152/UCD.2014.2518.

192. Brandao LF, Autorino R, Laydner H, et al. Robotic versus laparoscopic adrenalectomy: a systematic review and meta-analysis. *Eur Urol*. 2014;65(6):1154–1161. https://doi.org/10.1016/j.eururo.2013.09.021.

193. Agcaoglu O, Aliyev S, Karabulut K, Mitchell J, Siperstein A, Berber E. Robotic versus laparoscopic resection of large adrenal tumors. *Ann Surg Oncol*. 2012;19(7):2288–2294. https://doi.org/10.1245/s10434-012-2296-4.

194. Pineda-Solís K, Medina-Franco H, Heslin MJ. Robotic versus laparoscopic adrenalectomy: a comparative study in a high-volume center. *Surg Endosc*. 2013; 27(2):599–602. https://doi.org/10.1007/s00464-012-2496-9.

195. Wu JC-H, Wu H-S, Lin M-S, Chou D-A, Huang M-H. Comparison of robot-assisted laparoscopic adrenalectomy with traditional laparoscopic adrenalectomy — 1 year follow-up. *Surg Endosc*. 2008;22(2):463–466. https://doi.org/10.1007/s00464-007-9488-1.

196. You JY, Lee HY, Son GS, Lee JB, Bae JW, Kim HY. Comparison of robotic adrenalectomy with traditional laparoscopic adrenalectomy with a lateral transperitoneal approach: a single-surgeon experience. *Int J Med Robot*. 2013;9(3):345–350. https://doi.org/10.1002/rcs.1497.

197. Winter JM, Talamini MA, Stanfield CL, et al. Thirty robotic adrenalectomies. *Surg Endosc*. 2006;20(1): 119–124. https://doi.org/10.1007/s00464-005-0082-0.

198. Brunaud L, Bresler L, Ayav A, et al. Robotic-assisted adrenalectomy: what advantages compared to lateral transperitoneal laparoscopic adrenalectomy? *Am J Surg*. 2008;195(4):433–438. https://doi.org/10.1016/j.amjsurg.2007.04.016.

199. Probst KA, Ohlmann C-H, Saar M, Siemer S, Stöeckle M, Janssen M. Robot-assisted vs open adrenalectomy: evaluation of cost-effectiveness and peri-operative outcome. *BJU Int*. 2016;118(6):952–957. https://doi.org/10.1111/bju.13529.

CHAPTER 24

Advances in Transoral Endoscopic Thyroidectomy Vestibular Approach (TOETVA)

GUSTAVO G. FERNANDEZ RANVIER, MD, PHD • ARYAN MEKNAT, MD

INTRODUCTION

The earliest account of thyroid surgery dates back to the 12th century, but thyroid surgery was extremely dangerous with mortality rates greater than 40% until the latter half of the 1800's. This preceded progress in both general anesthesia and antisepsis, as well as advances in hemostasis and the surgical approaches to the thyroid gland. Traditional thyroid surgery is done via an open approach, with a cervical collar incision to expose the gland. In experienced hands, dissection with the open technique is very safe with low morbidity and mortality rates.[1] However, the inevitable result of using this technique is that some, if not most, patients are left with a cosmetically displeasing scar. Born from the desire to avoid disfigurement and scarring, approaches were developed that would relocate the conventional Kocher incision to more discreet or concealed locations.[1,2] Truly minimally invasive techniques were sought that would provide the same degree of visualization and access to both lobes, with minimal tissue trauma. Both endoscopic and robotic approaches have been developed, with their own respective risks and benefits. Avoiding a potentially disfiguring scar is the main benefit to the remote access approach. A cervical scar can be especially distressing to patients with darker skin pigmentation and with a history of hypertrophic and/or keloid scars.[3] Robotic thyroidectomy includes breast, bilateral axillo-breast, axillary, and face-lift, among the most popular approaches. Although they may not be cervical, these approaches leave significant scarring at their respective access sites and require extensive tissue dissection to reach the thyroid gland. Therefore, these are not ideal minimally invasive approaches, given the amount of tissue disruption required to reach the thyroid gland when compared to

the open approach. The transoral endoscopic thyroidectomy (TOETVA) represents the latest remote access endoscopic technique for the excision of the thyroid gland. The TOETVA is considered the ideal remote access approach because it applies all of the good principles that minimally invasive thyroidectomy should include: (1) decreased distance from the oral vestibule to the gland that limits the amount of tissue dissection needed to reach the surgical target, thus also decreasing risk for instrument collision; (2) good operative and anatomic views of vital structures for patient safety; (3) visualization and access to both thyroid lobes; (4) a lack of residual cutaneous scarring postoperatively, due to a hidden intraoral incision; (5) ability to obtain oncological resection margins along with the ability to cleanly remove tissue specimens; (6) economically efficient, with respect to operative costs by keeping operative times down and using conventional low-cost instruments; (7) a simple technique for widespread adaptation and applicability. It is for these reasons that the transoral route is considered truly minimally invasive.[2–5] The safety and efficacy has been demonstrated in the literature by a number of investigators.[6–8]

The transoral thyroidectomy was first approached through a sublingual route but later this technique was abandoned due to complications related to the violation of the floor of the mouth.[9–11] Richmond et al. later described a vestibular approach and modifications of this technique gained popularity for the treatment of thyroid disease.[12] This route entails the placement of three endoscopic ports in the vestibular area of the mouth as described by A. Anuwong.[6,13,14] Dissection is carried out beneath the platysma muscle, first over the chin, then down between the two strap

Advances in Treatment and Management in Surgical Endocrinology. https://doi.org/10.1016/B978-0-323-66195-9.00024-8

muscles. Complete dissection of the thyroid gland can be done completely endoscopically, with operative times comparable to the open technique.[10,15] One of the biggest hurdles to widespread applicability has been the need for specialized training. Even before training, the surgeon should have a baseline mastery of robotic, laparoscopic, and endocrine surgery to avoid a steep learning curve. The safety profile and exposure that the typical open technique provides has set a standard that had initially dissuaded surgeons from adopting this new approach. With that being said, as minimally invasive surgery training becomes the norm, and as the demand for a cosmetically pleasing approach becomes greater, TOETVA is in position to become the standard of care in appropriate circumstances.[1,15] Another reason remote access thyroidectomies have not become mainstreamed is attributed to the inevitable increase in cost. With a relative increase in operative times, there are anesthesia costs that come into play on top of the costs involved with the instruments necessary in remote access surgery, particularly robotic surgery. On the other hand, the transoral endoscopic route uses conventional laparoscopic equipment that can help to keep costs down. Transoral thyroidectomies are performed worldwide, and as experience increases and with technical refinement, operation time will decrease.[2] Ultimately, it is patient satisfaction

and subsequent quality of life that is most important, second only to alleviating a patient's underlying pathology. Studies have shown that a cervical incision can be burdensome and that a cosmetically pleasing result enhances patient satisfaction[1,3,4] (Fig. 24.1).

TRANSORAL ENDOSCOPIC THYROIDECTOMY VESTIBULAR APPROACH
Surgical Technique

The patient is placed in the supine position on the operating table, with the neck mildly hyperextended. General anesthesia is administered after nasotracheal intubation is established. After induction, the oral cavity and upper neck are prepped and draped in sterile fashion. The use of nerve monitoring system is highly recommended. Three incisions are made through the alveolar mucosa of the lower lip vestibule, opposite to the incisors—a 15−20 mm transverse medial incision along with two vertical 5 mm incisions (the two lateral incisions are just medial to the canines and just in the inner aspect of the inferior lip to avoid injury to the mental nerve—as depicted in Fig. 24.2). Three ports, a central 10−12 mm and two lateral 5 mm ports, are utilized. Before port placement, a working space is created by tissue dissection through the mentalis muscle with the use of electrocautery and/or blunt dissection.

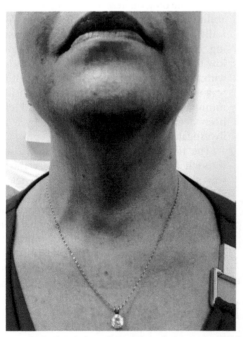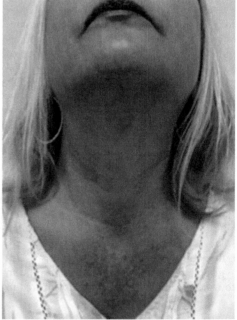

FIG. 24.1 A postoperative photograph, highlighting the absence of any postoperative scars.

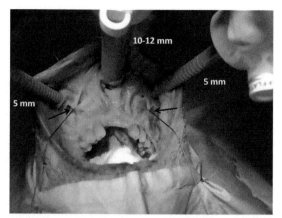

FIG. 24.2 Cadaveric dissection identifying anatomical landmarks for port placement in TOETVA. Central 10–12 mm port and lateral 5 mm ports have been placed. Bilateral mentalis nerve depicted with black arrows.

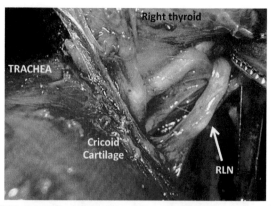

FIG. 24.3 Depiction of the oral vestibule and the closure of the two lateral 5 mm incisions (light blue arrows), and closed central incision (black arrow).

Subsequently, hydrodissection is performed with a Veress needle where about 60 cc of a mixture of NaCl containing epinephrine (1 mg in 500 cc NaCl) is injected to create a space beneath the platysma, which is then dilated with a blunt dissector (Anuwong dilator, KellyWick tunneler or Hegar dilators).[16] A 10–12 mm port is the first placed, through the central incision and then over the mandible advancing the port about 2 cm distally to the chin, taking care to avoid penetration of mentum skin. Next, the two lateral 5 mm ports are placed through the lateral. The surgical space is then maintained with insufflation of CO_2 at a pressure of 6 mm Hg. A 30-degree 5 or 10 mm camera is then placed through the central port. A Maryland dissector and bipolar energy or ultrasonic energy device is used on either side of the camera for further development of the surgical space.[17] Dissection is carried out in the caudal direction toward the sternal notch, always staying beneath the platysma muscle. Laterally, dissecting to bilateral sternocleidomastoid muscles further enhances exposure. Once the strap muscles are visualized, they are divided in the midline to expose the thyroid gland. The strap muscles are then retracted laterally by placing stay sutures preferably using monofilament sutures. The thyroid vessels are ligated and divided in sequence, starting with the middle thyroid veins to allow medialization of the thyroid lobe and then with the superior thyroid vessels, taking care to avoid injuring the external branch of the superior laryngeal nerve. The superior lobe is then mobilized and the recurrent laryngeal nerve is identified (Fig. 24.3). The use of a nerve monitoring system is encouraged and a good adjunct but not a mandatory tool to perform this procedure. The inferior thyroid vessels are divided and the rest of the lobe is then mobilized. The parathyroid glands are meticulously sought and preserved, along with their blood supply. The same approach and technique is then applied to the contralateral lobe, if a total thyroidectomy is undertaken. The gland is then placed in an endocatch bag and brought out through the central port.[14,16–19] The mentalis muscle is approximated with absorbable 3-0 sutures and the mucosa closed with 5-0 absorbable sutures (Fig. 24.4).

Patient Eligibility

Despite early success with the transoral thyroidectomy technique, measured by low morbidity and mortality rates, it is important to note that not every patient or any thyroid pathology is amenable to the transoral approach. Uniform indications and contraindications for the TOETVA have not officially been established.[5,19,20] Here, we present a compilation of inclusion and exclusion criteria from different individual authors, with the differences mediated. Without sufficient universal experience, the following recommendations have been structured based on our personal experience and all the literature available to date.[3,6,8,13,20,21] Instead of outlining the "indications" for the transoral thyroidectomy, we determine whether individual patients have "favorable features" for this technique to assess feasibility of the procedure. In a similar manner, patients with a disease process of the thyroid gland or having characteristics where there is controversy or contraindications for surgery would be considered to have "nonfavorable features" for a transoral thyroidectomy. Ultimately, the approach of the surgical procedure is based on the patient's preference

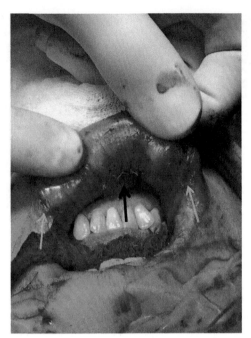

FIG. 24.4 Depiction of anatomical landmarks during dissection of the right thyroid lobe with identification of the trachea, cricoid cartilage, right thyroid lobe, and the insertion of the right recurrent laryngeal nerve (RLN).

after details of their clinical findings, risks, and benefits as well as the technical aspects of the transoral technique have been discussed thoroughly with the patient. The following are the indications based on the patient's favorable features: the patient's own motivation to avoid a cervical scar, symptomatic benign nodules ≤6 cm (benign nodules >6 cm < 10 cm are possible but may require significant expertise in TOETVA), cytologically indeterminate nodules (Bethesda three or four lesions) < 6 cm, an estimated thyroid diameter ≤ 10 cm on ultrasound, an estimated gland volume ≤ 45 mL on ultrasound, symptomatic Hashimoto's thyroiditis, Grave's disease (with the patient being euthyroid when possible), and differentiated thyroid cancer < 3 cm without extrathyroidal extension or lymph node metastasis on preoperative ultrasonography. Contraindications are based on the lack of favorable features or the presence of these nonfavorable features: the presence of a substernal goiter, previous neck and/or chin surgery, or previous neck radiation. Table 24.1 summarizes patients that are suitable for the TOETVA approach. More important than cosmetics is the correct management of the patient's thyroid pathology. Therefore, guidelines set forth by the American Thyroid Association should

coincide with the recommendations we laid out, when deciding to utilize the TOETVA.

Safety Profile and Complications

When the use of remote access surgery for the thyroid gland began, complications arose that were previously undocumented with the traditional open technique. These ranged from brachial plexopathy to esophageal perforation. Although these predominantly occurred with the trans-axillary or bilateral axillo-breast robotic approaches, they brought to light the fact that all new remote access techniques must be compared to the safety profile that we have come to expect with the traditional open technique.[20] The initial experience with the transoral endoscopic thyroidectomy vestibular approach demonstrated that the procedure was safe and feasible with complication rates comparable to the open thyroidectomy.[6] The transoral endoscopic vestibular approach has since been shown by many investigators to be an excellent alternative to the traditional cervical thyroidectomy for those patients

TABLE 24.1
Patient Eligibility for Transoral Endoscopic Thyroidectomy Vestibular Approach.

Favorable Features	Patient's own motivation to avoid a cervical scar
	Symptomatic benign nodules ≤6 cm (benign nodules >6 cm < 10 cm is possible but may require surgical expertise in TOETVA)
	Cytologically indeterminate nodules (Bethesda 3 or 4 lesions) < 6 cm
	Estimated thyroid diameter ≤ 10 cm on ultrasound
	Estimated gland volume ≤ 45 mL, on ultrasound
	Symptomatic Hashimoto's thyroiditis
	Grave's disease (well controlled when possible)
	Differentiated thyroid cancer < 3 cm without extrathyroidal extension or lymph node metastasis on preoperative ultrasonography
Nonfavorable Features	Substernal goiters
	Previous neck and chin surgery
	Previous neck radiation

who have favorable features and are highly motivated to avoid a cervical scar.[3,6,7,13,16,20–24] One of the critical improvements of the transoral endoscopic vestibular technique has been the port placement in the vestibule. Early experiences with this endoscopic procedure demonstrated high rates of mental nerve injury as demonstrated by the postoperative sensory disorder around the chin that persisted for more than 6 months after surgery in an early report of eight patients.[25] This problem was addressed by adjusting the placement of the lateral 5 mm ports. The two vertical incisions for the 5 mm ports were repositioned to the vestibular mucosa medial to the level of the canines and just in the inner aspect of the inferior lip, to avoid contact or damage to the mental nerve.[17] In a series of 425 patients, three (0.7%) had transient mental nerve injury and recovered their lip and chin sensation within 4 months.[13] In our experience, transient mental nerve injury is not unusual,[3,6,7,13,16,19–24,26–30] but a full recovery of the inferior lip and chin sensation should be expected within 6 months from the surgery.

A major concern with the transoral approach has been the risk of a surgical site infection. The mucosa of the oral cavity is colonized with a diverse bacterial flora, including gram positive and anaerobic bacteria. Previously, via the open route, thyroidectomies had a clean wound classification. Because of the violation of the oral mucosa, transoral thyroidectomies are classified as a clean contaminated case; assuming that there is no concomitant infectious process at the time the surgery (e.g., tooth abscess, etc.).[2] To combat this risk, appropriate preoperative prophylactic antibiotic coverage is recommended to cover against the polymicrobial flora of the mouth. Amoxicillin-clavulanic acid or cefazolin + an anaerobic covering antibiotic (clindamycin or metronidazole) would provide adequate coverage.[31] Fortunately, to date, there have been no reports of wound infection with the oral vestibular approach. Injuries to the recurrent laryngeal nerve have been reported in some series, with a full recovery of the vocal cords function before 6 months after surgery in all cases.[6,14,20] Hypocalcaemia, as in the traditional open thyroidectomy, is more common when a total thyroidectomy is performed. Fortunately, there has not been a report of permanent hypoparathyroidism but temporary hypoparathyroidism has been observed in up to 22% of the patients in a series of total thyroidectomies for the treatment of Grave's disease.[19] Not so much a complication as much as postoperative changes that training surgeons and patients should be made aware of is the potential cutaneous lesion as a result of intraoperative injuries to the skin. A very common finding,

and more frequently noticed in the immediate postoperative period, is ecchymosis of the chin and the anterior neck that may be associated with bruising, but in general they resolve at 1–2 weeks or sooner after surgery.[23,30] Full thickness injury or piercing of the skin has also been reported, and this is commonly seen under the chin secondary to use of the Veress needle during hydrodissection, electrocautery, or even the use of clamps during dissection of the superior neck flap.[3,30] Other skin injuries observed are skin tears that may be seen at the lip commissures from traction or burns that may be caused by the energy devices used during the procedure.[3,30] Postoperative hematoma may also be seen as in the traditional open thyroidectomy. To date, a very limited number of postoperative hematomas have been reported in the literature but the underestimation of this complication may be related to the limited cases reported in the literature.[13] There was a subset of patients[20] that developed postoperative seromas, observed in the largest series published to date (a series of 425 patients undergoing TOETVA). Five percent of them[10] had complete resolution with simple aspiration.[13] A small number of conversions to an open procedure have been reported with the reason for conversion being excessive intraoperative bleeding.[13,19] There was even case reported where conversion from a transoral robotic to the endoscopic technique was reported.[20] In comparison to the gold standard open thyroidectomy, TOETVA has been proven that it can be done as safely and efficiently as the traditional approach.[1,13]

Evolution and Applicability of TOETVA

The traditional open thyroidectomy has provided excellent anatomic and operative views for adequate oncological resections, with limited morbidity and mortality; therefore, any new technique must at least meet these standards.[5,20] Robotic and endoscopic surgery for head and neck pathologies, specifically for the thyroid gland, have evolved from being novel procedures to the favored approach for certain cases. Endoscopic techniques were first used for the parathyroid glands. Improvements in endoscopic technology and greater understanding of endoscopic cervical anatomy allowed for endoscopic techniques to also be applied to the thyroid gland. It has now expanded further to utilization for the dissection of the central lymph nodes. Early roadblocks, like limited exposure and the need for excessive tissue dissection to reach surgical targets, have been overcome with the transoral endoscopic vestibular approach. This can be attributed to improved cervical anatomic views that the endoscope provides.[5,13,20] The transoral endoscopic thyroidectomy vestibular approach is to head and neck surgery what the laparoscopic cholecystectomy was to hepatobiliary surgery.[16] The early challenges encountered by transoral thyroidectomies mirror those encountered by the laparoscopic cholecystectomy. Similar to the latter procedure, the earliest challenges have been resolved and the technique is being widely adopted. The TOETVA is currently being performed at multiple institutions around the world. The international hospitals embracing the procedure are high volume academic centers that have the financial means to support an endoscopic approach. Here, in the United States, there are seven centers performing TOETVA.[4] This technique requires specialized training of surgeons having a background in traditional thyroidectomies, endoscopic and robotic procedures, and endocrine disease for safe introduction. A steep learning curve can be overcome by increased volume, in the appropriate setting. With approximately 130,000 cases a year done for thyroid nodular disease, there is potential for widespread applicability. This caseload does not include surgeries that are done for Grave's hyperthyroidism or hyperparathyroidism, both of which are indications. Even if conservative estimates were to be used, the transoral approach could be utilized for thousands of cervical endocrine pathologies per year in the United States.[16] Especially, when the safety and outcomes are the same, when compared to the current gold standard, and patients are presented the option of a cosmetically appealing scarless surgery. Given the minimally invasive nature of the procedure, one drawback of the TOETVA is the need to remove the specimen from a 1 cm incision. Various techniques have been employed to facilitate extraction without removal from the endocatch bag. It is this drawback that has limited oncological resection to 1–2 cm cancer nodules. A large randomized control trial is still necessary to evaluate the benefits of TOETVA for thyroid cancer patients.

SUMMARY

The traditional open thyroidectomy has been the standard of care for thyroid pathologies requiring surgery, due to its efficacy and safety profile. The scarring and potential for disfigurement in certain patient populations lead to the development of minimally invasive techniques. This form of remote access surgery allows for the relocation of the typical cervical incision, and subsequent scar, to more discreet location. Both endoscopic and robotic techniques have been developed, with their own risks and benefits. However, it has been the TOETVA that leads the charge, in terms of being the most ideal minimally invasive technique. Different from the other robotic approaches, TOETVA applies most, if not all of the good principles that minimally invasive thyroidectomy should include: (1) minimal distance from access point to surgical target, thereby limiting tissue dissection; (2) good operative and anatomic views of vital structures for patient safety; (3) visualization and access to both thyroid lobes; (4) a lack of residual cutaneous scarring; (5) ability to obtain oncological resection margins; (6) economically efficient; (7) a simple technique for widespread adaptation and applicability. When compared to the gold standard open thyroidectomy, the efficacy and safety of the TOETVA have been demonstrated in the literature by a number of investigators to be on par. Studies have shown that a cervical incision can be burdensome and that a cosmetically pleasing result enhances patient satisfaction in the postoperative period. The transoral route allows motivated patients, given they have favorable features for the procedure, to have options outside of the typical scar inducing transcervical route. The transoral thyroidectomy was first approached through a sublingual route but this was abandoned due to complications related to violating the floor of the mouth. The technique that is applied now involves the placement of three endoscopic ports in the vestibular area of the mouth, in specific anatomical locations to avoid injuring the mental nerve. Preceding placement of these ports, a plane is dissected beneath the platysma muscle, first over the chin, then down between the two strap muscles. The camera is placed through the central 10–12 mm port while dissection, ligation, and mobilization of the thyroid gland carried out through the two lateral 5 mm ports. The thyroid nodule, lobe, or entire gland is removed from the central port, after placement into an endocatch bag. Operative times, for the endoscopic technique, have been shown to be comparable to the open technique. This approach requires specialized training of surgeons with baseline mastery in endocrine surgery and minimally invasive surgery. The steep learning curve can be attenuated by increased volume in the appropriate setting. As demand for a cosmetically pleasing approach becomes more prominent, even if conservative estimates were to be used, the transoral approach could be utilized for thousands of cervical endocrine pathologies per year in the United States. Not every patient, nor is every thyroid pathology a candidate for the TOETVA. Uniform indications and contraindications for this technique have not yet been established. Based on our personal experience and literature to date, we have compiled a list of inclusion and exclusion criteria. However, instead of outlining indications and contraindications, we determine whether individual patients have "favorable features" for this technique to assess feasibility of the procedure. In a similar manner, patients with a disease process of the thyroid gland or having characteristics where there is controversy or contraindications for surgery would be considered to have "nonfavorable features" for a transoral thyroidectomy. The following are the indications based on the patient's favorable features: the patient's own motivation to avoid a cervical scar, symptomatic benign nodules ≤6 cm (benign nodules >6 cm < 10 cm are possible but may require significant expertise in TOETVA), cytologically indeterminate nodules (Bethesda three or four lesions) < 6 cm, an estimated thyroid diameter ≤ 10 cm on ultrasound, an estimated gland volume ≤ 45 mL on ultrasound, symptomatic Hashimoto's thyroiditis, Grave's disease (with the patient being euthyroid when possible), and differentiated thyroid cancer < 3 cm without extrathyroidal extension or lymph node metastasis on preoperative ultrasonography. Contraindications are based on the lack of favorable features or the presence of these nonfavorable features: the presence of a substernal goiter, previous neck and/or chin surgery, or previous neck radiation. In the end, it is the patient's choice as to whether they want to proceed with the transoral route, given all the risks and benefits of all the surgical choices at their disposal. Initial experiences with TOETVA have shown to have similar complications and rates to the gold standard technique. Early on, this novel endoscopic procedure was encountering a complication that had never been seen with the open thyroidectomy: high rates of mental nerve injury as demonstrated by the postoperative sensory disorder around the chin that persisted for more than 6 months after surgery. With adjustments in port placement the rate of transient nerve injury has dramatically decreased, with one study showing rates as low as 0.7%. Because of the violation of the oral mucosa, transoral thyroidectomies are classified as a clean contaminated case, assuming that there is no concomitant infectious process at the time of the surgery (e.g., tooth abscess, etc.). With appropriate perioperative prophylactic coverage, there have been no reports of wound infection with the oral vestibular approach. Improvements in endoscopic technology and greater understanding of endoscopic cervical anatomy have led to the ability to overcome early roadblocks, such as limited exposure and the need for excessive tissue dissection to reach surgical targets. With approximately 130,000 cases a year done for thyroid nodular disease, there is potential for widespread applicability. This caseload does not include surgeries that are done for Grave's hyperthyroidism or hyperparathyroidism, both of which are indications. Especially when the safety and outcomes are the same, when compared to the current gold standard, and patients are presented the option of a cosmetically appealing scarless surgery.

CONCLUSION

TOETVA should no longer be considered an experimental operation. Its safety profile and efficacy have been proven with limited morbidity, when compared to the standards set by the open thyroidectomy.[5] Although widespread adoption of remote access surgery in the United States has been slow due to technical, population, and financial considerations, the endoscopic technique has shown to be a standalone in these respects.[20] Operative times and costs are comparable to the gold standard technique and still have more room for improvement. Its increase in popularity can be attributed to the cosmetic results of this "scarless surgery," all while accomplishing surgical goals. TOETVA is the best minimally invasive scarless approach to the thyroid gland. The endoscopic technique applies all of the principles necessary to make for a good minimally invasive surgery. Highlighted by but not limited to the short distance from the oral incision to the gland, the lack of any postoperative residual cutaneous scarring, and the ability to keep costs down by using conventional equipment.

Deciding between an open thyroidectomy versus a transoral thyroidectomy starts with the surgeon determining whether the patient has "favorable features" or "nonfavorable features" for a transoral procedure. A cosmetically pleasing approach for a disfiguring or dysfunctional pathology is an attractive option for motivated patients. With adverse events and complications being similar, or else no worse than the open approach, the utilization of the transoral procedure will inevitably become more widespread. A large randomized prospective trial is still necessary to definitively compare the risks and benefits of a transoral approach versus an open one. Such a study would also help to delineate long-term morbidity and mortality.

DISCLOSURES

The authors have identified no financial disclosures.

REFERENCES

1. Russell JO, Noureldine SI, Al Khadem MG, Tufano RP. Minimally invasive and remote-access thyroid surgery in the era of the 2015 American Thyroid Association guidelines. *Laryngoscope Investig Otolaryngol.* 2016;1(6):175–179.
2. Chai YJ, Chung JK, Anuwong A, et al. Transoral endoscopic thyroidectomy for papillary thyroid microcarcinoma: initial experience of a single surgeon. *Ann Surg Treat Res.* 2017;93(2):70–75.
3. Richmon JD, Kim HY. Transoral robotic thyroidectomy (TORT): procedures and outcomes. *Gland Surg.* 2017; 6(3):285–289.
4. Dionigi G, Lavazza M, Wu C-W, et al. Transoral thyroidectomy: why is it needed? *Gland Surg.* 2017;6(3):272–276.
5. Transoral Endoscopic Thyroidectomy Using Vestibular Approach: Updates and Evidences – Anuwong – Gland Surgery [Internet]. [cited 2017 Dec 17]. Available from: http://gs.amegroups.com/article/view/14691/15501.
6. Anuwong A. Transoral endoscopic thyroidectomy vestibular approach: a series of the first 60 human cases. *World J Surg.* 2016;40(3):491–497.
7. Wang Y, Xie QP, Yu X, et al. Preliminary experience with transoral endoscopic thyroidectomy via vestibular approach: a report of 150 cases in a single center. *Zhonghua Wai Ke Za Zhi.* 2017;55(8):587–591.
8. Dionigi G, Bacuzzi A, Lavazza M, et al. Transoral endoscopic thyroidectomy: preliminary experience in Italy. *Updates Surg.* 2017;69(2):225–234.
9. Witzel K, von Rahden BHA, Kaminski C, Stein HJ. Transoral access for endoscopic thyroid resection. *Surg Endosc.* 2008;22(8):1871–1875.
10. Benhidjeb T, Wilhelm T, Harlaar J, Kleinrensink G-J, Schneider TAJ, Stark M. Natural orifice surgery on thyroid gland: totally transoral video-assisted thyroidectomy (TOVAT): report of first experimental results of a new surgical method. *Surg Endosc.* 2009;23(5):1119–1120.
11. McHenry CR. Endoscopic minimally invasive thyroidectomy: a prospective proof-of-concept study in humans. *World J Surg.* 2011;35(3):552.
12. Richmon JD, Holsinger FC, Kandil E, Moore MW, Garcia JA, Tufano RP. Transoral robotic-assisted thyroidectomy with central neck dissection: preclinical cadaver feasibility study and proposed surgical technique. *J Robot Surg.* 2011;5(4):279–282.
13. Anuwong A, Ketwong K, Jitpratoom P, Sasanakietkul T, Duh Q-Y. Safety and outcomes of the transoral endoscopic thyroidectomy vestibular approach. *JAMA Surg.* 2018; 153(1):21–27.
14. Anuwong A, Sasanakietkul T, Jitpratoom P, et al. Transoral endoscopic thyroidectomy vestibular approach (TOETVA): indications, techniques and results. *Surg Endosc.* 2018;32(1):456–465.
15. Yeh MW. Thyroid surgery through the mouth might not be as crazy as it sounds [Internet] *JAMA Surg.* 2017;15(153):28. [cited 2017 Dec 17]. Available from: https://jamanetwork.com/journals/jamasurgery/fullarticle/2653284.
16. Udelsman R, Anuwong A, Oprea AD, et al. Trans-oral vestibular endocrine surgery: a new technique in the United States. *Ann Surg.* 2016;264(6):e13–e16.
17. Kahramangil B, Mohsin K, Alzahrani H, et al. Robotic and endoscopic transoral thyroidectomy: feasibility and description of the technique in the cadaveric model. *Gland Surg.* 2017;6(6):611–619.
18. Dionigi G, Lavazza M, Bacuzzi A, et al. Transoral endoscopic thyroidectomy vestibular approach (TOETVA): from A to Z. *Surg Technol Int.* 2017;30:103–112.
19. Jitpratoom P, Ketwong K, Sasanakietkul T, Anuwong A. Transoral endoscopic thyroidectomy vestibular approach (TOETVA) for Graves' disease: a comparison of surgical results with open thyroidectomy. *Gland Surg.* 2016;5(6): 546–552.
20. Russell JO, Clark J, Noureldine SI, et al. Transoral thyroidectomy and parathyroidectomy – a North American series of robotic and endoscopic transoral approaches to the central neck. *Oral Oncol.* 2017;71:75–80.
21. Park J-O, Sun D-I. Transoral endoscopic thyroidectomy: our initial experience using a new endoscopic technique. *Surg Endosc.* 2017;31(12):5436–5443.
22. Razavi CR, Russell JO. Indications and contraindications to transoral thyroidectomy [Internet] *Ann Thyroid.* 2017; 2(5):12. [cited 2018 Feb 19]. Available from: https://www.ncbi.nlm.nih.gov/pmc/articles/PMC5788189/.
23. Wang C, Zhai H, Liu W, et al. Thyroidectomy: a novel endoscopic oral vestibular approach. *Surgery.* 2014; 155(1):33–38.
24. Inabnet WB, Suh H, Fernandez-Ranvier G. Transoral endoscopic thyroidectomy vestibular approach with intraoperative nerve monitoring. *Surg Endosc.* 2017;31(7):3030.
25. Nakajo A, Arima H, Hirata M, et al. Trans-Oral Video-Assisted Neck Surgery (TOVANS). A new transoral technique of endoscopic thyroidectomy with gasless premandible approach. *Surg Endosc.* 2013;27(4):1105–1110.
26. Park J-O, Kim M-R, Kim DH, Lee DK. Transoral endoscopic thyroidectomy via the trivestibular route. *Ann Surg Treat Res.* 2016;91(5):269–272.
27. Pai VM, Muthukumar P, Prathap A, Leo J, Rekha A. Transoral endoscopic thyroidectomy: a case report. *Int J Surg Case Rep.* 2015;12:99–101.
28. Kim HY, Chai YJ, Dionigi G, Anuwong A, Richmon JD. Transoral robotic thyroidectomy: lessons learned from an initial consecutive series of 24 patients. *Surg Endosc.* 2018;32(2):688–694.
29. Zeng Y-K, Li Z-Y, Xuan W-L, He J-X. Trans-oral glasses-free three-dimensional endoscopic thyroidectomy-preliminary single center experiences. *Gland Surg.* 2016;5(6):628–632.
30. Yang J, Wang C, Li J, et al. Complete endoscopic thyroidectomy via oral vestibular approach versus areola approach for treatment of thyroid diseases. *J Laparoendosc Adv Surg Tech.* 2015;25(6):470–476.
31. Salmerón-Escobar JI, del Amo-Fernández de Velasco A. Antibiotic prophylaxis in oral and maxillofacial surgery. *Med Oral, Patol Oral Cirugía Bucal.* 2006;11(3):E292–E296.

CHAPTER 25

Advances in Perioperative Management: Nursing Care, Anesthesia Considerations, and Nurse Navigation for Endocrine Surgical Patients

SVETLANA L. KRASNOVA, BSN, RN, CNOR •
MAUREEN MCCARTNEY-ANDERSON, DNP, CRNA, APN-ANESTHESIA •
JOAN HALLMAN, BSN, RN, OCN •
ALEXANDER SHIFRIN, MD, FACS, FACE, ECNU, FEBS (ENDOCRINE), FISS

PERIOPERATIVE NURSING CONSIDERATIONS FOR THYROID, PARATHYROID, AND ADRENAL SURGERY

Thorough assessment of the patient preoperatively is paramount to ensure favorable outcomes. Patients' hemodynamic status, medication regimen, and physical limitations are factors that should be discussed. These are all important to consider and will provide the plan of care specific to the patient. Patients should be questioned about limited range of motion and their ability to lie comfortably in a supine position with their neck hyperextended. If questions arise, it is best to place the patient in the anticipated position as a trial before induction of anesthesia.

Physical limitations will be important in patient positioning in an effort to avoid unfavorable and disabling outcomes such as nerve damage, pressure-induced injury, ulceration, or compartment syndrome. Positioning the patient for a surgical procedure is a shared responsibility among all surgical staff including the surgeon, anesthesia provider, and the nurses in the operating room. The optimal position may require a compromise between the best position for surgical access and the position the patient can tolerate in an effort to avoid physiologic changes that can result in soft tissue injury. In addition, it is important to remember supine position affects pulmonary physiology, primarily related to cranial displacement of the diaphragm by abdominal contents. A decrease in functional residual capacity occurs in the supine position and is compounded by anesthesia. Reduction in lung compliance, airway closure, and atelectasis can result. Ventilation perfusion mismatch may occur during mechanical ventilation. Perfusion increases in dependent lung regions, while ventilation is more evenly distributed. Such changes are usually well tolerated by healthy patients but may be problematic for patients with obesity, pulmonary disease, and older patients.

Positioning includes focusing on the brachial plexus the ulnar nerve and the radial nerve to avoid debilitating injury. The brachial nerve is a group of nerves that come from the spinal cord in the neck and travel down the arm. These nerves are responsible for controlling the muscles of the shoulder, elbow, wrist, and hands, and their functions also involve providing feeling in the arms. The nerve can be damaged by stretching, for example, when the head and neck are forced away from the shoulder; if severe, these nerves can actually tear out of the spinal cord in the neck. Generally accepted recommendations supported by the American Society of Anesthesiology Task Force and Prevention include positioning of the arms abducted less than 90 degrees, to avoid stretching the brachial plexus across the head of the humerus in the axilla.[1] Although adducting the arms in both parathyroidectomy as well as thyroidectomy is preferred over abduction for both nerve considerations and better proximity to the surgical field by the surgical team. Ulnar nerve is one of the three main nerves in the arm;

Advances in Treatment and Management in Surgical Endocrinology. https://doi.org/10.1016/B978-0-323-66195-9.00025-X

it originates at the C8-T1 nerve roots that form the medial cord of the brachial plexus. The ulnar nerve runs down the arm and passes behind the medial epicondyle of the humerus at the elbow. To mitigate injury to the ulnar nerve arms should be positioned to decrease pressure on the postcondylar groove of the humerus (ulnar groove): adducting the arms along the patient's side and placing in a neutral position, with the palm facing the patient. A way to maintain the "thumb up" position is to place a piece of foam or a roll of Kerlex in the patient's hands bilaterally. The radial nerve is rarely injured but is theoretically at risk for compression as it runs in the spiral groove of the humerus in the posterior upper arm, between the heads of the triceps muscle. Arms adducted with enough space and support of the arms at the sides of the patient to decrease risk for compression should be considered. In addition, intravenous poles and devices attached to the operating table should be positioned away from the patient's upper arm.

In the supine position, prolonged pressure to the bony prominences in contact with the operating table mattress, arm boards, and head supports are at risk for skin pressure damage. Areas such as the back of the head, heels, and sacrum are all target areas for pressure sores. Protective measures should be implemented. Those include placing a pillow under the knees bilaterally and foam under the heels. The feet should be supported without pressure on the Achilles tendon and without the knee hyperextended. The head should be supported with foam resting in a head cradle or with a gel donut to minimize the pressure on the occiput. With the arms in the adducted position, they should be secured next to the patient's body using the draw sheet to achieve this goal by tucking the sheet between the bedframe and mattress for stability. Wrinkles should be avoided. The elbows should be slightly flexed with wrists in neutral position and palms facing inward. Bony prominences should be padded to avoid pressure on the ulnar groove. Lastly, extension in or hyperextension of the neck is often required for procedures on the neck such as the thyroid and the parathyroid surgeries. A roll is placed under the patient's shoulders after intubation, to extend the neck and facilitate exposure, importantly the head should not float but rather should be supported under the occiput by resting in a head cradle and if needed adding sheets/foam or blanket underneath the head cradle.

The use of perioperative antibiotics is at the discretion of the surgeon. In a comprehensive literature review consisting with meta-analyses, randomized control trials, prospective and retrospective cohort studies, case-control studies, and case series. The use of the antibiotics was not supported in clean head and neck surgeries such as thyroidectomy or parathyroidectomy. Furthermore, the frequency of surgical site infections was low in patients who received and those who had not received preoperative antibiotics prophylaxis based on randomized control trial of 807 patients who underwent clean neck surgery. Therefore, antibiotic prophylaxis was not recommended in routine clean thyroid or parathyroid surgeries.[2] One key point that cannot be overlooked is the use of antibiotics is patient specific, some conditions or metal implants such as a knee or hip replacement would warrant antibiotic prophylaxis. Again that would be at the discretion of the surgeon and patient allergy considerations.

The use of graduated compression stockings should be implemented on patients with parathyroid and thyroid surgeries. Venous thromboembolism (VTE) is common in the postoperative setting with over half of this population at moderate risk for VTE.[3] PE is one of the most common preventable causes of in-hospital deaths following surgery. Patients with Cushing's disease or syndrome have 10 times increase in incidence of venous thromboembolism due to the increase in procoagulant factors and impaired fibrinolysis. Studies showed that those patients have shortened activated partial thromboplastin time and higher levels of fibrinogen, Factor VIII, and protein S activity. Their fibrinolytic capacity was impaired with prolonged clot lysis time and higher levels of plasminogen activator inhibitor type 1, thrombin-activatable fibrinolysis inhibitor, and α2-antiplasmin.[4] Increased risk in cardiovascular complications are also noted in the literature.

ANESTHETIC CONSIDERATIONS FOR THYROID, PARATHYROID, AND ADRENAL SURGERY

Preoperative Considerations

All patients undergoing endocrine surgery should have a thorough preoperative evaluation and physical assessment. Blood work should be assessed for electrolyte abnormalities and vital signs reviewed. Pending the patient's medical history, a 12 lead EKG, chest X-ray, and specialty consultation reports may also be necessary. A physical assessment should assess patients' neck mobility in flexion and extension and the general cervical range of motion. This will be important for the positioning of the patient in the perioperative period. If the patient is unable to extend their neck, positioning can be challenging for necessary surgical exposure. Attempting to extend the patient's neck after induction of anesthesia can be unsafe for the patient and should be done with caution.

The presence and size of a goiter should be noted as well as thyromental distance. The airway assessment would include identifying the Mallampati score and any possible oropharyngeal swelling. Tracheal deviation can be observed through assessment and palpation of the patient's neck while reviewing any chest X-ray results and CT scans of the neck and chest. Open communication with the surgeon is valuable for the assessment and possibility of a difficult airway for intubation. Should a goiter be present, it should also be identified if the airway is being displaced or compressed and if the patient is able to assume the supine position with ease. The presence of a large goiter or a compressed airway will dictate the anesthetic approach for induction and advanced airway establishment. This may be inclusive of the utilization of a video laryngoscope or fiberoptic bronchoscope.[5] However, if intraoperative neural monitoring is to be performed through the utilization of a neural integrity monitoring (NIM) endotracheal tube, the use of topical local anesthetics, nebulized or transtracheal lidocaine, or superior laryngeal nerve blocks should be avoided as they will interfere with surgical localization of the laryngeal nerves.[6]

Risk stratification for postoperative nausea and vomiting should be identified with the possible application of a scopolamine patch in the preoperative setting. An intravenous catheter should be initiated with intravenous fluid running at a set rate. If possible, it is advantageous to attain a larger bore intravenous catheter, such as an 18 gauge as intraoperative blood samples may be necessary.

The patients' history and endocrine disorder should be considered throughout the preoperative assessment. Electrolyte optimization should be achieved in elective, nonemergent cases. The patient should be optimized from a medical perspective and may need a medical or cardiac consultation with optimization before surgery. Sequela from endocrine disorders needs to be thoroughly evaluated and considered in the anesthetic approach and maintenance for patient safety and improved perioperative outcomes.

Anesthetic Set up

When performing anesthesia for patients undergoing endocrine surgery, a general anesthesia set up is necessary. This would include an anesthesia machine and advanced airway equipment. Airway equipment would include an endotracheal tube, laryngoscope handle and blade, and various sized oropharyngeal airways. Pending the patient's preoperative assessment, a video laryngoscope or flexible bronchoscope should be readily available for the possibility of a difficult airway. A neural integrity monitor (NIM) electromyogram endotracheal tube is frequently utilized for endocrine surgery in the head and neck for monitoring laryngeal nerves. The NIM tubes are generally available in 6.0, 7.0, and 8.0 sizes for the adult population.

Induction agents would include a hypnotic, often midazolam, propofol, or etomidate; an analgesic, often fentanyl, hydromorphone, or remifentanil; and a paralytic, often succinylcholine, rocuronium, or vecuronium. Special consideration should be given if the patient has any cortisol insufficiency as etomidate can interfere with cortisol synthesis. General anesthetic maintenance can be achieved with an inhalational agent, usually sevoflurane or desflurane or a continuous propofol and remifentanil infusion. Additional analgesics to be available may include Ketorolac and Ofirmev. Medication for the prevention of postoperative nausea and vomiting should also be available, which may include Zofran, Decadron, Reglan, and Famotidine. A scopolamine patch can be advantageous, but should be applied in the preoperative setting.

Other set-up to consider is an additional intravenous line with a large bore angiocatheter. This is a consideration when intraoperative blood work needs to be performed. In some instances, an arterial line may be necessary for blood draws or if the patient's medical and endocrine history dictates the need. An esophageal temperature probe can be utilized to monitor patient temperature as well as assist the surgeon during a neck dissection. A lower body Baer Hugger blanket for thermoregulation and a foam head rest or gel donut for patient head positioning should also be accessible.

Perioperative Management

The anesthetic plan is a direct result of a thorough and vigilant preoperative assessment and open collaboration with the surgeon. Depending on the type of surgery being performed, the anesthetic maintenance plan can vary, but general anesthesia will be the consistent approach. If neural monitoring is being performed, the NIM tube needs to be utilized. This tube is placed on the induction of anesthesia with the color-coded contact band appropriately placed between the vocal cords.[6] The proper placement can be achieved through direct laryngoscopy and verified with a video laryngoscope or flexible laryngoscopy. The tube should not be secured until the contact band placement is verified.

The purpose of the NIM tube is to monitor laryngeal nerves in the intraoperative period at the surgical field. If the NIM tube is to be utilized with neural monitoring, the patient cannot receive any long-acting muscle relaxation on induction. This can be achieved by using a short acting, depolarizing paralytic medication or a subtherapeutic dose of long-acting nondepolarizing paralytic. Alternatively, a full dose of long-acting nonpolarizing paralytic can be used with subsequent reversal agent before surgical incision.

A second intravenous access can be achieved following induction. This access may be necessary for intraoperative blood sampling. If blood sampling is necessary, a larger bore angiocatheter is helpful in which you can draw back on. Verification of blood return after the patient is positioned is vital. This can be achieved by having the second IV connected to a continuous infusion with a stop cock and extension tubing to the angiocatheter. The blood pressure cuff can intermittently act as a tourniquet for blood sampling, which will dictate its position on the patient in coordination with the IV.

Patient positioning is generally supine with the arms tucked at the sides. A shoulder roll is utilized for neck extension and the head rests on a foam headrest or gel donut. Careful consideration should be given when extending the patients neck after the induction of anesthesia. The weight of the head should rest on the designated headrest and not hang above. When tucking and securing the arms, they should always be maintained in a neutral thumb up or supinated position. The legs are often positioned with the knees slightly flexed resting on pillows to alleviate lower lumbar pressure.[7] The endotracheal tube (ETT) should be directed toward the top of the patient to avoid interference in the surgical field. Extra eye protection is necessary as the surgeon and surgical instruments will be near the patient's eyes.

Anesthetic maintenance is achieved with inhalational agent (sevoflurane or desflurane with or without nitrous oxide) or continuous propofol and remifentanil infusion. Decadron given at or immediately after induction is beneficial for swelling, postoperative nausea, and vomiting prevention and decreased opioid consumption in the postoperative period.[8] Intermittent analgesic with narcotic is patient specific and may or may not be necessary. Nonnarcotic options may include Ofirmev and Ketorolac for intraoperative and postoperative pain management.

At the conclusion of the surgery, the patient should ideally be emerged from anesthesia smoothly with little to no coughing. Extubation criteria should be met before the removal of the endotracheal tube.

Immediately following extubation, the surgeon may assess the vocal cords through flexible laryngoscopy to assure bilateral symmetric movement. This can confirm the intraoperative monitoring through the NIM tube and give reassurance of recurrent laryngeal nerve activity. A flexible laryngoscopy following extubation requires patient cooperation and phonation.

Postoperative Considerations

Postoperative complications can occur due to the shift in electrolytes during the surgical intervention. Patient presentation could include stridor, tetany, laryngospasm, or seizures. This presentation can be secondary to acute hypocalcemia, recurrent laryngeal nerve injury, or hematoma development. Should the development of a hematoma develop and the patient need to be reintubated for neck exploration, a video laryngoscope should be readily available. Vigilant patient observation and monitoring should occur in the postanesthesia care unit in the immediate postoperative period.

NURSE NAVIGATION FOR ENDOCRINE SURGICAL PATIENTS

For patients with a new cancer diagnosis, navigating a complex and often fragmented healthcare system can be daunting. In the 1990s, Dr. Harold Freeman found that many of the patients he was treating at Harlem Hospital were presenting with late-stage disease. In his research, Dr. Freeman found that economically underserved population were diagnosed later and had poorer outcomes than individuals that had better access to care. Dr. Freeman introduced the concept of patient navigation for these cancer patients, and found that these patients' outcomes improved when they had access to a patient navigator. By implementing a dedicated trained individual or patient navigator, patients were provided with access to resources to which they otherwise would not have access. This improved access provided linkages to financial and support resources, thereby empowering the patients in their decision-making related to their care, as well as a coordinating their care among multiple healthcare providers.[9–11]

The patient newly diagnosed with a thyroid cancer or another endocrine malignancy faces similar challenges and barriers. These patients often are required to have multiple diagnostic or biochemical testing, and often need connection to other specialists such as an endocrinologist, nuclear medicine physician, or oncologists. Having an oncology nurse navigator dedicated to this population allows the patient to have a coordinated care experience, with timely access to specialists, before the surgical intervention. The oncology nurse navigator often facilitates and coordinates the multidisciplinary cancer conferences (tumor board) whereby the multidisciplinary team can discuss and develop a treatment plan for these patients. Once a treatment plan is established, and during the pre- and postoperative phase of care, the patient also has an educational resource regarding their diagnosis as well as resources for psychosocial support throughout their treatment trajectory.

REFERENCES

1. American Society of Anesthesiology Task Force and Prevention. *Practice Advisory for the Prevention of Perioperative Peripheral Neuropathies: A Report by the American Society of Anesthesiologists Task Force on Prevention of Perioperative Peripheral Neuropathies*; 2000. Retrieved from: http://anesthesiology.pubs.asahq.org/article.aspx?articleid=1945948.
2. Patel PN, Jayawardena ADL, Walden RL, Penn EB, Francis DO. Evidence-based use of perioperative antibiotics in otolaryngology. *Otolaryngol Head Neck Surg.* 2018;158(5):783–800.
3. Anderson Jr FA, Zayaruzny M, Heit JA, Fidan D, Cohen AT. Estimated annual numbers of US acute-care hospital patients at risk for venous thromboembolism. *Am J Hematol.* 2007;82(9):777.
4. Barbot M, Daidone V, Zilio M, et al. Perioperative thromboprophylaxis in Cushing's disease: what we did and what we are doing? *Pituitary.* 2015;18(4):487–493.
5. Nagelhout JJ, Sadd E. *Preoperative Evaluation and Preparation of the Patient.* Vol. 6. 2018.
6. Atlas G, Lee M. The neural integrity monitor electromyogram tracheal tube: anesthetic considerations. *J Anaesthesiol Clin Pharmacol.* 2013;29(2):403–404.
7. Cassoria L, Lee JW. Patient positioning and associated risks. *Miller's Anestheisa.* 2015;41:1240–1265.
8. Kaye AD, Chalabi J, Creel JB, Paetzold JR, Beakley BD. Pharmacology of antiemetics: update and current consideration in anesthesia practice. *Anesthesiol Clin.* 2017;35(2):e41–e54.
9. Freeman HP, Muth BJ, Kerner JF. Expanding access to cancer screening and clinical follow up among the medically underserved. *Cancer Pract.* 1995;3:19–30.
10. http://www.ascopost.com/issues/february-15-2013/the-doctor-who-championed-patient-navigation-in-harlem/.
11. http://www.cancer.org/Cancer/news/Features/navigating-difficultwaters-the-history-of-the-patient-navigators.

Index

'*Note:* Page numbers followed by "f" indicate figures, "t" indicate tables.'

Printed and bound by CPI Group (UK) Ltd, Croydon, CR0 4YY

03/10/2024

01040349-0004